DRUGS, BEHAVIOUR, AND SOCIETY

SECOND CANADIAN EDITION

Carl L. Hart
Columbia University

Charles Ksir
University of Wyoming

Andrea L. O. Hebb
Saint Mary's University

Robert W. Gilbert
Dalhousie University

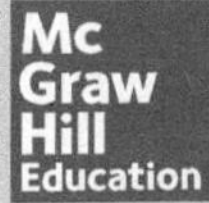

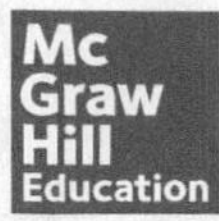

DRUGS, BEHAVIOUR, AND SOCIETY
Second Canadian Edition

ISBN-13: 978-1-25-902463-4
ISBN-10: 1-25-902463-6

1 2 3 4 5 6 7 8 9 10 WEB 1 9 8 7 6 5

Printed and bound in Canada.

Director of Product Management: *Rhondda McNabb*
Product Manager: *Jason Chih*
Senior Marketing Manager: *Margaret Greenfield*
Product Developer: *Daphne Scriabin*
Senior Product Team Associate: *Marina Seguin*
Supervising Editor: *Stephanie Gay*
Photo/Permissions Editor: *Alison Lloyd Baker / Alison Derry*
Copy Editor: *Kelli Howey*
Plant Production Coordinator: *Tammy Mavroudi*
Manufacturing Production Coordinator: *Sheryl MacAdam*
Cover Design: *Dianne Reynolds*
Interior Design: *Lightbox Visuals*
Cover Image: *Helen Cathcart/ Getty Images*
Page Layout: *SPi Global*
Printer: *Webcom*

ABOUT THE AUTHORS

Dr. Carl Hart is an associate professor of psychology in both the Departments of Psychiatry and Psychology at Columbia University. A major focus of his research is to understand complex interactions between drugs of abuse and the neurobiology and environmental factors that mediate human behaviour and physiology. He is the author or coauthor of dozens of peer-reviewed scientific articles in the area of neuropsychopharmacology and a member of the National Advisory Council on Drug Abuse. He has lectured on the topic of psychoactive drug use throughout the world and has been awarded Columbia University's highest teaching award.

Dr. Charles Ksir is professor emeritus of psychology and neuroscience at the University of Wyoming. Now retired after 35 years of research and teaching, he has authored or coauthored *Drugs, Society & Human Behavior* since 1984. He continues to teach a class based on this text via the Internet.

Dr. Andrea L. O. Hebb received her bachelor's degree at Dalhousie University and her M.Sc. and Ph.D. in Neuroscience from Carleton University. She pursued postdoctoral training in Neurobiology and Pharmacology at the Universities of Ottawa and Dalhousie. Her research investigated putative therapeutic genetic targets for the diagnosis and treatment of neurobiological disease. Dr. Hebb is the inventor on two patents and has published more than 20 papers and several major review papers and book chapters. Dr. Hebb is a research scientist with the Division of Neurosurgery at Dalhousie University and holds a faculty position at Saint Mary's University, where she teaches undergraduate classes in development, neuroscience, pharmacology, and addiction.

Dr. Robert Gilbert is an Associate Professor in the Faculty of Health Professions at Dalhousie University. He received his M.Sc. in Medicine from Memorial University and a Ph.D. in Pharmacology and Neurosciences from Dalhousie University. His research interests focus on the development of tools for assessing health care professionals' knowledge of the principles of evidence-based medicine and skills essential to applying those principles. This interest in knowledge translation blends well with his applied research initiatives that have, through clinical trial, investigated purported outcomes of several popular treatment approaches in addictions. In recent years Dr. Gilbert's efforts have also focused on the development of educational resources and programs that support the development of members of Canada's substance abuse workforce.

BRIEF CONTENTS

Preface xi

SECTION ONE **Drug Use in Modern Society** 1

Chapter 1 Drug Use: An Overview 2
Chapter 2 Drug Use as a Social Problem 25
Chapter 3 Drug Policy 44

SECTION TWO **How Drugs Work** 63

Chapter 4 The Nervous System 64
Chapter 5 The Actions of Drugs 87

SECTION THREE **Uppers and Downers** 119

Chapter 6 Stimulants 120
Chapter 7 Other Depressants and Inhalants 151
Chapter 8 Psychotherapeutic Drugs: Medication for Mental Disorders 174

SECTION FOUR **Alcohol** 207

Chapter 9 Alcohol 208

SECTION FIVE **Familiar Drugs** 243

Chapter 10 Tobacco 244
Chapter 11 Caffeine 269
Chapter 12 Natural Health Products and Over-the-Counter Drugs 292

SECTION SIX **Restricted Drugs** 311

Chapter 13 Opioids 312
Chapter 14 Hallucinogens 339
Chapter 15 Cannabis 369
Chapter 16 Performance-Enhancing Drugs 395

SECTION SEVEN **Prevention and Treatment** 411

Chapter 17 Preventing Substance Abuse 412
Chapter 18 Treating Substance Abuse and Dependence 429

CONTENTS

Preface xi

SECTION ONE
Drug Use in Modern Society 1

1 Drug Use: An Overview 2
"The Drug Problem" 2
Talking about Drug Use 2
Four Principles of Psychoactive Drugs 4
How Did We Get Here? 7
Have Things Really Changed? 7
Drugs and Drug Use Today 9
Extent of Drug Use 9
Trends in Drug Use 10
Correlates of Drug Use 16
Risk and Protective Factors 17
Gender, Socioeconomic Status, and Level of Education 18
Personality Variables 19
Genetics 19
Antecedents of Drug Use 19
Motives for Drug Use 21
Summary 23
Review Questions 24

2 Drug Use as a Social Problem 25
Laissez-Faire 25
Toxicity 26
Categories of Toxicity 26
Determining the Toxicity of Drugs of Abuse and Misuse 27
How Dangerous Is the Drug? 29
Intravenous Drug Use and the Spread of Blood-Borne Diseases 30
Substance Dependence: What Is It? 33
Three Basic Processes 33
Changing Views of Dependence 34
Which Is More Important: Physical Dependence or Psychological Dependence? 36
Broad Views of Substance Dependence 36
Is Dependence Caused by the Substance? 37
Is Dependence Biological? 38
Is There an "Addictive Personality"? 38
Is Dependence a Family Disorder? 39
Is Substance Dependence a Disease? 39
Crime and Violence: Does Drug Use Cause Crime? 40
Why We Try to Regulate Drugs 42
Summary 42
Review Questions 43

3 Drug Policy 44
The History of Drug Regulations 44
The Opium Act of 1908 45
Patent Medicine Act of 1909 46
Narcotic Control Act of 1961 46
The Le Dain Commission 47
Canada's Drug Strategies 47
Controlled Drugs and Substances Act 48
Sentencing 48
Drug Paraphernalia Laws 48
Regulation of the Sale of Alcohol and Tobacco 49
Impaired Driving 49
Diversion to Treatment 49
International Conventions 49
Bill S-10: An Act to Amend the Controlled Drugs and Substances Act 51
Regulation of Pharmaceuticals 52
New-Drug Submission Processes 52
Provincial and Territorial Responsibilities 52
Compulsory Licences 53
Developing and Introducing a New Drug 53
The Pharmaceutical Industry in Canada 54
The Compendium of Pharmaceuticals and Specialties 56
Medicinal Marijuana Regulations 56
Canadian Marihuana Medical Access Regulations (MMAR) 56
New Marihuana for Medical Purposes Regulations (MMPR) 58
Natural Health Products 60
Summary 60
Review Questions 61

SECTION TWO
How Drugs Work 63

4 The Nervous System 64
Homeostasis 64

Components of the Nervous System 65
Glia 65
Neurons 67
Neurotransmission 67
Action Potential 68
The Peripheral Nervous System 69
Somatic Nervous System 69
Autonomic Nervous System 69
Central Nervous System 70
The Brain 70
Major Structures 70
Chemical Pathways 73
Drugs and the Brain 78
Life Cycle of a Neurotransmitter 78
Examples of Drug Actions 82
Chemical Theories of Behaviour 83
Brain Imaging Techniques 84
Summary 85
Review Questions 86

5 The Actions of Drugs 87
Sources and Names of Drugs 87
Names of Drugs 88
Categories of Drugs 89
Pharmacodynamics 92
Drug Effects 92
Nonspecific (Placebo) Effects 93
Dose-Response Relationships 95
Potency 100
Pharmacokinetics of Drug Action 101
Time-Dependent Factors in Drug Actions 101
Mechanisms of Drug Action: Getting the Drug to the Brain 103
A Little Chemistry 103
Routes of Administration 103
Drug Distribution and Transport in the Blood 107
More about the Blood-Brain Barrier 107
Mechanisms of Drug Actions 107
Effects on All Neurons 108
Effects on Specific Neurotransmitter Systems 108
Drug Metabolism and Deactivation 109
Drug Half-Life 111
Mechanisms of Tolerance and Withdrawal Symptoms 112
Drug Disposition Tolerance 112
Behavioural Tolerance 112
Pharmacodynamic Tolerance 113
Drug Classifications 114
Summary 116
Review Questions 117

SECTION THREE
Uppers and Downers 119

6 Stimulants 120
Cocaine 120
History 120
Coca Wine 121
Local Anaesthesia 121
Early Psychiatric Uses 121
Legal Controls on Cocaine 122
Supplies of Illicit Cocaine in Canada 123
Pharmacology of Cocaine 124
Forms of Cocaine 124
Mechanism of Action 125
Absorption and Elimination 126
Medical Uses of Cocaine 126
Causes for Concern 127
Current Patterns of Cocaine Use 128
Cocaine's Future 129
Amphetamines 130
History 130
Supplies of Illicit Methamphetamine in Canada 134
Pharmacology of Amphetamines 134
Mechanism of Action 135
Absorption and Elimination 136
Medical Uses of Amphetamines 136
Causes for Concern 147
Summary 149
Review Questions 150

7 Other Depressants and Inhalants 151
History and Pharmacology 152
Before Barbiturates 152
Barbiturates 152
Meprobamate 153
Methaqualone 154
Benzodiazepines 155
Nonbenzodiazepine Hypnotics 158
Mechanism of Action of Benzodiazepines 158
Beneficial Uses of Depressants 159
As Anxiolytics 159
As Sleeping Pills 160
As Anticonvulsants 163
Causes for Concern 163
Dependence Liability 163
Toxicity 163
Patterns of Abuse 164
Benzodiazepine Use in First Nation and Inuit Populations 164

Drugs Used to Facilitate Sexual Assault 166
Inhalants 167
Gaseous Anaesthetics 169
Nitrites 170
Volatile Solvents 171
Rates of Volatile Solvent Abuse in Canada 172
GHB (Gamma-Hydroxybutyric Acid) 172
Summary 173
Review Questions 173

8 Psychotherapeutic Drugs: Medication for Mental Disorders 174
Mental Illness 174
Concurrent Disorders 175
The Medical Model 175
Classification of Mental Disorders 177
Treatment of Mental Disorders 184
Before 1950 184
Antipsychotics 186
Antidepressants 194
Electroconvulsive Therapy 201
Mood Stabilizers 201
Consequences of Drug Treatments for Mental Illness 203
Summary 206
Review Questions 206

SECTION FOUR
Alcohol 207

9 Alcohol 208
Alcoholic Beverages 208
Fermentation and Fermentation Products 208
Distilled Products 208
Beer 210
Wine 210
Distilled Spirits 211
Alcohol Use and "The Alcohol Problem" 212
The Temperance Movement 213
Prohibition 213
Prohibition Worked! 215
Prohibition Is Repealed 215
Regulation after 1933 215
Who Drinks? And Why? 216
Cultural Influences on Drinking 216
Prevalence and Patterns of Alcohol Use in Canada 216
Canadian Alcohol and Drug Use Monitoring Survey (CADUMS) 216
Alcohol Use among Postsecondary Students 216
Regional Differences in Alcohol Use in Canada 220
Alcohol Pharmacology 220
Absorption 220
Distribution 221
Metabolism 223
Mechanism(s) of Action 223
Behavioural Effects 225
Time-Out and Alcohol Myopia 227
Driving under the Influence 227
Sexual Behaviour 229
Blackouts 230
Crime and Violence 230
Physiological Effects 231
Alcohol Toxicity 231
Hangover 231
Chronic Disease States 232
Brain Damage 232
Liver Disease 233
Heart Disease 233
Cancer 234
The Immune System 234
Canadian Recommended Guidelines for Low-Risk Drinking 234
Fetal Alcohol Syndrome 236
Alcohol Dependence 238
Withdrawal Syndrome 238
Dependent Behaviours 238
Summary 241
Review Questions 241

SECTION FIVE
Familiar Drugs 243

10 Tobacco 244
Tobacco History 244
Early Medical Uses 245
Chewing Tobacco 246
Cigars 246
Cigarettes 247
Tobacco under Attack 247
The Quest for "Safer" Cigarettes 250
Current Cigarette Use 252
Smokeless Tobacco 253
Are Cigars Back? 257
Adverse Health Effects 257
Passive Smoking: The Danger of Second-Hand Smoke 257
Smoking and Pregnancy 260

Pharmacology of Nicotine 261
Absorption and Metabolism 261
Physiological Effects 261
Behavioural Effects 263
Nicotine Dependence 263
How to Stop Smoking 265
Summary 267
Review Questions 268

11 Caffeine 269
Caffeine: The World's Most Common Psychostimulant 269
Coffee 269
Tea 273
Chocolate 276
Other Sources of Caffeine 278
Soft Drinks 278
"Energy" Drinks 279
Over-the-Counter Drugs 282
Caffeine Pharmacology 282
Time Course 283
Mechanism of Action 284
Physiological Effects 285
Behavioural Effects 287
Causes for Concern 289
Cancer 289
Pregnancy and Conception 289
Heart Disease 290
Caffeinism 290
Summary 291
Review Questions 291

12 Natural Health Products and Over-the-Counter Drugs 292
Natural Health Products 292
Some Natural Health Products Have Psychoactive Properties 293
St. John's Wort 293
SAMe 294
Ginkgo Biloba 294
Caffeine 295
Weight-Control Products 296
Sleep Aids 297
Over-the-Counter Drugs 297
Regulation of Over-the-Counter Products 297
Improved Labelling of Over-the-Counter Drugs 298
Over-the-Counter versus Prescription Drugs 298
Behind-the-Counter Nonprescription Drugs 299
Sleep Aids 299
Analgesics 300
People and Pain 300
Aspirin 300
Acetaminophen 303
Ibuprofen and Other NSAIDs 304
Products Containing Codeine 304
Cold and Allergy Products 305
The All-Too-Common Cold 305
Treatment of Cold Symptoms 306
Allergy and Sinus Medications 307
Choosing an OTC Product 307
Summary 308
Review Questions 309

SECTION SIX
Restricted Drugs 311

13 Opioids 312
History of Opioids 312
Opium 312
Morphine 315
Heroin 315
Opium and Heroin Supply, Distribution, and Trafficking in Canada 317
The Changing Profile of Opioid Users 318
Abuse of Prescription Opioids 319
Pharmacology of Opioids 321
Chemical Characteristics 321
Mechanism of Action 324
Beneficial Uses 326
Pain Relief 326
Intestinal Disorders 327
Cough Suppressants 327
Causes for Concern 327
Dependence Potential 327
Toxicity Potential 329
Patterns of Abuse 331
Research Studies and Pilots Addressing the Needs of Injection Drug Users in Canada 332
Insite: Vancouver's Supervised Injection Facility 333
North American Opiate Medication Initiative (NAOMI) 336
Study to Assess Long-Term Opioid Maintenance Effectiveness (SALOME) 336
Summary 338
Review Questions 338

14 Hallucinogens 339
Animism and Religion 339
Terminology and Types 340
Phantastica 341
Indole Hallucinogens 341
Catechol Hallucinogens 354
Deliriants 359
PCP 359
Anticholinergic Hallucinogens 362
Amanita Muscaria 364
Salvia Divinorum 366
Summary 367
Review Questions 368

15 Cannabis 369
Cannabis, the Plant 369
Cannabis Preparations 370
History of Cannabis 371
Early History 371
The Nineteenth Century: Romantic Literature and the New Science of Psychology 371
History of Cannabis Policy in Canada 372
Supply, Distribution, and Trafficking 372
Marijuana Supply, Distribution, and Trafficking in Canada 372
Hashish and Hash Oil Supply, Distribution, and Trafficking in Canada 373
Prevalence Rates of Cannabis Use 373
What Canadian Youth Think about Cannabis 374
Worldwide Use of Cannabis 376
Compassion Clubs 376
Pharmacology 377
Cannabinoid Chemicals 377
Absorption, Distribution, and Elimination 377
Mechanism of Action 378
Physiological Effects 379
Behavioural Effects 379
Medical Uses of Cannabis in Canada 382
Nausea and Vomiting 382
Wasting Syndrome in AIDS and Cancer 383
Multiple Sclerosis and Amyotrophic Lateral Sclerosis 383
Epilepsy 383
Pain 384
Psychiatric Disorders 384
Other Diseases and Symptoms 384
Contraindications 386
Causes for Concern 386
Abuse and Dependence 386
Toxicity Potential 386
Cannabis and Psychosis 391
Cannabidiol 392
Summary 393
Review Questions 394

16 Performance-Enhancing Drugs 395
Historical Use of Drugs in Athletics 395
Ancient Times 396
Early Use of Stimulants 396
Amphetamines 397
International Drug Testing 397
North American Football 398
Steroids 398
The BALCO Scandal 399
The Battle over Testing 400
Stimulants as Performance Enhancers 401
Steroids 403
Mechanism of Action 404
Prevalence of Illicit Steroid Use in Canada 405
Psychological Effects of Steroids 405
Adverse Effects on the Body 406
Regulation 407
Other Hormonal Manipulations 407
Beta-2 Agonists 408
Blood Doping 408
Creatine 408
Getting "Cut" 408
Summary 409
Review Questions 410

SECTION SEVEN
Prevention and Treatment 411

17 Preventing Substance Abuse 412
Defining Goals and Evaluating Outcomes 412
Types of Prevention 413
Prevention Programs in Schools 415
Why Invest in Young People? 415
The Knowledge-Attitudes-Behaviour Model 415
Affective Education 416
Antidrug Norms 418
Development of the Social Influence Model 419
Prevention Programs That Work 420
School-Based Prevention Programs 420
Project ALERT 421
Drug Abuse Resistance Education (DARE) 421
Project Life Skills Training 423

Programs That Target Peers, Parents, and the Community 423
Peer Programs 424
Parent and Family Programs 424
Strengthening Families for the Future 424
Community Programs 425
Prevention in the Workplace 425
What Should We Be Doing? 427
Summary 428
Review Questions 428

18 Treating Substance Abuse and Dependence 429
The Social and Economic Costs of Alcohol and Other Drugs in Canada 429
Pharmacotherapies (Medication Treatments) 430
Detoxification (Withdrawal Management) and Maintenance Phase 430
Alcohol 431
Nicotine 432
Opioids 434
Cocaine 438
Cannabis 439
Management of Problematic Substance Use in Pregnancy 440
Pharmacotherapies for Adolescents with Substance-Related Disorders 441
Behavioural and Psychosocial Treatments 442
Defining Treatment Goals 442
Motivational Enhancement Therapy 442
Contingency Management 443
Relapse Prevention 443
Transtheoretical Model (Stages of Change) and Substance Abuse Treatment 444
Harm Reduction 445
Substance Abuse in Canada: Concurrent Disorders 449
Treatment and Rehabilitation: The Big Picture in Canada 449
Is Treatment Effective? 450
Alcoholics Anonymous 450
A Systems Approach to Substance Use in Canada 452
Summary 453
Review Questions 454

Glossary GL-1
Credits CR-1
References RE-1
Available Online:
Appendix A: Drug Names
Appendix B: Resources for Information and Assistance

PREFACE TO THE SECOND CANADIAN EDITION

Today's media-oriented postsecondary students are aware of many issues relating to drug use. Nearly every day we hear new concerns about methamphetamine, club drugs, prescription opioids, and the effects of tobacco and alcohol, and most of us have had some personal experience with these issues through family, friends, or co-workers. This course is one of the most exciting that students will take because it will help them relate the latest information on drugs to their effects on human behaviour and Canadian society. Not only will students be in a better position to make decisions to enhance their own health and well-being, but they will also have a deeper understanding of the individual problems and social conflicts that arise when others misuse and abuse psychoactive drugs.

Practices and patterns of psychoactive drug use, and their effects on human behaviour and Canadian society, are in a continual state of flux. The 1960s through 1970s was a period of widespread experimentation with marijuana and hallucinogens, while the 1980s brought increased concern about illegal drugs and conservatism, along with decreased use of alcohol and all illicit drugs. Not only did drug-using behaviour change, but so did attitudes and knowledge. And, of course, in each decade the particular drugs of immediate social concern changed: LSD gave way to heroin, then to cocaine and crack and today to prescription medications.

A recent trend is the increased misuse of prescription opioid pain relievers, such as OxyContin and Dilaudid. These pharmaceuticals have now joined methamphetamine and ecstasy as leading causes of concern about drug misuse and abuse. Methamphetamine, ecstasy, GHB, and the misuse of prescription opioids and performance enhancers are the big news items.

Meanwhile, our old standbys alcohol and tobacco remain with us and continue to create serious health and social problems. Regulations undergo frequent changes, new scientific information becomes available, and new approaches to prevention and treatment are tested, but the reality of substance use and abuse always seems to be with us.

This text examines drugs and drug use from a variety of perspectives–behavioural, pharmacological, historical, social, legal, and clinical–which will help students connect the content to their own interests.

What's New in the Second Canadian Edition?

In developing this edition we considered the outlook and experiences of Canadian students.

Throughout each chapter, we have included the latest Canadian statistics, and the Drugs in the Media feature has allowed us to include breaking news right up to press time. Additionally, we have introduced many timely topics and have highlighted cutting-edge research by and practices of Canadians. Collectively these will pique students' interest and stimulate class discussion.

- Chapter 1 and throughout: Statistics on rates and patterns of drug use and the societal consequences of drug abuse and dependency from a variety of Canadian sources, such as the *Canadian Alcohol and Drug Use Monitoring Survey*, the *Ontario Student Drug Use and Health Survey*, and other Canadian sources.
- Chapter 2 and throughout: Updated criteria for the diagnosis of substance-related and addictive disorders, as defined by the DSM-5.
- Chapter 3: Chapter title changed to "Drug Policy"; new box material "Canadian Police Chiefs Propose Ticket System for Pot"; new material on Canada's national drug strategy; updated information on the sales of patented and nonpatented drugs in Canada, 2001–2012, and the top ten pharmaceuticals sold in Canada, 2012; new box material "Expanding Drug Treatment Courts in Canada"; updated information on trends in authorizations to possess and licences to produce marijuana in Canada by region, 2013; new section on the Marihuana for Medical Purposes Regulations (MMPR); new section on Bill S-10, an act to amend the Controlled Drugs and Substances Act and to make related and consequential amendments to other acts; and new box material "Federal Court Reverses Ban on Grow-Your-Own Medical Marijuana."
- Chapters 3 and 15: The evolution of the Canadian Marihuana Medical Access Regulations has been introduced.
- Chapter 4: In Chapter 4 we present new information on the functions of glia in the nervous system. We have also included new Canadian information

on drug-induced Parkinson's disease (parkinsonism), and new material on Parkinson's research. We attribute this to the Michael J. Fox Foundation and neurologists Dr. Ali Rajput and Dr. Alex Rajput, who have dedicated their work at Royal University Hospital.

- Chapter 5: In this chapter we present new statistics on Ritalin abuse by Canadian youth. We have added updated data on the Canadian pharmaceutical trade as well as new data and Canadian statistics on prescription amphetamine abuse. We have extended our discussion on placebo effects compared to therapeutic effects of drugs on depression and pain. We have extended our discussion on dose-response curves for better understanding of the pharmacokinetic and pharmacodynamic effects of drugs in the body. We have touched on the practice of vaginal and rectal administration of drugs, referred to as "booty bumping" or "butt bongs," as well as the introduction of topical administration of drugs. We have furthered our explanation on drug classifications. We have also briefly discussed the social implications of legalization of marijuana.
- Chapter 6: In Chapter 6 we present new material on "bath salts" and their implications for Canadians.
- Chapter 7: Title changed to "Other Depressants and Inhalants"; new material on chloral hydrate; new material on drugs used to facilitate sexual assault in Canada; new section on rates of inhalant abuse in Canada.
- Chapter 8: In Chapter 8 we have included a discussion of concurrent disorders and their increase in Canada including descriptions of the strong links between mental health and substance abuse. We have included discussion of the drug Abilify, the first and only medication in Canada approved to treat schizophrenia in adolescents, and updated data on the placebo effect of antidepressant treatment. We acknowledge the positive effects of the transition from acute care to community-based services for some individuals, and provide coverage of the mentally ill and the Ashley Smith incarceration.
- Chapter 9: New material on the *Canadian Alcohol and Drug Use Monitoring Survey* (CADUMS); new section on alcohol use among postsecondary students; updated information on sales of alcoholic beverages per capita 15 years and over for the year 2013; new box material "Heavy Drinking a Problem at Most Canadian Campuses"; new material on the mechanisms of action of alcohol; new section on cross-Canada student alcohol and drug use; new section on Canadian Recommended Guidelines for Low-Risk Drinking.
- Chapter 10: In Chapter 10 we have included new trends in cigarette consumption in Canada, with specific province and territory data. We provide new data on smoking prevalence from 1985 to 2012 for Canadians aged 15 years and older, youth aged 15–19, and young adults aged 20–24. We have included new data from *Canadian Tobacco Use Monitoring Survey* (CTUMS), 2012, as well as a new timeline for key Canadian facts related to tobacco. We have also included a new box on "The Adverse Effects of Shisha Consumption or Hookah Use."
- Chapter 11: In Chapter 11 we outline new data on coffee drinking habits of Canadians, including the growth of Tim Hortons restaurant outlets. We describe new information on the health benefits of tea. We further our discussion by examining Canadians' energy drink consumption, both alone and in combination with alcohol. Finally, we outline differences between DSM-IV and DSM-5 with regard to caffeine abuse and misuse, and include the DSM-5 boxes "Caffeine Intoxication" and "Caffeine Withdrawal Disorder."
- Chapter 12: Presents current evidence regarding the efficacy of alleged natural health product sleep aids.
- Chapter 13: New section on opioid formulations designed to resist or deter abuse; new box material from the Canadian Community Epidemiology Network on Drug Use (CCENDU) on "Increasing Availability of Counterfeit Oxycodone Tablets Containing Fentanyl"; new box material "Take Home Naloxone: Backgrounder"; new box material with Gabor Maté's comments on media coverage of Cory Monteith's death; new section on the North American Opioid Medication Initiative (NAOMI); new box material "B.C. Addicts Get Injunction to Continue Using Prescription Heroin."
- Chapter 14: New data profiling the patterns of hallucinogen use by students in Canadian high schools and postsecondary institutions.
- Chapter 15: New box material "Health Canada Statement: Changes to the Reporting Requirements in the MMPR"; additional information on cannabis use in Canada (*Canadian Alcohol and Drug Use Monitoring Survey*, 2012); added content from a Canadian Centre on Substance Abuse study examining youth's perceptions of driving while under the influence of cannabis; updated surveys on Canadians who drove after using cannabis;

key findings from a CCSA study on what Canadian youth think about cannabis; updated information on global estimates of illicit drug users; new box material "Bring the Prince of Pot, Marc Emery, Back to Canada to Serve His Time, Say 3 MPs"; new box material "Canadian Bar Association, British Columbia Branch: Possession of Marijuana"; new box material "Justin Trudeau Says Canada Should 'Draw on Best Practices' from Marijuana Legalization in Colorado, Washington."

- Chapter 16: Updated material on the regulation of and testing for performance-enhancing drugs in Canadian athletes.
- Chapter 17: Evidence demonstrating why youth-focused prevention initiatives are of paramount importance to Canada's National Anti-Drug Strategy.
- Chapter 18: New material on electronic smoking; new box material "Insite Survives 10 Years On: Supervised Injection Site Opened as Three-Year Experiment Sept. 21, 2003"; new box material "Crack Pipe Vending Machines Draw Ire of Tory Minister Who Wants to Limit 'Access to Drug Paraphernalia'"; added clinical practice guidelines developed by the Society of Obstetricians and Gynecologists of Canada for clinical management of problematic substance use during pregnancy; included study of efficacy of nicotine replacement therapies; referenced recent study that suggests nicotine replacement may essentially not be a worthwhile approach.

Focus Boxes

Boxes are used in *Drugs, Behaviour, and Society* to explore a wide range of current topics in greater detail than is possible in the text itself. The boxes are organized around key themes.

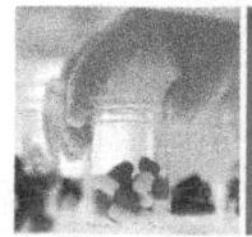

DRUGS IN THE MEDIA

Our world revolves around media of all types: TV, films, radio, print media, and the Web. To meet students on familiar ground, the Drugs in the Media boxes take an informative and critical look at these media sources of drug information. Students can build their critical thinking skills while reading about such topics as alcohol advertising, media coverage of prescription drugs, and the presentation of cigarette smoking in films.

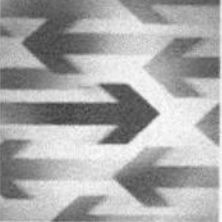

TAKING SIDES

These boxes discuss a particular drug-related issue or problem and ask students to take a side in the debate. This thought-provoking material will help students apply what they have learned in the chapter to real-world situations. Taking Sides topics include potential medical uses of marijuana, current laws relating to drug use, and the issue of government funding for research on hallucinogens.

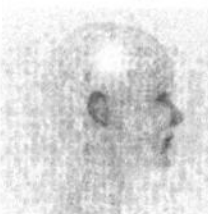

MIND/BODY CONNECTION

The Mind/Body Connection boxes highlight the interface between the psychological and the physiological aspects of substance use, abuse, and dependence. These boxes help students consider influences on their own attitudes toward drug use. Topics include religion and drug use, the social and emotional costs of smoking, and the nature of dependence.

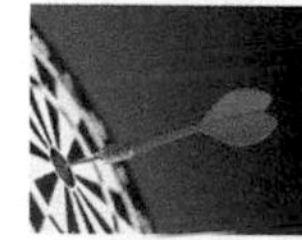

TARGETING PREVENTION

The Targeting Prevention boxes offer perspective and provoke thought regarding which drug-related behaviours we, as a society, want to reduce or prevent. Topics include syringe exchange programs, criminal penalties for use of date-rape drugs, and nondrug techniques for overcoming insomnia. These boxes help students better evaluate prevention strategies and messages.

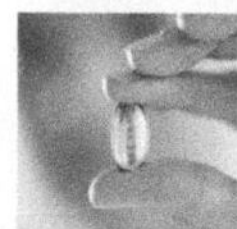

DRUGS IN DEPTH

These boxes examine specific, often controversial, drug-related issues, such as the growing number of people in prison for drug-related offences. Drugs in Depth boxes are a perfect starting point for class or group discussion.

DSM-5

The *Diagnostic and Statistical Manual of Mental Disorders* (*DSM*), the handbook used by health care professionals as the authoritative guide to the diagnosis of mental disorders, has been updated. DSM-5 boxes and content throughout the text reflect current recommendations and concepts presented in the DSM-5.

Pedagogical Aids

Although all the features of *Drugs, Behaviour, and Society* are designed to facilitate and improve learning, several specific learning aids have been incorporated into the text:

- **Chapter Objectives:** Chapters begin with a list of numbered objectives that identify the major concepts and help guide students in their reading and review of the text.
- **Definitions of Key Terms:** Key terms are set in boldface type and are defined in corresponding boxes. Other important terms in the text are set in italics for emphasis. Both approaches facilitate vocabulary comprehension.
- **Chapter Summaries:** Each chapter concludes with a bulleted summary of key concepts. Students can use the chapter summaries to guide their reading and review of the chapters.
- **Review Questions:** A set of questions appears at the end of each chapter to aid students in their review and analysis of chapter content.
- **Appendices:** The appendices include handy references on brand and generic names of drugs and on drug resources and organizations. These will be available online in Connect.
- **Summary Drugs Chart:** A helpful chart of drug categories, uses, and effects appears on the back inside cover of the text.

Mc Graw Hill Education connect®

McGraw-Hill Connect™ is a web-based assignment and assessment platform that gives students the means to better connect with their coursework, with their instructors, and with the important concepts that they will need to know for success now and in the future.

With Connect, instructors can deliver assignments, quizzes and tests online. Nearly all the questions from the text are presented in an auto-gradeable format and tied to the text's learning objectives. Instructors can edit existing questions and author entirely new problems. Track individual student performance–by question, assignment or in relation to the class overall–with detailed grade reports. Integrate grade reports easily with Learning Management Systems (LMS).

By choosing Connect, instructors are providing their students with a powerful tool for improving academic performance and truly mastering course material. Connect allows students to practise important skills at their own pace and on their own schedule. Importantly, students' assessment results and instructors' feedback are all saved online–so students can continually review their progress and plot their course to success.

Connect also provides 24/7 online access to an eBook–an online edition of the text–to aid them in successfully completing their work, wherever and whenever they choose.

Key Features

Simple Assignment Management With Connect, creating assignments is easier than ever, so you can spend more time teaching and less time managing.

- Create and deliver assignments easily with selectable end-of-chapter questions and test bank material to assign online.
- Streamline lesson planning, student progress reporting, and assignment grading to make classroom management more efficient than ever.
- Go paperless with the eBook and online submission and grading of student assignments.

Smart Grading When it comes to studying, time is precious. Connect helps students learn more efficiently by providing feedback and practice material when they need it, where they need it.

- Automatically score assignments, giving students immediate feedback on their work and side-by-side comparisons with correct answers.
- Access and review each response; manually change grades or leave comments for students to review.
- Reinforce classroom concepts with practice tests and instant quizzes.

Instructor Library The Connect Instructor Library is your course creation hub. It provides all the critical resources you'll need to build your course, just how you want to teach it.

- Assign eBook readings and draw from a rich collection of textbook-specific assignments.
- Access instructor resources, including ready-made PowerPoint presentations and media to use in your lectures.
- View assignments and resources created for past sections.
- Post your own resources for students to use.

eBook Connect reinvents the textbook learning experience for the modern student. Every Connect subject area is seamlessly integrated with Connect eBooks, which are designed to keep students focused on the concepts key to their success.

- Provide students with a Connect eBook, allowing for anytime, anywhere access to the textbook.
- Merge media, animation and assessments with the text's narrative to engage students and improve learning and retention.
- Pinpoint and connect key concepts in a snap using the powerful eBook search engine.
- Manage notes, highlights, and bookmarks in one place for simple, comprehensive review.

Instructor Resources

The following instructor resources are available for download from *Connect*. To obtain a password to download these teaching tools, please contact your local sales representative.

- Instructor's Manual: Organized by chapter, the Instructor's Manual includes chapter outlines, key points, suggested class discussion questions and activities, and video suggestions. These have been prepared by text author Robert Gilbert.
- Test Bank: Test bank questions are available as Word files and with the EZ Test computerized testing software. EZ Test provides a powerful, easy-to-use test maker to create printed quizzes and exams. For secure online testing, exams created in EZ Test can be exported to WebCT, Blackboard, and EZ Test Online. EZ Test comes with a Quick Start Guide, user's manual, and Flash tutorials. Additional help is available online at www.mhhe.com/eztest.
- Microsoft® PowerPoint® Slides: With figures and exhibits from the text, the PowerPoint slides include key lecture points and images from the text and other sources.
- Image Bank: Contains more than 200 full-colour figures and images from the text.

Additional Resources Online

- Appendix A: Drug Names
- Appendix B: Resources for Information and Assistance

Mc Graw Hill Education connect

Superior Learning Solutions and Support

The McGraw-Hill Ryerson team is ready to help you assess and integrate any of our products, technology, and services into your course for optimal teaching and learning performance. Whether it's helping your students improve their grades or putting your entire course online, the McGraw-Hill Ryerson team is here to help you do it. Contact your Learning Solutions Consultant today to learn how to maximize all of McGraw-Hill Ryerson's resources!

For more information on the latest technology and Learning Solutions offered by McGraw-Hill Ryerson and its partners, please visit us online: www.mheducation.ca/he/solutions.

ACKNOWLEDGMENTS

For this Canadian edition of *Drugs, Behaviour, and Society,* acknowledgment must first be given to Oakley Stern Ray, Carl Hart, and Charles Ksir, who over the past 40 years have worked to ensure the high standards and attention to detail seen in previous editions. We are indebted to these individuals for a strong foundation to build on.

It has been a pleasure to work with the team at McGraw-Hill Ryerson, and we appreciate their considerable patience and guidance throughout this process. The editorial and production staff were directed by Marcia Siekowski, Product Manager, Jason Chih, Product Manager, Daphne Scriabin, Product Developer, and Stephanie Gay, Supervising Editor. Without their support this project would have been insurmountable. We would also like to thank Kelli Howey for the careful copyedit of the text.

We recognize the diverse backgrounds and levels of expertise of our readers and encourage you to send any comments or suggestions about this Canadian edition to us at rgilbert@dal.ca (Robert Gilbert). Your input is essential to the development of future editions.

Finally, we are extremely grateful to our colleagues from across Canada who reviewed this book and provided insightful suggestions for improvement. Their contributions of time and expertise have enhanced our knowledge and enriched the content of this book in a valuable way. We acknowledge these individuals in the list that follows.

Review of the First Edition:

Anastasia Bake
St. Clair College

W. Bourque
University of New Brunswick

Martin Davies
University of Alberta

Derek Leduc
Dalhousie University

Kenneth Lomp
Durham College

Bruce McKay
Wilfrid Laurier University

Laurain Mills
University of Victoria

Amanda Shand
St. Lawrence College

Todd Sojonky
University of Regina

Nicole Vittoz
Kwantlen Polytechnic

Manuscript Review:

Stasi Bake
St. Clair College

Martin Davies
University of Alberta

Anna Hicks
Memorial University

Noel Quinn
Sheridan College

Zachary Walsh
University of British Columbia

Andrea L. O. Hebb
Robert W. Gilbert

SECTION

1

CHAPTER 1
Drug Use: An Overview
Which drugs are being used and why?

CHAPTER 2
Drug Use as a Social Problem
Why does our society want to regulate drug use?

CHAPTER 3
Drug Policy
What are the regulations, and what is their effect?

DRUG USE IN MODERN SOCIETY

The interaction between drugs and behaviour can be approached from two general perspectives. Certain drugs, the ones we call *psychoactive*, have profound effects on behaviour. Part of what a book on this topic should do is describe the effects of these drugs on behaviour, and later chapters do that in some detail. Another perspective, however, views drug taking as behaviour. The psychologist sees drug-taking behaviours as interesting examples of human behaviour that are influenced by many psychological, social, and cultural variables. In the first section of this text, we focus on drug taking as behaviour that can be studied in the same way that other behaviours, such as aggression, learning, and human sexuality, can be studied. You will also be given information on the pharmacological and social aspects of recreational drugs so that you will be able to make informed choices on drug use.

CHAPTER 1

DRUG USE: AN OVERVIEW

OBJECTIVES

When you have finished this chapter, you should be able to

- **LO1** Develop an analytical framework for understanding any specific drug-use issue.
- **LO2** Apply four general principles of psychoactive drug use to any specific drug-use issue.
- **LO3** Explain the differences among misuse, abuse, and dependence.
- **LO4** Describe the concepts of dependence, tolerance, and withdrawal.
- **LO5** Explain correlates and antecedents of adolescent drug use.
- **LO6** Explain risk factors and protective factors for drug use.
- **LO7** Discuss motives that people may have for illicit or dangerous drug-using behaviour.

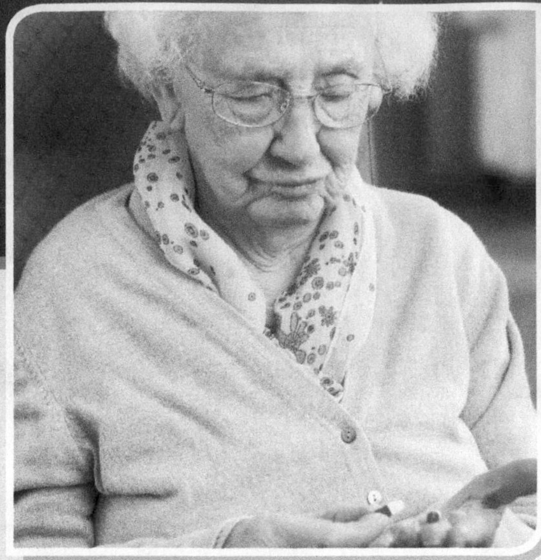

Drug use is on the rise among older adults in Canada. The use of multiple medications (*polypharmacy*) increases the risks of adverse drug events and interactions.

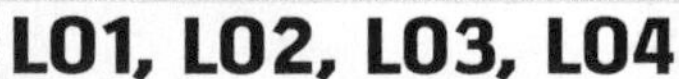

"The Drug Problem"

"Drug use on the rise" is a headline that has been seen quite regularly over the years. It gets our attention. At any given time the unwanted use of some kind of drug can be found to be increasing, at least in some group of people. How big a problem does the current headline represent?

Talking about Drug Use

Before we can evaluate the extent of a drug problem or propose possible solutions, we need to be more specific about just what the problem is. It's obvious that not all types of drug use demand our concern. If your Aunt Margie has a headache and takes two Tylenol tablets, that's drug use, but most of us don't see it as a problem. However, Uncle John's continued need for pain medication even though his injury has healed, and your best friend Karren's dependence on alcohol for social interactions at parties, may be viewed as problem drug use. Whether prescription or illicit, some drugs being used by some people in some situations are a problem our society must deal with. Let's look at some of the factors that determine whether a particular kind of drug use is a problem that we should attend to.

Journalism students are told that an informative news story must answer the questions who, what, when, where, why, and how. Let's see how answering the same questions, and one more question—how much—can help us analyze problem drug use.

- Who is taking the drug? The majority of Canadians perceive drug and alcohol abuse to be very or somewhat serious problems in Canada, their province or territory, and their community.[1] However, we are more concerned about a 15-year-old girl drinking a beer than we are about a 21-year-old woman doing the same thing. We worry more about a 10-year-old boy chewing tobacco than we do about a 40-year-old man chewing it (unless we happen to be riding right behind him when he spits out the window). Images on YouTube of children as young as two years of age in other parts of the world smoking, whether real or not, are especially disturbing. And although we don't like the idea of anyone taking heroin, we undoubtedly get more upset when we hear about the girl next door becoming a user.

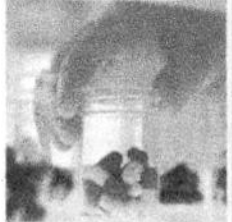

DRUGS IN THE MEDIA

Reporting on the "Drug du Jour"

In 2000, newspaper and television stories about drugs were dominated by the so-called club drugs, such as ecstasy and GHB. Ecstasy grew to become the most popular designer drug in Canada, and its use extended beyond the rave culture and into schools, homes, and the streets. In a 2011 survey of students in Ontario, 3.3% of students in grades 9 through 12, some 24 200 students, self-reported using ecstasy in the previous 12 months.[2] Fortunately, the use of ecstasy, in Canada, has been in decline since then.[3,4,5] Before ecstasy, there was a wave of media reports about crystal meth and other forms of methamphetamine. Before that, in the mid-1980s, it was crack cocaine. Recent media attention in Canada has focused on the use of the psychoactive drug Desomorphine ("krokodil"/"crocodile").[6] Whether such waves of media attention are true reflections of the extent or reality of drug use is sometimes debated. What is clear, however, is that when the news media jump on the latest *drug du jour* (drug of the day), they generally do so en masse.

One question that we should continue to ask is, What role does media attention play in popularizing a current drug fad, perhaps making it spread farther and faster than it would without the publicity? About 40 years ago, in a chapter titled "How to Create a Nationwide Drug Epidemic," journalist E. M. Brecher described a sequence of news stories that he believed were the key factor in spreading the practice of sniffing the glues sold to kids for assembling plastic models of cars and airplanes (see the section on volatile solvents in Chapter 7). He argued that, without the well-meaning attempts to warn people of the dangers of this practice, it would probably have remained isolated to a small group of youngsters in Pueblo, Colorado. Instead, sales of model glue skyrocketed across North America, leading to widespread restrictions on sales to minors. The 2012 *Ontario Student Drug Use and Health Survey* showed that 2.8% of males and 4.1% of females, grades 7–12, reported having used an inhalant (glue or solvents) in the past year. The highest rates of use were reported by students in grades 7 and 8 at 5.9% and 7.6% respectively.[2]

Thinking about the kinds of things such articles often say about the latest drug problem, are there components of those articles that you would include if you were writing an advertisement to promote use of the drug? Do you think such articles actually do more harm than good, as Brecher suggested? If so, does the important principle of a free press mean there is no way to reduce the impact of such journalism?

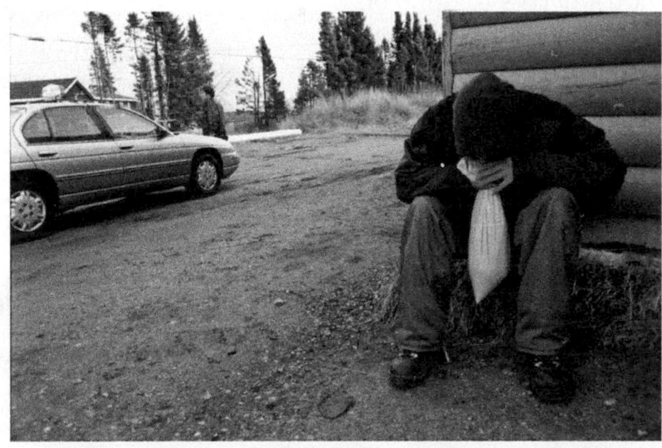

Gas inhalation among children in Davis Inlet, 15 kilometres south of Natuashish, Labrador, attracted worldwide media attention in the 1990s. While seen in all ethnic groups in Canada, solvent use is especially prevalent among street youth, inner city youth, and some First Nations and Inuit youth in selected rural or remote areas of Canada.[7] Solvent use, involving the inhalation of volatile substances such as gasoline, glue, and cleaning products, has been increasingly reported in isolated Aboriginal communities. A survey carried out on reserves in Canada reported that most youth who have tried solvents did so by the time they were 11 years old. Most (43%) said they tried it only once, followed by social users (38%), and chronic users (19%).[8] Inhaled solvent use among First Nations and Inuit youth has been linked to high rates of poverty, boredom, unemployment, family breakdown, loss of self-respect, and poor social and economic structures.[9]

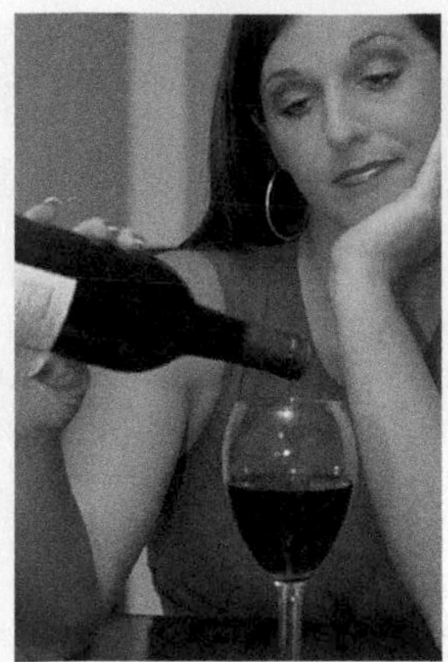
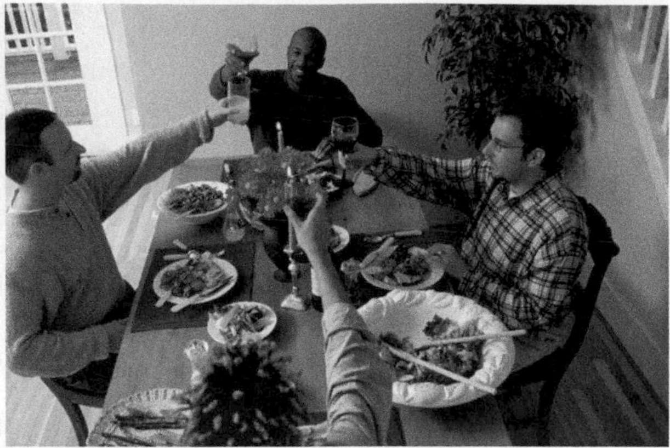

Our concern about the use of a substance often depends on who is using it, how much is being used, and when, where, and why it is being used.

- What drug are they taking? This question should be obvious, but often it is overlooked. A simple claim that a high percentage of students are "drug users" doesn't tell us if there has been an epidemic of methamphetamine use or if the drug is alcohol (which is more likely). If someone begins to talk about a serious "drug problem" at the local high school, the first question should be, What drug or drugs?
- When and where is the drug being used? The situation in which the drug use occurs often makes all the difference. The clearest example is the drinking of alcohol; if it is confined to appropriate times and places, most people accept drinking as normal behaviour. When an individual begins to drink on the job, at school, or in the morning, that behaviour may be evidence of a drinking problem. Even subcultures that accept the use of illegal drugs might distinguish between acceptable and unacceptable situations; some university-age groups might accept marijuana smoking at a party but not just before going to a psychology class!
- Why a person takes a drug or does anything else is a tough question to answer. Nevertheless, it is important in some cases. If a person takes Vicodin because her doctor prescribed it for the knee injury she got while skiing, most of us would not be concerned. If, however, she takes that drug on her own, just because she likes the way it makes her feel, then we should begin to worry about possible abuse of the drug. The motives for drug use, as with motives for other behaviours, can be complex. Even the person taking the drug might not be aware of all the motives involved. One way a psychologist can try to answer *why* questions is to look for consistency in the situations in which the behaviour occurs (when and where). If a person drinks only with other people who are drinking, we may suspect social motives; if a person often drinks alone, we may suspect that the person is trying to deal with personal problems by drinking.
- How the drug is taken can often be critical. Indigenous South Americans who chew coca leaves absorb cocaine slowly over a long period. The same total amount of cocaine snorted into the nose produces a more rapid, more intense effect of shorter duration and probably leads to much stronger dependence. Smoking cocaine in the form of "crack" produces an even more rapid, intense, and brief effect, and dependence occurs very quickly.
- How much of the drug is being used? This isn't one of the standard journalism questions, but it is important when describing drug use. Often the difference between what is considered normal use and what is considered abuse of, for example, alcohol or a prescription drug comes down to how much a person takes.

Four Principles of Psychoactive Drugs

Now that we've seen how helpful it can be to be specific when talking about drug use, let's look for some organizing principles.

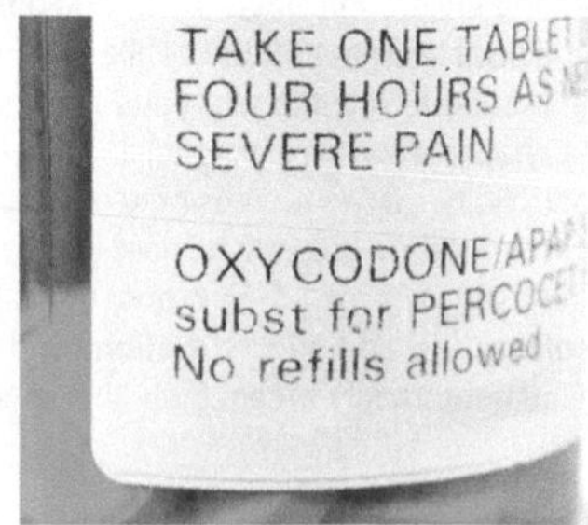

Ontario's minister of health has repeatedly spoken about the issue of OxyContin abuse in that province.

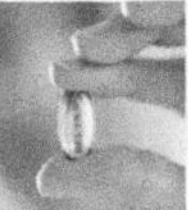

DRUGS IN DEPTH

Important Definitions—and a Caution!

Some terms that are commonly used in discussing drugs and drug use are difficult to define with precision, partly because they are so widely used for many different purposes. Therefore, any definition we offer should be viewed with caution because each represents a compromise between leaving out something important and including so much that the defined term is watered down.

The word **drug** will be defined as any substance, natural or artificial, other than food, which by its chemical nature alters structure or function in the living organism. A drug may be loosely defined as any chemical substance that has an effect on a living organism. If you accept that broad definition, can you think of other substances that you may now classify as a drug? What about food? One obvious difficulty is that we haven't defined *food*, and how we draw that line can sometimes be arbitrary. Alcoholic beverages, such as wine and beer, may be seen as drug, food, or both. Are we discussing how much sherry wine to include in beef Stroganoff, or are we discussing how much wine can be consumed before becoming intoxicated? Since this is not a cookbook but, rather, a book on the use of psychoactive chemicals, we will view all alcoholic beverages as drugs. Psychoactive drugs have their effect on the central nervous system, the brain in particular, with their resultant expression in behaviour.

Illicit drug is a term used to refer to a drug that is unlawful to possess or use. Many of these drugs are available by prescription, but when they are manufactured or sold illegally, they are illicit. Traditionally, alcohol and tobacco have not been considered illicit substances even when used by minors, probably because of their widespread legal availability to adults. Common household chemicals, such as glues and paints, take on some characteristics of illicit substances when people inhale them to get high.

Harm reduction is an initiative of Canada's Drug Strategy to use public education programs to significantly reduce the damage associated with alcohol and other drugs. The term *harm reduction* has become controversial in part because some people equate it with advocating for legalization of all drugs. The most commonly accepted definition of harm reduction is "measures taken to address drug problems that are open to outcomes other than abstinence or cessation of use."[10] Measures may include programs, policies, or interventions that seek to reduce or minimize the adverse social and health consequences associated with drug use.

Examples of harm reduction measures applied to injection drug use in Canada include safe injection sites, syringe exchange programs, and methadone maintenance therapy for heroin intravenous drug users. As applied to alcohol use, harm reduction measures include introduction of earlier opening hours for a liquor outlet in downtown Edmonton to reduce the use of Lysol and other nonbeverage alcohol, changes to space and the padding of furniture in licensed establishments to minimize the harm that may result from fights, and designated driver and alternative transportation programs for drinkers. Harm reduction focuses on lowering the risk and severity of adverse consequences arising from drinking without necessarily trying to reduce consumption. The key message in population-based approaches is that drinking less is better; the key message in harm reduction is to avoid problems when you drink.[10] An elaborated discussion of the principles that guide harm reduction initiatives in Canada is provided in the document "Harm Reduction: What's in a Name?" published by the Canadian Centre on Substance Abuse and available at www.ccsa.ca.

Drug misuse generally refers to the use of prescribed drugs in greater amounts than, or for purposes other than, those prescribed by a physician or dentist. For nonprescription drugs or chemicals, such as paints, glues, or solvents, misuse might mean any use other than the use intended by the manufacturer.

Abuse consists of the use of a substance in a manner, amounts, or situations such that the drug use causes problems or greatly increases the chances of problems occurring. The problems may be social (including legal), occupational, psychological, or physical. Once again, this definition gives us a good idea of what we're talking about, but it isn't precise. For example, some would consider any use of an illicit drug to be abuse because of the possibility of legal problems, but many people who have tried marijuana would argue that they had no problems and therefore didn't abuse it. Also, the use of almost any drug, even under the orders of a physician, has at least some potential to cause problems. The question might come down to how great the risk is and whether the user is recklessly disregarding the risk. How does cigarette smoking fit this definition? Should all cigarette smoking be considered drug abuse? For someone to receive a diagnosis of having a *substance use disorder* (see the DSM-5 feature in Chapter 2), the use must be recurrent, and the problems must lead to significant impairment or distress.

continued

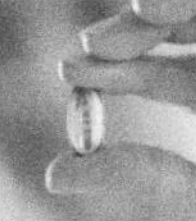

DRUGS IN DEPTH

Important Definitions—and a Caution! *continued*

Addiction is a chronic relapsing condition characterized by compulsive drug seeking and abuse and by long-lasting chemical changes in the brain. Addiction is the same irrespective of whether the drug is alcohol, amphetamines, cocaine, heroin, marijuana, or nicotine. Every addictive substance induces pleasant states or relieves distress. Continued use of the addictive substance induces adaptive changes in the brain that lead to tolerance, physical dependence, uncontrollable craving, and, all too often, relapse. Addiction is a controversial and complex term that has different meanings for different people. Because the term is so widely used in everyday conversation, it is risky for us to try to give it a precise, scientific definition, and then have our readers use their own long-held perspectives whenever we use the term. Therefore, we have avoided using this term where possible, instead relying on more precisely defined terms, such as *dependence.*

Drug **dependence** refers to a state in which the individual uses the drug so frequently and consistently that it appears it would be difficult for the person to get along *without* using the drug. Stopping is very difficult and may cause severe physical and psychological withdrawal. Some drugs and some users have clear withdrawal signs when the drug is not taken, implying a *physiological dependence.* Dependence can take other forms, as shown in the DSM-5 feature in Chapter 2. If a great deal of the individual's time and effort is devoted to getting and using the drug, if the person often winds up taking more of the substance than he or she intended, and if the person has tried several times without success to cut down or control the use, then the person meets the criteria for dependence.

Tolerance is a condition that may follow repeated ingestion of a drug. Drug tolerance occurs when a person's reaction to a psychopharmaceutical drug (such as a painkiller or an intoxicant) decreases so that larger doses are required to achieve the same effect. Drug tolerance can involve both psychological and physiological factors. The resulting pattern of uncontrolled escalating doses may lead to drug overdose and death.

Withdrawal symptoms are abnormal physical or psychological effects that occur after stopping a drug. They may include sweating, tremors, vomiting, anxiety, insomnia, and muscle aches and pains.

Can any general statements be made about **psychoactive** drugs–those compounds that alter consciousness and affect mood? Four basic principles seem to apply to all these drugs.

1. *Drugs, per se, are not good or bad.* There are no "bad drugs." When drug abuse, drug dependence, and risky drug use are talked about, it is the behaviour, the way the drug is being used, that is being referred to. This statement sounds controversial and has angered some prominent political figures and drug educators. It therefore requires some defence. For a pharmacologist, it is difficult to view the drug, the chemical substance itself, as somehow possessing evil intent. It sits there in its bottle and does nothing until we put it into a living system. From the perspective of a psychologist who treats drug users, it is difficult to imagine what good there might be in heroin or cocaine. However, heroin is a perfectly good painkiller, at least as effective as morphine, and it is used medically in many countries. Cocaine is a good local anaesthetic and is still used for medical procedures, even in Canada and the United States. Each of these drugs can also produce bad effects when people abuse them. In the cases of heroin and cocaine, our society has weighed its perception of the risks of bad consequences against the potential benefits and decided that we should severely restrict the availability of these substances. It is wrong, though, to place all the blame for these bad consequences on the drugs themselves and to conclude that they are simply "bad" drugs. Many people tend to view some of these substances as possessing an almost magical power to produce evil. When we blame the substance itself, our efforts to correct drug-related problems tend to focus exclusively on eliminating the substance, perhaps ignoring all the factors that led to the abuse of the drug.
2. *Every drug has multiple effects.* Although a user might focus on a single aspect of a drug's effect, we do not

psychoactive: having effects on thoughts, emotions, or behaviour.

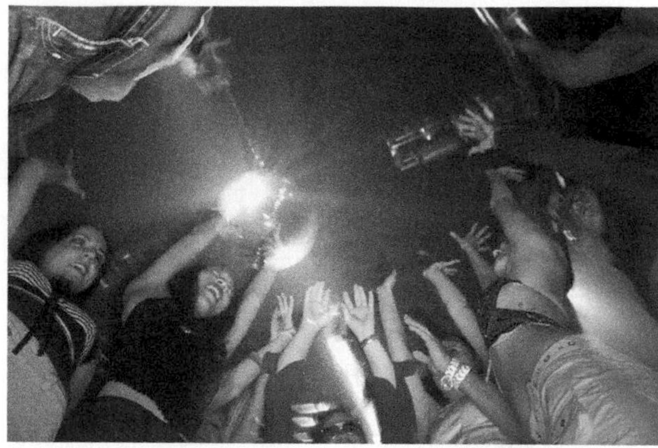

The setting and the expectations of the user influence the effects of drugs.

yet have compounds that alter only one aspect of consciousness. All psychoactive drugs act on more than one place in the brain, so we might expect them to produce complex psychological effects. Also, virtually every drug that acts in the brain also has effects on the rest of the body, influencing blood pressure, intestinal activity, or other functions.

3. *Both the size and the quality of a drug's effect depend on the amount the individual has taken.* The relationship between dose and effect works in two ways. An increase in the dose usually causes an increase in the same effects noticed at lower drug levels. Also, at different dose levels there is often a change in the kind of effect, an alteration in the character of the experience.
4. *The effect of any psychoactive drug depends on the individual's history and expectations.* Because these drugs alter consciousness and thought processes, the effect they have on an individual depends on what was there initially. An individual's attitude can have a major effect on his or her perception of the drug experience. The fact that relatively inexperienced users can experience a high when smoking oregano and dry oak tree leaves–thinking it's good **marijuana**–should come as no surprise to anyone who has arrived late at a party and felt a "buzz" after one drink rather than the usual two or three. It is not possible, then, to talk about many of the effects of these drugs independent of the user's history and attitude and the setting.

How Did We Get Here?

Drug use is not new. Humans have been using alcohol and plant-derived drugs for thousands of years–as far as we know, since *Homo sapiens* first appeared on the planet. A truly "drug-free society" has probably never existed, and might never exist. Psychoactive drugs were used in rituals that we might classify today as religious in nature and where their use was believed to enhance spiritual experiences. A common belief in many early cultures was that illness results from invasion by evil spirits, so in that context it makes sense that psychoactive drugs were often used as part of a purification ritual to rid the body of those spirits. In these early cultures, the use of drugs to treat illness likely was intertwined with spiritual use so that the roles of the priest and that of the *shaman* (medicine man) often were not separate. In fact, the earliest uses of many of the drugs that we now consider to be primarily recreational drugs or drugs of abuse (nicotine, caffeine, alcohol, cocaine, and marijuana) were as treatments for various illnesses. Today many such drugs are either restricted or tightly regulated through the Controlled Drugs and Substances Act.

Have Things Really Changed?

What happens when the regulation or restriction of a drug conflicts with religious practices and freedoms? One example can be seen in the actions of the Santo Daime church in Quebec. Santo Daime is a syncretic spiritual practice founded in the 1930s in Brazil and now practised worldwide. Syncretism combines different systems of philosophical or religious belief or practice, in this case, Folk Catholicism, Kardecist Spiritism, African animism, and South American Shamanism. An important part of its religious ceremony includes the drinking of a tea that contains psychoactive harmala alkaloids. The use of these alkaloids is restricted in Canada. To address this restriction on their religious practice, the Santo Daime church officials applied for an exemption to the Controlled Drugs and Substances Act. In 2006 they were granted an exemption in principle, under section 56 of the Act, thereby allowing the importation and use of harmala alkaloids by the church's members. In a related example the hallucinogen peyote (described in Chapter 14), which is listed as a Schedule III drug in the Controlled Drug and Substances Act, is exempt from restriction when used in religious ceremonies by members of the Native American Church of Canada.

Psychoactive drugs have also played significant roles in the economies of societies in the past. Chapter 10

marijuana: also spelled "marihuana." Dried leaves of the *Cannabis* plant.

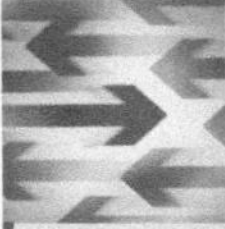

TAKING SIDES

Can We Predict or Control Trends in Drug Use?

Looking at the overall trends in drug use, it is clear that significant changes have occurred in the number of people using marijuana, cocaine, alcohol, and tobacco. However, while it's easy to describe the changes once they have happened, it's much tougher to predict what will come next. Maybe even harder than predicting trends in drug use is knowing what social policies are effective in controlling these trends. The two main kinds of activities that we usually look to as methods to prevent or reduce drug use are legal controls and education (including advertising campaigns). How effective do you think laws have been in helping prevent or reduce drug use? Be sure to consider in your analysis laws regulating sales of alcohol and tobacco to minors. What about the public advertising campaigns you are familiar with? How about school-based prevention programs? As you read this book, these questions will come up again, along with more information about specific laws, drugs, and prevention programs. For now, choose which side you would rather take in a debate on the following proposition: Broad changes in drug use reflect shifts in society and are not greatly influenced by drug-control laws, antidrug advertising, or drug-prevention programs in schools.

describes the importance of tobacco in the early days of European exploration and trade around the globe, as well as its importance in the establishment of English colonies in North America; Chapter 6 discusses the significance of the coca plant (from which cocaine is derived) in the foundation of the Mayan empire in South America; and Chapter 13 points out the importance of the opium trade in opening China's doors to trade with the West in the 1800s.

One area in which enormous change has occurred over the past 100-plus years is in the development and marketing of legal pharmaceuticals. The introduction of vaccines to eliminate smallpox, polio, and other communicable diseases, followed by the development of antibiotics that are capable of curing some types of otherwise deadly illnesses, laid the foundation for our current acceptance of medicines as the cornerstone of our health care system. Some of the scientific and medical discoveries, problems, and laws associated with these changes are outlined in Chapter 3. The many kinds of legal pharmaceuticals designed to influence mental and behavioural functioning are discussed in Chapter 8.

Another significant development in the past 100 years has been government efforts to limit access to certain kinds of drugs that are deemed too dangerous or too likely to produce dependence to allow them to be used in an unregulated fashion. The enormous growth, both in illegal trade and in the number of controlled substances, has led many to refer to this development as a "war on drugs." Canada's National Anti-Drug Strategy outlines the government's heightened focus on illicit drug law enforcement. Critics of the strategy cite that it overlooks a critical element of Canada's substance abuse problem in that the majority of our health and social consequences stem from the use of drugs that are legally produced. These laws are also outlined in Chapter 3, but we will trace their effect on different drug classes throughout the chapters.

With both of these developments, the proportion of our economy devoted to psychoactive drugs, both legal and illegal, and to their regulation, has also expanded considerably. Drug use is an important topic for us to understand if only for that fact. In addition, drug use and its regulation are reflective of changes in our society and in how we as individuals interact with that society. Finally, drug problems and our attempts to solve them have in turn had major influences on us as individuals and on our perceptions of appropriate roles for government, education, and health care.

In May 2003, the Government of Canada underscored its commitment to addressing the ongoing public health concern of substance abuse with its renewed Canada's Drug Strategy (CDS). The goal of the CDS was to significantly reduce the harm associated with alcohol and other drugs by using a broad four-component approach that includes education, prevention, harm reduction, and enforcement. The CDS initiative balances a population-based approach, with the goal of decreasing consumption and related risks, with harm reduction measures that focus on reducing the risks and severity of adverse consequences arising from drug and alcohol use while not necessarily reducing consumption. Harm reduction strategies, unlike population-based approaches, normalize drug-taking behaviour and focus on the avoidance of problems. Numerous harm reduction strategies have been employed in Canada. Examples include needle exchange programs and supervised injection sites to reduce the transmission of blood-borne disease in intravenous drug users and the regulation of cheap drink promotions (e.g., happy hours) to reduce the incidence of alcohol-related poisonings, violence, and drunk driving. Discussions of evidence-based harm reduction strategies are provided throughout subsequent chapters.

Drugs and Drug Use Today

In trying to get an overall picture of drug use in today's society, we quickly discover that it's not easy to get accurate information. It's not possible to measure with great accuracy the use of, let's say, cocaine in Canada. We don't really know how much is imported and sold, because most of it is illegal. We don't really know how many cocaine users there are in the country, because we have no good way of counting them. For some things, such as prescription drugs, tobacco, and alcohol, we have a wealth of legal sales information and can make much better estimates of rates of use. Even there, however, our information might not be complete (e.g., home-brewed beer and wine, which accounts for a portion of consumed alcohol and is shown in Figure 1.1, might not be counted, illegal tobacco sales are difficult to estimate, and prescription drugs might be bought and then resold or left unused in the medicine cabinet).

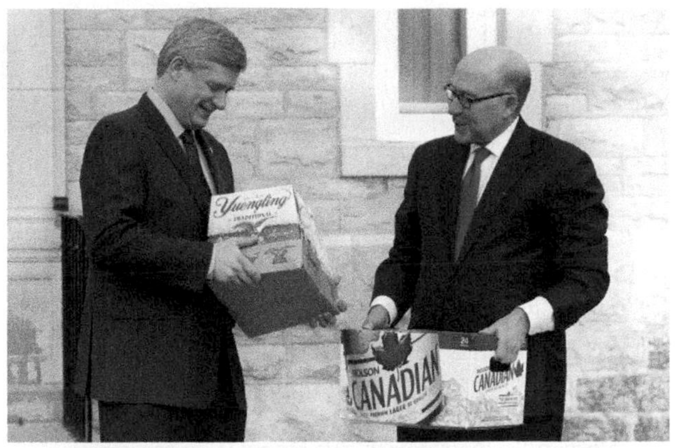

Prime Minister Stephen Harper, shown here with the former U.S. Ambassador to Canada David Jacobson.

Extent of Drug Use

Let us look at some of the kinds of information we do have. A large number of survey questionnaire studies have been conducted in junior highs, high schools, and

Figure 1.1 Homemade Beer and Wine Production in Canadian Provinces, 2004

According to the 2004 ***Canadian Addiction Survey*** a minority of Canadians (6.7%) produce their own wine or beer at home. The figure shows the average number of bottles of homemade beer and wine produced in the provinces in 2004.

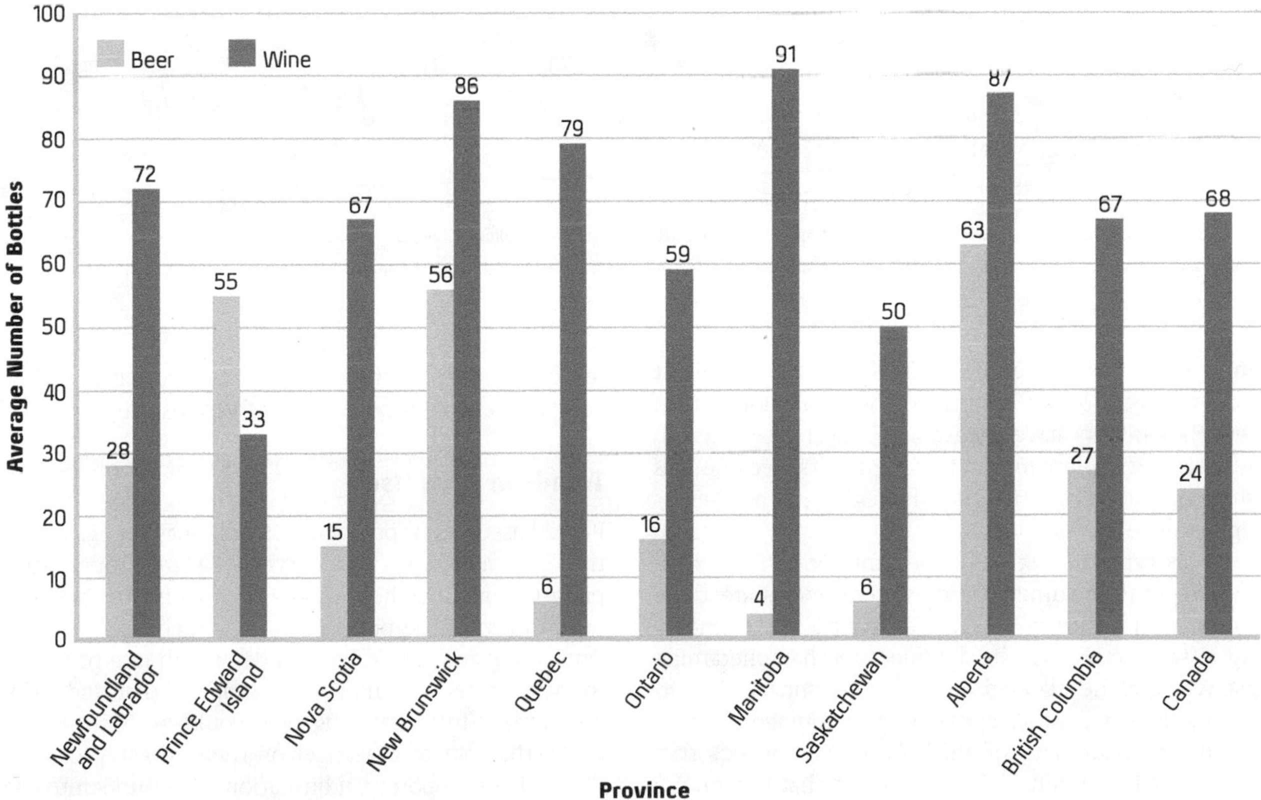

Source: Adlaf, E. M., P. Begin, and E. Sawka, eds. *Canadian Addiction Survey (CAS): A National Survey of Canadians' Use of Alcohol and Other Drugs: Prevalence of Use and Related Harms: Detailed Report.* Ottawa: Canadian Centre on Substance Abuse, 2005.

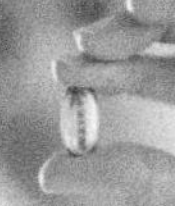

DRUGS IN DEPTH

Methamphetamine Use in Your Community

Assume that you have just been appointed to a community-based committee that is looking into drug problems. A high school student on the committee has just returned from a residential treatment program and reports that methamphetamine use has become "very common" in local high schools. Some members of the committee want to call in experts immediately to give school-wide assemblies describing the dangers of methamphetamine. You have asked for a little time to check out the student's story to find out what you can about the actual extent of use in the community and report back to the group in a month. Make a list of potential information sources and the type of information each might provide. How close do you think you could come to making an estimate of how many current methamphetamine users there are in your community? Do you think it would be above or below the national average? How would it compare with the prevalence of daily intravenous drug users in Vancouver as described in Figure 1.2?

Figure 1.2 Intravenous Drug Users in Vancouver, British Columbia, 1996–2011

The figure illustrates the percentage of individuals from a cohort of injection drug users ($n = 1979$) who self-reported injecting crystal methamphetamine in the past year.

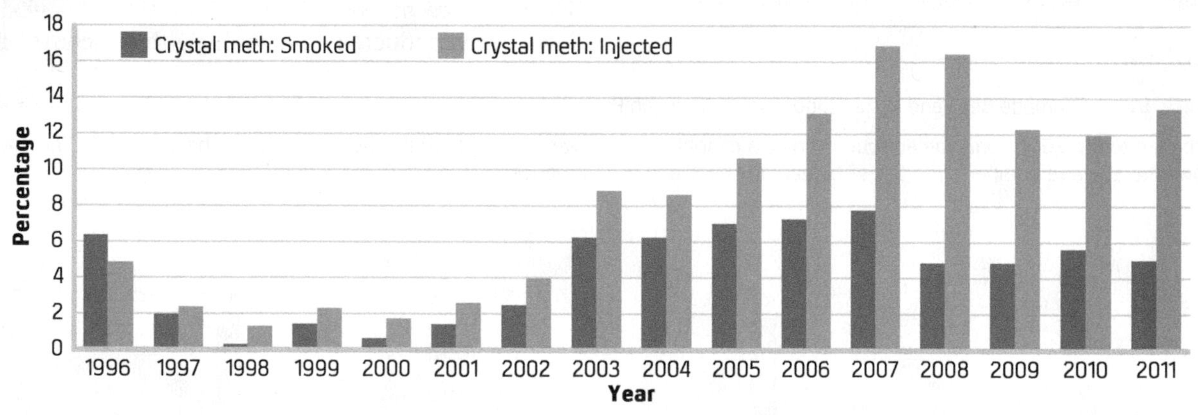

Source: Drug Situation in Vancouver Report prepared by the Urban Health Research Initiative of the British Columbia Centre for Excellence in HIV/AIDS, Second Edition, June 2013. Available at: http://www.cfenet.ubc.ca/sites/default/files/uploads/news/releases/war_on_drugs_failing_to_limit_drug_use.pdf.

universities, partly because this is one of the easiest ways to get a lot of information with a minimum of fuss. Researchers have always been most interested in drug use by adolescents and young adults, because this is the age when drug use usually begins and reaches its highest levels.

This type of data has some limitations. For example, we must assume that most self-reports are done honestly. In reality, however, we have no way of checking to see if Johnny really did inject methamphetamine last week, as he claimed on the questionnaire. Nevertheless, if every effort is made to encourage honesty (including assurances of anonymity), we expect that this factor is minimized. To the extent that tendencies to overreport or underreport drug use are relatively constant from one year to the next, we can use such results to reflect trends in drug use over time and to compare relative reported use of various drugs.

Trends in Drug Use

Broad-based self-report information may be gathered through house-to-house surveys. With proper sampling techniques, these studies can estimate the drug use in most of the population. This technique is time-consuming and expensive and has a high rate of refusal to participate. We must also suspect that individuals engaged in illegal drug use would be reluctant to reveal that fact to a stranger on their doorstep or telephone. Despite potential limitations, snapshots into the general Canadian public use of alcohol and drugs have been provided through the *Canadian Addiction Survey*

(CAS), last performed in 2004, and more recently through the *Canadian Alcohol and Drug Use Monitoring Survey* (CADUMS), conducted annually since 2008.[3] The intent of these surveys is to measure how Canadians aged 15 years and older use alcohol, cannabis, and other drugs, and the impact that use has on their physical, mental, and social well-being. This information, when compared with past studies, indicates trends in drug use and harms associated with use.[3,11]

These surveys, which are collaborative initiatives by Health Canada, the Canadian Executive Council on Addictions–which includes the Canadian Centre on Substance Abuse; the provinces of Nova Scotia, New Brunswick, and British Columbia; the Alberta Alcohol and Drug Abuse Commission; the Addictions Foundation of Manitoba; the Centre for Addiction and Mental Health; the Prince Edward Island Provincial Health Services Authority; and the Kaiser Foundation–and the Centre for Addictions Research of BC, have four key objectives:

1. To determine the prevalence, incidence, and patterns of drug and alcohol use
2. To measure the personal (e.g., physical health, home life and marriage, work and studies, financial position, legal problems, housing, learning) and social harms (e.g., friendships and social life) associated with patterns of use of alcohol, tobacco, and illicit drugs, including opiates, cocaine and crack, amphetamines, hallucinogens (including MDMA), and inhalants, during a person's lifetime and during the 12 months before the survey
3. To assess the context of use and identify risk and protective factors related to drug use and consequences of such use in specific subgroups and the general Canadian population
4. To establish baseline data against which to evaluate the effectiveness of CDS and harm reduction efforts focused on alcohol and other drug use in the Canadian population aged 15 years and older

The 2004 CAS, a national telephone survey based on a random sample, collected information on drug use and its consequences from 13 909 respondents 15 years of age and older. Data collected represented 1000 respondents, on average, for each province, but with 2200 from Alberta, 3000 from British Columbia, and 1500 from Manitoba. One limitation of this study is that it excludes groups that often contain a disproportionally high number of drug and alcohol users: people in prisons, hospitals, and military bases, and transient populations, such as the homeless.

Comparisons of the key findings from the 1994 and 2004 CAS and 2012 CADUMS are presented in Table 1.1.

Data collected through tools like the CAS and the CADUMS provide a wealth of information about trends in drug and alcohol use in Canada. We strongly recommend that you visit the Web sites for these surveys to gain a full appreciation of the uses and limitations of the information these surveys provide.[12,13]

At the beginning of this chapter we discussed that we may be more concerned with young adults and children using alcohol and drugs. Three surveys, the *Canadian Campus Survey* (CCS), the *American College Health Association* (ACHA) *National College Health Assessment*, and the *Ontario Student Drug Use and Health Survey* (OSDUHS), provide insight into the alcohol and drug use practices of Canadian youth.

Table 1.2 compares past-year use of alcohol and other drugs among Canadian undergraduates measured in the 1998 and 2004 CCS. Only two drugs, hallucinogens and LSD, showed small, albeit statistically significant, decreases. Alcohol use showed little change. Among all students, the past-year use of cannabis remained similar in 1998 and 2004, 28.8% versus 32.1%. Between 1998 and 2004, the CCS also showed that cannabis use declined among students in the Prairies, from 24.1% to 19.4%, and increased in the Atlantic region, from 26.5% to 36.9%.[14] The CCS has not been implemented since 2004. However, in 2013 the Canadian Association of College and University Student Services published results of the ACHA National College Health Assessment survey, which reported selected drug use trends among 34 039 students from 32 postsecondary Canadian institutions.[15]

A difference in the categorization of specific drugs in the respective surveys prevents trend comparison between the 2004 and 2013 surveys. The 2013 ACHA National College Health Assessment data do, however (as shown in Table 1.3), provide a snapshot of current use patterns among postsecondary students. For example, past-30-day use of alcohol was 70.8%, while 16.4% of students self-reported as lifetime abstainers. By far the most commonly used illicit drug was cannabis, used by 16.0% of students during the past 30 days and 30.9% during their lifetime.

Now let's look at the epidemiological trends in drug use among students in grades 7 through 12. The OSDUHS, which began in 1977, is the longest ongoing school-based survey in Canada. The OSDUHS interviews thousands of students every second year from 150 elementary and secondary schools across Ontario. The purpose of the survey is to identify epidemiological trends in student drug use, harmful consequences of use, and risk and protective factors.[16]

In Figure 1.3, two numbers are presented for each drug: the percentage of students (grades 7 to 12) who

Table 1.1 Lifetime and 12-Month Prevalence of Alcohol and Other Drug Use, Canadians Ages 15+, 1994, 2004, and 2012

Report of Use	Lifetime			12-Month		
Drug	**1994**	**2004**	**2012**	**1994**	**2004**	**2012**
Alcohol	n/a	92.8	91.0	72.3	79.3	78.4
Males	n/a	94.6	92.9	n/a	82	82.7
Females	n/a	91.1	89.3	n/a	76.8	74.4
Cannabis	28.2	44.5	41.5	7.4	14.1	10.2
Males	33.5	50.1	47.9	10	18.2	13.7
Females	23.1	39.2	35.5	4.9	10.2	7.0
Cocaine/Crack	3.8	10.6	7.3	0.7	1.9	1.1
Males	4.9	14.1	9.9	0.8	2.7	1.5
Females	2.7	7.3	4.7	0.5	1.1	S
Hallucinogens	5.2	11.4	12.5	0.9	0.7	0.9
Males	7.2	16	16.6	1.3	1.0	1.5
Females	3.3	7.1	8.6	0.6	0.3	S
Speed	2.1	6.4	4.1	0.2	0.8	S
Males	3.1	8.7	5.7	0.4	1.0	S
Females	1.2	4.1	2.5	s	0.6	S
Heroin	0.5	0.9	0.5	s	S	S
Males	0.8	1.3	0.7	s	S	S
Females	s	0.5	s	s	S	S
Ecstasy	n/a	4.1	4.4	n/a	1.1	0.6
Males	n/a	5.2	5.6	n/a	1.5	s
Females	n/a	3.0	3.2	n/a	0.7	s
Inhalants	0.8	1.3	n/a	n/a	n/a	n/a
Males	1.2	1.9	n/a	n/a	n/a	n/a
Females	0.3	0.7	n/a	n/a	n/a	n/a
Steroids	0.3	0.6	n/a	n/a	n/a	n/a
Males	0.4	1.0	n/a	n/a	n/a	n/a
Females	s	s	n/a	n/a	n/a	n/a
Non Medicinal Prescription Opioids	n/a	n/a	n/a	n/a	n/a	5.2
Males	n/a	n/a	n/a	n/a	n/a	6.9
Females	n/a	n/a	n/a	n/a	n/a	3.9

Notes: s = estimate suppressed due to high sampling variability; n/a = data not available

Sources: Adapted from Adlaf, E. M., P. Begin, and E. Sawka, eds. *Canadian Addiction Survey (CAS): A National Survey of Canadians' Use of Alcohol and Other Drugs: Prevalence of Use and Related Harms: Detailed Report.* Ottawa: Canadian Centre on Substance Abuse, 2005; Health Canada. *Canadian Alcohol and Drug Use Monitoring Survey. Detailed Tables for 2012.* Ottawa: Author, 2013. To obtain a copy of this document, please send an e-mail request to CADUMS-ESCCAD@hc-sc.gc.ca.

have ever used the drug (% Lifetime Use) and the percentage who report having used it within the past year (% Past-Year Use). Note that most of these students have tried alcohol at some time in their lives. Twenty-seven percent have tried marijuana, and 15% have reported non-medical use of prescription opioid pain relievers. It is interesting to note that the lifetime and daily use of many of these drugs can be considered rare.[17]

The OSDUHS results allow us to see changes over time in the rates of drug use. Figure 1.4 shows rates of marijuana use among students in grades 7 through 12. In 1977, fewer than 25% of students reported having previously used marijuana. This proportion rose in 1979 to just fewer than 30% and then declined each year until 1991, when only 10% of students reporting having used marijuana. In 1993 the trend reversed, with

Table 1.2 Changes in Past-Year Alcohol and Other Drug Use, Canadian Undergraduates, 1998, 2004

Drug	1998	2004
Alcohol	86.5	85.7
Cannabis	28.8	32.1
Any illicit drug use (excluding cannabis)	10.3	8.7
Hallucinogens	8.2	5.7
Ecstasy (MDMA)	2.4	2.5
Amphetamines	1.8	2.6
LSD	1.8	<1.0
Cocaine	1.6	2.1
Anabolic steroids	s	s
Crack	s	s
Heroin	s	s

Notes: s = no reliable data

Sources: Adlaf, E. M., A. Demers, and L. Gliksman, eds. *Canadian Campus Survey 2004.* Toronto: Centre for Addiction and Mental Health, 2005.

Table 1.3 Prevalence of Alcohol and Other Drug Use among Canadian Postsecondary Institution Students (*N* = 34 039), 2013

Report of Use	Lifetime	30 Days
Drug		
Alcohol	83.6	70.8
Cannabis	30.9	16.0
Cigarettes	29.2	11.6
Hallucinogens (LSD, PCP)	5.7	0.6
Opiates (heroin, smack)	1.3	0.3
Ecstasy (MDMA)	8.8	1.4
Methamphetamine (crystal, meth, ice, crank)	1.6	0.2
Inhalants (glue, solvents, gas)	1.0	0.2
Cocaine (crack, rock, freebase)	5.4	1.1
Anabolic steroids (Testosterone)	0.8	0.2
Club drugs (GHB, Ketamine, Rohypnol)	2.4	0.3

Source: American College Health Association. American College Health Association—National College Health Assessment II: Canadian Reference Group Data Report Spring 2013. Hanover, MD: American College Health Association, 2013.

the percentage of students trying marijuana increasing steadily to 2003, when it once again was just below 30%. By 2005, the percentage of students who had ever tried marijuana had decreased to approximately 22%; by 2009 it was at 20%. Because marijuana is by far the most commonly used illicit drug, we can use this graph to make a broader statement: Illicit drug use among students in grades 7 through 12 slowly declined between 2003 and 2013. In 2013 marijuana use among students in grades 7 through 12 was just slightly lower

Figure 1.3 Percentage Reporting Lifetime and Past-Year Drug Abuse, 2013 OSDUHS (Grades 7–12)

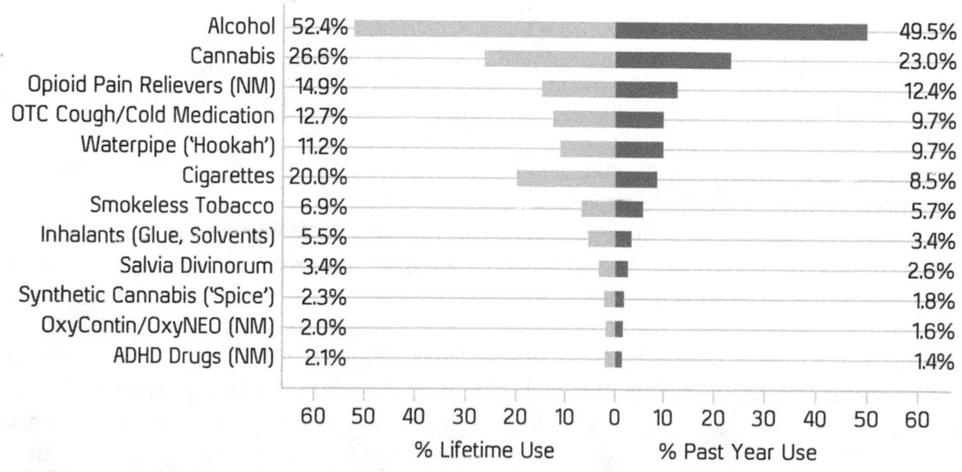

Source: Paglia-Boak, A., and others. (2013). *Drug Use among Ontario Students, 1977–2013: Detailed OSDUHS Findings* (CAMH Research Document Series No. 36). Toronto: Centre for Addiction and Mental Health. Retrieved December 12, 2013, from http://www.camh.ca/en/research/news_and_publications/ontario-student-drug-use-and-health-survey/Documents/2013%20OSDUHS%20Docs/2013OSDUHS_Detailed_DrugUseReport.pdf.

Figure 1.4 Long-Term Trends in Drug Use, 1977–2013 OSDUHS

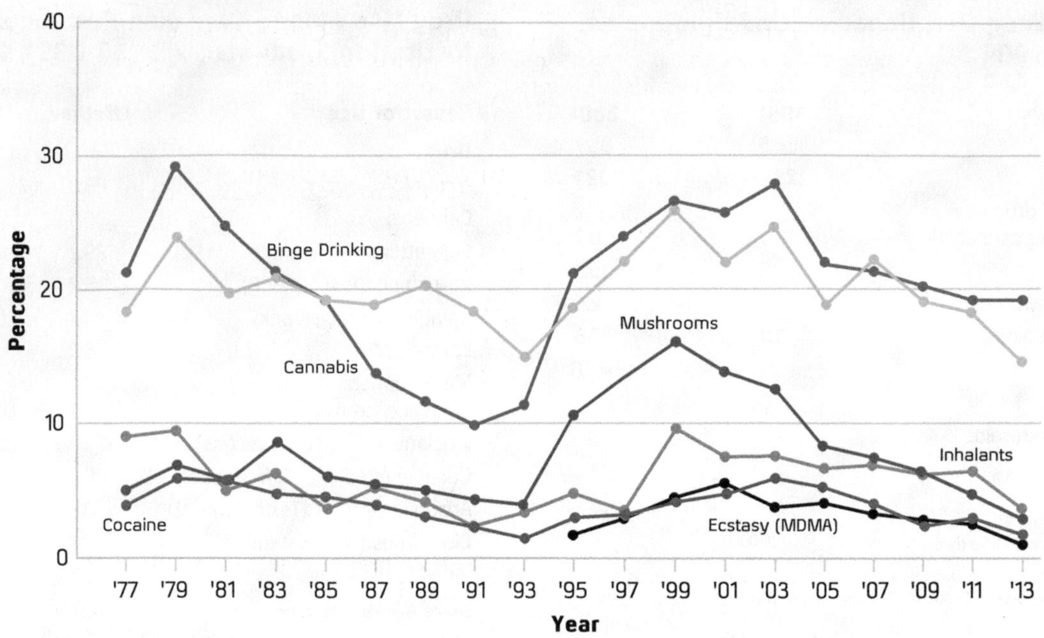

Note: (1) binge drinking refers to drinking 5 or more drinks on one occasion at least once in the past month; (2) estimates for mushrooms and cocaine exclude Grade 7 students

Source: Adapted from Paglia-Boak, A., and others. *Drug Use among Ontario Students, 1977–2013: Detailed OSDUHS Findings* (CAMH Research Document Series No. 36). Toronto: Centre for Addiction and Mental Health, 2009, Table 3.2.4 (binge drinking, cocaine, mushrooms), 3.2.5 (cannabis) and 3.2.6 (ecstasy). Retrieved December 12, 2013, from http://www.camh.ca/en/research/news_and_publications/ontario-student-drug-use-and-health-survey/Documents/2013%20OSDUHS%20Docs/2013OSDUHS_Detailed_DrugUseReport.pdf.

than it was in 1977, but it was more common than it was at its lowest point in 1991. Interestingly, the trend for binge drinking follows the same pattern as that for cannabis. It is tempting to speculate that these drugs are used in combination, but we don't have data to support such statements. Evidence like that described above is important because some groups say that drug use is increasing among young people or that people are starting to use drugs at younger and younger ages, but the best data we have provide no support for such statements.

How can we explain these very large changes in rates of marijuana use over time? Maybe marijuana was easier to obtain in 1977, less available in 1991, and so on. Each year the same students were asked their opinion about how easy they thought it would be to get marijuana if they wanted to do so. In 1977 about 90% of senior students said that it would be fairly easy or very easy for them to get marijuana. In 2013, the substance most readily available to students was alcohol (65% reported that it would be fairly easy or very easy to obtain), followed by cigarettes (61%), marijuana (51%), OxyContin or other prescription pain relievers (19%), ecstasy (14%), cocaine (14%), and LSD (9%). Trend data on perceived availability indicate that alcohol, cannabis, cocaine, LSD, and ecstasy were more difficult to obtain in 2013 compared with a decade before, yet this is not reflected in their levels of use.[16] Thus, the perceived availability does *not* appear to explain differences in rates of use over time. This result is important because it implies that large changes in rates of drug use can occur even when the supply of the drug does not appear to change much. What might have a stronger influence is the perceived risk of drug use and its social acceptability (i.e., approval of use), as shown in Figure 1.5.

Comparing Figure 1.4 with Figure 1.5 shows that a correlation may exist between the perception of risk and the reported use of alcohol and other drugs. In Figure 1.6, we can see that alcohol has the least perceived harm. This result is important because it seems to say that the best way to achieve low rates of alcohol and other drug use is by convincing students that it is risky to use alcohol and other drugs and that efforts to control the availability of alcohol and other drugs (supply reduction) might have less influence. However, keep in

Figure 1.5 Percentage of Students Reporting Great Risk of Harm with Drug-Using Behaviours

In 2013, the OSDUHS asked students in grades 7–12 their perceptions of the risks associated with selected drug use behaviours. Students identified the greatest risk of physical harm to be associated with regular marijuana use, followed by trying cocaine, trying non-medicinal prescription opioids, trying ecstasy, cigarettes, binge drinking on weekends, and trying marijuana. Perceptions of risk significantly increase with grade level for trying non-medicinal prescription opioids and cigarettes, but decrease with grade level for marijuana use (trying it and regular use).[16]

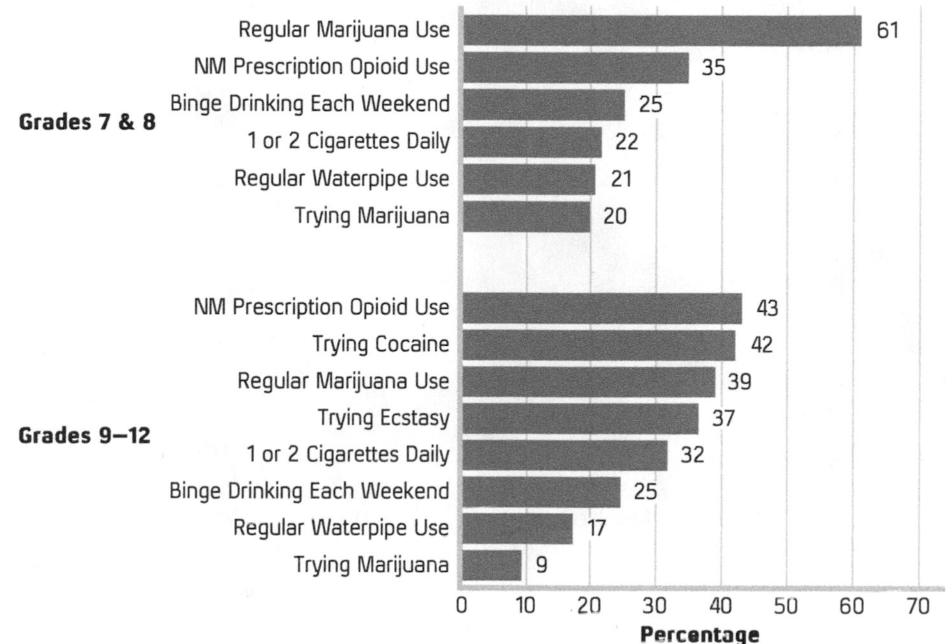

Notes: (1) NM = nonmedical use, without one's own prescription; (2) Binge Drinking = 5+ drinks of alcohol on one occasion; (3) Grade 7 and 8 students were not asked about trying cocaine or trying ecstasy

Source: Used with permission from Centre for Addiction and Mental Health.

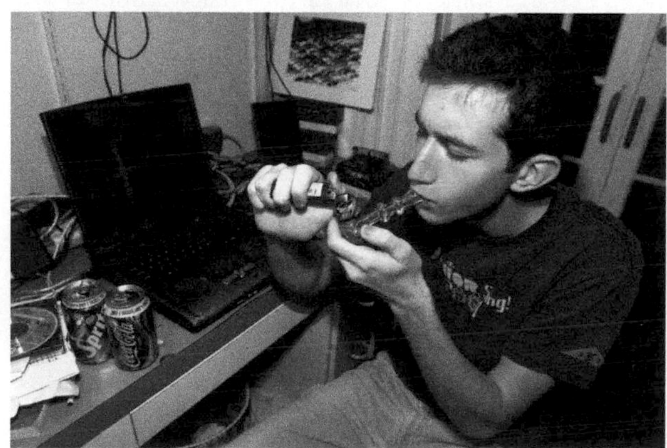

Marijuana is the most commonly used illicit drug, and major surveys, including the CCS and OSDUHS in Canada and the *Monitoring the Future* project in the United States, track trends in its use by students.

mind that a cause-and-effect relationship has not been proven, and Canadians do see the availability of drugs as being linked to Canada's problems with drugs (see Figure 1.7). Changes in both rates of use and perceptions of risk could be caused by something else that isn't being directly measured.

A comparison of Canadian students, surveyed through the 2004 CCS, and American students, surveyed in 2003 by the *Monitoring the Future* study, revealed that Canadian university students are more likely than American students to have drunk alcohol in the past month (77.1% versus 66.2%) and less likely (30.2% versus 38.5%) to have been binge drinking (consuming five or more drinks on a single occasion). Canadian students were also less likely than Americans to have used cocaine (2.1% versus 5.4%) or ecstasy (2.5% versus 4.4%) in the past year. Past-year cannabis use did not differ (32.1% versus 33.7%), nor did hallucinogens

Figure 1.6 Perceived Harms from Various Substance Use Behaviours

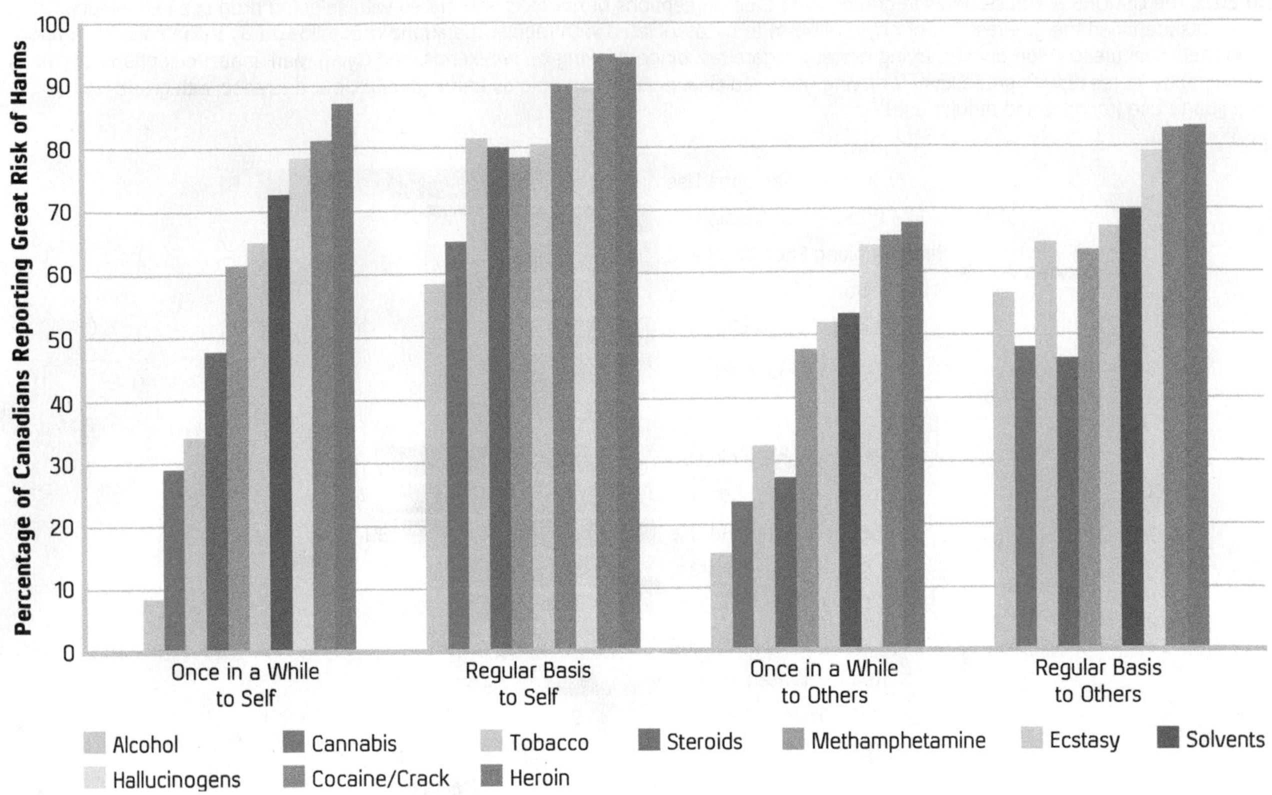

Source: Canadian Addiction Survey (CAS). Health Canada, 2006. Reproduced with permission from the Minister of Health, 2014.

use (5.6% versus 5.4%) or alcohol consumption (85.7% versus 81.7%).[18,19]

We have seen fairly dramatic trends over time in marijuana use, but what about other substances? We saw in Table 1.1 that the percentage of drinkers remained the same from 2004 to 2012. We will look more closely at specific drug-taking trends in subsequent chapters.

Survey data have shown us that patterns and rates of drug and alcohol use change with time. What accounts for these changes? Are they reflective of political legislation? The current consensus is that government's policies might have helped to amplify the effects of underlying social change, but they do not create it. If we can't point to government policies as the cause of change, how can we explain them? The short answer is that for now, we can't. We are left with saying that changes in rates and patterns of illicit drug use and in alcohol use probably reflect changes over time in a broad range of attitudes and behaviours among Canadians–what we can refer to as *social trends*. This isn't much of an explanation, and that is somewhat frustrating. After all, if we understood why these changes were taking place, it might allow us to influence rates of substance use among the general population or at least to predict what will happen next. Perhaps some of today's university students will be the ones to develop this understanding over the next few years.

LO5, LO6, LO7

Correlates of Drug Use

Once we know that a drug is used by some percentage of a group of people, the next logical step is to ask about the characteristics of those who use the drug, as compared with those who don't. Often the same questionnaires that ask each person which drugs they have used include several questions about the people completing the questionnaires. The researchers might then use computer programs to prospect through the data, looking for any personal characteristics that can be correlated with drug use. But these studies rarely

Figure 1.7 Factors Seen as the Main Cause of Drug Problems by Canadians

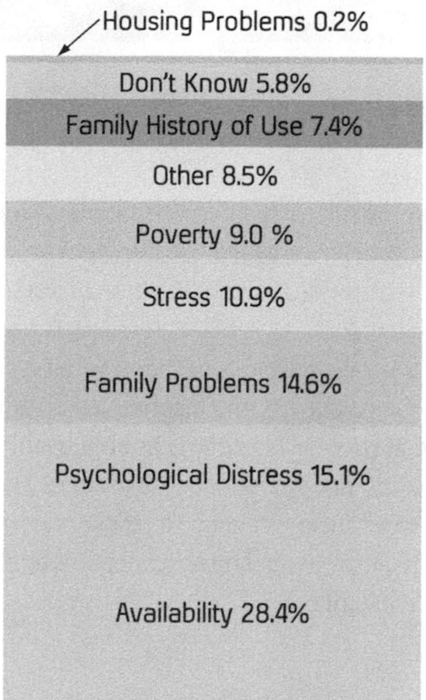

Source: © All rights reserved. Canadian Addiction Survey (CAS). Health Canada, 2006. Reproduced with permission from the Minister of Health, 2014.

reveal much about either very unusual or very common types or amounts of drug use. For example, if we used a computer to comb through the data from 1000 questionnaires, looking for characteristics correlated with heroin use, only one or two people in that sample might report heroin use, and we can't correlate much based on one or two people. Likewise, it would be difficult to identify the distinguishing characteristics of the people who have "ever tried" alcohol, because that group usually represents more than 90% of the sample.

Much of the research on **correlates** of drug use has used marijuana smoking as an indicator, partly because marijuana use has been a matter of some concern and partly because enough people have tried it so that meaningful correlations can be done. Other studies focus on early drinking or early cigarette smoking.

Risk and Protective Factors

Increasingly, researchers are analyzing the correlates of drug use in terms of risk factors and protective factors. Risk factors are correlated with higher rates of drug use, while protective factors are correlated with lower rates of drug use. A study based on data obtained from the U.S. *National Survey on Drug Use and Health* examined risk and protective factors regarding use of marijuana among adolescents (ages 12–17).[20] This large-scale study provides some of the best information we have about the correlates of marijuana use among American adolescents. The Canadian Centre on Substance Abuse and the Canadian *National Longitudinal Survey of Children and Youth* (ages 10–15 years) report similar findings among Canadian adolescents.[21] The most significant factors are reported in Table 1.4.

In some ways, the results confirm what most people probably assume: The kids who live in rough neighbourhoods, whose parents don't seem to care what they do, who have drug using friends, who steal and get into fights, who aren't involved in religious activities, and who don't do well in school are the most likely to smoke marijuana. The same study analyzed cigarette smoking and alcohol use, with overall similar results.

correlate: a variable that is statistically related to some other variable, such as drug use.

Table 1.4 Risk and Protective Factors Associated with Marijuana Use by Adolescents

The likelihood of substance use or abuse increases with the *cumulative number* of risk factors rather than with any one specific risk factor. Risk and severity of outcome increase as risk factors multiply.[21]

Risk Factors (in order of importance)

1. Having friends who use marijuana or other substances
2. Engaging in frequent fighting, stealing, or other antisocial activities
3. Perceiving that substance use is prevalent at your school
4. Knowing adults who use marijuana or other substances
5. Having a positive attitude toward marijuana use

Protective Factors (in order of importance)

1. Perceiving that there are strong sanctions against substance use at school
2. Having parents as a source of social support
3. Being committed to school and sports
4. Believing that religion is important and frequently attending religious services
5. Participating in two or more extracurricular activities

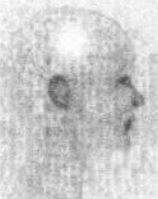

MIND/BODY CONNECTION

Religion and Drug Use

In study after study, those young people who report more involvement with religion (they attend services regularly and say their religion influences how they make decisions) are less likely to smoke cigarettes, drink alcohol, or use any type of illicit drug. In Canada the *National Population Health Survey*, which interviewed more than 20 000 Canadian households, similarly revealed that attendance at religious services for both male and female adolescents was linked with lower levels of multiple-risk behaviour, including smoking and binge drinking.[22] Such results are not surprising given that studies of Canadian adolescents have shown that those with a definite belief in God are consistently more likely than teens who hold an atheistic position to place a high value on such traits as trust, honesty, concern for others, and working hard.[23] Today approximately 13% of Canadian adolescents report that religion plays an important part in their lives.

Consider your own feelings about religion and about drug use. Why do you think this relationship between religiosity and lower rates of drug use is such a consistent finding? If you have friends from different religious backgrounds, discuss this relationship with them. Some religions have specific teachings against any alcohol use or tobacco use, but the general relationship seems to hold even for those religions that do not forbid these behaviours (at least for adults). What other factors related to religious involvement in general might serve as protective factors against the use of these substances?

There are some surprising results, however. Those adolescents who reported that their parents frequently monitored their behaviour (checking homework, limiting TV watching, and requiring chores, for example) were actually a little *more* likely to report using marijuana than adolescents who reported less parental monitoring. This finding points out the main problem with a correlational study: We don't know if excessive parental monitoring makes adolescents more likely to smoke marijuana, or if adolescents' smoking marijuana and getting in fights makes their parents more likely to monitor them (the latter seems more likely).

Another example of the limitation of correlational studies is the link between marijuana smoking and poor academic performance. Does smoking marijuana cause the user to get lower grades? Or is it the kids who are getting low grades anyway who are more likely to smoke marijuana? One indication comes from the analysis of risk and protective factors for cigarette smoking in this same study. The association between low academic performance and cigarette smoking was even stronger than the association between low academic performance and marijuana smoking. This leads most people to conclude that it's the kids who are getting low grades anyway who are more likely to be cigarette smokers, and the same conclusion can probably be reached about marijuana smoking.

The overall picture that emerges from studies of risk and protective factors is that the same adolescents who are likely to smoke cigarettes, drink heavily, and smoke marijuana are also likely to engage in other risk behaviours, such as vandalism, stealing, fighting, and early sexual behaviour. We all can think of individual exceptions to this rule, but correlational studies over many years all come to the same conclusion: If you want to find the greatest number of young people who use illicit drugs, look among the people who are getting in trouble in other ways.

Gender, Socioeconomic Status, and Level of Education

Table 1.5 shows how some demographic variables are related to current use of some drugs of interest. The first thing to notice is something that has been a consistent finding over many kinds of studies: Males are more likely to drink alcohol, smoke marijuana, and use illicit drugs than are females. Second, education level is powerfully related to two common behaviours: People with some postsecondary education and university degrees (compared with those who completed only high school) are more likely to drink alcohol, and people with higher levels of education are somewhat less likely to use marijuana. This probably doesn't surprise most people, but

Table 1.5 Drug Use among 15- to 75-Year-Olds: Percentage Reporting Use in the Past Year

Drug	Alcohol	Marijuana	Other Illicit Drug Use†
Male	82.0%	18.2%	4.3%
Female	76.8	10.2	1.8
High school graduate*	79.2	14.2	3.6
Some postsecondary education*	84.2	16.5	3.8
University graduate*	84.1	10.9	1.7
Low income (<30K)*	66.2	17.0	4.5
Middle income (<60K)*	80.9	13.7	2.9
High income (>80K)*	88.7	15.9	3.0

*Females and males combined.

†Cocaine, speed, ecstasy, hallucinogens, heroin

Source: Adapted from Adlaf, E. M., P. Begin, and E. Sawka, eds. *Canadian Addiction Survey (CAS): A National Survey of Canadians' Use of Alcohol and Other Drugs, Prevalence of Use and Related Harms: Detailed Report.* Ottawa: Canadian Centre on Substance Abuse, 2005.

it is good to see that in many cases the data do provide support for what most people would expect.

Personality Variables

The relationships between substance use and various indicators of individual differences in personality variables have been studied extensively over the years. In general, large-scale survey studies of substance use in the general population have yielded weak or inconsistent correlations with most traditional personality traits as measured by questionnaires. For example, it has been difficult to find a clear relationship between measures of self-esteem and rates of using marijuana. More recently, several studies have found that various ways of measuring a factor called *impulsivity* can be correlated with rates of substance use in the general population.[24] Impulsivity is turning out to be of much interest to drug researchers but also hard to pin down in that different laboratories have different ways of measuring it. In general, it seems to relate to a person's tendency to act quickly and without consideration of the longer-term consequences. We can expect to see more research on this concept over the next few years.

Instead of looking at any level of substance use within the general population, we can look for personality differences between those who are dependent on substances and those who are not. When we do that, we find many personality differences associated with being more heavily involved in substance abuse or dependence. The association with impulsivity, for example, is much stronger in this type of study. Likewise, if we look at groups of people who are diagnosed with personality disorders, such as conduct disorder or antisocial personality disorder, we find high rates of substance use in these groups. Overall, it seems that personality factors may play a small role in whether someone decides to try alcohol or marijuana but a larger role in whether that use develops into a serious problem. Because the main focus of this first chapter is on rates of drug use in the general population, we will put off further discussion of personality variables to the next chapter.

Genetics

There is increasing interest in genetic influences on drug use. Again, studies that look at the general population and ask simply about recent use are less likely to produce significant results than are studies that focus on people diagnosed with substance use disorders. As with personality, genetic factors (phenotypes) may also play a significant role in determining whether use of alcohol or marijuana might develop into a serious problem. Studies of genetic variability in impulsivity and related traits are beginning to show clear association with substance use disorders.[25] Students interested in further reading on genetic phenotype associated with increased risk of dependence are directed to Chapter 2 where a number of excellent references on this subject are identified.

Antecedents of Drug Use

Finding characteristics that tend to be associated with drug use doesn't help us understand causal relationships very well. For example, do adolescents first become involved with a peer group and then use drugs, or do they first use drugs and then begin to hang around with others who do the same? Does drug use cause them to become poor students and to fight and steal? To answer such questions, we might interview the same individuals at different times and look for **antecedents**, characteristics that predict later initiation of drug use. One such study conducted in Finland found that future initiation of substance use or heavy alcohol use can be predicted by several of the same risk factors we have already discussed: aggressiveness, conduct problems, poor academic performance, "attachment to bad company," and parent and community norms more supportive of drug use.[26] Because these factors were measured before the increase in substance use, we are more likely to conclude that they may be causing substance use. But some other, unmeasured, variables might be causing both the antecedent risk factors and the subsequent substance use to emerge in these adolescents' lives.

A few scientists have been able to follow the same group of people at annual intervals for several years in what is known as a **longitudinal study**. One such study has tracked more than 1200 participants from a predominantly Black community in Chicago from ages 6 through 32.[27] Males who had shown a high "readiness to learn" in grade 1 were less likely to be cocaine users as adults, but females with poor academic performance in grade 1 had lower rates of cocaine use than females with higher scores in grade 1. Males who were either "shy" or "aggressive" in grade 1 were more likely to be adult drug users than were the students who had been considered neither shy nor aggressive 26 years earlier. It is much more difficult to obtain this type of data, and it is somewhat surprising that any variables measured at age six could reliably predict adult drug use.

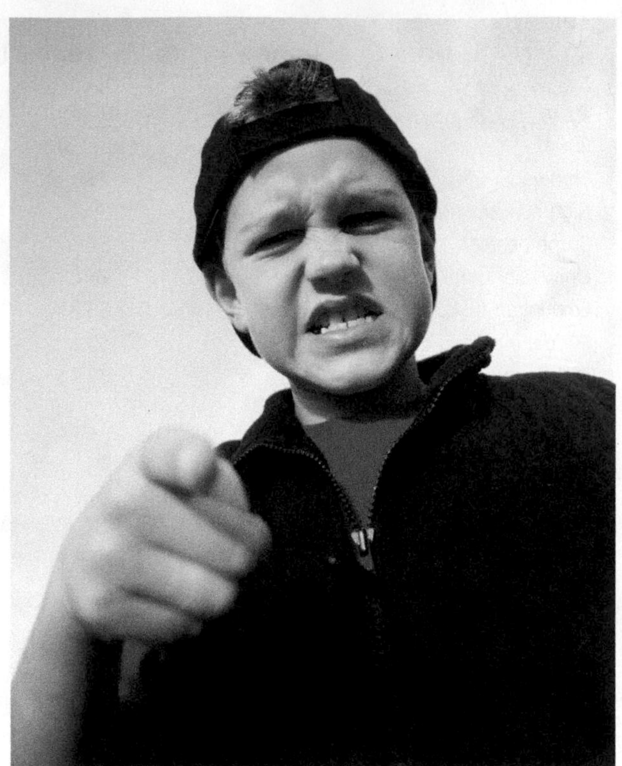

Males who are aggressive in early elementary school are more likely to be drug users as adults.[28,29]

Gateway Substances One very important study from the 1970s pointed out a typical sequence of involvement with drugs.[30] Most of the high school students in that group started their drug involvement with beer or wine. The second stage involved hard liquor, cigarettes, or both; the third stage was marijuana use; and only after going through those stages did they try other illicit substances. Not everyone followed the same pattern, but only 1% of the students began their substance use with marijuana or another illicit drug. It is as though they first had to go through the **gateway** of using alcohol and, in many cases, cigarettes. The students who had not used beer or wine at the beginning of the study were much less likely to be marijuana smokers at the end of the study than the students who had used these substances. The cigarette smokers were about twice as likely as the nonsmokers to move on to smoking marijuana.

If the gateway theory can explain something about later drug use, then perhaps looking at those people who followed the traditional order of substance use (alcohol or cigarettes, followed by marijuana, followed by other illicit drugs) and comparing them with people who followed different orders of use might tell us something useful about the importance of particular orders of initiation. One recent study examined 375 homeless street youth, ages 13–21, in Seattle.[31] They were asked at what age they first started using various substances and then

antecedent: a variable that occurs before some event, such as the initiation of drug use.

longitudinal study: a study done over time (months or years).

gateway: one of the first drugs (e.g., alcohol or tobacco) used by a typical drug user.

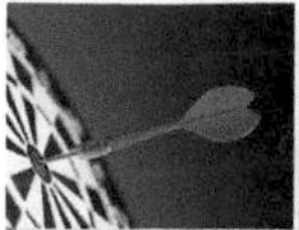

TARGETING PREVENTION

Preventing What?

Chapter 1 provides an overview of psychoactive drug use, primarily based on data from Canada. As we look toward the topic of prevention, it's appropriate to think about what aspects of psychoactive drug use we would most like to reduce. Following are some perspectives:

- We should work to prevent any use of tobacco or alcohol by those under age 25, as well as any use of drugs, such as marijuana, cocaine, and LSD. These drugs are all illegal, and we know that early use of tobacco and alcohol is associated with a greatly increased risk of dependency and illicit drug use in the future.
- Focusing only on drug use ignores the fact that illicit drug use is usually part of a larger pattern of risk-taking or antisocial behaviour. Therefore, our efforts would be more effective if we were to target younger people and work to prevent poor academic performance, fighting, shoplifting, and other early indicators of this lifestyle, in addition to early experimentation with tobacco and alcohol.
- Wait a minute! We're confusing what might be desirable with what might be possible. We can't prevent everyone from doing things we don't like. For example, as adults most people will drink alcohol at least once in a while, yet perhaps only 10% of drinkers have most of the problems. Trying to prevent all drug use and other undesirable behaviour is just too big a job, and it violates our sense of individual freedom. We need to focus our efforts on preventing abuse and the risk that goes with it. That's a much smaller problem, and we have a better chance of success.

With which of these perspectives do you most agree at this point? Are there other perspectives not represented by these three?

grouped into categories depending on whether they followed the traditional gateway order or some other order of initiation. The order of use did not predict current levels or types of drug use in this population, leading the study's authors to conclude that knowing which substances people use first might not be very important in helping to prevent future escalation of drug use.

One possible interpretation of the gateway phenomenon is that young people are exposed to alcohol and tobacco and that these substances somehow make people more likely to go on to use other drugs. Because most people who use these gateway substances do not go on to become cocaine users, we should be cautious about jumping to that conclusion. More likely is that early alcohol use and cigarette smoking are common indicators of the general deviance-prone pattern of behaviour that also includes an increased likelihood of smoking marijuana or trying cocaine. Because beer and cigarettes are more widely available to a deviance-prone young person than are marijuana or cocaine, it is logical that beer and cigarettes would most often be tried first. The socially conforming students are less likely to try even these relatively available substances until they are older, and they are less likely ever to try the illicit substances. Let's ask the question another way: If we developed a prevention program that stopped all young people from smoking cigarettes, would that cut down on marijuana smoking? Most of us think it might, because people who don't want to suck tobacco smoke into their lungs probably won't want to inhale marijuana smoke either. Would such a program keep people from getting D averages or getting into other kinds of trouble? Probably not. In other words, we think of the use of gateway substances not as the cause of later illicit drug use but, instead, as an early indicator of the basic pattern of risk-taking behaviour resulting from a variety of psychosocial risk factors.

Motives for Drug Use

To most of us, it doesn't seem necessary to find explanations for normative behaviour; we don't often ask why someone takes a pain reliever when she has a headache. Our task is to try to explain the drug-taking behaviour that frightens and infuriates–the risk-taking drug use. We should keep one fact about human conduct in mind throughout this book: Despite good, logical evidence telling us we "should" avoid certain things, we all do some of them anyway. We know that we shouldn't eat that second piece of pie or have that third drink on an empty stomach. Cool-headed logic tells us so. We would be hard pressed to find good, sensible reasons why we should smoke cigarettes, drive faster than the speed limit, go skydiving, sleep late when we have work to do, flirt with someone and risk an established relationship, or use cocaine. Whether one labels these behaviours sinful or just stupid, they don't seem to be designed to maximize our health or longevity.

But humans do not live by logic alone; we are social animals who like to impress each other, and we are pleasure seekers. These factors help explain why people do some of the things they shouldn't, including using drugs.

The research on correlates and antecedents points to a variety of personal and social variables that influence our drug taking, and many psychological and sociological theorists have proposed models for explaining illegal or excessive drug use. We have seen evidence for one common reason that some people begin to take certain illegal drugs: Usually young, and somewhat more often male than female, they have chosen to identify with a risk-taking subculture. These groups frequently engage in a variety of behaviours not condoned by the larger society. Within that group, the use of a particular drug might, in fact, be expected. Occasionally the use of a particular drug becomes such a fad among a large number of youth groups that it seems to be a nationwide problem. However, within any given community there will still be people of the same age who don't use the drug.

Rebellious behaviour, especially among young people, serves important functions not only for the developing individual but also for the evolving society. Adolescents often try very hard to impress other people and may find it especially difficult to impress their parents. An adolescent who is unable to gain respect from people or who is frustrated in efforts to go his or her own way might engage in a particularly dangerous or disgusting behaviour as a way of demanding that people be impressed or at least pay attention.

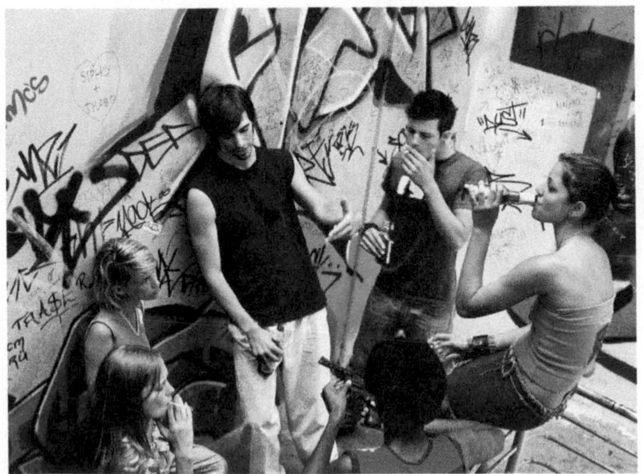

People who use drugs and who identify with a particular subculture are more likely to engage in a variety of behaviours not condoned by society.

One source of excessive drug use may be found within the drugs themselves. Many of these drugs are capable of reinforcing the behaviour that gets the drug into the system. **Reinforcement** means that, everything else being equal, each time you take the drug you increase slightly the probability that you will take it again. Thus, with many psychoactive drugs there is a constant tendency to increase the frequency or amount of use. Some drugs (such as intravenous heroin or cocaine) appear to be so reinforcing that this process occurs relatively rapidly in a large percentage of those who use them. For other drugs, such as alcohol, the process seems to be slower. In many people, social factors, other reinforcers, or other activities prevent an increase. For some, however, the drug-taking behaviour does increase and consumes an increasing share of their lives.

Most drug users are seeking an altered state of consciousness, a different perception of the world than is provided by normal, day-to-day activities. Many of the high school students in the nationwide surveys report that they take drugs "to see what it's like," or "to get high," or "because of boredom." In other words, they are looking for a change, for something new and different in their lives. This aspect of drug use was particularly clear during the 1960s and 1970s, when LSD and other perception-altering drugs were popular. We don't always recognize the altered states produced by other substances, but they do exist. A man drinking alcohol might have just a bit more of a perception that he's a tough guy, that he's influential, that he's well liked. A cocaine user might get the seductive feeling that everything is great and that she's doing a great job (even if she isn't). Many drug-abuse prevention programs have focused on efforts to show young people how to feel good about themselves and how to look for excitement in their lives without using drugs.

Another thing seems clear: Although societal, community, and family factors (the outer areas of Figure 1.8) play an important role in determining whether an individual will first try a drug, with increasing use the individual's own experiences with the drug become increasingly important. For those who become seriously dependent, the drug and its actions on that individual become central, and social influences, availability, cost, and penalties play a less important role in the continuation of drug use.

reinforcement: a procedure in which a behavioural event is followed by a consequent event, such that the behaviour is then more likely to be repeated. The behaviour of taking a drug may be reinforced by the effect of the drug.

Figure 1.8 Influences on Drug Use

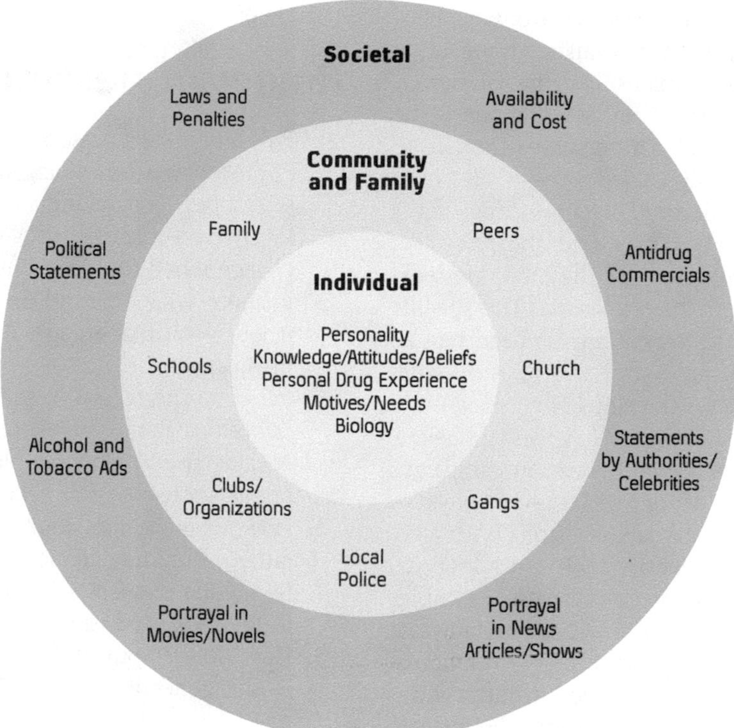

Summary

- In discussing a drug-use issue, we must consider who is using the drug, what drug is being used, when and where the drug use is occurring, why the person is using the drug, how the person is taking the drug, and how much drug is being used.
- No drug is either entirely good or bad, and every drug has multiple effects. The size and type of effect depends on the dose of the drug and the user's history and expectations.
- Risky drug use includes those forms of drug use not considered acceptable by the society at large. Drug *misuse* is using a drug in a way that was not intended by its manufacturer. Drug *abuse* is drug use that causes problems. (If the problems are frequent and serious, then a diagnosis of substance use disorder is applied.) Drug *dependence* involves using the substance more often or in greater amounts than the user intended and having difficulty stopping or cutting down on its use. *Tolerance* can occur with repeated ingestion of a drug and requires the user to use increasingly larger doses to achieve the same effect. *Withdrawal* symptoms are abnormal physical or psychological effects that occur after stopping a drug.
- Among Canadian postsecondary institution students, 71% can be considered current (within the past 30 days) users of alcohol, 12% current smokers of tobacco cigarettes, 17% current marijuana users, and fewer than 3% current users of other illicit drugs. Both alcohol and illicit drug use reached an apparent peak around 1980, then decreased until the early 1990s, with a slower increase after that. Current rates of use are lower than at the peak.
- The correlates and antecedents of adolescent drug use include risk and protective factors: genetics, race, gender, and level of education, personality variables (which may in part reflect genetics), and the use of other drugs.
- Adolescents who use illicit drugs (mostly marijuana) are more likely to know adults who use drugs, less likely to believe that their parents would object to their drug use, less likely to see their parents as a source of social support, more likely to have friends who use drugs, more likely to engage in

other antisocial activities, less likely to be religious, and more likely to have academic problems.

- A typical progression of drug use starts with cigarettes and alcohol, then marijuana, then other drugs, such as amphetamines, cocaine, or heroin. However, no evidence shows that using one of the gateway substances causes a person to escalate to more risky forms of drug use.
- People may use illicit or dangerous drugs for a variety of reasons: They may find the effects of the drugs to be reinforcing, or they may be seeking an altered state of consciousness. The specific types of drugs and the ways they are used will be influenced by the user's social and physical environment. If dependence develops, then these environmental factors may begin to have less influence.
- Harm reduction uses public education campaigns or facilities that aim to reduce substance-related harms to lessen the damage associated with alcohol and other drugs. It doesn't try to stop drug use, just to lessen the harm done by that use. Examples of harm reduction measures in Canada include safe injection sites, syringe exchange programs, methadone maintenance therapy for heroin intravenous drug users, earlier opening hours for a liquor outlet in downtown Edmonton, changes to space and the padding of furniture in licensed establishments to minimize the harm that may result from fights, and designated driver and alternative transportation programs.

Review Questions

1. Besides asking a person the question directly, what is one way a psychologist can try to determine why a person is taking a drug?
2. What two characteristics of a drug's effect might change when the dose is increased?
3. In about what year did drug use in Canada peak?
4. About what percentage of university students use marijuana?
5. What do the results of the *Canadian Addiction Survey* tell us about the overall rates of marijuana and cocaine use among people of different socioeconomic status?
6. How does having a university degree influence rates of drinking alcohol? Using tobacco?
7. Name one risk factor and one protective factor for drug use related to the family or parents.
8. How does impulsivity relate to rates of drug use in the general population? How does impulsivity relate to substance dependence?
9. Comment on Canada's new initiative for harm reduction. Do harm reduction strategies promote drug use?

CHAPTER 2

DRUG USE AS A SOCIAL PROBLEM

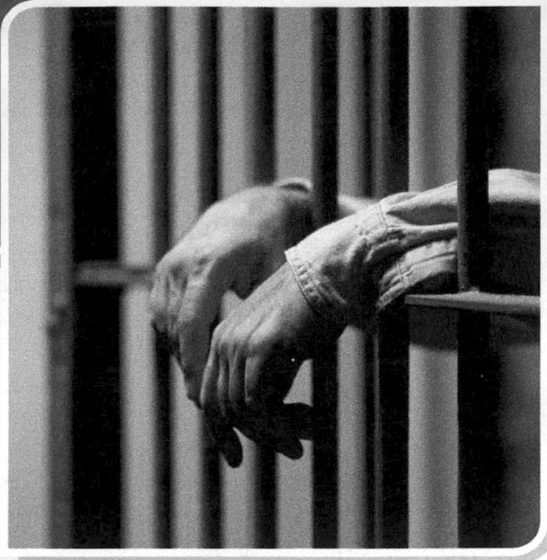

OBJECTIVES

When you have finished this chapter, you should be able to

- **LO1** Describe the federal government's regulatory approach before the early 1900s and now.
- **LO2** Explain the difference between acute and chronic toxicity and between physiological and behavioural toxicity.
- **LO3** Provide examples of how data collected through drug monitoring systems can be used to estimate the toxicity of drugs of abuse and misuse.
- **LO4** Define tolerance, physical dependence, and behavioural dependence.
- **LO5** Examine how the scientific perspective on substance dependence has changed in recent years.
- **LO6** Describe criteria used in the diagnosis of substance-related and addictive disorders.
- **LO7** Debate the various theories on the cause of dependence.
- **LO8** List four ways it has been proposed that drug use might cause an increase in crime.
- **LO9** Debate possible consequences of drug regulation.

As we look into the problems experienced by society as a result of the use of psychoactive drugs, we need to consider two broad categories. In the first category are the problems directly related to actually taking the drug, such as the risk of developing dependence or of overdosing. Second, because the use of certain drugs is considered a deviant act, the continued use of those drugs by some individuals represents a different set of social problems, apart from the direct dangers of the drugs themselves. These problems include arrests, fines, jailing, and the expenses associated with efforts to prevent misuse and to treat abuse and dependence. We begin by examining the direct drug-related problems that first raised concerns about opium, cocaine, and other drugs. Problems related to law enforcement, prevention, and treatment will be examined more thoroughly in Chapters 3, 17, and 18.

LO1 Laissez-Faire

Before the early 1900s, the Canadian government, like the majority of countries around the world, had virtually no laws governing the sale or use of drugs. The idea seemed to be that if the seller wanted to sell it and the buyer wanted to buy it, let them do it—**laissez-faire**, in French. Consider, for example, the use of opiates. Between 1871 and 1908 the government of Canada viewed opium as an economic opportunity, regulating its production, and deriving profit, through the creation of licensing fees for Canadian opium factories. What happened to cause governments to believe it was necessary to create especially restrictive regulations for some drugs?

Factors that precipitated the creation of drug laws have varied from country to country (a historical account of events that led to the creation of Canada's first drug law, the Opium Act of 1908, is presented in Chapter 3). Despite different beginnings throughout the twentieth century, three principal concerns have universally driven the development of drug laws:

1. *Toxicity*. Some drug sellers were considered to be endangering the public health and victimizing individuals because they were selling dangerous, toxic chemicals, often without labelling them or putting appropriate warnings on them.

laissez-faire: a hands-off approach to government interference in the workings of the market.

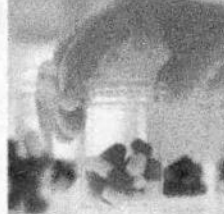

DRUGS IN THE MEDIA

Pharm Parties?

As evidence from various sources points to an increasing problem with misuse of prescription medications, especially opioids such as OxyContin and Vicodin, it should not be surprising that sometimes drug "experts" and news organizations will sensationalize the issue. In 2006, *USA Today* reported that drug counsellors across the country were beginning to hear about "pharm" or "pharming" parties, at which young people bring whatever prescription pills they can acquire, put them all into a large bowl, and then just take pills at random from the bowl. The problem with the story was that no actual data on these practices were presented, leading Jack Shafer, a columnist for the online magazine *Slate*, to respond with an article, "Pharfetched Pharm Parties: Real or a Media Invention?" After looking into the origins of these stories, Shafer became even more convinced that this was just a sensationalistic story with little or no basis in fact. It's not to say that such a party has never happened anywhere—indeed, those of us who have been watching the drug scene for decades recall similar media stories in the early 1970s. But is this really something that has become as frequent as implied? One concern about such media reports is that they might encourage some young people to try this, because it is reported to be a craze that's currently sweeping the nation. Despite Shafer's attempts to prevent the ongoing publication of unsubstantiated stories they continue to be reported in the Canadian and U.S. press. You can read Shafer's articles online at www.slate.com. Can you think of any recent drug media stories that have played out in a similar fashion? What about bath salts or krokodil?

2. *Dependence*. Some sellers were seen as victimizing individuals and endangering their health by selling them habit-forming drugs, again often without appropriate labels or warnings.
3. *Crime*. The drug user came to be seen as a threat to public safety–the attitude became widespread that drug-crazed individuals would often commit horrible, violent crimes. In Chapter 3, we will look at the roots of these concerns and how they have influenced the development of our legal structures.

For now, let's look at each issue and develop a knowledge base for future discussion related to toxicity, dependence, and drug-induced criminality.

LO2, LO3 Toxicity

The word **toxic** means "poisonous, deadly, or dangerous." All the drugs we discuss in this text can be toxic if misused or abused. We will use the term to refer to those effects of drugs that interfere with normal functioning in such a way as to produce dangerous or potentially dangerous consequences. Seen in this way, for example, alcohol can be toxic in high doses because it suppresses respiration–this can be dangerous if breathing stops long enough to induce brain damage or death. But we can also consider alcohol to be toxic if it causes a person to be so disoriented that, for them, otherwise normal behaviours, such as driving a car or swimming, become dangerous. This is an example of something we refer to as **behavioural toxicity**. We make a somewhat arbitrary distinction, then, between behavioural toxicity and "physiological" toxicity–perhaps taking advantage of the widely assumed mind-body distinction, which is more convenient than real. The only reason for making this distinction is that it helps remind us of some important kinds of toxicity that are unique to psychoactive drugs and that are sometimes overlooked.

Categories of Toxicity

Why do we consider physiological toxicity to be a "social" problem? One view might be that if an individual chooses to take a risk and harms his or her own body, that's the individual's business. But impacts on hospital emergency rooms, increased health care costs, lost productivity, and other consequences of physiological toxicity mean that social systems also are affected

toxic: poisonous, dangerous.

behavioural toxicity: toxicity resulting from behavioural effects of a drug.

when an individual's health is put at risk, whether by drug use or failure to wear seat belts.

Another distinction we make for the purpose of discussion is acute versus chronic. Most of the time when people use the word **acute**, they mean "sharp" or "intense." In medicine an acute condition is one that comes on suddenly, as opposed to a **chronic** or long-lasting condition. When talking about drug effects, we can think of the acute effects as those that result from a single administration of a drug or are a direct result of the actual presence of the drug in the system at the time. For example, taking an overdose of heroin can lead to acute toxicity. By contrast, the chronic effects of a drug are those that result from long-term exposure and can be present whether or not the substance is actually in the system at a given point. For example, smoking cigarettes can eventually lead to various types of lung disorders. If you have emphysema from years of smoking, that condition is there when you wake up in the morning and when you go to bed at night, and whether your most recent cigarette was five minutes ago or five days ago doesn't make much difference.

Using these definitions, Table 2.1 can help give us an overall picture of the possible toxic consequences of a given type of drug. However, knowing what is possible is different from knowing what is likely. How can we get an idea of which drugs are most likely to produce adverse drug reactions?

Table 2.1 Examples of Four Types of Drug-Induced Toxicity

Acute (immediate)	
Behavioural	"Intoxication" from alcohol, marijuana, or other drugs that impair behaviour and increase danger to the individual
Physiological	Overdose of heroin or alcohol causing the user to stop breathing
Chronic (long-term)	
Behavioural	Personality changes reported to occur in alcoholics and suspected by some to occur in marijuana users (amotivational syndrome)
Physiological	Heart disease, lung cancer, and other effects related to smoking; liver damage resulting from chronic alcohol exposure

Determining the Toxicity of Drugs of Abuse and Misuse

Today many countries operate systems for the surveillance of drugs of abuse and misuse. Such systems can provide a profile of a nation's substance abuse or misuse problems and help to guide the development of prevention, intervention, and treatment programs. In the United States the toxicity of drugs other than alcohol is monitored through the Drug Abuse Warning Network (DAWN). The **DAWN** was established in 1972 and collects data on drug-related emergency room visits from hospital emergency departments in major metropolitan areas around the United States. When an individual goes to an emergency room with any sort of problem related to drug misuse or abuse, each drug involved (up to six) is recorded. For each drug or drug type, staff members can add up the number of visits associated with that particular drug. The visit could be for a wide variety of reasons, such as injury caused by an accident, accidental overdose, a suicide attempt, or a distressing panic reaction that is not life-threatening to the patient. The emergency room personnel who record these incidents do not need to determine that the drug actually caused the visit, only that some type of drug misuse or abuse was involved. This avoids many of the subjective judgments that would vary from place to place and from day to day, especially when (as is often the case) more than one drug is involved. If someone is in an automobile accident after drinking alcohol, smoking marijuana, and using some cocaine, rather than trying to say which one of these substances was responsible for the accident, each of them is counted as being involved in that emergency room visit.

Because not every emergency room in the United States participates in the DAWN system, for many years the sampled data were used to estimate the overall number of emergency room visits for the entire country. Because of concerns about the accuracy of those estimates, more recent results are not used in

acute: referring to drugs, the short-term effects of a single dose.

chronic: referring to drugs, the long-term effects from repeated use.

DAWN: Drug Abuse Warning Network. System for collecting data on drug-related deaths or emergency room visits.

Table 2.2 Toxicity Data from the Drug Abuse Warning Network (DAWN)

Drug-Related Emergency Room Visits (2011)			Drug-Related Deaths (2009)		
Rank	**Drug**	**Number**	**Rank**	**Drug**	**Rate/100 000**
1.	Alcohol in combination	606 653	1.	Prescription opioids	7.1
2.	Cocaine	505 224	2.	Alcohol in combination	3.7
3.	Prescription Opioids	488 004	3.	Benzodiazepines	3.1
4.	Marijuana	455 668	4.	Cocaine	2.6
5.	Benzodiazepines	357 836	5.	Methadone	2.5
6.	Heroin	258 482	6.	Antidepressants	2.0
7.	Methamphetamine	102 961	7.	Heroin	1.8
8.	Antidepressants	88 965	8.	Sedative-hypnotics	1.0
9.	Antipsychotics	61 951	9.	Stimulants (includes methamphetamine)	0.7
10.	Acetaminophen	39 783	10.	Antipsychotics	0.3

Sources: Substance Abuse and Mental Health Services Administration. *Drug Abuse Warning Network, 2011: National Estimates of Drug-Related Emergency Department Visits.* Rockville, MD: U.S. Department of Health and Human Services, 2013. Retrieved January 3, 2014, from http://www.samhsa.gov/data/2k13/DAWN2k11ED/DAWN2k11ED.htm#2.1; and Substance Abuse and Mental Health Services Administration. *Drug Abuse Warning Network, 2009: Area Profiles of Drug-Related Mortality.* Rockville, MD: Author, 2011. Retrieved January 3, 2014, from http://www.samhsa.gov/data/2k11/dawn/2k9dawnme/html/dawn2k9me.htm.

that way. The numbers for emergency room visits for 2011 shown on the left side of Table 2.2 are the totals from the sampled hospitals.[1]

The DAWN system also collects data on drug-related deaths, with the reports being completed by medical examiners (coroners) in the same metropolitan areas around the United States. The agency responsible for the DAWN data (the Office of Applied Studies from the Substance Abuse and Mental Health Services Administration) became so concerned about the accuracy of national estimates that it has stopped providing overall national totals and rankings by drug type. The numbers on the right side of Table 2.2 were derived calculating the rate of drug-associated deaths in 2009 related to each drug type from the 13 states that get reports from all of their medical examiners.[2]

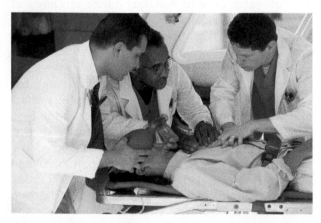

The Drug Abuse Warning Network (DAWN) uses data from hospital emergency rooms to monitor drug toxicity.

Alcohol is treated somewhat differently from other drugs in the sample. Whenever an emergency room visit or a death is related only to alcohol use by an adult, the DAWN system does not keep track of that. Alcohol-related problems are only counted when alcohol in combination with some other drug is reported (alcohol in combination) or if alcohol alone is recorded in an individual under 21 years of age. Notice that alcohol in combination is at or near the top ranking in both types of data, a place it has held for many years. In fact, if alcohol were counted alone, its numbers would be large enough to make the other drugs seem much less important beside it. This seems to indicate that alcohol is a fairly toxic substance. It can be, but let us also remember that in the United States about half of all adults drink alcohol at least once a month, whereas only a small percentage of the adult population uses cocaine, a drug that is also at the top of both lists. The DAWN system does not correct for differences in rates of use but rather gives us an idea of the relative impact of a substance on medical emergencies and drug-related deaths. Cocaine vied with alcohol in combination for the top spot on these lists since the mid-1980s, however in recent years the number of cocaine-related deaths has decreased. Legal drugs are found on both lists, with prescription opioids now at the top of the mortality data. Including the widely prescribed hydrocodone (Vicodin) and oxycodone (OxyContin), these drugs are increasingly marketed through Internet pharmacies that might be contributing to the increased number of toxic reactions. Other groups of prescription drugs, such as benzodiazepine sedatives (e.g., Xanax) and sleeping pills (e.g., Ativan) and the antidepressants, are relatively important, especially in the category of drug-related deaths.

The importance of drug combinations, particularly combinations with alcohol, in contributing to these numbers cannot be overstressed. Typically about half of the emergency room visits involve more than one substance, and about three-fourths of the drug-related deaths include multiple drugs. By far the most common "other" drug is alcohol. The most dramatic case is for the benzodiazepines. In 2003, only 16 of the 1611 benzodiazepine-related deaths were reported as single-drug deaths, implying that the real danger lies in combining sedatives or sleeping pills with alcohol.

Canada does not have a plan for providing regular description of the incidence and causes of drug-related emergency room visits or deaths nationally. However, this type of information can be obtained through analysis of data collected by the Canadian Institute for Health Information (CIHI). The CIHI is a federally chartered institution established to provide health information for health services and research initiatives in Canada. Since 1994 the CIHI has collected information on all patient hospital separations (discharge, sign out, death, or transfer of the patient to another facility) from all acute in-patient institutions, in all provinces and territories except Quebec. Data collected by CIHI include demographic (e.g., age, gender, province or territory of residence) and administrative and clinical elements (status at discharge, the most responsible diagnosis and secondary diagnoses). Diagnoses are recorded in the CIHI database by using codes defined in the International Classification of Diseases and Related Health Problems system (ICDs). The ICD is maintained by the World Health Organization and includes codes for a variety of drug-related disorders and conditions.[3] The CIHI also collects data on diagnostic, therapeutic, and support intervention performed while in hospital (coded according to the Canadian Classification of Health Interventions). Although the CIHI can provide a means for obtaining national profiles on drug-related emergency room visits, it has yet to be used for this purpose. It should be noted, however, that before such work could be done, the accuracy, specificity, and completeness of drug-related data collected for this system would have to be verified.[4]

Although Canada does not have a system for providing regular descriptions of the incidence and causes of drug-related deaths it has on occasion produced such information. In 2006 the Canadian Centre on Substance Abuse published the results of a study on mortality attributable to alcohol, illicit drugs, and tobacco.[4] As described in Table 2.3, in 2002, 1695 deaths were attributed to illicit drug use (including cocaine and crack; opioids, such as heroin; and other injectable drugs) and 39 deaths were attributed to cannabis use. Collectively this accounted for 0.8% of all deaths in 2002. The leading causes of illicit-drug-related deaths included overdose (57%), followed by drug-attributed suicide (17%), hepatitis C infection (10%), and HIV (5%). The incidence of illicit-drug-related death was highest in males, all ages. In that same year 4258 deaths were attributed to alcohol, and 37 209 deaths were attributed to cigarette smoking.

It should be noted that the Canadian Vital Statistics system collects national data on the underlying cause of all deaths and classifies those causes by using ICD codes. This system has the potential to serve as a source for information on drug-related deaths in Canada, but to our knowledge it has never been used for this purpose. Similar to the CIHI data, the accuracy, specificity, and completeness of drug-related data collected for this system have yet to be verified.[4]

How Dangerous Is the Drug?

The DAWN and systems like it can be used to determine the relative toxicities of drugs of abuse and misuse within a society. Let's consider how DAWN data can be used to determine the relative toxicity of one drug versus another. Data presented in Table 2.2 give us some idea of the drugs contributing to the largest numbers of toxic reactions in these two sets of data. We mentioned that the DAWN data do not correct for frequency of use. However, researchers in the United States also collect sets of data that provide information on the relative rates of use of different drugs. The *National Survey on Drug Use and Health* (NSDUH) publishes rates of current use of alcohol and cocaine alongside marijuana use for Americans between 18 and 25 years of age.[5] As demonstrated in Figure 2.1 many more people are current users of alcohol (about two-thirds of adults), and many fewer use cocaine in any given year. But overall, the trends over time are generally similar, with the peak year for all three substances being around 1980, lower rates of use in the early 1990s, and less dramatic changes after that.

The populations and sampling methods for DAWN and NSDUH are different, so it is not possible to make fine distinctions with any degree of accuracy. But we

Table 2.3 Mortality Attributable to Alcohol, Illicit Drugs, and Tobacco by Age and Sex, Canada, 2002

	Alcohol	Illicit Drugs*	Cannabis	Tobacco†
Males				
0–14 years	50	24	1	58
15–29 years	682	238	9	40
30–44 years	842	379	6	522
45–59 years	1 045	408	5	3 708
60+ years	875	134	5	19 438
Total all males	3 494	1 183	26	23 766
Males as a % of all causes of death	3.08%	1.04%	0.02%	20.98%
Females				
0–14 years	26	10	1	33
15–29 years	124	95	3	29
30–44 years	218	163	2	293
45–59 years	386	153	2	1 782
60+ years	9	92	4	11 305
Total females	764	512	13	13 443
Females as % of all causes of death total	0.69%	0.46%	0.01%	12.18%
Total	4 258	1 695	39	37 209
Total as a % of all causes of death	1.90%	0.76%	0.02%	16.64%

*Including cannabis (traffic accidents only)

†Including active and passive smoking

Source: Rehm, J. D., and others. *The Cost of Substance Abuse in Canada, 2002.* Ottawa: Canadian Centre on Substance Abuse, 2006. Retrieved December 10, 2010, from http://www.ccsa.ca/2006CCSADocuments/ccsa-011332-2006.pdf.

know from the data summarized in Figure 2.1, for example, that roughly eight times as many people report current use of marijuana as report current use of cocaine. The 2007 DAWN mortality report shows roughly ten times as many cocaine-related deaths as marijuana-related deaths. If one-eighth as many users experience ten times as many deaths, can we say that the risk of death to an individual cocaine user is 80 times the risk of death to an individual marijuana user? That's too precise an answer, but it seems pretty clear that cocaine is relatively much more toxic than marijuana.

Is it possible to gain a true measure of the relative toxicities of drugs of abuse and misuse drugs in Canada? The answer is yes. As discussed above the frameworks of established national systems, such as the CIHI and Canadian Vital Statistics, provide the platform for the collection of data required for determining incidence and causes of drug-related emergency room visits or deaths. However, as noted, what is not clear is whether the data being collected are, in their current form, sufficiently accurate, specific, and complete. What was missing in Canada was a system like the NSDUH, one that would provide annual estimates of the behaviours and outcomes of alcohol and illicit drug users. Before 2008 collection of such data was sporadic and only two national surveys had been completed in 20 years. Fortunately, with the development of the *Canadian Alcohol and Drug Use Monitoring Survey* in 2008, we now have such a system.[6]

Intravenous Drug Use and the Spread of Blood-Borne Diseases

In Canada, it is estimated that there are between 75 000 and 125 000 intravenous drug users (IDUs).[7] Almost any legal or illicit psychoactive drug that can be liquefied can be injected. The drugs most commonly used

Figure 2.1 Trends in Reported Drug Use within the Past 30 Days for Young Adults Ages 18–25

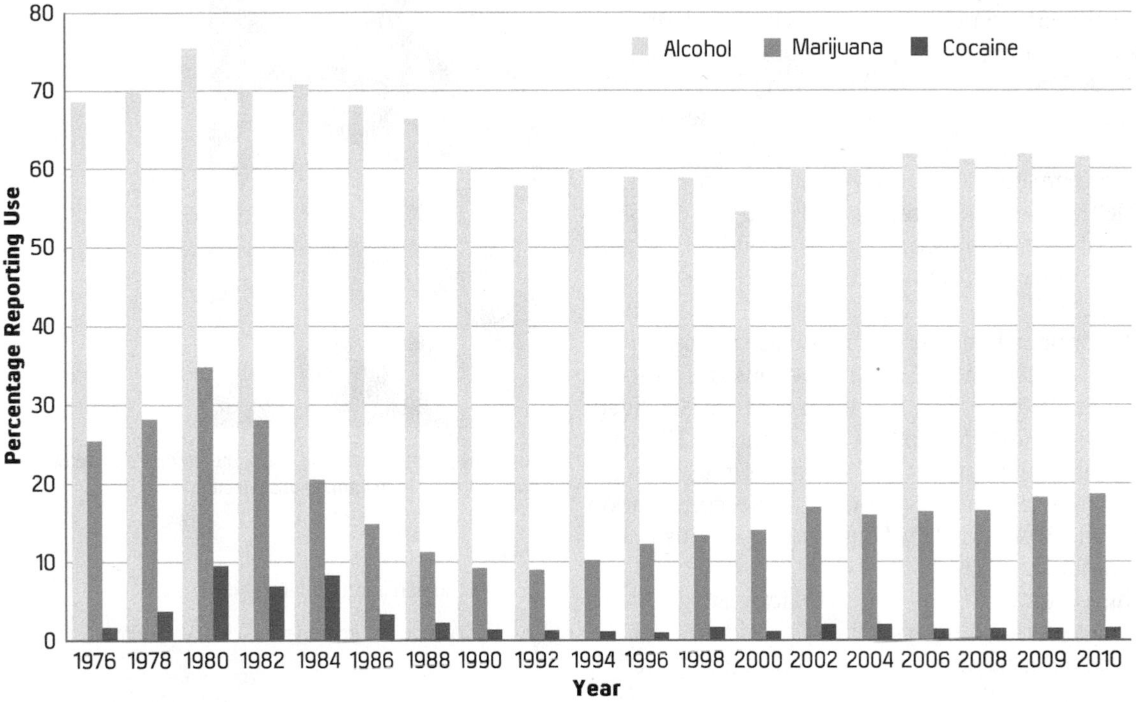

Source: Substance Abuse and Mental Health Services Administration. *Results from the 2008 National Survey on Drug Use and Health: National Findings.* Rockville, MD: Author, 2009. Retrieved September 12, 2011, from http://oas.samhsa.gov/nsduh/2k8nsduh/2k8Results.cfm.

MIND/BODY CONNECTION

Fear and Decision Making

Fear is a useful emotion. Being afraid of something that threatens you helps you to avoid the real dangers that do exist in our world. But, of course, fear also can be irrational, far out of proportion to any real threat. When that happens, as individuals we might be hampered by being unable to use elevators or ride in airliners, or fear of contamination might seriously interfere with our social lives. Fear is also a favourite tool of many politicians. If they can convince us that there is a real threat of some kind and they offer to protect us from it, we are likely to elect them and to give them the power or funding they seek to provide that protection. Again, this is a rational and perfectly appropriate governmental response to the extent that the threat is both real and likely to harm us, but sometimes it is difficult to get it right. Maybe the Canadian government has underestimated the threat of global climate change. Maybe because of the horrible televised images of the World Trade Center attack we overestimate the threat of Al Qaeda. Raising fears about specific types of drugs has been a staple of politics and government in Canada and the United States for more than 100 years, from the age of Demon Rum through heroin, marijuana, LSD, PCP, cocaine, MDMA (ecstasy), and methamphetamine. How do we get it right?

On an individual level, most of us are sufficiently afraid of the possible consequences of using illicit drugs that we avoid using them at all. If those fears are overblown, so what? As long as we avoid using dangerous drugs, we can see those fears as being useful. But a politician can easily amplify fears about a drug and use that fear to help get elected, and to pass laws that go too far, compared with the actual magnitude of the threat. Think about frightening things you have heard about specific drugs. For example, there has been a lot of talk about "meth" labs exploding and about the toxic effects of exposure to the harsh chemicals used in making methamphetamine. How can you evaluate such stories other than to go look up statistics on the actual occurrences of such events? Remember to use your common sense. If a story seems to be outrageous, there's a pretty good chance that someone is overstating the actual risk.

by IDUs include pharmaceutical opioids, cocaine, heroin, amphetamines, Ritalin, and anabolic steroids.[8] One specific toxicity concern for users who inject drugs is the potential for spreading blood-borne diseases, such as **HIV**, **AIDS**, and the life-threatening liver infection hepatitis C virus (HCV). These viral diseases can be transmitted through the sharing of needles.

Approximately 250 000 Canadians are infected with HCV and 65 000 are infected with HIV.[9,10] Sixty percent of persons infected with HCV and 17% of people living with HIV were likely infected when injecting drugs.[9,10,11] The incidence of new HIV infections among Aboriginal people is of particular concern, with 63% of infections caused by intravenous drug use.[9,10] In a recent study of IDUs in Canada, rates of HIV infection ranged from a low of 3% to a high of 22%. Rates of HCV infection among injecting drug users were higher, ranging from 62% to 69%.[12] The combination of IDUs and HIV and HCV constitutes a serious public health hazard.

This type of drug-associated toxicity is not due to the action of the drug itself but is incidental to the sharing of needles, no matter which drug is injected or

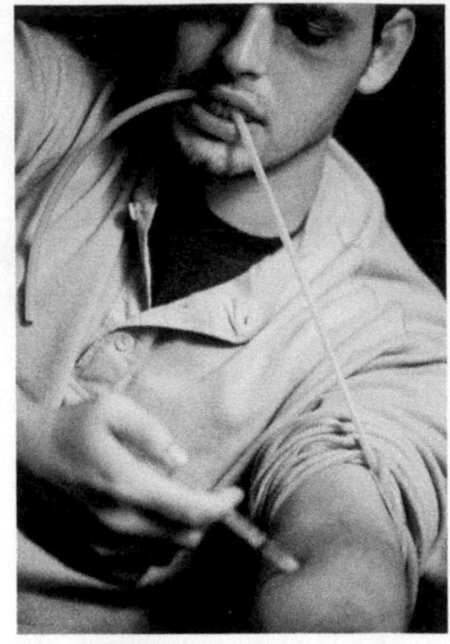

For many psychoactive drug users, the preferred route of administration is by intravenous injection.

HIV: human immunodeficiency virus.

AIDS: acquired immune deficiency syndrome.

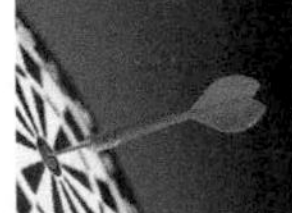

TARGETING PREVENTION

Clean Needles?

The spread of the human immunodeficiency virus (HIV) among drug users is associated primarily with the sharing of the needles used for injecting heroin and other drugs. Evidence from several studies indicates that HIV transmission can be reduced if clean syringes and needles are made readily available to IDUs.[13] Do you know whether a user of illicit drugs in your community can get access to clean syringes and needles?

You might start learning about this by asking a local pharmacist to see how easy it is to obtain these items and how expensive they are. It will also be interesting to see how the pharmacist reacts to your questions about this topic. How do you react to the idea of possibly being looked at as a user of illicit drugs? You might take this book along to show that you do have an academic reason for asking!

Once you find out what the situation is with direct purchasing, see if you can discover if your community has a needle exchange program. This will be a little harder, but you can start by looking up "public health" in the phone book and calling that office.

Are there steps your community could take to make clean needles more readily available to users of illicit drugs? Do you believe that such programs encourage or condone drug use? Would the program help prevent the spread of HIV in your community? Visit Connect for links to more information on needle exchange programs.

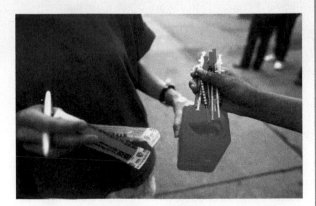

Needles are collected through an exchange program in an effort to prevent the spread of HIV among intravenous drug users.

whether the injection is intravenous or intramuscular. An individual drug user may inject 1000 times a year, and that takes a lot of needles. Data from Canadian population-specific surveillance systems suggest that approximately 15% of IDUs borrow needles that have been used by someone else and 31% borrowed other injectable equipment that had already been used by someone else.[12]

In an attempt to curb the spread of blood-borne infections, many countries have developed needle exchange programs, in which new, clean syringes are traded for used syringes. The first official needle exchange program in Canada began in 1989 in Vancouver. Today more than 100 such programs operate across the country. Evidence shows that given the opportunity, IDUs increase their use of clean syringes, rates of HIV and hepatitis C infection are lowered, and the programs more than pay for themselves in the long run.[13,14,15] Despite occasional bouts of public uncertainty, syringe exchange currently represents one of the most practical ways to prevent the spread of these blood-borne diseases among drug users and from them to the non-drug-using population.

LO4, LO5, LO6

Substance Dependence: What Is It?

All our lives we have heard people talk about *alcoholics* and *addicts*, and we're sure we know what we're talking about when one of these terms is used. Years ago when people first became concerned about some people being frequent, heavy users of cocaine or morphine, the term *habituation* was often used. If we try to develop scientific definitions, such terms as *alcoholic* or *addict* are actually hard to pin down. For example, not everyone who is considered an alcoholic drinks every day—some drink in binges, with brief periods of sobriety in between. Not everyone who drinks every day is considered an alcoholic—a glass of wine with dinner every night doesn't match most people's idea of alcoholism. The most extreme examples are easy to spot: the homeless man dressed in rags, drinking from a bottle of cheap wine, or the heroin user who needs a fix three or four times a day to avoid withdrawal symptoms. No hard-and-fast rule for quantity or frequency of use can help us draw a clear line between what we want to think of as a *normal drinker* or a *recreational user* and someone who has developed a dependence on the substance, who is compelled to use it, or who has lost control over use of the substance. It would be nice if we could separate substance use into two distinct categories: In one case, the individual controls the use of the substance; in the other case, the substance seems to take control of the individual. However, the real world of substance use, misuse, abuse, and dependence does not come wrapped in such convenient packages.

Three Basic Processes

The extreme examples mentioned above, of the homeless wine drinker or the frequent heroin user, typically exhibit three characteristics of their substance use that distinguish them from first-time or occasional users. These appear to represent three processes that may occur with repeated drug use, and each of these processes can be defined and studied by researchers interested in understanding drug dependence.

Tolerance **Tolerance** refers to a phenomenon seen with many drugs, in which repeated exposure to the same dose of the drug results in a lesser effect. This diminished effect can occur in many ways, and some examples are given in Chapter 5. For now, it is enough for us to think of the body as developing ways to compensate for the chemical imbalance caused by introducing a drug into the system. As the individual experiences less and less of the desired effect, often the tolerance can be overcome by increasing the dose of the drug. Some regular drug users might eventually build up to taking much more of the drug than it would take to kill a nontolerant individual.

Physical Dependence Physical dependence is defined by the occurrence of a **withdrawal syndrome**. Suppose a person has begun to take a drug and a tolerance has developed. The person increases the amount of drug and continues to take these higher doses so regularly that the body is continuously exposed to the drug for days or weeks. With some drugs, when the person stops taking the drug abruptly, a set of symptoms begins to appear as the drug level in the system drops. For example, as the level of heroin drops in a regular user, that person's nose might run and he or she might begin to experience chills and fever, diarrhea, and other symptoms. When we have a drug that produces a

tolerance: the reduced effect of a drug after repeated use.

withdrawal syndrome: a consistent set of symptoms that appears after discontinuing use of a drug.

consistent set of these symptoms in different individuals, we refer to the collection of symptoms as a withdrawal syndrome. These withdrawal syndromes vary from one class of drugs to another. Our model for why withdrawal symptoms appear is that the drug initially disrupts the body's normal physiological balances. These imbalances are detected by the nervous system, and over a period of repeated drug use the body's normal regulatory mechanisms compensate for the presence of the drug. When the drug is suddenly removed, these compensating mechanisms produce an imbalance. Tolerance typically precedes physical dependence. To continue with the heroin example, when it is first used, it slows intestinal movement and produces constipation. After several days of constant heroin use, other mechanisms in the body counteract this effect and get the intestines moving again (tolerance). If the heroin use is suddenly stopped, the compensating mechanisms produce too much intestinal motility. Diarrhea is one of the most reliable and dramatic heroin withdrawal symptoms.

Because of the presumed involvement of these compensating mechanisms, the presence of a withdrawal syndrome is said to reflect **physical** (or physiological) **dependence** on the drug. In other words, the individual has come to depend on the presence of some amount of that drug to function normally; removing the drug leads to an imbalance, which is slowly corrected over a few days.

Psychological Dependence **Psychological dependence** (also called behavioural dependence) can be defined in terms of observable behaviour. It is indicated by the frequency of using a drug or by the amount of time or effort an individual spends in drug-seeking behaviour. Often it is accompanied by reports of craving the drug or its effects. A major contribution of behavioural psychology has been to point out the scientific value of the concept of **reinforcement** for understanding psychological dependence.

The term *reinforcement* is used in psychology to describe a process: A behavioural act is followed by a consequence, resulting in an increased tendency to repeat that behavioural act. The consequence may be described as pleasurable or as a "reward" in some cases (e.g., providing a tasty piece of food to someone who has not eaten for a while). In other cases, the consequence may be described in terms of escape from pain or discomfort. The behaviour itself is said to be strengthened, or reinforced, by its consequences. The administration of certain drugs can reinforce the behaviours that led to the drug's administration. Laboratory rats and monkeys have been trained to press levers when the only consequence of lever pressing is a small intravenous injection of heroin, cocaine, or another drug. Because some drugs but not others are capable of serving this function, it is possible to refer to some drugs as having "reinforcing properties" and to note that a general correlation exists between those drugs and the ones to which people often develop psychological dependence.

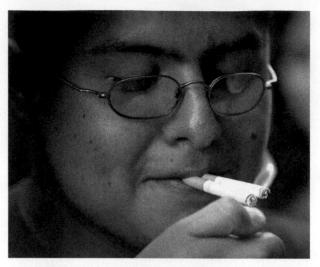

Frequent drug use, craving for the drug, and a high rate of relapse after quitting indicate psychological dependence.

Changing Views of Dependence

Until the twentieth century, the most common view was probably that dependent individuals were weak willed, lazy, or immoral (the "moral model"). Then medical and scientific studies began of users of alcohol and opioids. It seemed as if something more powerful than mere self-indulgence were at work, and the predominant view began to be that dependence is a drug-induced illness.

Early Medical Models If heroin dependence is induced by heroin, or alcohol dependence by alcohol, then why do some users develop dependence and others not? An early guess was simply that some people,

physical dependence: drug dependence defined by the presence of a withdrawal syndrome, implying that the body has become adapted to the drug's presence.

psychological dependence: behavioural dependence; indicated by a high rate of drug use, craving for the drug, and a tendency to relapse after stopping use.

reinforcement: a procedure in which a behavioural event is followed by a consequent event such that the behaviour is then more likely to be repeated. The behaviour of taking a drug may be reinforced by the effect of the drug.

DSM-5

Substance-Related Disorders

Substance-related disorders, defined by the DSM-5, encompass 10 separate classes of drugs: alcohol; cannabis; hallucinogens; inhalants; opioids; sedatives, hypnotics and anxiolytics; stimulants; tobacco; caffeine; and other substances. Substance-related disorders are divided into two groups: substance use disorders and substance-induced disorders. A number of conditions may be classed as substance-induced disorders including: withdrawal, intoxication, and other substance/medication-induced mental disorders. The essential feature of a substance use disorder is the cluster of physiological, behavioural, and cognitive symptoms indicating that the individuals continue using despite significant substance-related problems. The diagnosis of a substance use disorder is based on a person's demonstration of a pathological pattern of behaviours related to use of the substance. To assist in the diagnosis of substance use disorders these behaviours have been categorized into four themes with 11 criteria.

Diagnostic Criteria for Substance Use Disorder

Impaired Control over Substance Use:

1. The substance is often taken in larger amounts or over a longer period than was intended.
2. There is a persistent desire or unsuccessful efforts to cut down or discontinue substance use.
3. A great deal of time is spent in using the substance, obtaining the substance, or recovering from its effects.
4. Craving or an intense desire or urge to use a substance

Social Impairment:

5. Recurrent substance use resulting in failure to fulfill major role obligations at work, school, or home
6. Continued substance use despite having persistent or recurrent social or interpersonal problems caused or exacerbated by the effects of the substance
7. Withdrawal from family activities and hobbies in order to use the substance.

Risky Use of the Substance:

8. Recurrent substance use in situations in which it is physically hazardous
9. Failure to abstain from using a substance despite knowledge that use is having a persistent or recurrent physical or psychological problem that is likely to have been caused or exacerbated by the substance

Pharmacokinetic/Pharmacodynamic Changes:

10. Tolerance, as defined by either of the following:
    a. A need for a markedly increased dose of the substance to achieve the desired effect
    b. Markedly diminished effect when the usual dose is consumed
11. Withdrawal, as manifested by either of the following:
    a. The characteristic withdrawal syndrome for the substance
    b. The same (or a closely related) substance is taken to relieve or avoid withdrawal symptoms

Substance use disorders can vary widely in severity and range from mild to severe. Mild substance use disorder is suggested by the presence of two to three symptoms. Moderate substance use is suggested by the presence of four to five symptoms, and severe by the presence of 6 or more.

Source: Reprinted with permission from the Diagnostic and Statistical Manual of Mental Disorders, Fourth Edition (Copyright © 2000) and the Diagnostic and Statistical Manual of Mental Disorders, Fifth Edition (Copyright © 2013). American Psychiatric Association.

for whatever reasons, were exposed to large amounts of the substance for a long time. This could happen through medical treatment or self-indulgence. The most obvious changes resulting from long exposure to large doses are the withdrawal symptoms that occur when the drug is stopped. Both alcohol and the opioids can produce rather dramatic withdrawal syndromes. Thus, the problem came to be associated with the presence of physical dependence (a withdrawal syndrome), and enlightened medically oriented researchers went looking for treatments based on reducing or eliminating withdrawal symptoms. According to the narrowest interpretation of this model, the dependence itself was cured when the person had successfully completed withdrawal and the symptoms disappeared.

Pharmacologists and medical authorities continued into the 1970s to define addiction as occurring only when physical dependence was seen. Based on this view, public policy decisions, medical treatment, and individual drug-use decisions could be influenced by the question "Is this an addictive drug?" If some drugs produce dependence but others do not, then legal restrictions on specific drugs, care in the medical use of those drugs, and education in avoiding the recreational use of those drugs are appropriate. The determination of whether a drug is or is not addictive was therefore crucial.

In the 1960s, some drugs, particularly marijuana and amphetamines, were not considered to have well-defined, dramatic, physical withdrawal syndromes. The growing group of interested scientists began to refer to such drugs as marijuana, amphetamines, and cocaine as "merely" producing psychological dependence, whereas heroin produced a "true addiction," which includes physical dependence. The idea seemed to be that psychological dependence was "all in the head," whereas with physical dependence actual bodily processes were involved, subject to physiological and biochemical analysis and possibly to improved medical treatments. This was the view held by most drug-abuse experts in the 1960s.

Positive Reinforcement Model In the 1960s, a remarkable series of experiments began to appear in the scientific literature–experiments in which laboratory monkeys and rats were given intravenous **catheters** connected to motorized syringes and controlling equipment so that pressing a lever would produce a single brief injection of morphine, an opioid very similar to heroin. In the initial experiments, monkeys were exposed for several days to large doses of morphine, allowed to experience the initial stages of withdrawal, and then connected to the apparatus to see if they would learn to press the lever, thereby avoiding the withdrawal symptoms. These experiments were based on the predominant view of drug use as being driven by physical dependence. The monkeys did learn to press the levers.

As these scientists began to publish their results and as more experiments like this were done, interesting facts became apparent. First, monkeys would begin pressing and maintain pressing without first being made physically dependent. Second, monkeys who had given themselves only fairly small doses and who had never experienced withdrawal symptoms could be trained to work very hard for their morphine. A history of physical dependence and withdrawal didn't seem to have much influence on response rates in the long run. Clearly, the small drug injections themselves were working as positive reinforcers of the lever-pressing behaviour, just as food can be a positive reinforcer to a hungry rat or monkey. Thus, the idea spread that drugs can act as reinforcers of behaviour and that this might be the basis of what had been called psychological dependence. Such drugs as amphetamines and cocaine could easily be used as reinforcers in these experiments, and they were known to produce strong psychological dependence in humans. Animal experiments using drug self-administration are now of central importance in determining which drugs are likely to be used repeatedly by people, as well as in exploring the basic behavioural and biological features associated with drug dependence.[16]

catheters: plastic or other tubing implanted into the body.

Which Is More Important: Physical Dependence or Psychological Dependence?

The animal research that led to the positive reinforcement model implies that psychological dependence is more important than physical dependence in explaining repeated drug use, and this has led people to examine the lives of heroin users from a different perspective. Stories were told of users who occasionally stopped taking heroin, voluntarily going through withdrawal so as to reduce their tolerance level and get back to the lower doses of drug they could more easily afford. When we examine the total daily heroin intake of many users, we see that they do not need a large amount and that the agonies of withdrawal they experience are no worse than a case of food poisoning. We have known for a long time that heroin users who have already gone through withdrawal in treatment programs or in jail have a high probability of returning to active heroin use. In other words, if all we had to worry about was users avoiding withdrawal symptoms, the problem would be much smaller than it actually is.

Psychological dependence, based on reinforcement, is increasingly accepted as the real driving force behind repeated drug use, and tolerance and physical dependence are now seen as related phenomena that sometimes occur but probably are not critical to the development of frequent patterns of drug-using behaviour.

LO7 Broad Views of Substance Dependence

If we define drug dependence not in terms of withdrawal but in more behavioural or psychological terms, as an overwhelming involvement with getting and using the drug, then might this model also be used to describe other kinds of behaviour? What about a man who visits prostitutes several times a day; someone who eats large amounts of food throughout the day; or someone who places bets on every football and basketball game, every horse race or automobile race, and who spends hours each day planning these bets and finding money to bet again. Shouldn't these also be considered examples of dependence? Do the experiences of overeating, gambling, sex, and drugs have something in common–a common change in physiology or brain chemistry or a common personality trait that leads to any or many of these compulsive behaviours? Are all these filling an unmet social or spiritual need? Increasingly, researchers are looking for these common threads and discussing "dependencies" as a varied set of behavioural manifestations of a common dependence process or disorder.

Table 2.4 Dependence Potential of Psychoactive Drugs

Very high	Heroin (IV)
	Crack cocaine
High	Morphine (injected)
	Opium (smoked)
Moderate/high	Cocaine powder (snorted)
	Tobacco cigarettes
	PCP (smoked)
Moderate	Diazepam (Valium)
	Alcohol
	Amphetamines (oral)
Moderate/low	Caffeine
	MDMA* (ecstasy)
	Marijuana
Low	Ketamine (see Chapter 14)
Very low	LSD†
	Mescaline
	Psilocybin

* MDMA, methylenedioxymethamphetamine

† LSD, lysergic acid diethylamide

Is Dependence Caused by the Substance?

Especially with chemical dependence, many people speak as though the substance itself is the cause of the dependence. Certainly some drugs are more likely than others to result in dependence. For example, it is widely believed that heroin and crack cocaine are both extremely likely to lead to compulsive use. In contrast, most users of marijuana report occasional use and little difficulty in deciding when to use it and when not to. We also know that some methods of taking a drug (e.g., intravenous injection) are more likely to result in repeated use than other methods of taking the same drug (by mouth, for instance). We can determine which drugs, or which methods of using those drugs, pose the greatest risk for dependence. One major study reviewed 350 published articles to come up with relative ratings and then had the preliminary tables reviewed by a panel of psychopharmacologists for suggested changes.[17] Based on that report, we can classify psychoactive drugs into seven categories of dependence potential. Smoked or injected methamphetamine would probably be in one of the top two categories in such a ranking (see Table 2.4). The range of risk of dependence depends to some extent on the drug itself and also on its method of use (as well as a variety of other biological, psychological, and social factors). Thus, the substance itself cannot be seen as the entire cause of the problem, even though some people would like to put all the blame on alcohol or on heroin or on crack cocaine.

When we extend the concept of dependence to other activities, such as gambling, sex, or overeating, it seems harder to place the entire blame on the activity, again because many people do not exhibit compulsive patterns of such behaviours. Some activities might be more of a problem than others–few people become dependent on filling out income tax forms, whereas a higher proportion of all those who gamble become overwhelmingly involved. Still, it is wrong to conclude that any activity is by its nature always habit forming.

When a chemical is seen as causing the dependence, there is a tendency to give that substance a personality and to ascribe motives to it. When we listen either to a practising user's loving description of his interaction with the drug or to a recovering alcoholic describe her struggle against the bottle's attempts to destroy her, the substance seems to take on almost human characteristics. We all realize that is going too far, yet the analogy is so powerful that it pervades our thinking. **Alcoholics Anonymous (AA)** members often describe alcohol as being "cunning, baffling, and powerful" and admit that they are powerless against such a foe. And those seeking the prohibition of alcohol,

Alcoholics Anonymous (AA): a worldwide organization of self-help groups based on alcoholics helping one another achieve and maintain sobriety.

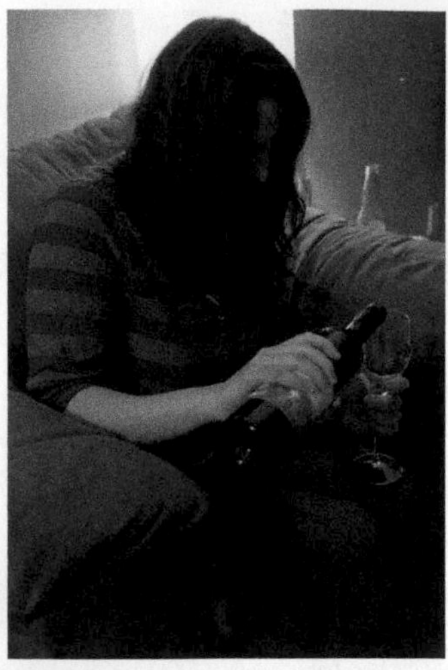

Alcohol causes serious dependence in perhaps one in ten drinkers.

cocaine, marijuana, heroin, and other drugs have over the years tended to demonize those substances, making them into powerful forces of evil. The concept of a "war on drugs" reflects in part such a perspective—that some drugs are evil and war must be waged against the substances themselves.

Is Dependence Biological?

In recent years, interest has increased in the possibility that all compulsive behaviours might have some common physiological or biochemical action in the brain. For example, many theorists have recently focused on dopamine, one of the brain's important neurotransmitters, which some believe to play a large role in positive reinforcement. The idea is that any drug use or other activity that has pleasurable or rewarding properties spurs dopamine activity in a particular part of the brain. This idea is discussed more fully in Chapter 4. Although this theory has been widely tested in animal models and much evidence is consistent with it, considerable evidence also shows that this model is too simple and that other neurotransmitters and other brain regions are also important. A great deal of attention has been given to reports from various brain-scanning experiments done on drug users. For example, cues that stimulate craving for cocaine activate many areas that are widely separated in the brain, including some that are known to be dopamine-rich areas and some that are not.[18] Although these studies show some of the physiological consequences produced by cocaine or by even thinking about cocaine, they have not yet been useful in examining the possible biological causes of dependence. One important question that remains is whether the brains of people who have used cocaine intermittently show different responses, compared with the brains of dependent cocaine users. Ultimately, the strongest demonstration of the power of such techniques would be if it were possible to know, based on looking at a brain scan, whether a person had developed dependence. Many previous biological theories of dependence have failed this test: So far, no genetic, physiological, or biochemical marker has been found that definitively predicts drug dependence.

Is There an "Addictive Personality"?

Perhaps the explanation for why some people become dependent but others do not lies in the personality—that complex set of attributes and attitudes that develops over time, partly as a result of particular experiences. Is there a common personality factor that is seen in compulsive drug users but not in others? We've known for some time that people who are diagnosed with certain types of personality disorders, such as antisocial personality or conduct disorder, are more likely to also have one of the substance-related or addictive disorder diagnoses. We've also known that people who have a long history of alcohol dependence or heroin dependence will demonstrate a variety of differences from the normal population on personality tests. But neither of these findings tells us anything about what caused these relationships. Conduct disorder and antisocial personality disorder reflect a general tendency for a person to violate social norms. Perhaps drug use is just one of many ways this person might choose to break the rules? And someone who has been drinking heavily for many years, who has had health problems, and who has perhaps lost a job and family might well have developed personality differences because of the consequences of years of substance abuse. So we have not had much good information until fairly recently about personality differences that might predispose individuals to develop a substance use disorder.

One personality trait that has frequently been associated with greater risk for abuse of stimulants, such as amphetamine or cocaine, is called "sensation seeking." The sensation-seeking scale measures the person's preference for variety, risk, and various physical sensations. People who score higher on this scale tend to report a greater "high" and a greater "liking" for the drug when given amphetamine in a laboratory setting.[19]

Another, possibly related, personality factor is often referred to as impulsivity—the tendency to act quickly without as much regard to long-term consequences. The relationships between impulsivity and drug use are complex, and researchers are becoming more sophisticated in trying to understand the relationships among impulsivity, specific types of drug use, and the setting in which the drug is used. In other words, being impulsive might have more to do with whether a person drinks heavily when away from home on a weekend night than it does with whether a person has a glass of wine with dinner.[20]

Is Dependence a Family Disorder?

Although few scientific studies have been done, examination of the lives of alcohol-dependent individuals reveals some typical patterns of family adaptation to the problem. A common example in a home with an alcohol-dependent father is that the mother enables this behaviour, by calling her husband's boss to say he is ill or by making excuses to family and friends for failures to appear at dinners or parties and generally by caring for her incapacitated husband. The children might also compensate in various ways, and all conspire to keep the family secret. Thus, it is said that alcohol dependence often exists within a dysfunctional family–the functions of individual members adjust to the needs created by the presence of excessive drinking. This new arrangement can make it difficult for the drinker alone to change his or her behaviour, because doing so would disrupt the family system. Some people suspect that certain family structures actually enhance the likelihood of alcohol abuse or dependence developing. For example, the *co-dependent* needs of other family members to take care of someone who is dependent on them might facilitate drunkenness.

Much has been written about the effects on children who grow up in an "alcoholic family," and there is some indication that even as adults these individuals tend to exhibit certain personality characteristics. The "adult children of alcoholics" are then perhaps more likely to become involved in dysfunctional relationships that increase the likelihood of alcohol abuse, either in themselves or in another family member. Again, the evidence indicates that such influences are statistical tendencies and are not all-powerful. It is perhaps unfortunate that some people with alcoholic parents have adopted the role of "adult children" and try to explain their entire personalities and all their difficulties in terms of that status.

Is Substance Dependence a Disease?

The most important reason for adopting a disease model for dependence is based on the experiences of the founders of AA and is discussed in Chapter 9. Psychiatrists had commonly assumed that alcohol dependence was secondary to another disorder, such as anxiety or depression, and often attempted to treat the presumed underlying disorder while encouraging the drinker to try to "cut down." The founders of AA believed that alcohol dependence itself was the primary problem and needed to be recognized as such and treated directly. This is the reason for the continued insistence that alcohol dependence is a disease–that it is often the primary disturbance and deserves to stand in its own right as a recognized disorder requiring treatment.

On the other hand, Peele[21] and others have argued that substance dependence does not have many of the characteristics of some classic medical diseases, such as tuberculosis or syphilis: We can't use an X-ray or a blood test to reveal the underlying cause, and we don't have a way to treat the underlying cause and cure the symptoms–we don't really know that there is an underlying cause, because all we have are the symptoms of excessive involvement. Furthermore, if substance dependence itself is a disease, then gambling, excessive sexual involvement, and overeating should also be seen as diseases. This in turn weakens our normal understanding of the concept of disease. The disease model is perhaps best seen as an analogy–substance dependence is like a disease in many ways, but that is different from insisting that it is a disease. One reason for the conflict over the disease model of dependence may be differences in how we think of the term disease. For example, many would agree that high blood pressure and lung cancer are considered diseases–they are each certainly viewed as a medical disorder. We know that these diseases are multifactorial, produced by a combination of genetic factors, cigarette smoking, diet, lack of exercise, or other risk factors. In that context, the idea that alcohol or drug dependence is like a disease doesn't seem so far-fetched. This is taking a broad, **biopsychosocial** perspective that dependence might be related to dysfunctions of biology, personality, social interactions, or a combination of these factors. Such debate will undoubtedly continue for some time. However, debate should not be taken lightly and entered into only after a thorough review of relevant and current evidence. In preparation for such debate we recommend careful consideration of the works of Dr. Nora Volkow[22] and others.[23–28]

biopsychosocial: a theory or perspective that relies on the interaction of biological, individual psychological, and social variables.

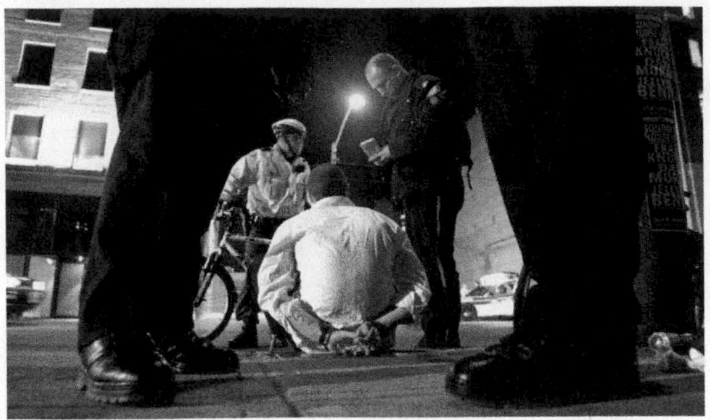

More than 100 000 police-reported drug offences are recorded every year in Canada. The belief that a causal relationship exists between many forms of drug use and criminality probably forms the basis for many of our laws concerning drug use and drug users. The relationship between crime and illicit drug use is complex, and only recently have data-based statements become possible. Facts are necessary because laws are enacted on the basis of what we believe to be true.

LO8 Crime and Violence: Does Drug Use Cause Crime?

It might seem obvious to a reader of today's newspapers or to a viewer of today's television that drugs and crime are linked. There are frequent reports of killings attributed to warring gangs of drug dealers. Our prisons house a significant population of people convicted of drug-related crimes, and several reports have revealed that a large fraction of arrestees for nondrug felonies have positive results from urine tests for illicit substances.

The basis for concern was the belief that drug use causes crime. The fact that drug users engage in robberies or that car thieves are likely to also use illicit drugs does not say anything about causality. Both criminal activity and drug use could well be caused by other factors, producing both types of deviant behaviour in the same individuals. There are several senses in which it might be said that drugs cause crime, but the most frightening possibility is that drug use somehow changes the individual's personality in a lasting way, making him or her into a "criminal type." For example, during the 1924 debate that led to prohibition of heroin sales in the United States, a testifying physician asserted, regarding users, that heroin "dethrones their moral responsibility." Another physician testified that some types of individuals will have their mental equipment "permanently injured by the use of heroin, and those are the ones who will go out and commit crimes." Similar beliefs are reflected in the introductory message in the 1937 film *Reefer Madness,* which referred to marijuana as "The Real Public Enemy Number One!" and described its "soul-destroying" effects as "emotional disturbances, the total inability to direct thought, the loss of all power to resist physical emotions, leading finally to acts of shocking violence . . . ending often in incurable insanity."

Such verbal excesses seem quaint and comical these days, but the underlying belief that drug use changes people into criminals still can be detected in much current political rhetoric. Remember from Chapter 1 that longitudinal research on children and adolescents has led to the conclusion that indicators of criminal or antisocial behaviour usually occur before the first use of an illicit drug. The interaction over time between developing drug-use "careers" and criminal careers is complex and interactive, but it is incorrect to conclude that using any particular drug will turn a person into a criminal.[29]

A second sense in which drug use might cause criminal behaviour occurs when the person is under the influence of the drug. Do the acute effects of a drug make a person temporarily more likely to engage in criminal behaviour? There is little good evidence for this with most illicit substances. In most individuals, marijuana produces a state more akin to lethargy than to crazed violence (see Chapter 15), and heroin tends to make its users more passive and perhaps sexually impotent (see Chapter 13). Stimulants, such as amphetamine and cocaine, can make people paranoid and jumpy, and this can contribute to violent behaviour in some cases (see Chapter 6). The hallucinogen PCP causes disorientation and blocks pain, so users are sometimes hard to restrain (see Chapter 14). This has led to a considerable amount of folklore about the dangerousness of PCP users, although actual documented cases of excessive violence are either rare or nonexistent. A recent study of homicide cases found that every year about 5% are considered to be drug-related. However, most of these are murders that occur in the context of drug trafficking, so it cannot be said that increased violence results from the pharmacological actions of the drugs.[30]

Although there is some question as to whether the direct influence of illicit drugs produces a person more likely to engage in criminal or violent behaviour, there has been less doubt about one commonly used substance: alcohol. In a recent study investigating the cost of substance abuse in Canada, it was estimated that 30% of all criminal offences were attributable to alcohol.[31] Many studies indicate that alcohol is clearly linked with violent crime. In many assaults and sexual

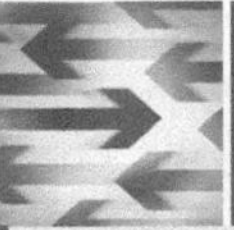

TAKING SIDES

Are Current Laws Fair?

People do things all the time that are potentially dangerous for them and potentially messy and expensive for others. Driving faster than the speed limit, driving without a seat belt, and eating while driving are examples, some of which may not be illegal where you live. In what ways are these behaviours similar to a person snorting cocaine or injecting heroin into his or her veins? In what ways are they different? Do you feel that the laws as they currently exist in your area are appropriate and fair in dealing with these behaviours? If it were up to you, would you outlaw some things that are now legal, legalize some things that are now controlled, or some of each?

assaults, alcohol is present in both assailant and victim. Most homicides are among people who know each other–and alcohol use is associated with half or more of all murders. Drinking at the time of the offence was reported in about 25% of assaults and more than one-third of all rapes and sexual assaults, with drinking rates closer to two-thirds for cases of domestic violence.[32] Victims of violent crime report that they believed the offender had been using alcohol in 25% of the cases, compared with about 5% of the cases in which they believed the offender had been using drugs other than alcohol.[30] Even with such strong correlational evidence linking alcohol use with crime and violence, debate continues about how much of the effect is related to the disinhibitory pharmacological action of alcohol and how much is related to other factors. For example, several studies that have controlled for age, sex, and a generalized tendency to engage in problem behaviours have concluded that both drinking and criminal violence are associated with young males who exhibit a range of antisocial behaviours and that the immediate contribution of being intoxicated might be small.

A third sense in which drug use may be said to cause crime refers to crimes carried out for the purpose of obtaining money to purchase illicit drugs. Research in Canada has shown that not only are many crimes committed by persons under the influence of drugs and/or alcohol but crime, in particular property crime, is often committed to obtain money to purchase illicit drugs.[33] Among jail inmates who had been convicted of property crimes, about one-fourth reported that they had committed the crime to get money for drugs. Also, about one-fourth of those convicted of drug crimes reported that they had sold drugs to get money for their own drug use.[31]

From 1987 through 2003, the U.S. Justice Department collected data on drug use from people arrested and booked into jails for serious crimes. The interviewers tried not to sample too many people who were arrested for drug sale or possession so that usually fewer than 20% of those in the study had been arrested on drug charges. All interviews and urine tests were anonymous; about 90% of arrestees who were asked agreed to an interview, and about 90% of those agreed to provide urine specimens. In 2003, in 39 sites around the country, a median figure of 67% of the adult male arrestees tested positive for the presence of at least one of the five drugs of interest (cocaine, marijuana, methamphetamine, opiates, and PCP). Marijuana was the drug most frequently detected (44%), followed by cocaine (30%).[34] This level of drug use among those arrested for nondrug crimes is quite high; how can we account for it? First, those who adopt a deviant lifestyle might engage in both crime and drug use. Second, because most of these arrests were for crimes in which profit was the motive, the arrestees might have been burglarizing a house or stealing a car to get money to purchase drugs.

The commission of crimes to obtain money for expensive illicit drugs is due to the artificially high cost of the drugs, not primarily to a pharmacological effect of the drug. The inflated cost results from drug controls and enforcement. Both heroin and cocaine are inexpensive substances when obtained legally from a licensed manufacturer, and it has been estimated that if heroin were freely available it would cost no more to be a regular heroin user than to be a regular drinker of alcohol. The black-market cost of these substances makes the use of cocaine or heroin consume so much money.

The fourth and final sense in which drug use causes crime is that illicit drug use is a crime. At first that may seem trivial, but there are two senses in which it is not. First, we are now seeing more than 100 000 police-reported drug offences in Canada annually.[35] In 2007, 63% of these reported drug offences were for cannabis, 22% for cocaine, and 15% for other drugs (heroin, crystal meth, ecstasy, date rape, LSD, etc.). Sixty-eight percent of those offences were for possession, 23% for trafficking, and 9% for production, importation, and exportation of illicit drugs. Currently incarcerated drug offenders account for one-fifth of our federal inmate population.[36] Thus, drug-law violations are one of the major types of crime in Canada. Second, it is likely that the relationship between drug use and other forms of deviant behaviour is strengthened by the fact that drug use is a crime. A person willing to commit one type of crime might be more willing than the average person to commit another type of crime. Some of the people who are actively trying to impress others by living dangerously and committing criminal acts might be drawn to illicit drug use as an obvious way to demonstrate their alienation from society. To better understand this relationship, imagine what might happen if the use of marijuana were legalized. Presumably, a greater number of otherwise law-abiding citizens might try using the drug, thus reducing the correlation between marijuana use and other forms of criminal activity. The concern over possibly increased drug use is, of course, one major argument in favour of maintaining legal controls on the illicit drugs.

LO9 Why We Try to Regulate Drugs

We can see that there are reasonable concerns about the potential toxicity and habit-forming nature of some drugs and even the criminality of some drug users. But the drugs that have been singled out for special controls, such as heroin, cocaine, and marijuana, are not unique in their association with toxicity, dependence, or criminal behaviour. Tobacco, alcohol, and many legally available prescription drugs are also linked to these same social ills. At the beginning of the chapter we mentioned another important source of social conflict over drug use. Once a substance is regulated in any way, those regulations will be broken by some. This produces enormous social conflict and results in many problems for society. From underage drinking to injecting heroin, from Internet sales of prescription narcotics to "date-rape" drugs, the conflicts resulting from particular kinds of drug use lead to additional costs to Canadian society (police, courts, prisons, treatment, etc.) beyond the direct drug effects of toxicity, dependence, and links to other kinds of criminal behaviour. Our current laws do not represent a rationally devised plan to counteract the most realistic of these concerns in the most effective manner. In fact, most legislation is passed in an atmosphere of emotionality, in response to a specific set of concerns. Often the problems have been there for a long time, but public attention and concern have been recently aroused and Parliament must respond. Sometimes members of Parliament or government officials play a major role in calling public attention to the problem for which they offer the solution: a new law, more restrictions, and a bigger budget for some agency. This is what is known in political circles as "starting a prairie fire." As we will see in Chapter 3, often the prairie fires include a lot of emotion-arousing rhetoric that borders on the irrational, and sometimes the results of the prairie fire and the ensuing legislation are unexpected and undesirable.

Summary

- Canadian society has changed from being one that tolerated a wide variety of individual drug use to being one that attempts strict control over some types of drugs. This has occurred in response to social concerns about drug toxicity, dependence potential, and drug-related crime and violence.
- Toxicity can refer either to physiological poisoning or to dangerous disruption of behaviour. Also, we can distinguish acute toxicity, resulting from the presence of too much of a drug, from chronic toxicity, which results from long-term exposure to a drug.
- Heroin and cocaine have high risks of toxicity per user, but their overall public health impact is low compared with tobacco and alcohol. Prescription drugs are also important contributors to overall drug toxicity figures.
- Needle exchange programs reduce the rates of HIV infection by enabling IDUs to use clean syringes.
- Drug dependence does not depend solely on the drug itself, but the use of some drugs is more likely to result in dependence than is the use of other drugs.
- *Physical dependence* is defined by the presence of withdrawal symptoms, implying that the body has adapted to the drug's presence. *Behavioural dependence* is indicated by a high rate of drug use, craving for the drug, and a tendency to relapse after stopping use. *Tolerance* is defined as a reduced effect of a drug after repeated exposure.
- Until the twentieth century, people with a substance dependence were believed to be

self-indulgent or immoral. Scientific research now supports the view that substance dependence is a disease with multiple etiologies.

- The DSM-5, a publication of the American Psychiatric Association, provides tools for use in the diagnosis of substance-related and addictive disorders.
- Drug use might be said to cause crime in several ways: (1) changing the individual's personality in a way that makes him or her into a criminal type; (2) making a person under the influence of drugs temporarily more likely to engage in criminal behaviour; (3) leading a person to commit a crime to obtain money to purchase illicit drugs; and (4) using illicit drugs is itself a crime.
- More than 100 000 police-reported drug offences occur each year in Canada. The idea that opioid drugs or marijuana can produce violent criminality in their users is an old and largely discredited idea. Opioid users seem to engage in crimes mainly to obtain money, not because they are made more criminal by the drugs they take. One drug that is widely accepted as contributing to crimes and violence is alcohol.
- Laws that have been developed to control drug use have a legitimate social purpose, which is to protect society from the dangers caused by some types of drug use. Whether these dangers have always been viewed rationally, and whether the laws have had their intended results, can be better judged after we have learned more about the drugs and the history of their regulation.

Review Questions

1. The French term *laissez-faire* is used to describe what type of relationship between a government and its people?
2. What three major concerns about drugs contributed to the creation and development of laws controlling their availability?
3. Long-term, heavy drinking can lead to permanent impairment of memory. What type of toxicity is this (acute or chronic; physiological or behavioural)?
4. What two kinds of data are recorded by the DAWN system?
5. Why does Canada not produce data similar to those provided through the DAWN system?
6. Why have HIV and HCV been of particular concern for users of illicit drugs?
7. What drugs and methods of using them are considered to have very high dependence potential?
8. What is the apparent dependence potential of hallucinogenic drugs, such as LSD and mescaline?
9. What are four ways in which drug use might theoretically cause crime?
10. About how many offences are reported each year in Canada for violations of drug laws?

CHAPTER 3

DRUG POLICY

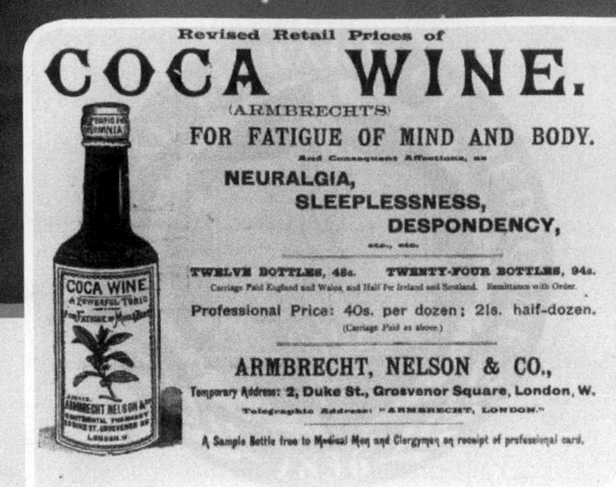

OBJECTIVES

When you have finished this chapter, you should be able to

LO1 Summarize the history of and influences on the creation of drug regulations in Canada.

LO2 Describe the Controlled Drugs and Substances Act.

LO3 Discuss Bill S-10 and its potential impacts.

LO4 Explain how pharmaceuticals are regulated in Canada.

LO5 Discuss the pharmaceutical industry in Canada.

LO6 Explain the Marihuana Medical Access Regulations (MMAR) of July 2001.

LO7 Discuss the Marihuana for Medical Purposes Regulations (MMPR) of April 2014.

LO8 Describe how natural health products are regulated in Canada.

In Chapter 2, we saw that drug regulations are passed mainly for what is perceived to be the public good. As the story of the laws and regulations about drugs unfolds, it will become clear that most of the debate centres on the question, "What is the public good?" Issues of fact, morality, health, personal choice, and social order are intertwined–and sometimes confused. If we want to understand our current drug laws, we must see how they have evolved over the years. In this chapter we will look at the drug regulations and acts in Canada.

LO1 The History of Drug Regulations

Prior to 1908 Canada did not have regulations, federal or provincial, for governing the use of drugs. Tobacco and especially alcohol were considered to be more of a threat to society and personal health than was the use of opium.[1]

It can reasonably be argued that the beginnings of drug regulation in Canada were not driven by concerns for the health of the population or the dangers that the drugs presented but rather had more to do with public fear of Chinese and Japanese immigrants–fuelled, at least in part, by monetary and political agendas. Chinese workers began immigrating to British Columbia in the 1850s. These immigrants, predominantly single males, were willing to work for wages that were much lower than their Euro-Canadian counterparts. These immigrants typically lived in isolated communities where opium dens were known but not perceived as harmful by either the government or the public. In fact, prior to the twentieth century government saw opium not as a health or safety issue, but as an opportunity for financial gain. Government received tax revenue from opium factories in the Chinese immigrant communities, and the federal government also received revenue through a $500 licensing fee obtained from these factories.[1]

Two factors are believed to have contributed to an escalation of the public's fear and resentment of Asiatic immigrants and consequently the movement toward an era of drug regulation and antidrug policies.[2] First, associations between certain elements of Euro-Canadian society (e.g., actors and gamblers) and Chinese immigrants began to develop. Respectable citizens viewed this mixing of races with disdain.[3] Second, Chinese immigrant workers began to be perceived as an "economic threat" to Euro-Canadians. With a decline in the railroads and the gold rush came fewer employment opportunities for all Canadians. The willingness of Chinese labourers to work for lower wages made them more marketable and affected overall wage rates. Euro-Canadian workers, with families to support, could not compete with Chinese labourers.[1] As economic conditions worsened, Chinese immigrants became a growing target for Euro-Canadian resentment and fear.

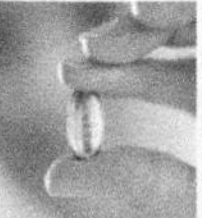

DRUGS IN DEPTH

Opioid Contracts: Mandatory Drug Testing for Chronic Pain Patients. Who Benefits?

In a recent article published in the *Chronicle Herald*, patients that are being seen at the Centre for Pain Management in Halifax are being asked to subject to a urinary toxicology screen to determine what, if any, drugs (illicit or legal) the patient is consuming. "Shelley Brown, a former patient at the Centre for Pain Management, said the requirement violates her rights. The Mahone Bay woman, who has a form of leukemia that causes severe pain, was upset at being told last week that she wouldn't be treated unless she provided a sample."[4] This mandatory drug test is being proposed necessary to determine whether or not patients receiving an opioid for pain, in conjunction with medications/drugs presently consumed, are at increased risk of harm both from an overdose and from an addiction perspective. Does the patient really benefit, or is it a means of discrimination? There is a hum of information on social media,[5] and reference to its utility on PubMed. A question emerges in light of this recent news media: "Is it ethical to subject patients to mandatory drug tests and what will be done with this information? In a quantitative design, what number of clients that receive opioids also test positive for other drugs, legal or illicit? What evidence exists that these 'opioid contracts' improve care and possess efficacy to reduce opioid addiction?"[6] These are all questions that may be answered by prospective clinical studies following patients being treated for chronic pain.

In addition to gathering data, clinical measures need to be put in place by the interdisciplinary team for methods of treating pain other than with the administration of opioids. On the team would be a social worker/counsellor to talk with the client about population studies, a physician to be involved in establishing proper (non-judgmental) guidelines for the prescription of opioids,[7,8] a nurse trained to recognize signs of addiction as well as pain, a psychologist to assess for depression or anxiety disorders that might exacerbate pain syndromes, a physiotherapist to initiate non-pharmacological strategies for pain (e.g. massage, heat), and a toxicologist trained in drug testing to rule out false positive and negative results.[9] With well controlled studies the factors leading to addiction in these patients may be identified, the care of individuals with a higher risk for opioid misuse improved,[10] and the costs and dangers of drug use could be greatly reduced.[11]

Resentment turned to hostility, which subsequently was reflected in legislation designed to end Chinese immigration and drive the Chinese out of Canada's economic mainstream. By 1904 the tax on Chinese immigrants had risen to $500 per person, which slowed Chinese immigration. However, between 1904 and 1907 Japanese immigration into British Columbia rose dramatically, fuelling an increase in Asiatic resentment and hostility.[12] Subsequently, a major labour demonstration in 1907 (directed against Japanese immigrants) resulted in a riot and caused serious property damage in Vancouver's Chinese community. The investigation of the event and recommendations that were made resulted in the passing of the Opium Act of 1908.

The Opium Act of 1908

In 1908, then Canadian Deputy Minister of Labour Mackenzie King travelled to British Columbia to gather information pertaining to the 1907 labour demonstrations and riots. During this visit King interviewed two Vancouver opium merchants, who revealed to him the extent to which opium was being traded and consumed in British Columbia.[1] Based on these interviews, King drew four conclusions: (1) that opium smoking was growing in popularity among white people, (2) that Chinese merchants were making considerable profits through the opium trade, (3) that the opium trade was in violation of current provincial pharmacy legislation, and (4) that as a Christian nation, Canada had a moral responsibility to serve as a leader in the then-international campaign against opium use.[1] On his return to Ottawa King made the elimination of the "opium menace" an immediate goal, and through his actions led Parliament to enact Canada's first prohibitionist drug policy, the 1908 Opium Act.[12]

Canada's 1908 Opium Act made it an indictable offence to import, manufacture, and offer to sell or possess to sell opium for non-medical purposes. It did not, however, prohibit simple possession or use, and the demand for opium continued.[1] As a result, the 1908 Opium Act led to the development of a black market for opium. Law enforcement opinion was that the best way to curb the demand for opium was to create harsher penalties (including imprisonment) and to expand enforcement powers. Consequentially, three years after its creation the Opium Act was repealed and replaced with a harsher legislation, the 1911 Opium and Drug Act. This Act began the enforcement era of Canadian drug policy, one that would continue unchallenged until the 1950s.[12] Advocates for the treatment of drug users lacked power and momentum prior to the 1950s, so it was easy for law enforcement interests to effect the implementation of harsh antidrug legislation. Sadly, this also meant that even though drug users were thought of as being sick, imprisonment was a priority over treatment.[3] In addition, because habitual drug use was most often associated with Chinese immigrants, many Canadians felt they were "immune from the effects of harsh drug legislation."[2]

Patent Medicine Act of 1909

Canada's first effort toward federal drug regulation came in the form of the Patent Medicine Act of 1909. This legislation required the documentation and approval of selected drugs that were then formulated and issued by doctors.[13] This Act prohibited the use of cocaine in medicines and required pharmaceutical companies to include a list of ingredients on the label of any medicine containing heroin, morphine, or opium. Following the creation of the federal Department of Health, the Patent Medicine Act was superseded, in 1920, by the Food and Drugs Act. Under this Act regulations were created that defined specific requirements for licensing drugs for use in Canada. This Act also gave the Minister of Health authority to cancel or suspend a drug licence for violations of requirements. In 1947 the Food and Drug Act underwent revisions that laid the foundation for the regulations in place today.[13]

Narcotic Control Act of 1961

In the 1950s illegal drug use was on the decline in Canada. However, media publications of highly sensational accounts of drug-addicted youth created recognition of the need to treat habitual drug users in Canada.[1] During this period of discourse many physicians came to see drug addiction as a responsibility that fell within their scope of practice. In other words, perhaps drug addiction was a social and medical problem, not a crime.[2] This change in perspective resulted in a call from the medical community for the treatment of addictions. In response, in 1955 the federal government established the Senate Special Committee on the Traffic of Narcotic Drugs in Canada.[1] Unfortunately, after holding hearings across Canada the committee ended up favouring the view of the law enforcement community, and this was eventually reflected in the highly punitive 1961 Narcotic Control Act.

Criminalization of drugs happened in Canada because many people held to the belief that certain drugs had the ability to enslave users.[14] With time,

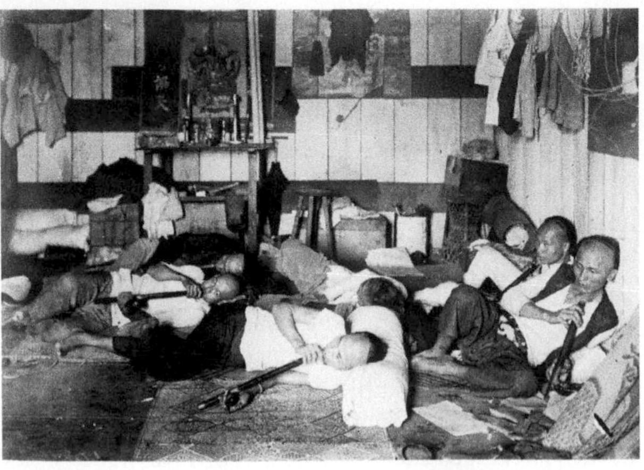

Opium smoking spread widely following its introduction in the nineteenth century.

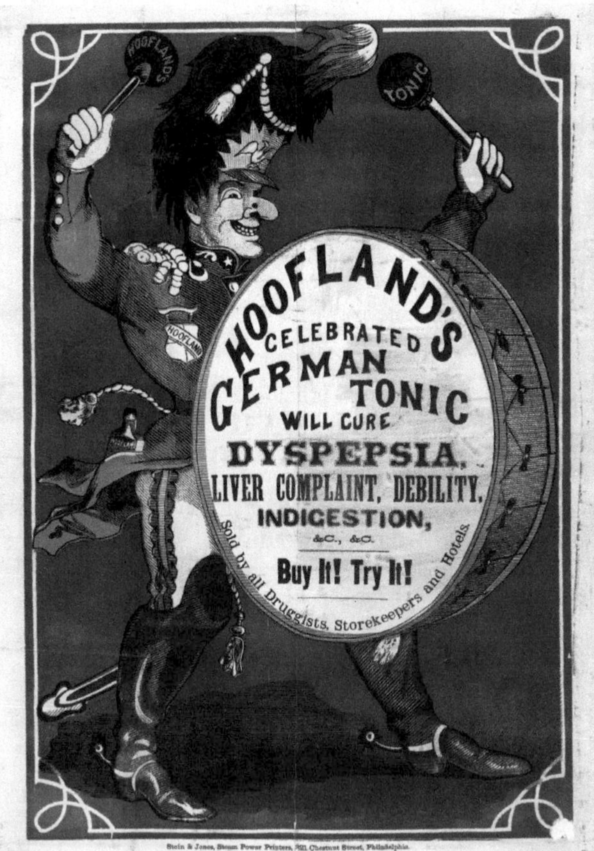

Many patent medicines contained habit-forming drugs. This tonic from the 1860s was about 30% alcohol.

however, people began to question their beliefs and the criminalization of drugs came under challenge. The "dope fiend" mythology, used by law enforcement interests to justify strict laws, became discredited because large numbers of middle-class youth were using illicit drugs recreationally without turning into "dangerous lunatics." During the 1960s and 1970s the social distance between drug users and mainstream society narrowed considerably, and laws began to draw criticism for making criminals out of white middle-class youth.

The Le Dain Commission

In 1969, the Government of Canada established a Commission of Inquiry to evaluate and debate the non-medical (illicit) use of drugs in Canada. This Commission (also known as the Le Dain Commission) was chaired by Dean Gerald Le Dain and worked from 1969 to 1973. All in total 365 submissions were presented at Commission hearings, with approximately 12 000 people in attendance. In completion of the Commission's work, four reports were produced. Paramount among the reports' recommendations was a call for a gradual decriminalization of illegal drugs. The reports also recommended greater leniency for the crime of possession including the abolishment of imprisonment.[15] The Commission further recommended that the possession of cannabis not be considered an offence and that the federal government conduct research to evaluate changes in the extent and patterns of cannabis use, and explore possible health, personal, and social changes consequential to its controlled legal distribution. Despite the Le Dain Commission's recommendations, Canada's drug policies, 40 years later, remained relatively unchanged.

Canada's Drug Strategies

In 1986, U.S. President Ronald Reagan declared war on drugs in the United States. Canada followed suit and a new era of drug prohibition and law enforcement began.[14] The fear of drugs, perpetuated in the 1980s by politics and the media, led to the development of Canada's first "National Drug Strategy," introduced in 1987.[16] Although the Strategy acknowledged that substance-related disorders were predominantly a health issue, it continued the enforcement-based approach that began with the 1908 Opium Act. In 1992, the Government of Canada

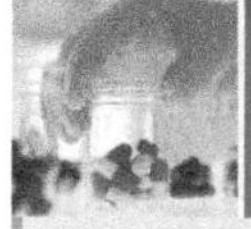

DRUGS IN THE MEDIA

Canadian Police Chiefs Propose Ticket System for Pot: Proposal Would Give Officer Discretion, Free Up Court Time, Chiefs Say

Canada's police chiefs have voted overwhelmingly in favour of reforming drug laws in the country. The Canadian Association of Chiefs of Police, meeting in Winnipeg this week, wants officers to have the ability to ticket people found with 30 grams of marijuana or less.

Kentville, N.S., police Chief Mark Mander, chair of the association's drug-abuse committee, said Tuesday officers currently have only two choices: turn a blind eye or lay down the law. Mander said officers could "either to caution the offender or lay formal charges resulting in [a] lengthy, difficult process, which results in a criminal charge if proven, a criminal conviction, and a criminal record." Mander said ticketing the offender would be far less onerous and expensive. However, federal Justice Minister Peter MacKay said there are no plans in the works to legalize or decriminalize marijuana. Though MacKay had no follow up on the chiefs' recommendation, he said he appreciates their input.

"We don't support legalization or decriminalization," Mander said. "Clearly there are circumstances where a formal charge for simple possession is appropriate. However, the large majority of simple possession cases would be more effectively, efficiently dealt with [by issuing a ticket]," he added, noting the move would free up court time. The president of the association and Vancouver police Chief Jim Chu said the plan offers a good compromise. "It's a middle ground there, right? Nothing is nothing. All is a criminal record," Chu said. Bill Vandegraaf, an advocate for marijuana use, said the ticket system amounts to decriminalization.

"They are diminishing the seriousness of the offence," said the former Winnipeg police officer, a member of the group Law Enforcement Against Prohibition who is currently licensed to grow and use marijuana for medical purposes. "They are turning it into a common offence where they issue tickets on the street." Vandergraaf called the proposal a good first step, but said it doesn't go far enough. "If it's going to be a common offence notice, they might as well end prohibition altogether," he said.

Source: Drugs in the Media: Canadian Police Chiefs Propose Ticket System for Pot: Proposal Would Give Officer Discretion, Free Up Court Time, Chiefs Say http://www.cbc.ca/news/canada/manitoba/canadian-police-chiefs-propose-ticket-system-for-pot-1.1335493. Used with permission from the CBC.

approved Canada's Drug Strategy calling for an approach that would reduce the demand for and the supply of drugs through such activities as control and enforcement, prevention, treatment and rehabilitation, and harm reduction. Furthermore, as part of the 1987 National Drug Strategy, a committee was formed to draft new legislation.[12] Almost 10 years later, in 1996, the Controlled Drugs and Substances Act (Bill C8) was voted into law.

Canada's Drug Strategy was renewed in 2003. In the renewal process focus was placed on the reduction of harms associated with the use of narcotics and controlled substances and the abuse of alcohol and prescription drugs. It is important to note that the renewed Strategy recognized underlying factors associated with substance-related disorders. Therefore, it is not surprising that in addition to enhanced enforcement measures the Strategy also supported education, prevention, and health promotion initiatives. In 2007, the Government of Canada introduced its National Anti-Drug Strategy. The goal of this strategy is to reduce the supply and demand for illicit drugs. Key priorities of the Strategy include preventing illicit drug use, treating substance-related disorders, and combatting illicit drug production and distribution.

LO2 Controlled Drugs and Substances Act

Provisions within the Controlled Drugs and Substances Act (CDSA) govern importation, production, distribution, and possession of various drugs and substances in Canada.[17] This Act replaced the Narcotic Control Act and Parts III and IV of the Food and Drugs Act. All drugs and substances prohibited under the CDSA may not be imported, exported, produced, sold, provided, or possessed within Canada, except where permitted by regulations. Controlled drugs and substances used in medical treatments may be legally obtained but only with a prescription from a health care practitioner with a licence to do so (e.g., medical doctors, dentists, nurse practitioners, and veterinarians). A controlled drug may be legally possessed and used by the person for whom it was prescribed. Sharing prescribed controlled drugs and substances is illegal and can result in convictions for trafficking, unlawful possession, export, import, or trade of a drug. Such convictions may result in imprisonment, a fine, or both.

Not all offences under the CDSA result in a criminal record upon conviction. For example, conviction of a *summary conviction only* offence generally does not result in a criminal record. Simple possession of 30 grams or less of cannabis or 1 gram or less of cannabis resin (hashish) might constitute a summary conviction only offence. (A criminal record refers to a conviction entered in a register maintained by the RCMP and known as the Canadian Police Information Centre.) In contrast, the simple possession of more than 30 grams of cannabis (i.e., 31 grams) or 1 gram of cannabis resin is an example of a dual offence under the CDSA. Such possessions can lead to either a *summary conviction* or an *indictable offence* which, upon conviction, will result in a criminal record. Offences that are *indictable offences only*, such as trafficking or the possession of cannabis for the purposes of trafficking, will also result in a criminal record upon conviction. Those convicted of a summary offence resulting in a criminal record may apply for a pardon five years after conviction, while those convicted of an indictable offence may apply for a pardon ten years after conviction.

It is an offence under the CDSA to seek or obtain a controlled substance from a medical practitioner without disclosing to that practitioner all other controlled substances obtained from other practitioners within the previous 30 days. The maximum punishment for this offence on indictment is seven years. However, for a first offence on summary conviction, the maximum punishment is a fine of up to $1000 and up to six months in prison.

Canada's CDSA is a comprehensive and complex document, under constant scrutiny and challenge. A wide variety of components are defined within this Act, including but not limited to sentencing, drug paraphernalia laws, regulation of the sale of alcohol and tobacco, impaired driving, and diversion to treatment.

Sentencing

Under the CDSA judges are afforded considerable discretion in sentencing offenders. Aggravating factors that often influence sentencing decisions include selling drugs to children, involving children under 18 years of age in the commission of an offence, or selling drugs in or near schools or public places frequented by youth.

Drug Paraphernalia Laws

Under section 462.2 of the Criminal Code of Canada the import, export, manufacturing, promoting, or selling of instruments or literature for illicit drug use is a summary conviction offence. The consequences of conviction are severe (e.g., for a first offence, to a fine not exceeding $100 000 or to imprisonment for a term not exceeding six months or both). It is interesting to note that patients prescribed medical marijuana often use devices such as bongs, pipes, vapourizers, water pipes, or hookahs when consuming their medicine. Some of these devices have been categorized by the government as medical devices and are covered for reimbursement by provincial health insurance plans.

Regulation of the Sale of Alcohol and Tobacco

The sale and use of alcohol and tobacco is subject to both federal and provincial/territorial legislation. Extended review of the regulation of these substances is provided in Chapters 9 and 10, respectively.

Impaired Driving

The Criminal Code of Canada includes offences related to driving while impaired by alcohol or other drugs. A historical review of regulation pertaining to impaired driving is presented in Chapter 9.

Diversion to Treatment

Components of the CDSA allow for diversion of people from the criminal justice system into treatment. In addition to the obvious benefit for persons with substance-related disorders, such programs also have the potential to expand collaboration between the police and justice system and the health and social service system. Diversion to treatment also addresses issues of prison and court overcrowding and the lack of available services to support recovery during incarceration. Many provinces and territories also require those convicted of impaired driving offences to attend substance abuse education or treatment programs.

International Conventions

In addition to its own laws Canada has also ratified a number of international conventions to control drugs, including the 1961 Single Convention on Narcotic Drugs, as amended by the 1972 Protocol; the 1971 Convention on Psychotropic Substances; and the 1988 Convention against Illicit Traffic in Narcotic Drugs and Psychotropic Substances.

Table 3.1 details the schedules in the Controlled Drugs and Substances Act, with examples of the drugs in each schedule.

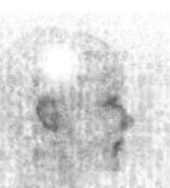

MIND/BODY CONNECTION

Expanding Drug Treatment Courts in Canada

A drug treatment court (DTC) provides judicially supervised treatment in lieu of prison time for individuals who have a substance use problem related to their criminal activities (e.g., drug-related offences, such as drug possession, use, or noncommercial trafficking or property offences committed to support their drug use, such as theft or shoplifting). The eligible accused must decide between the DTC program and customary criminal justice processing that ranges from fines to incarceration. Typically, formal admission into a DTC program requires the individual to plead guilty to the charges. If an individual fails to comply or participate in all aspects of the program, consequences range from an official reprimand or revocation of bail to expulsion from the program.

DTC participants are required to attend both individual and group counselling sessions and receive appropriate medical attention (such as methadone treatment) and are subject to random drug tests. Participants must also appear regularly in court, where a judge reviews their progress and can then either impose sanctions or provide rewards (ranging from verbal commendations to a reduction in court appearances). DTC staff work with community partners to address participants' other needs, such as safe housing, stable employment, and job training. Once a participant gains social stability and can exhibit control over their substance use problem, criminal charges are either stayed (suspended or postponed judgment) or the offender receives a noncustodial sentence (restrictions other than jail, including house arrest).

The first Canadian DTC was established in Toronto in 1998 as collaboration among the Centre for Addiction and Mental Health, the Provincial Court of Ontario, Justice Canada, the Toronto Police Service, and other community-based organizations. The DTC of Vancouver was opened in December 2001 to address the high rates of heroin use and cocaine and crack cocaine use in Vancouver. In 2003, the federal government underscored its support for the use of DTCs in Canada by dedicating $23 million over five years to support the continued operation of the two existing Canadian DTCs and to facilitate the development, implementation, and operation of four additional sites in Ottawa, Winnipeg, Regina, and Edmonton.

Table 3.1 Controlled Drugs and Schedules

Schedule	Description	Examples
I	Those drugs already listed in the Narcotic Control Act, including opium, heroin, morphine, coca leaves, cocaine, methadols, moramides, and fentanyl.	• coca (leaves, cocaine, ecgonine, crack) • flunitrazepam (Rohypnol) • GHB • ketamine • methamphetamine • opioids (heroin, morphine, oxycodone, pethidine, etc.) • phencyclidine
II	All forms of cannabis, cannabis resin, and "similar synthetics," such as nabilone. Specifically excludes nonviable seed and a stalk that has been stripped of leaves and branches.	• hashish • cannabis
III	Stimulants and hallucinogens listed in the Food and Drug Act, including amphetamine, Quaaludes, psilocybe, LSD, DMT, MDA.	• amphetamines (excluding methamphetamine) • barbiturates • cathinone • MDMA • LSD • methaqualone (Quaaludes) • methcathinone • psilocybin • temazepam (Restoril)
IV	Some prescribed drugs, anabolic steroids, weight-reduction drugs (anorexiants), sedatives, such as barbiturates and benzodiazepines (better known as Valium and Ativan), and khat.	• anabolic steroids (testosterone, etc.) • benzodiazepines (except flunitrazepam and temazepam)
V	Ingredients that may appear in nonprescription medication, including phenylpropanolamine and propylhexedrine.	• propylhexedrine
VI	Certain precursors (substances commonly used to manufacture some of the other listed drugs).	**Class A** • ephedrine (easily reduced into methamphetamine) • isosafrole (used in making MDMA) • lysergic acid • potassium permanganate • pseudoephedrine (easily reduced into methamphetamine) • 1,4-butanediol • red phosphorus • white phosphorus **Class B** • acetone • ethyl ether • hydrochloric acid • sulphuric acid • toluene
VII		• 3 kilograms or more of hashish • 3 kilograms or more of cannabis
VIII		• 1 gram of hashish • 30 grams of cannabis

Source: Based on Canada. *The Controlled Drugs and Substances Act (S.C. 1996, c. 19)*. 2011. Retrieved September 20, 2011, from http://laws-lois.justice.gc.ca/eng/acts/C-38.8/.

LO3 Bill S-10: An Act to Amend the Controlled Drugs and Substances Act

Bill S-10, otherwise known as the "Safe Streets and Communities Act," was an omnibus Bill that included amendments to Canada's Controlled Drugs and Substances Act (CDSA). It was created by Stephen Harper's government and proposed minimum penalties for serious drug offences, such as dealing drugs for organized crime purposes or when a weapon or violence is involved.[18,19]

Bill S-10 received Royal Assent and became law during the 41st Parliament, which ended in September 2013. This law made jail time for serious drug offence convictions mandatory, and where "aggravating factors" are present such as:

- production;
- trafficking;
- possession for the purpose of trafficking or exporting; and
- importing and exporting.

The amendments in Bill C-10 prescribe mandatory prison terms for offences related to drugs listed in Schedule I (e.g., heroin, cocaine, and methamphetamine) and in Schedule II (e.g., marijuana). Generally, the minimum sentence would apply if the offence occurred in combination with an "aggravating factor" such as:

- for the benefit of organized crime;
- involving use or threat of violence;
- involving use or threat of use of weapons;
- by a person who has been previously convicted (in the past 10 years) of a serious drug offence;
- in a prison;
- by abusing a position of authority or access to restricted areas;
- in or near a school, in or near an area normally frequented by youth or in the presence of youth;
- involving a youth in the commission of the offence; and,
- in relation to a youth (e.g., selling to a youth).

The amendments contained within Bill C-10 contain an exception for allowing leniency in sentencing if an offender successfully completes a drug treatment court (DTC) or related program. Drug Treatment Court programs are designed to assist eligible individuals who are charged with drug-related offences to overcome their substance-related disorder and, by association, avoid future conflict with the law. Treatment programs must be approved by a province and participants remain under judicial supervision throughout their course of treatment. Approved treatment programs typically include social services support, incentives for refraining from drug use, and sanctions for failure to comply with the orders of the court. Leniency in sentencing following successful program completion is permitted under subsection 720(2) of the Criminal Code.

With the Royal Assent for Bill S-10 mandatory minimum jail sentences for marijuana offences became law. For example, a conviction for growing as few as five marijuana plants requires a six-month sentence, while a conviction for extracting hash or making pot edibles, and sharing them, requires an 18-month sentence. This means medical marijuana users who share their home-baked pot cookies or chocolates are at risk of arrest, as there is no protection for such activities under current medical marijuana laws. Some of the mandatory sentences increase to two years for growing or dealing near schools, and even more time when combined with additional "aggravating factors."

Through this Bill, mandatory minimum sentences are now required for low-level, non-violent drug transactions if they are associated with an "aggravating factor" (e.g., if the activity occurred in or near an area normally frequented by youth). Aggravating factors are very broadly defined, and the amounts of drugs involved so small that the law may be destined to target marginalized individuals whose offences are often related to their drug-related disorder. This potential for targeting marginalized Canadians has created great debate within our society.[20] Advocates for marginalized people contend that the poor and members of minority groups, particularly Indigenous people, are already incarcerated in disproportionate numbers, many for substance-related offences. Their belief is that this significant human rights issue will now worsen with the Bill's passage. There is also debate as to whether mandatory minimum sentences do more harm than good. Imprisonment creates health risks and often leaves those who serve time unemployable and more likely to be entrenched in a life of crime. Compounding these concerns is the fact that opportunities for treatment of substance-related disorders oftentimes are lacking in prisons and jails.

One might ask whether the changes to the CDSA contained in Bill S-10 are intended to protect society or to punish people for having substance-related disorders.

LO4 Regulation of Pharmaceuticals

Ensuring the efficacy, safety, and quality of pharmaceutical drugs, vitamins, vaccines, and medical devices sold in Canada is the responsibility of Health Canada. Their mandate to provide this oversight is contained within the Food and Drugs Act and Regulations. Consequentially, Health Canada's Health Products and Food Branch (HPFB) has the daunting task of evaluating and monitoring thousands of human and veterinary drugs, medical devices, natural health products, and other therapeutic products available to Canadians.[21] More than 22 000 pharmaceutical products and 40 000 medical devices currently fall under their jurisdiction.

New-Drug Submission Processes

If results of clinical trial studies indicate that a new drug has potential therapeutic value, and that the value outweighs the risks associated with its proposed use (e.g., adverse effects or toxicity), the manufacturer may seek authorization to sell the product in Canada. To do this they must file a New Drug Submission (NDS) with HPFB. New Drug Submissions must present scientific evidence attesting to the product's safety, efficacy, and quality. They include the results of both the preclinical and the clinical studies, details on the production of the drug and its packaging and labelling, and information about its claimed therapeutic value, conditions for use, and side effects.

New drugs are commonly referred to as brand-name products. They have been created and patented by companies and therefore cannot then be reproduced by competitors. Generic products must demonstrate the same quality standards as brand names (i.e., they must be shown to be as safe and efficacious as the brand-name product). This comparison is usually done through comparative bioavailability studies. If, post-approval, a manufacturer would like to make some change to a previously approved product, it must submit a Supplemental NDS (SNDS). Product changes requiring an SNDS include but are not limited to changes in the dosage, form, or strength of the drug, the formulation, the method of manufacture, the labelling, or the recommended route of administration.

If, upon completion of a new-drug review, the HPFB concludes that the benefits outweigh the risks and that the risks can be mitigated or managed, the manufacturer receives a Notice of Compliance (NOC) and the product is issued an eight-digit Drug Identification Number (DIN). The DIN allows the manufacturer to sell the product in Canada. Product DINs must be present on the label of all prescription and nonprescription drug products sold in Canada.

Provincial and Territorial Responsibilities

Health Canada, through the HPFB, is responsible for regulating the manufacture, sale, and import of therapeutic products. However, it is the responsibility of provincial/territorial governments to do the following:

- Manage and deliver health care services
- Plan and evaluate the provision of hospital care and allied health care services
- Provide public drug benefit plans to certain segments of their population (e.g., all provinces and territories provide coverage to seniors and those receiving social assistance)

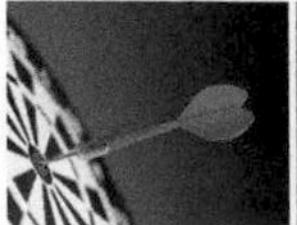

TARGETING PREVENTION

Prescribing Practices

Under Canada's Controlled Drugs and Substances Act, scheduled drugs for medical treatment may be legally obtained only with a prescription from a licensed medical practitioner (including dental and veterinary practitioners). However, many of these scheduled prescription medications (i.e., opioids, benzodiazepines, amphetamines) have the potential for patients to abuse them or to become dependent on them. Prescribing rules vary, but one of the most common limitations is that the prescriptions may not be automatically refilled. In other words, the physician must write a new prescription if the patient wants to get more of the drug. Despite these rules, we are hearing more and more about people who develop dependence on prescription drugs. Do you think the current limitations are effective? Could changes be made that would effectively reduce the chances of patients becoming dependent?

- Assess drug or medical device eligibility for inclusion in drug formularies (lists of drugs for which public reimbursement from government drug plans is available), including consideration of the financial consequences
- Manage drug formularies
- Oversee the practice of medicine and pharmacy and the regulation of health professionals
- Assess whether a brand-name drug and its generic competitor are interchangeable. If they are, public reimbursements from government drug plans are typically limited to the lower-cost generic.

Drug benefit programs for certain client groups within Canada are managed by the federal government. These include:

- Veterans
- Members of the Canadian Forces
- Canada's First Nations and Inuit peoples
- Members of the Royal Canadian Mounted Police
- Certain designated classes of migrant peoples
- Inmates of federal penitentiaries and some former inmates on parole

Compulsory Licences

Canada's Patent Act was amended in 1969 to permit compulsory licences to import medicines into Canada. This allowed generic drug manufacturers to import a medicine's active ingredients and process them for sale. Eighteen years later Bill C-22 amended the Patent Act to guarantee patent owners a period of protection, 20 years from the date on which a patent application was filed, from compulsory licences.[22]

A 2003 Trade-Related Aspects of Intellectual Property Rights agreement permitted World Trade Organization (WTO) member countries to issue compulsory licences for patented pharmaceuticals. Compulsory licensing authorized the production and sale of generic drugs that are therapeutically equivalent to their patented, brand-name counterparts, without the consent of patent holders. It was generally believed that by breaking the patent monopoly and introducing competition, the prices of medicines would be reduced. This agreement also permitted pharmaceutical manufacturers to produce generic pharmaceutical products solely or primarily for export to countries with insufficient capacity to produce their own. The Jean Chrétien Pledge to Africa Act implemented the WTO decision in 2005. Regulations within this Act also define a formula for calculating royalty payments to patent-holders when issuing a compulsory licence for export. The maximum royalty is 4% of the total value of the contract between the generic manufacturer and the purchaser.[23]

Developing and Introducing a New Drug

The history of new-drug introduction into the Canadian marketplace can be reliably traced to the 1960s, when regulations on Investigational New Drug Applications (INDs) were developed. INDs assisted government in the review of applications for drugs to be distributed for clinical trials. In 1987, a 60-day default review period was introduced to help the pharmaceutical industry in their planning and to encourage new research opportunities. These regulations remained unchanged until 2001. On September 1, 2001, regulatory amendments to the Food and Drug Regulations (Drugs for Clinical Trials Involving Human Subjects) came into force, with the primary goals of strengthening protection for subjects participating in clinical trials and attracting and sustaining investment in research and development in Canada.[24]

The HPFB of Health Canada's mandate is to take an integrated approach to the management of the risks and benefits to the health of Canadians. It is responsible for review and approval of clinical trials in humans. Table 3.2 provides a description of the three phases of the clinical trial process required in Canada before a product can reach the marketplace. The fourth phase of the clinical trial process refers to all studies performed after the drug has been approved. Clinical trials pertaining to drugs and medical devices are under

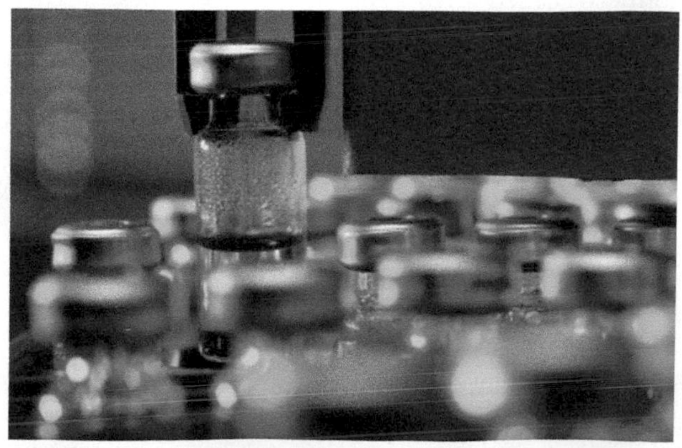

A new drug must move through three phases of clinical investigation before it reaches the market in Canada. All studies performed after the drug has been approved are considered Phase IV and are designed to optimize the drug's therapeutic effects.

Table 3.2 Clinical Trial Phases

Phase	Description
I	Initial safety studies on a new drug, including the first administration of the drug into humans, usually conducted in healthy volunteers. These trials may be conducted in patients when administration of the drug to healthy volunteers is not ethical. Phase I trials are designed mainly to determine the pharmacological actions of the drug and the side effects associated with increasing doses. Pharmacokinetic and drug–drug interaction studies are usually considered as Phase I trials regardless of when they are conducted during drug development as these are generally conducted in healthy volunteers. Phase I trials also include trials in which new drugs are used as research tools to explore biological phenomena or disease processes.
II	Clinical trials to evaluate the efficacy of the drug in patients with medical conditions to be treated, diagnosed, or prevented and to determine the side effects and risks associated with the drug. If a new indication for a marketed drug is to be investigated, then those clinical trials may generally be considered Phase II trials.
III	Controlled or uncontrolled trials conducted after preliminary evidence suggesting efficacy of the drug has been demonstrated. These are intended to gather the additional information about efficacy and safety that is needed for further risk-benefit assessment of the drug. In this phase, clinical trials are also conducted in special patient populations (e.g., people with renal failure), or under special conditions dictated by the nature of the drug and disease.
IV	All studies performed after the drug has been approved by the regulator for the market and related to the approved indication. These studies are often important for optimizing the drug's use. They may be of any type but must have valid scientific objectives. Commonly conducted studies include safety studies and studies designed to support use under the approved indication, such as mortality and morbidity studies or epidemiological studies.

Source: *Clinical Trials, Abbreviations/Definitions.* Health Canada, 2008. Reproduced with the permission of the Minister of Health, 2011.

the jurisdiction of the Therapeutic Product Directorate (TPD). Clinical trials with biological and radiopharmaceutical drugs, including blood and blood products, viral and bacterial vaccines, gene therapy products, cells, tissues, organs, and xenografts are the responsibility of the Biologics and Genetic Therapies Directorate (BGTD).

With the 2001 amendments to the Food and Drug Regulations (Drugs for Clinical Trials Involving Human Subjects), changes to clinical trial applications (CTA, formerly called IND) came into place. These regulations were based on best clinical practices and were intended to enable internationally competitive review timelines. The most significant changes to the regulations were a 30-day default review period for Phases I to III CTAs and a new inspection program to ensure adherence to good clinical practices. In addition, TPD established a shorter review target of seven days for bioequivalence (BE) and Phase I trials in healthy volunteers. However, this seven-day assessment target was not adopted by BGTD.[25]

HPFB also created a new organization, the HPFB Inspectorate. The Inspectorate has the mandate to manage, inspect, investigate, and monitor activities and enforce strategies related to the fabrication, packaging, labelling, testing, importation, distribution, and wholesaling of regulated health products. The number of CTA submissions in 2002 to the BGTD, by classification and quarter, are shown in Table 3.3 and to the TPD in Table 3.4.

In 2002, the TPD received 1291 CTAs, while the BGTD received 183. The number of CTAs increased after the new regulation took effect. In 2000, the TPD received approximately 600 CTAs, and the BGTD approximately 150. Similar numbers were submitted to TPD and BGTD for the first nine months of 2001.

LO5 The Pharmaceutical Industry in Canada

More than 22 000 pharmaceutical products are available in the Canadian market. In 2005, 63 new drugs were submitted for evaluation to Health Canada. Also submitted were 139 new generic drugs and 227 submissions for new uses or new formulations of existing drugs.[21] Brand-name pharmaceutical manufacturers primarily engaged in the development of innovative prescription and over-the-counter products that are used to prevent or treat illnesses in humans or animals. Brand-name drugs are products that are patentable and therefore protected from competition. Generic pharmaceutical manufacturers develop bioequivalent

Table 3.3 Clinical Trial Applications Submitted to the Biologics and Genetic Therapies Directorate, 2002

Classification	Target Review Time (days)	2002 Q1	2002 Q2	2002 Q3	2002 Q4
Phase 1, BE	Not applicable				
Phase 1, healthy humans	Not applicable				
Phase 1, healthy humans, others	30	0	2	1	1
Phase 1, other	30	5	3	7	12
Phase 2	30	15	18	11	17
Phase 3	30	20	14	17	21
Phase 1/2	30	3	0	1	1
Phase 2/3	30	2	1	1	2
Phase unassigned	30	3	2	2	1
Approvals					
No Objection Letter		37	42	28	48
Not Satisfactory Notice		5	3	4	4

Source: Boisvert, J. (2003). "The Canadian Clinical Trial Regulation Overview and Update." *GOR* Vol. 5, No. 2, Summer 2003, pp. 35–39. Retrieved December 26, 2010, from http://www.touchbriefings.com/pdf/15/ACF6EE9.pdf.

copies of brand-name drugs whose patents have expired. Pharmaceutical sales in Canada account for a 3% share of the global market, making Canada the ninth-largest world market. A 7% average annual growth over 2004–2008 makes Canada the fourth fastest-growing market globally, after Brazil, China, and Spain. Brand-name companies account for 78% of Canadian sales and 52% of volume. Generics account for the rest.[26]

From 2001 to 2012, total pharmaceutical sales in Canada approximately doubled to $21.6 billion (see Table 3.5), with 89% sold to retail drug stores and 11% sold to hospitals. Governments account for 42% of drug expenditures and private payers the remaining 58%.

Table 3.4 Clinical Trial Applications Submitted to the Therapeutic Product Directorate, 2002

Classification	Target Review Time (days)	2002 Q1	2002 Q2	2002 Q3	2002 Q4
Phase 1, BE	7	150	136	171	175
Phase 1, healthy humans	7	11	13	9	12
Phase 1, healthy humans, others	30	2	4	1	0
Phase 1, other	30	5	5	10	12
Phase 2	30	49	43	63	55
Phase 3	30	69	93	88	79
Phase 1/2	30	2	0	1	3
Phase 2/3	30	1	4	5	4
Phase unassigned	30	3	4	6	3
Approvals					
No Objection Letter		282	270	335	340
Not Satisfactory Notice		1	0	1	2
Cancelled (Withdrawn)		10	10	2	0

Source: Boisvert, J. (2003). "The Canadian Clinical Trial Regulation Overview and Update." *GOR*, Vol. 5, No. 2, Summer 2003, pp. 35–39. Retrieved December 26, 2010, from http://www.touchbriefings.com/pdf/15/ACF6EE9.pdf.

Table 3.5 Manufacturer's Sales of Patented and Nonpatented Drugs in Canada, 2001–2012

Year	Patented	Nonpatented	Total
2001	7.6	4.1	11.7
2002	8.9	4.3	13.2
2003	10.2	3.8	14.0
2004	11.0	4.2	15.2
2005	11.5	4.8	16.3
2006	11.9	5.7	17.6
2007	12.3	7.2	19.5
2008	12.6	7.8	20.4
2009	12.9	8.9	21.8
2010	12.4	9.7	22.1
2011	12.9	8.7	21.6
2012	12.8	8.8	21.6

Source: Manufacturer's Sales of Patented and Non-Patented Drugs, 2000–2009 (Table). From: Industry Canada. Canadian Pharmaceutical Industry Profile (2010). Reproduced with the permission of the Minister of Public Works and Government Services, 2014.

Cross-border Internet pharmacy sales between Canada and the United States grew swiftly from 2000 to 2003, but have since progressively declined to $103 million or 2% of total exports in 2011. The top ten pharmaceutical products sold in Canada account for 14% of 2012 industry sales. Leading therapeutic categories are neuro-therapies, cardiovascular, and gastrointestinal (see Table 3.6).

The Compendium of Pharmaceuticals and Specialties

The *Compendium of Pharmaceuticals and Specialties* (CPS) is published annually by the Canadian Pharmacists Association (CPhA) and has been providing health care professionals with a centralized source of Health Canada-approved product monographs since 1960. It contains 2500 current product monographs, including 129 drug or drug class monographs prepared by CPhA, quick reference drug information and clinical tools, directories of sources of drug and health care information, a list of discontinued products, and a comprehensive cross-referenced index of generic and brand names. The online version of the *Compendium of Pharmaceuticals and Specialties* (e-CPS) provides health care professionals with Web access to the most current Canadian drug information available.

LO6, LO7 Medicinal Marijuana Regulations

Canadian Marihuana Medical Access Regulations (MMAR)

Marijuana has not received approval as a therapeutic drug in any country. Although some evidence points to some prospective benefits, credible scientific evidence does not prove the safety and efficacy of cannabis to the extent necessary by the Food and Drug Regulations for marketed drugs in Canada. However, the Marihuana Medical Access Regulations (MMAR) provide a mechanism for patients to access

Table 3.6 Top Ten Pharmaceuticals Sold in Canada, 2012

Rank	Leading Products	Therapeutic Subclass	Total Sales ($millions)	2010 Growth (%)	Company
1	Remicade	Anti-arthritic	564.4	2.6	Schering
2	Crestor	Cholesterol reducer	411.6	1.9	AstraZeneca
3	Humira	Anti-arthritic	373.5	1.7	Nycomed
4	Enbrel	Anti-arthritic	315.8	1.4	Amgen
5	Lucentis	Ophthalmic Preps	286.4	1.4	Novartis
6	Lyrica	Neuropathic pain	235.8	1.0	Pfizer
7	Cipralex	Antidepressant	215.2	1.0	Purdue
8	Nexium	Stomach acid control	210.1	1.0	AstraZeneca
9	Advair	Asthma therapy	203.9	0.9	Abbott
10	Rituxan	Autoimmune	200.0	0.9	Roche

Source: Adapted from Industry Canada. *Canadian Pharmaceutical Industry Profile*. 2012. Retrieved June 6, 2014 from http://www.ic.gc.ca/eic/site/lsg-pdsv.nsf/eng/h_hn01703.html#sales

marijuana for medical purposes with the support of their physician.

On July 30, 2001, Health Canada implemented the MMAR, which clearly articulated the process through which access to marijuana for medical purposes was permitted. (Note that Health Canada uses the spelling *marihuana* instead of *marijuana*, which we use in this book.) Health Canada granted access to marijuana for medical use to individuals who have grave and debilitating illnesses. The MMAR dealt exclusively with the medical use of marijuana and did not address legalizing marijuana for general consumption. The Regulations contained three main components:

1. Authorizations to possess dried marijuana
2. Licences to produce marijuana, which include Personal-Use Production Licences
3. Designated-Person Production Licences and access to a supply of marijuana seeds or dried marijuana

Regulations further detailed two categories of people who could apply to possess marijuana for medical purposes:

Category 1: This category comprised any symptoms treated within the context of compassionate end-of-life care or the symptoms associated with the specified medical conditions listed in the schedule to the Regulations. These included the following:

- Severe pain or persistent muscle spasms from a spinal cord injury
- Severe pain or persistent muscle spasms from multiple sclerosis
- Severe pain or persistent muscle spasms from spinal cord disease
- Severe pain, cachexia, anorexia, weight loss, or severe nausea from cancer
- Severe pain, cachexia, anorexia, weight loss, or severe nausea from HIV/AIDS infection
- Severe pain from severe forms of arthritis
- Seizures from epilepsy

Applicants were required to provide a declaration from a physician in support of their application.

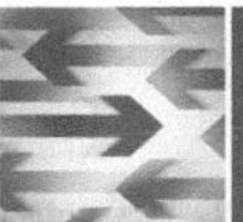

TAKING SIDES

History behind Canada's Medicinal Marijuana Access Regulations

Health Canada established the Marihuana Medical Access Program in 1999 to give Canadians with serious medical conditions access to a legal source of marijuana for medical purposes. Health Canada authorized these people to possess marijuana by giving exemptions to the Controlled Drugs and Substances Act (CDSA).

R. v. Parker (2000) was the momentous legal decision that invalidated the marijuana prohibition under the CDSA. It ruled the law prohibiting marijuana possession a violation of the Canadian Charter of Rights and Freedoms because it did not take users of medical marijuana into account. The Ontario Court of Appeal found fault with the way Health Canada used the CDSA as a means to grant exemptions.

Justice Marc Rosenberg wrote, "I have concluded that the trial judge was right in finding that Parker needs marihuana to control the symptoms of his epilepsy. I have also concluded that the prohibition on the cultivation and possession of marihuana is unconstitutional. . . . I would declare the prohibition on the possession of marihuana in the Controlled Drugs and Substances Act to be of no force and effect. However, since this would leave a gap in the regulatory scheme until Parliament could amend the legislation to comply with the Charter, I would suspend the declaration of invalidity for a year. During this period, the marihuana law remains in full force and effect." Justice Rosenberg's ruling challenged the federal government to change marijuana laws within one year to take medical users into account or risk having courts toss out charges against anyone found in possession of marijuana.

One year later, Canada became the first country with a regulatory system for medical marijuana through which Health Canada could grant any seriously ill Canadian authorization to possess or a licence to produce marijuana for personal medical use. However, the Marihuana Medical Access Regulations didn't address the issue of recreational use. In its decisions of December 23, 2003 (*R. v. Clay* and *R. v. Malmo-Levine; R. v. Caine*), the Supreme Court of Canada upheld Canada's laws against possessing small quantities of marijuana for recreational use.

Sources: *R. v. Parker*, 2000 CanLII 5762 (ON CA). Retrieved November 8, 2011, from http://canlii.ca/s/p2zn; *R. v. Clay*, 2003 SCC 75 (CanLII), [2003] 3 SCR 735. Retrieved November 8, 2011, from http://canlii.ca/s/pnwg; and *R. v. Malmo-Levine; R. v. Caine*, 2003 SCC 74 (CanLII), [2003] 3 SCR 571. Retrieved November 8, 2011, from http://canlii.ca/s/pnwk.

Category 2: This category applied to persons who had debilitating symptoms of medical conditions other than those described in Category 1. Under this category people could apply for authorization to possess dried marijuana for medical purposes if a specialist confirmed the diagnosis and conventional treatments failed or were judged inappropriate to relieve symptoms of the condition. Applications were submitted in writing to Health Canada and were required to include a declaration from a medical practitioner that supported the application.[27]

Under the MMAR authorized Canadians could choose to order marijuana from Health Canada. Through this option they could access a standardized and tested source of supply produced under contract for Health Canada. A second option was to cultivate their own marijuana or have a person designated to cultivate it for them. To cultivate their own marijuana a Personal-Use Production Licence (PUPL) was required. To have someone else grow it for them a Designated-Person Production Licence (DPPL) was needed. The number of marijuana plants a person could cultivate was based on the daily amount identified in the application. For instance, a person requiring a daily amount of 3 grams was permitted of 15 plants and a storage quantity of 675 grams of marijuana.

New Marihuana for Medical Purposes Regulations (MMPR)

Since its inception, stakeholder concerns about the Marihuana Medical Access Program (MMAP) have grown. Participants in the program expressed general dissatisfaction with the application process and that only a single strain of marijuana was available for purchase from Health Canada. Other stakeholders identified health, safety, and security issues relating to home and community-based marijuana production.[28] Included among their concerns are:

1. Potential for diversion of marijuana to illicit markets due to limited security requirements
2. Risk of violent home invasion by criminals attempting to steal marijuana
3. Creation of fire hazards resulting from faulty or overloaded electricity installations used to support marijuana cultivation

There has been a rapid expansion in the number of authorized users in the program (see Table 3.7). In 2002, 477 individuals had authorization to possess marijuana for medical purposes. By 2013, this number had grown to 29 888. By the end of 2014, it is expected that over 50 000 Canadians will have

Table 3.7 Authorizations to Possess and Licences to Produce Marijuana in Canada by Region, January 31, 2013 Compared to December 31, 2013

	Authorization to Possess		Personal-Use Production Licence		Designated-Person Production Licence	
Region	**Jan 31, 2013**	**Dec 31, 2013**	**Jan 31, 2013**	**Dec 31, 2013**	**Jan 31, 2013**	**Dec 31, 2013**
Yukon	–	–	–	–	–	–
Northwest Territories	–	–	–	–	–	–
Nunavut	–	–	–	–	–	–
Newfoundland and Labrador	87	145	31	48	–	–
Prince Edward Island	39	67	–	34	–	–
Nova Scotia	1,256	1,865	877	1,335	93	131
New Brunswick	358	571	256	436	–	–
Quebec	560	884	340	553	83	117
Ontario	5,368	8,765	3,211	5,147	427	645
Manitoba	141	430	80	268	–	67
Saskatchewan	338	680	151	278	32	58
Alberta	690	1,389	286	638	55	110
British Columbia	4,928	12,764	2,987	8,879	1,182	2,175
Totals	**13,765**	**27,560**	**8,219**	**17,616**	**1,872**	**3,303**

urce: Marihuana for Medical Purposes. Health Canada, 2014. Minister of Public Works and Government Services Canada, 2014.

received authorization to possess marijuana for medical purposes.

Under the new Marihuana for Medical Purposes Regulations (MMPR), Health Canada will no longer issue authorizations to possess marijuana for medical purposes. Persons who require marijuana for medical purposes will be able to legally possess dried marijuana if it was obtained from a pharmacist or licensed producer. Supporting medical documentation from an authorized health care practitioner is required. This change in the regulations is expected to:

- Make accessing marijuana for medical purposes more efficient for individuals,
- Give individuals more options with regards to obtaining the support of an authorized health care practitioner,
- Increase access to more choices of strains and suppliers, and
- Provide increased access to quality-controlled marijuana.

Individuals will no longer be licensed to produce marijuana. This will address the public health, safety, and security concerns raised by stakeholders. The MMPR will authorize three key activities:

- The possession of dried marijuana for medical purposes by individuals who have the support of an authorized health care practitioner;
- The production of dried marijuana by licensed producers; and
- The sale and distribution of dried marijuana by licensed producers and hospitals to individuals who can possess it.

As described above, objectives of the new MMPR aim to reduce risks to the health, security, and safety of Canadians. Proponents of the MMPR believe that one way to accomplish this is through the creation of a supply and distribution system for dried marijuana that relies on commercial and not home-based production. In this way security requirements can be defined and monitored for both production sites and key personnel of licensed producers. Under the new regulations, licensed producers become subject to regulatory requirements pertaining to security; good production practices; packaging, labelling, and shipping; record keeping and reporting; and distribution. To ensure public health, safety, and security production facilities will be subject to Health Canada inspections. In line with other controlled substances, personal and designated production will be phased out. All existing Authorizations to Possess (ATP), Personal-Use Production Licences (PUPL), or Designated-Person Production Licences (DPPL) will expire. Health Canada will no longer sell and distribute marijuana for medical purposes, and PUPL and DPPL holders

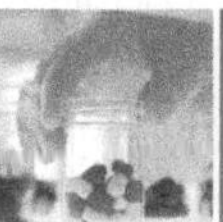

DRUGS IN THE MEDIA

Federal Court Reverses Ban on Grow-Your-Own Medical Marijuana

OTTAWA—A Federal Court judge in Vancouver issued an injunction Friday against the government's plans to end the practice of grow-your-own medical marijuana.

The order gave a coalition of people who use the drug for medicinal purposes an exemption from new Health Canada rules, which were set to eliminate 30,000 licences for home-grown pot on April 1 and force patients to buy what the feds say would be "quality-controlled" marijuana from approved commercial producers. "I am very stressed about the plan to take away my ability to produce my medicine," plaintiff Neil Allard said in his affidavit.

RCMP officer Shane Holmquist said in his sworn statement the current system is rife with crime. Holmquist testified that licence holders "are known to transport shipments of marijuana for sale under the guise of their authorized possession amount."

Health Minister Rona Ambrose said she's disappointed with the Federal Court's ruling. The marijuana access program has had "significant unintended consequences on public health, safety and security," including the risks of home invasion, fires and toxic mould for those growing the plant at home, their neighbours and community, the agency said in a statement late Friday. "Health Canada will review the decision in detail and consider its options."

Source: Daniel Proussalidis, Toronto Sun, March 21, 2014. Retrieved June 2, 2014, from http://www.torontosun.com/2014/03/21/federal-court-reverses-ban-on-grow-your-own-medical-marijuana *Copyright held by Sun Media Corporation.*

will be required to responsibly dispose of all dried marijuana and marijuana plants. This will reduce the health and safety risks to individuals and to the public while allowing for a quality-controlled and more secure product for medical use.

The process by which individuals access marijuana for medical purposes will also be improved. Individuals will no longer be required to apply to Health Canada but will be able to obtain marijuana with information similar to a prescription from an authorized health care practitioner (e.g., a physician or, potentially, a nurse practitioner, where supporting access to marijuana for medical purposes is included under their scope of practice or in legislation).

LO8 Natural Health Products

According to the Food and Drugs Act and Regulations, any substance "manufactured, sold or represented for use in the diagnosis, treatment, mitigation or prevention of a disease, disorder or abnormal physical state, or its symptoms, in human beings or animals" is a drug. Foods are defined as any article manufactured, sold, or represented for use as food or drink for human beings.

In the 1990s, officials at Health Canada became concerned with a rapidly growing market in natural health products (NHPs). The term NHP was used to represent a variety of substances that were being formulated, packaged, and/or promoted in a manner similar to drugs but that were classified and regulated as foods. These substances include vitamins and mineral supplements, herbal remedies (herb- and plant-based remedies), homeopathic medicines, traditional medicines such as traditional Chinese and Ayurvedic medicines, probiotics, amino acids, and essential fatty acids. Growth in the public awareness and demand for these products had been fuelled by a number of factors, including (1) an increased interest in foods that could be used in prevention and as a treatment of illness, (2) a growing belief that NHPs were better than conventional (chemical) drugs, and (3) the emergence of aggressive multi-level marketing organizations that became distributors of purported natural cures and preventions.

Health Canada's concerns lay in that fact that these natural products, while being promoted as therapeutic, were classified as foods. Recall from earlier in this chapter that drug manufacturers have to demonstrate, before marketing a drug, that it is (1) *safe* when used as intended, and (2) *effective* for its intended use. However, with foods Health Canada is concerned only with ensuring their purity and safety, not their efficacy. As such, when classified as foods, the manufacturers of NHPs had to provide evidence that the product was pure and safe, but they were not required to provide proof of any health claims made. Furthermore, because these NHPs were not considered drugs, the manufacturers were exempt from providing information on potential contraindications, side effects, or toxicities associated with the use of their products.

To address these concerns the Government of Canada established a regulatory authority, the Natural Health Products Directorate (NHPD). Beginning in January 2004 all natural products with associated claims of health benefits became subject to the regulations of the NHPD. A comprehensive discussion pertaining to the evolution and specifics of NHP regulation and use in Canada is provided in Chapter 12.

Summary

- Up until 1908, no regulations were established federally or provincially governing the use of drugs in Canada. The 1908 Opium Act made it an indictable offence to import, manufacture, offer to sell, sell, or possess to sell opium for non-medical purposes.
- Following the establishment of a federal Department of Health in 1919, the Food and Drugs Act was introduced in 1920. By the late 1920s, regula[illegible]ns developed under the Act established specific [illegible]irements for licensing drugs.
- The 1961 Narcotic Control Act focused on the criminalization of drugs because of the strongly held belief that certain drugs had the ability to enslave users.
- In 1969, the Le Dain Commission studied the illicit drug issue in Canada. It recommended greater leniency for the crime of possession, including the abolishment of imprisonment.
- Canada's first federal drug strategy was introduced in 1987 under the title National Drug Strategy. Parliament approved Canada's Drug Strategy in 1992, which tried to speak to both the demand for drugs and their supply through such actions

as control and enforcement, prevention, treatment and rehabilitation, and harm reduction. Canada's Drug Strategy was renewed in 2003 to address the core factors linked with substance use and abuse and included education, prevention, and health promotion initiatives as well as enhanced enforcement measures.

- In 2007 the Government of Canada introduced its National Anti-Drug Strategy with the goal of reducing the supply and demand for illicit drugs. The three key priorities of the Strategy are to prevent illicit drug use, treat illicit drug addiction, and combat illicit drug production and distribution.
- The Controlled Drugs and Substances Act replaced the Narcotic Control Act and Parts III and IV of the Food and Drugs Act on May 14, 1997. Controlled substances are placed on one of seven schedules.
- Bill S-10 received Royal Assent and became law in March 2013. This Bill amends the Controlled Drugs and Substances Act (CDSA) to provide for minimum penalties for serious drug offences, such as dealing drugs for organized crime purposes or when a weapon or violence is involved.
- The Food and Drugs Act and Regulations authorizes Health Canada to regulate the safety, efficacy, and quality of pharmaceutical drugs, vitamins, vaccines, and medical devices sold in Canada.
- If clinical trial results indicate that a new drug has potential therapeutic value that outweighs its risks, a drug manufacturer may seek authorization to sell the product by filing a New Drug Submission (NDS) with Health Canada's Health Products and Food Branch (HPFB). If the HPFB review process concludes that the benefits of a drug outweigh the risks, the product is issued a Notice of Compliance (NOC) letter and a Drug Identification Number (DIN), which allows the manufacturer to sell the product in Canada. All drugs marketed in Canada must have a DIN.
- On September 1, 2001, amendments to the Food and Drug Regulations (Drugs for Clinical Trials Involving Human Subjects) were introduced.
- More than 22 000 pharmaceutical products are available on the Canadian market. From 2000 to 2009 total Canadian pharmaceutical sales doubled to $21 billion, with 88% sold to retail drug stores and 12% sold to hospitals.
- In July 2001 Health Canada implemented the Marihuana Medical Access Regulations (MMAR), which clearly articulated the process in which access to marijuana for medical purposes was permitted. Health Canada granted access to marijuana for medical use to individuals who have grave and debilitating illnesses. The MMAR dealt exclusively with the medical use of marijuana and did not address legalizing marijuana for general consumption.
- In March 2014 the MMAR will be repealed and the Marijuana Medical Access Program (MMAP) ends. All Authorizations to Possess (ATP), Personal-Use Production Licences (PUPL), or Designated-Person Production Licences (DPPL) expire. In April 2014, Health Canada will no longer sell and distribute marijuana for medical purposes. Personal and designated production is no longer permitted. All PUPL or DPPL holders must safely dispose of all dried marijuana and marijuana plants. The only legal source to obtain marijuana for medical purposes for Canadians is from licensed producers under the new regime.
- The new Marihuana for Medical Purposes Regulations (MMPR) will try to treat dried marihuana like other narcotics used for medical purposes by creating a licensing scheme for its commercial production and distribution for medical purposes.
- Natural health products (NHPs) include vitamins and minerals; herbal remedies; homeopathic medicines; traditional medicines; probiotics; and other products such as amino acids and essential fatty acids. The Government of Canada established a regulatory authority, the Natural Health Products Directorate (NHPD), and beginning in January 2004 all natural products with associated claims of health benefits became subject to its regulations.

Review Questions

1. What type of drug use contributed significantly to the creation of the Opium Act of 1908?
2. Has the creation of Canada's drug regulations been based on protecting the health of the population, political agenda, enforcement concerns, or all three?
3. Is marijuana legal in Canada because there is access to it for medical reasons?
4. What are the symptoms or medical conditions listed in Category 1 and Category 2 under which a person can apply to possess marijuana for medicinal reasons?
5. What role does Health Canada's Health Products and Food Branch (HPFB) play in regulating pharmaceuticals?

6. What three phases of clinical drug testing are required before a new drug application can be approved?
7. What historic piece of federal legislation did the most to shape our overall approach to the control of habit-forming drugs in Canada?
8. What are drug paraphernalia laws, and why have they been subject to court challenges?
9. What products are included in the National Health Product Regulations?

SECTION 2

CHAPTER 4

The Nervous System

How do drugs interact with the brain and the nervous system?

CHAPTER 5

The Actions of Drugs

How do drugs move in the body, and what are the general principles of drug action?

HOW DRUGS WORK

A drug is nothing but a chemical substance until it comes into contact with a living organism. In fact, that's what defines the difference between drugs and other chemicals: drugs have specific effects on living tissue.

Because this book is about psychoactive drugs, the tissue we're most interested in is the brain. We want to understand how psychoactive drugs interact with brain tissue to produce effects on behaviour, thoughts, and emotions.

Obviously, we don't put drugs directly into our brains; usually we swallow them, inhale them, or inject them. In Section 2, we will find out how the drugs we take get to the brain and what effects they might have on the other tissues of the body.

CHAPTER 4

THE NERVOUS SYSTEM

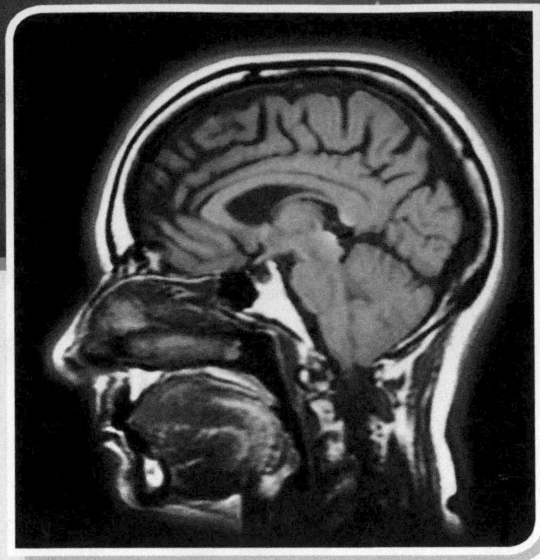

OBJECTIVES

When you have finished this chapter, you should be able to

- **LO1** Explain the concept of homeostasis.
- **LO2** List the general properties of glia and neurons.
- **LO3** Describe the action potential.
- **LO4** Describe the roles of the sympathetic and parasympathetic branches of the autonomic nervous system and associated neurotransmitters.
- **LO5** Match the major functions of the neurotransmitters with key brain structures and chemical pathways.
- **LO6** Describe the role of dopamine in Parkinson's disease.
- **LO7** Describe the life cycle of a neurotransmitter molecule.
- **LO8** Recognize the importance of receptor types in determining the action of a neurotransmitter at a particular site in the brain.
- **LO9** Describe brain imaging techniques.

Drugs are psychoactive, for the most part, because they alter ongoing functions in the brain. To understand how drugs influence behaviour and psychological processes, it is necessary to have some knowledge of the normal functioning of the brain and other parts of the nervous system and then to see how drugs can alter those normal functions.

LO1 Homeostasis

Psychoactive drugs can also influence homeostasis. **Homeostasis** can be loosely translated as "staying the same," and it describes the fact that many biological factors are maintained at or near certain levels. For example, most of the biochemical reactions basic to the maintenance of life are temperature dependent in that these reactions occur optimally at temperatures near 37° C. Because we cannot live at temperatures too much above or below this level, our bodies have many mechanisms to either raise or lower temperature: perspiring, shivering, altering blood flow to the skin, and others. Similar homeostatic mechanisms regulate the acidity, water content, and sodium content of the blood; glucose concentrations; and other physical and chemical factors that are important for biological functioning. Alcohol inhibits the release of the antidiuretic hormone vasopressin, which causes an increase in the excretion of urine. Two important lines of evidence suggest that homeostatic processes mobilize to counteract some alcohol-related effects: (1) following consumption of an alcoholic beverage, heavy drinkers have less urine output than do infrequent drinkers; and (2) during alcohol withdrawal, heavy drinkers exhibit an increased vasopressin release, resulting in greater water retention.[1] The goal of this chapter is not to turn you into a neuroscientist. Rather, the goal is to introduce basic concepts and terminology that will help you understand the effects of psychoactive drugs on the brain and on behaviour. The knowledge acquired in this chapter should also make you aware of the limitations of applying an exclusively biological approach to the study of psychoactive drug effects.

homeostasis: maintenance of an environment of body ...s within a certain range (e.g., temperature, blood

LO2 Components of the Nervous System

Although we often speak of the nervous system, several communication and control systems use nerve cells and chemical signals. Before discussing distinctions between these systems, we will describe the major components common to the entire nervous system.

Glia

The nervous system is composed of two types of cells: (1) glial cells, often referred to as glia (see Figure 4.1), and (2) nerve cells, often referred to as neurons. The nervous system has been reported to have 10 to 50 times as many glia as neurons (see Box 4.1). Historically, neurobiology dogma purported that glia lacked information-processing capabilities (i.e., they could not communicate with other cells). Recent evidence, however, demonstrates that glia not only communicate with one another but also communicate with neurons and modulate their activity.[2] Astrocytes, large, star-shaped cells found in the brain, like most glial cells, were long considered essential for their role in supporting and maintaining nerve tissue. For instance, it has long been known that astrocytes supply glucose needed for nerve activity. Glucose enters through the end feet of the astrocyte where the glucose is partially metabolized and sent to the neuron. More intense synaptic activity, it seems, promotes a better supply of glucose by activating this astrocytic metabolism. It is also known that astrocytes are connected with each other via *gap junctions*, through which they can pass various metabolites. It is through these junctions that astrocytes evacuate to the capillaries the excess extracellular potassium generated by intense neuronal activity. But what has been discovered is that this network of intercommunicating astrocytes forms a network that behaves like a single unitary entity. This network of astrocytes plays a major role in modulating neuronal activities.[3]

The details of glia-related information-processing capabilities are still being worked out, and many

Figure 4.1 Glial Cells

Glial cells have been reported to outnumber neurons at least 10 to 1. This was a "biased" histological result from half a century ago—modern techniques using "unbiased stereological methods" put the ratio at 2:1, or 3:1 at best (see Box 4.1). The main function of the five different types of glia cells is to support the neurons in place and provide insulation. Specifically, astrocytes provide physical and nutritional support for neurons, remove the debris of dead neurons (as do microglia), and regulate the extracellular fluid around the neuron. Oligodendroglia and Schwann cells (not shown) myelinate the neurons in the central nervous system (CNS) and peripheral nervous system (PNS) (see discussions of CNS and PNS later in this chapter), while satellite cells (not shown) provide physical support for neurons in the PNS.

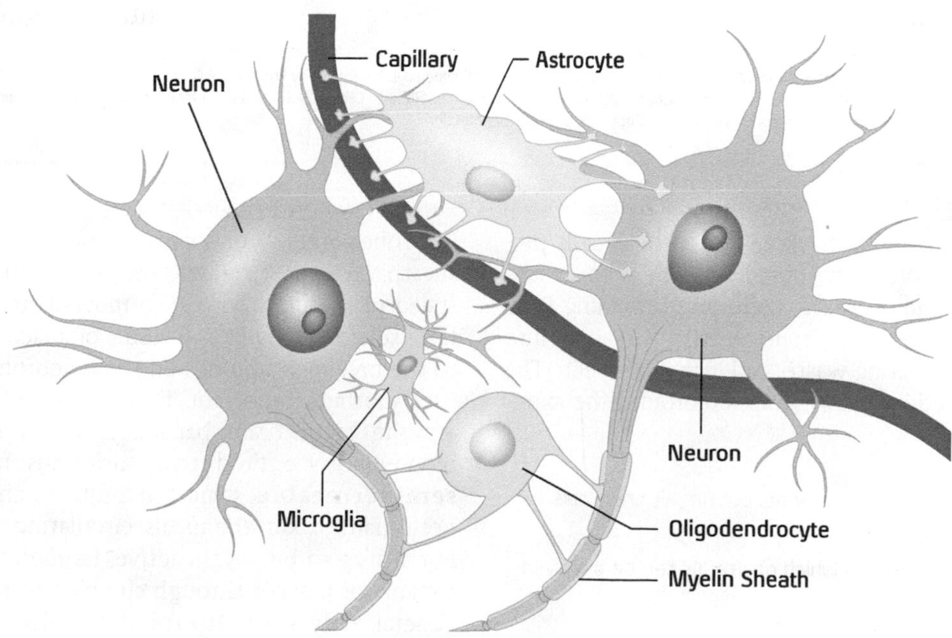

BOX 4.1

Glia to Neuron Ratio

The idea that glia "outnumber neurons by as much as 50 to one," from Eric Kandel's widely used textbook *The Principles of Neural Science,* has recently been challenged. The statement has been echoed not only in previous versions of this textbook but by other sources in the popular press. To date, we could not find a single published study that directly supports a 10:1 glia to neuron ratio in the whole human brain. There are areas where it approaches or surpasses a 10:1 ratio (e.g., 17:1 in the thalamus has been reported) in a specific area, and other areas such as the cerebellum have been reported to have more neurons than glia (4.3 neurons for every glia in this region). Why do we care? The 10:1 glia to neuron ratio may be a myth, and the ratio in human and other primate brains may be much closer to 2:1. The glia to neuron ratio may be one of the least important questions you can ask about the brain. Whatever the true glia to neuron ratio, functionally the glia are the brain's other half.[4–9]

Figure 4.2 Whole Brain

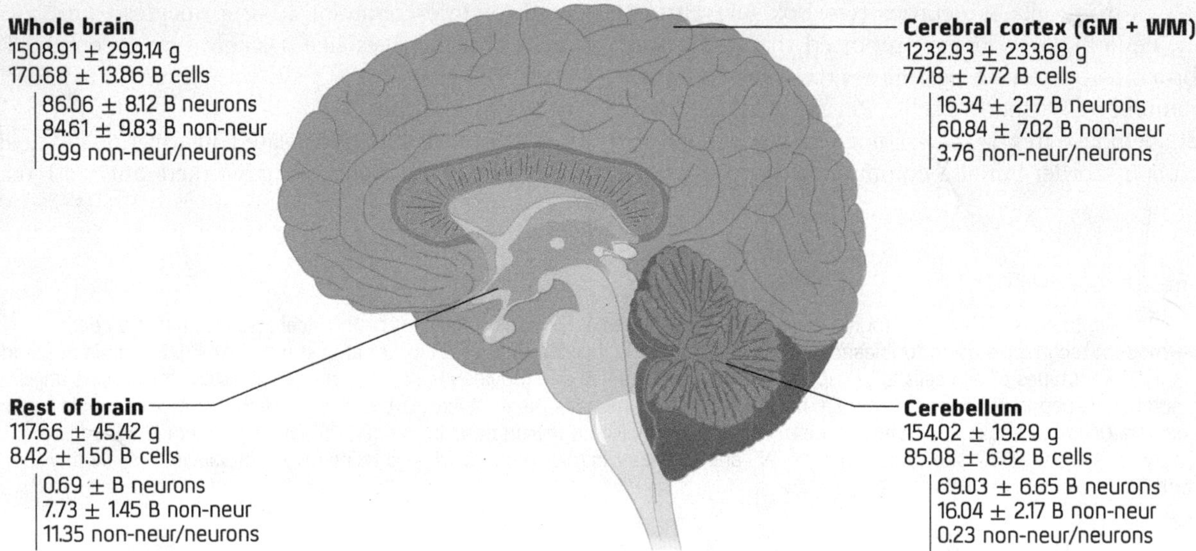

Source: Republished with permission of John Wiley and Sons Inc., from *The Journal of Comparative Neurology,* by Frederico A.C. Azevedo, Ludmila R.B. Carvalho, Lea T. Grinberg, José Marcelo Farfel, Renata E.L. Ferretti, Renata E.P. Leite, Wilson Jacob Filho, Roberto Lent, and Suzana Herculano-Houzel, Volume 513, Issue 5, pages 532–541, 10 April 2009; permission conveyed through Copyright Clearance Center, Inc.

questions remain. What is clear is that these cells provide several important functions that help to ensure the survival of the organism, including providing firmness and structure to the brain, getting nutrients into the system, eliminating waste, and forming myelin. The myelin produced by glia is wrapped around the axons (described below) of some neurons to form a myelin sheath, which increases the information-processing speed of these neurons. The movement disorder multiple sclerosis occurs as a result of a lack of or damage to the myelin wrappings on some neurons.

Another important function of glia is to create the blood-brain barrier, a barrier between the blood and the fluid that surrounds neurons. This **semipermeable** structure protects the brain from potentially toxic chemicals circulating in the blood. For a drug to be psychoactive, its molecules must be capable of passing through the blood-brain barrier. In general, only small **lipophilic** molecules enter the

semipermeable: allowing some, but not all, chemicals to pass.

lic: the extent to which chemicals can be dissolved
d fats.

brain. This feature has important implications for the effects of some psychoactive drugs on the brain, and ultimately on behaviour. Take, for example, the opioid drugs morphine and heroin. Heroin (also known as diacetylmorphine) was synthesized by adding two acetyl groups to the morphine chemical. This slight modification of the morphine structure made the new chemical more lipophilic, thereby facilitating its movement across the **blood-brain barrier** and into the brain. As a result, heroin has a more rapid onset of effects and is about three times as potent as morphine.

Neurons

Neurons are the primary elements of the nervous system responsible for analyzing and transmitting information. In other words, everything that we see and understand as behaviour is dependent on the functioning of these cells. The nervous system contains more than 100 billion neurons, and each can influence or be influenced by hundreds of other glia and neurons. Before we can understand how neurons produce behaviour, we must first become familiar with a few basic facts about neurons. Although neurons come in a variety of shapes and sizes, they all have four morphologically defined regions: a cell body, dendrites, an axon, and presynaptic terminals (see Figure 4.3). Each of these regions contributes to the neuron's ability to communicate with other neurons, and psychoactive drugs can exert effects within each of these regions. The cell body contains the nucleus and other substances that sustain the neuron.

The dendrites are treelike features extending from the cell body and contain within their membranes the specialized structures (**receptors**) that recognize and respond to specific chemicals' signals. (Some receptors are also found on cell regions other than dendrites.) Stimulation of specific receptors by psychoactive drugs can either activate or inhibit the neuron, depending on the type of receptor. The long, slender axon extends from the cell body and is responsible for conducting the electrical signal (action potential, described below) to the presynaptic terminals. Finally, the presynaptic terminals are the bulbous structures located at the end of the axon, where chemical messengers (neurotransmitters) are stored in small, round packages called vesicles. Psychoactive drugs can affect neurotransmission. Large doses of amphetamines, for example, can destroy axons and presynaptic terminals.

LO3 Neurotransmission

Have you ever wondered how local anaesthetics, such as those dentists use, can block the perception of pain? After a brief discussion of the basic concepts of

blood–brain barrier: structure that prevents many drugs from entering the brain.

receptors: recognition proteins that respond to specific chemical signals.

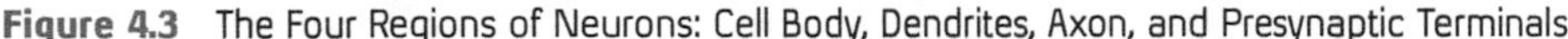

Figure 4.3 The Four Regions of Neurons: Cell Body, Dendrites, Axon, and Presynaptic Terminals

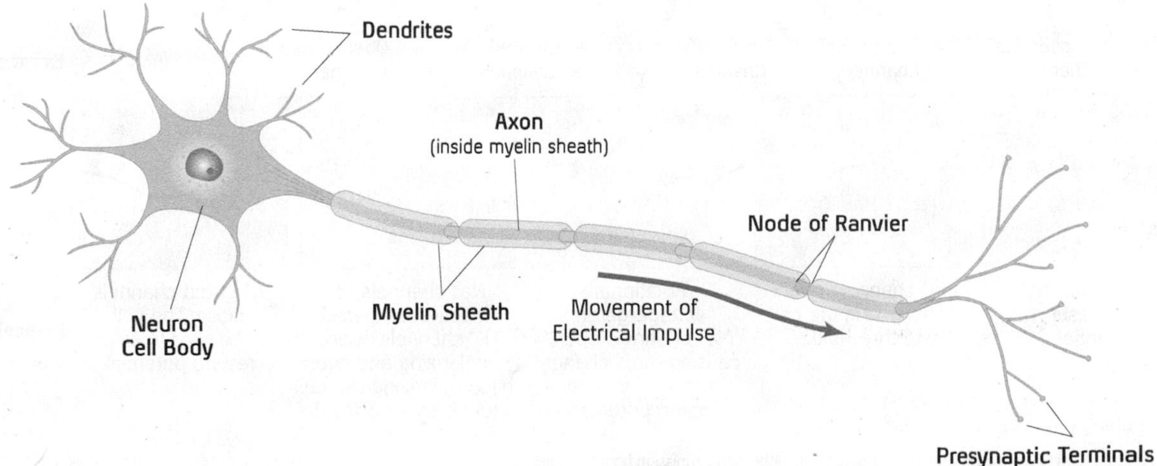

neurotransmission, you will be better able to understand how local anaesthetics and other drugs work to alter perception, mood, and behaviour.

Action Potential

The production of even simple behavioural acts requires complex interactions between the individual's environment and nerve cells. Here we focus on only one element of this complex interaction–the communication between neurons. Such communication is accomplished through a highly specialized, precise, and rapid method. An essential process for neuronal communication is the **action potential** (see Figure 4.4). This electrical signal initiates a chain of events that allows one neuron to communicate with another through the release of **neurotransmitters**. The action potential occurs as a result of opening ion channels (pores in the membrane) that allow electrically charged particles (ions) access to the inside of the cell. This change moves the cell's membrane away from its resting potential (about −65 mV to −70 mV) to a more positively charged voltage. When the cell membrane is at rest, it has an uneven distribution of ions between the inside (intracellular) and outside (extracellular) of the cell. Specifically, more potassium (K^+) ions and negatively charged organic anions are on the inside of the cell, while more sodium (Na^+) and chloride (Cl^-) ions are on the outside of the cell. This uneven distribution of ions is the source of the negative resting potential across the membrane. In this state, the neuron is **polarized**. **Hyperpolarization** refers to the

action potential: the electrical signal transmitted along the axon when a neuron fires.

neurotransmitters: chemical messengers released from neurons and having brief, local effects.

polarized: when the membrane potential is more negative.

hyperpolarization: occurs when the membrane potential is pushed below the resting potential.

Figure 4.4 Action Potential

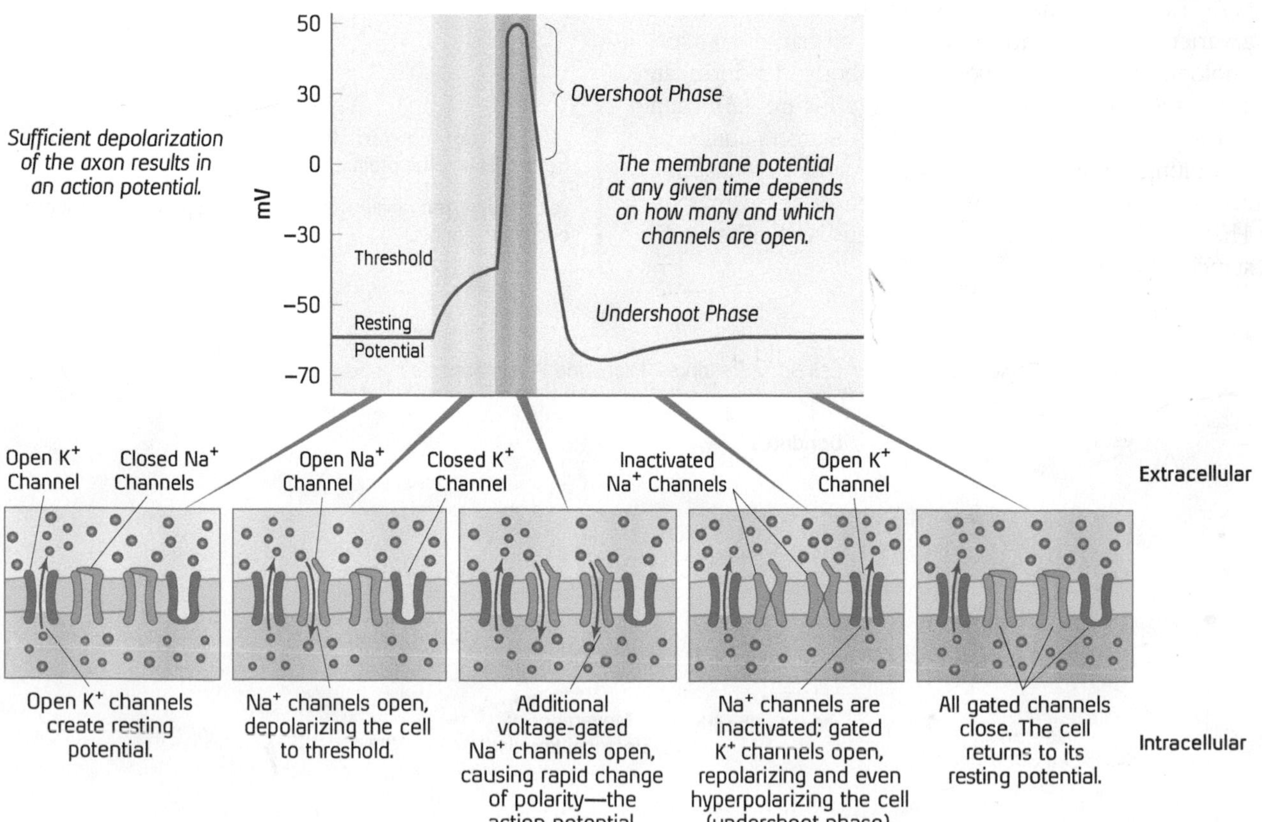

Source: Adapted from Rosenzweig, Leiman, and Breedlove, 1999, with permission from the publishers.

state that occurs when the membrane potential of a cell is pushed below the resting potential.

The action potential occurs when the neuron's membrane is **depolarized** to the threshold of excitation, during which time Na^+ channels open, allowing Na^+ ions to move across the membrane intracellularly and further depolarize adjacent regions of the neuron. Consequently, K^+ channels begin to open, allowing K^+ to leave the neuron to the extracellular space. It was once thought that these events allowed for propagation of an "all-or-none" action potential signal. The action potential was referred to as *all or none* because, once initiated, it was thought to travel without decrement to the end of the axon in the presynaptic terminals, where it will ultimately cause the release of a neurotransmitter. Recent evidence, however,[10] reveals that action potentials (1) are not all or none and (2) do not travel undiminished in height from one end of the axon to the other under all circumstances. The explanations are interesting and elegant.

Following the action potential, Na^+ channels and K^+ channels close. With the help of the sodium potassium pump (Na^+/K^+-ATPase), Na^+ and K^+ ions are returned to their original distribution inside (K^+) and outside (Na^+) the cell, and the neuron returns to its resting potential.

Suppose we selectively blocked Na^+ channels. What would be the effect? Selective blockade of Na^+ channels prevents the action potential and thus disrupts communication between neurons. Selective blockade of Na^+ channels is the mechanism through which drugs, such as cocaine and novocaine, reduce pain. Although many local anaesthetics are used in clinical practice today, cocaine was the first. More recent local anaesthetics are simple modifications of the cocaine molecule. In the case of novocaine, the chemical alteration of the cocaine structure yielded a compound that does not readily cross the blood-brain barrier (i.e., it does not produce cocaine-like psychoactive effects).

LO4 The Peripheral Nervous System

The **peripheral nervous system** (PNS) is made up of the nerves outside the brain and spinal cord and consists of the somatic and autonomic nervous system.

Somatic Nervous System

The nerve cells that are on the "front lines," interacting with the external environment, are referred to as the **somatic system**. These peripheral nerves carry sensory information into the central nervous system and carry motor (movement) information back out. The cranial nerves that relate to vision, hearing, taste, smell, chewing, and movements of the tongue and face are included, as are spinal nerves carrying information from the skin and joints and controlling movements of the arms and legs. We think of this system as serving voluntary actions. For example, a decision to move your leg results in activity in large cells in the motor cortex of your brain. These cells have long axons, which extend down to the spinal motor neurons. These neurons also have long axons, which are bundled together to form nerves and travel out directly to the muscles. The neurotransmitter at **neuromuscular junctions** in the somatic nerve system is **acetylcholine**, which acts on receptors that excite the muscle.

Autonomic Nervous System

Your body's internal environment is monitored and controlled by the **autonomic** nervous system (ANS), which regulates the visceral, or involuntary, functions of the body, such as heart rate and blood pressure. Many psychoactive drugs have simultaneous effects in the brain and on the ANS. The ANS is also where chemical neurotransmission was first studied. If the vagus nerve in a frog is electrically stimulated, its heart slows. If the fluid surrounding that heart is then withdrawn and placed around a second frog's heart, it too will slow. This is an indication that electrical activity in the vagus nerve causes a chemical to be released onto the frog's heart muscle. When Otto von Loewi first demonstrated this phenomenon in 1921, he named the unknown chemical "vagusstoffe." We now know that

depolarized: when the membrane potential is less negative than resting potential.

peripheral nervous system: a division of the nervous system containing all the nerves that lie outside the brain and spinal cord.

somatic system: nerve cells that interact with the external environment to carry sensory information into the central nervous system and carry motor (movement) information back out.

neuromuscular junction: the synapse between a muscle and a neuron.

acetylcholine: neurotransmitter found in the parasympathetic branch in the cerebral cortex.

autonomic: the part of the nervous system that controls "involuntary" functions, such as heart rate.

this is acetylcholine, the same chemical that stimulates muscle contraction in our arms and legs. Because a different type of receptor is found in the heart, acetylcholine inhibits heart muscle contraction.

The ANS is divided into **sympathetic** and **parasympathetic** branches. The inhibition of heart rate by the vagus nerve is an example of the parasympathetic branch; acetylcholine is the neurotransmitter at the end organ. In the sympathetic branch, norepinephrine is the neurotransmitter at the end organ. Norepinephrine increases heart rate. Table 4.1 gives examples of parasympathetic and sympathetic influences on various systems. Note that often, but not always, the two systems oppose each other.

Because the sympathetic system is interconnected, it tends to act more as a unit, to open the bronchi, reduce blood supply to the skin, increase the heart rate, and reduce stomach motility. This has been called the "fight-or-flight" response and is elicited in many emotion-arousing circumstances in humans and other animals. Amphetamines, because they have a chemical structure that resembles norepinephrine, stimulate these functions in addition to their effects on the brain. Those drugs that activate the sympathetic branch are referred to as sympathomimetic drugs.

sympathetic: the branch of the autonomic system involved in flight or fight reactions.

parasympathetic: the branch of the autonomic system that stimulates digestion, slows the heart, and has other effects associated with a relaxed physiological state.

central nervous system (CNS): the neurons and pathways of the brain and spinal cord.

basal ganglia: subcortical brain structures controlling muscle tone.

Central Nervous System

The **central nervous system (CNS)** consists of the brain and spinal cord. These two structures form a central mass of nervous tissue, with sensory nerves coming in and motor nerves going out. This is where most of the integration of information, learning, and memory and the coordination of activity occur.

LO5, LO6 The Brain

Knowing about a few of the major brain structures makes it easier to understand some of the effects of psychoactive drugs.

Major Structures

When looking at the brain of most mammals, and especially of a human, much of what we can see consists of cerebral cortex (also referred to as the cerebrum), a layer of tissue that covers the top and sides of the upper parts of the brain (see Figure 4.5 and Figure 4.6). Some areas of the cortex are known to be involved in processing visual information; other areas are involved in processing auditory or somatosensory information. Relatively smaller cortical areas are involved in the control of muscles (motor cortex), and large areas are referred to as association areas. Higher mental processes, such as reasoning and language, occur in the cerebral cortex. In an alert, awake individual, arousal mechanisms keep the cerebral cortex active. When a person is asleep or under the influence of sedating drugs, the cerebral cortex is much less active, whereas other parts of the brain might be equally active whether a person is awake or asleep.

Underneath the cerebral cortex on each side of the brain and hidden from external view are the **basal ganglia**, comprising three primary components: the

Table 4.1 Sympathetic and Parasympathetic Effects on Selected Structures

Structure or Function	Sympathetic Reaction	Parasympathetic Reaction
Pupil	Dilation	Constriction
Heart rate	Increase	Decrease
Breathing rate	Fast and shallow	Slow and deep
Stomach and intestinal glands	Inhibition	Activation
Stomach and intestinal wall	No motility	Motility
Sweat glands	Secretion	No effect
Skin blood vessels	Constriction	Dilation
Bronchi	Relaxation	Constriction

Figure 4.5 Major Subdivisions of the Human Cerebral Cortex

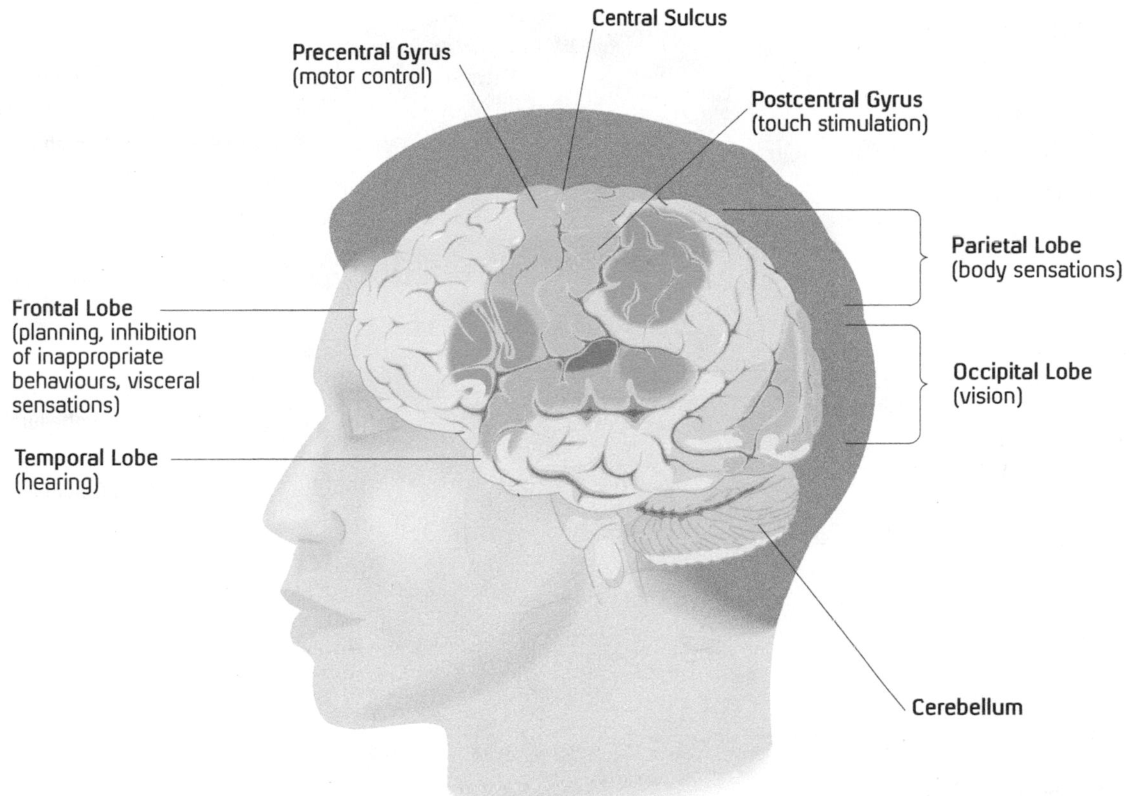

caudate nucleus, the putamen, and the globus pallidus (see Figure 4.7). The basal ganglia are important for the maintenance of proper muscle tone. For example, when you are standing still in a relaxed posture, your leg muscles are not totally relaxed. If they were, you would fall down in a slump. Instead, you remain standing,

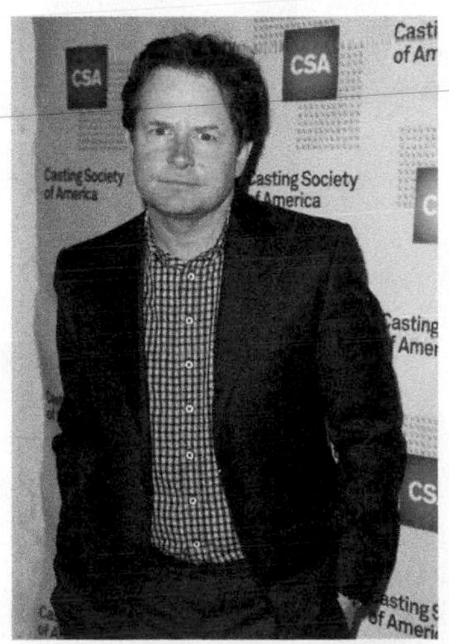

Canadian-born actor Michael J. Fox was diagnosed with Parkinson's disease in 1991. He has since become an activist for research toward finding a cure. He established the Michael J. Fox Foundation for Parkinson's Research and played an early role in supporting work in stem cell research for Parkinson's disease.

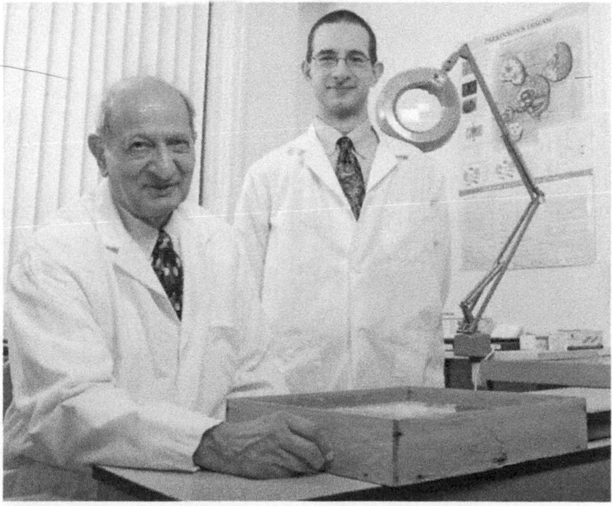

Neurologists Dr. Ali Rajput and Dr. Alex Rajput have dedicated their work at Royal University Hospital to the treatment and understanding of Parkinson's disease and other neurological movement disorders. The endowment for this important research was created in 2008 with a $1 million gift from an anonymous donor.

Figure 4.6 Cross-Section of the Brain: Major Structures

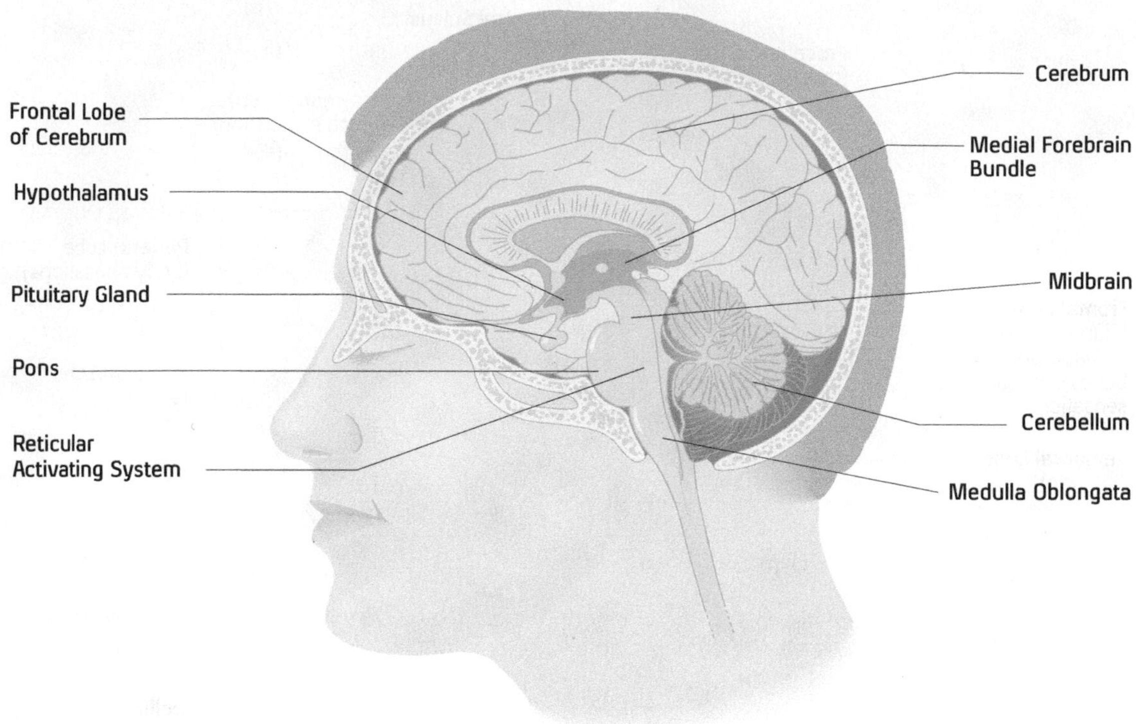

Figure 4.7 The Basal Ganglia

The basal ganglia, as the name suggests, consist of tightly interconnected clusters of neuronal cell bodies buried deep within the brain. The caudate nucleus, the putamen, and the globus pallidus are the main structures. The basal ganglia receive information from different regions of the cortex and, once processed, return this information to the motor cortex via the thalamus.

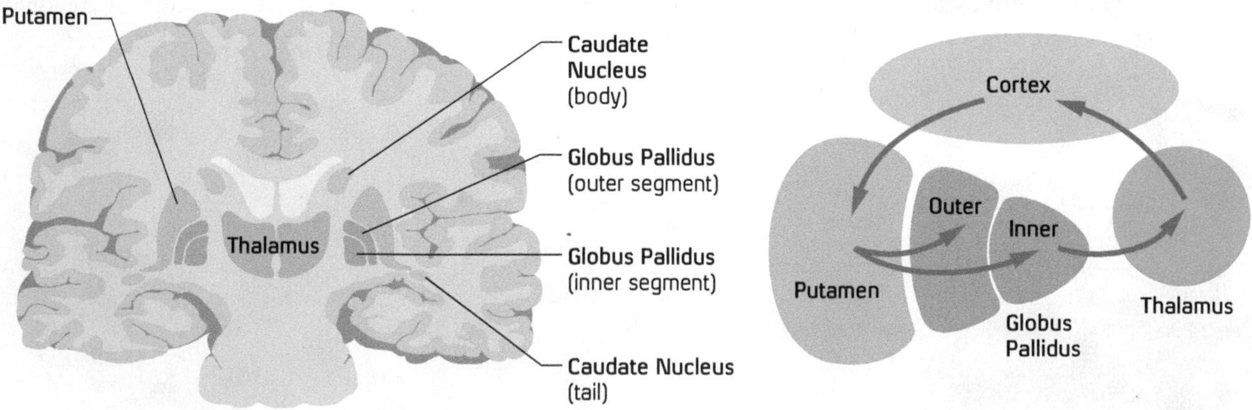

partly because of a certain level of muscular tension, or tone, that is maintained by the output of the basal ganglia. Too much output from these structures results in muscular rigidity in the arms, legs, and facial muscles. This can occur if **Parkinson's disease** damages the basal ganglia or as a side-effect of some psychoactive drugs that act on the basal ganglia.

Parkinson's disease: degenerative neurological disease involving damage to dopamine neurons in the basal ganglia.

The hypothalamus is a small structure near the base of the brain just above the pituitary gland (see Figure 4.6). The hypothalamus is an important link between the brain and the hormonal output of the

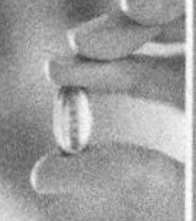

DRUGS IN DEPTH

Drug-Induced Parkinson's Disease

The drug 1-methyl-4-phenyl-1,2,3,6-tetrahydropyridine (MPTP), a potential by-product of illicitly produced opioids, causes neuronal death through inhibition of certain components located in the cell body. The conversion of MPTP, a potent neurotoxin that destroys nigrostriatal dopamine neurons (the nigrostriatal dopamine system is described later), resulting in irreversible idiopathic parkinsonism, to 1-methyl-4-phenylpyridine (MPP^+) is responsible for the generation of its neurotoxicity. Takada and colleagues at the University of Toronto report that this metabolism is mediated by the action of the enzyme monoamine oxidase B, which in the substantia nigra pars is localized specifically in astroglia. When rats were administered an astroglia-specific toxin, named l-α-aminoadipic acid (l-α-AA) and resulting in selective astroglial ablation, MPTP-induced nigrostriatal neuronal death in the rat was averted. These data provide clear morphological evidence for the critical importance of the presence of astroglia in the onset of MPTP neurotoxicity.[11]

Source: Takada, M., Z. K. Li, and T. Hattori. "Astroglial Ablation Prevents MPTP-Induced Nigrostriatal Neuronal Death." *Brain Research* 509, no. 1 (1990), pp. 55-61.

pituitary and is thus involved in feeding, drinking, temperature regulation, and sexual behaviour.

The limbic system consists of a number of connected structures that are involved in emotion, memory for location, and level of physical activity. The limbic system includes the amygdala, nucleus accumbens, and hippocampus, among others. Together with the hypothalamus, the limbic system involves important mechanisms for behavioural control at a more primitive level (sexual, eating behaviours, natural rewards) than that of the cerebral cortex or cerebrum.

The dopaminergic pathway from the ventral tegmental area to the nucleus accumbens is called the mesolimbic pathway, and it plays a key role in reward and reinforcement (see Figure 4.8). Pitchers and colleagues at the University of Western Ontario demonstrated with studies in rats that alterations in the mesolimbic system are commonly induced by rewards (natural and drug) and might play a role in general reinforcement in humans.[12]

The midbrain, pons, and medulla are the parts of the brain stem that connect the larger structures of the brain to the spinal cord. Within these brain stem structures are many groups of cell bodies (nuclei) that play important roles in sensory and motor reflexes, as well as coordinated control of complex movements. Within these brain stem structures also are the nuclei that contain most of the cell bodies for the neurons that produce and release the neurotransmitters dopamine, norepinephrine, and serotonin (see Figure 4.9). Virtually all the brain's supply of these important neurotransmitters is produced by a relatively small number of neurons (a few thousand for each neurotransmitter) located in these brain-stem regions.

The lower brain stem contains a couple of small areas of major importance. One area is the vomiting centre located in the medulla. Often when the brain detects foreign substances in the blood, such as alcohol, this centre is activated, and vomiting results. It is easy to see the survival value of such a system to animals, including humans, that have it. Another brainstem centre located in the pons and medulla regulates the rate of breathing. Various drugs that cause respiratory depression, which can lead to death, can suppress this respiratory centre.

These structures and their functions have been understood in general terms for many years. Knowledge about such things comes partly from people who have suffered accidental brain damage and partly from experiments using animals. These basic structures exist in mammals other than humans, with functions and connections that are basically the same, so it is possible to learn a great deal about human brain function from animal experiments. Animal research plays an important role in elucidating the effects of many psychoactive drugs and is regulated by the Canadian Council on Animal Care.[13]

Chemical Pathways

Although many neurotransmitters have been identified, we are concerned mostly with those few we believe to be associated with the actions of the psychoactive drugs we are studying. Those neurotransmitters include dopamine, acetylcholine, norepinephrine, serotonin, GABA, glutamate, and the endorphins.

Dopamine In some cases, groups of cells in a particular brain region contain a particular neurotransmitter, and

Figure 4.8 The Dopamine Pathways

Schematic diagram that represents the dopamine pathway projecting from the ventral tegmental area (VTA) to the nucleus accumbens (NAcc) (mesolimbic pathway), indicating how substances of abuse can alter the activity of this pathway to produce their rewarding effects.

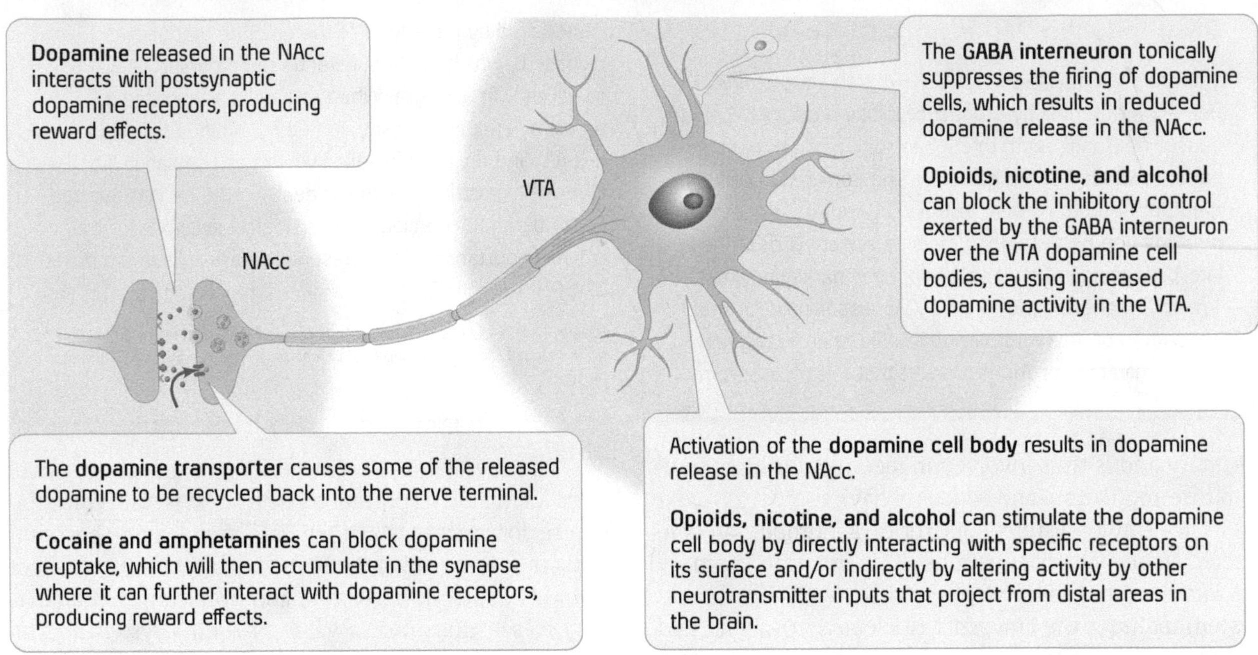

Dopamine released in the NAcc interacts with postsynaptic dopamine receptors, producing reward effects.
VTA
NAcc
The GABA interneuron tonically suppresses the firing of dopamine cells, which results in reduced dopamine release in the NAcc.
Opioids, nicotine, and alcohol can block the inhibitory control exerted by the GABA interneuron over the VTA dopamine cell bodies, causing increased dopamine activity in the VTA.
The dopamine transporter causes some of the released dopamine to be recycled back into the nerve terminal.
Cocaine and amphetamines can block dopamine reuptake, which will then accumulate in the synapse where it can further interact with dopamine receptors, producing reward effects.
Activation of the dopamine cell body results in dopamine release in the NAcc.
Opioids, nicotine, and alcohol can stimulate the dopamine cell body by directly interacting with specific receptors on its surface and/or indirectly by altering activity by other neurotransmitter inputs that project from distal areas in the brain.

Source: Tomkins, D.M. & Sellers, E.M. Addiction and the brain: the role of neurotransmitters in the cause and treatment of drug dependence. CMAJ. March 20, 2001; 164 (6).

axons from these cells are found grouped together and terminate in another brain region. We think of many psychoactive drug actions in terms of a drug's effect on one of these chemical pathways. For example, we know that cells in the **nucleus accumbens** receive input from **dopamine** fibres that arise in the ventral tegmental area in the midbrain to form the **mesolimbic dopamine pathway**. The mesocortical pathway also originates in the ventral tegmental area, but projects to the frontal cortex and surrounding structures. These pathways have been proposed to mediate some types of psychotic behaviour, such as that seen in **schizophrenia**. That is, overactivation of dopamine neurons in these pathways produces hallucinations, which are attenuated by dopamine-blocking drugs. This example highlights an important point and provides the basis for many neurochemical theories of behaviour: malfunctions of neurotransmitter systems lead to disease states, which can be effectively treated with drugs that target the affected system.

The most prominent neurochemical theory of drug abuse is based on the idea that all rewarding drugs, from alcohol to methamphetamine, stimulate dopamine neurons in the mesolimbic pathway. This pathway is proposed to be the main component responsible for the rewarding properties of electrical stimulation of the midbrain or limbic system. Thus, according to this theory, drugs lead to abuse because they stimulate this reward system, which is responsible for telling the rest of the brain "that's good–do that again."[14] Recent data, however, suggest this view may be overly simplistic. For example, it has been demonstrated that although initial depletion of dopamine

nucleus accumbens: a collection of neurons in the forebrain thought to play an important role in emotional reactions to events.

dopamine: neurotransmitter found in the basal ganglia and other regions.

mesolimbic dopamine pathway: one of two major dopamine pathways; may be involved in psychotic reactions and in drug dependence.

schizophrenia: a mental disorder characterized by chronic psychosis.

Figure 4.9 The Dopamine, Serotonin, and Norepinephrine Pathways

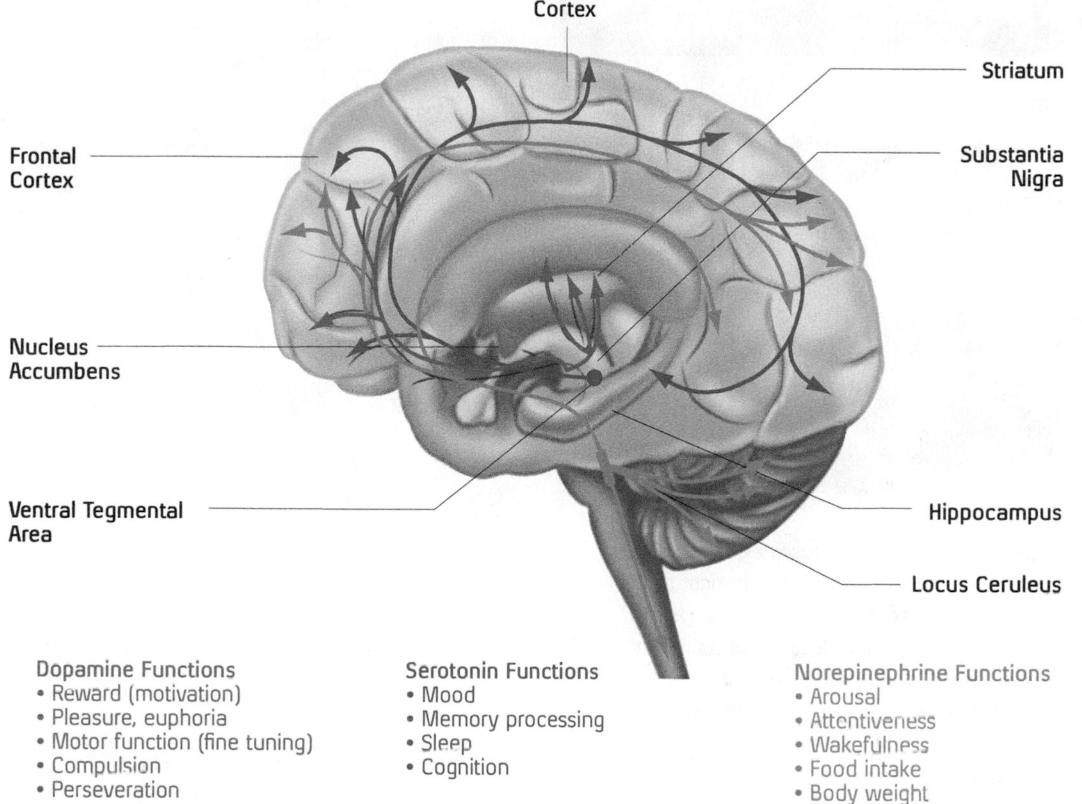

Dopamine Functions
- Reward (motivation)
- Pleasure, euphoria
- Motor function (fine tuning)
- Compulsion
- Perseveration

Serotonin Functions
- Mood
- Memory processing
- Sleep
- Cognition

Norepinephrine Functions
- Arousal
- Attentiveness
- Wakefulness
- Food intake
- Body weight

in the nucleus accumbens produces profound reductions in cocaine self-administration by rodents, cocaine self-administration recovers long before restoration of nucleus accumbens dopamine levels.[15] This suggests that other brain mechanisms play a role in the rewarding effects of cocaine and other drugs of abuse.

Another important dopamine pathway also begins in the midbrain–the **nigrostriatal dopamine pathway** (see Figure 4.10). Cells from the substantia nigra course together past the hypothalamus and terminate in the corpus striatum (part of the basal ganglia) to form this pathway. Substantial loss of cells along this pathway leads to Parkinson's disease; as a result, Parkinson's disease can be defined as a dopamine-deficiency disorder. Accordingly, the most popular and effective treatment of Parkinson's disease is the administration of the dopamine precursor L-dopa. Once in the brain, L-dopa is rapidly converted to dopamine, thereby restoring brain dopamine concentrations and relieving many symptoms related to Parkinson's disease. Dopamine itself is not administered as a treatment because it does not readily cross the blood-brain barrier. The fourth dopaminergic pathway, the tuberoinfundibular dopaminergic pathway, connects the hypothalamus to the pituitary gland, where it influences the secretion of hormones in the body.

Acetylcholine Pathways containing acetylcholine arise from cell bodies in the nucleus basalis in the lower part of the basal ganglia and project widely throughout the cerebral cortex. Nucleus basalis-cortex projections have been implicated in learning and memory storage. Indeed, in people who have Alzheimer's disease, a neurodegenerative condition that causes widespread cognitive deficits and personality changes, cells along these projections are reduced or damaged and the cortex contains much less acetylcholine than normal. Given this well-established acetylcholine deficiency and substantial experimental evidence demonstrating memory impairments following administration of drugs that block acetylcholine receptors, the predominant strategy used to treat Alzheimer's disease is to replace or

nigrostriatal dopamine pathway: one of two major dopamine pathways; damaged in Parkinson's disease.

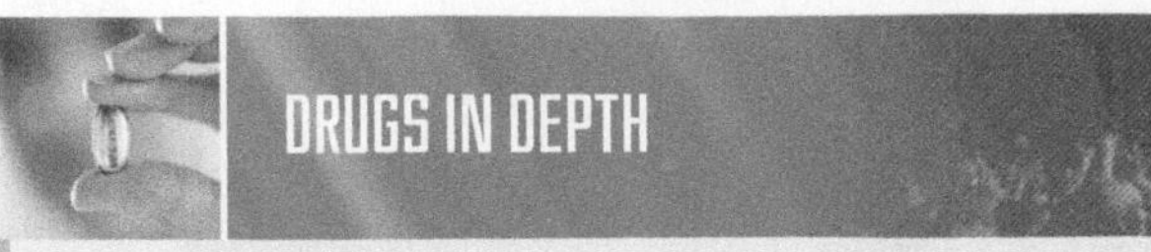

Rhodiola Rosea

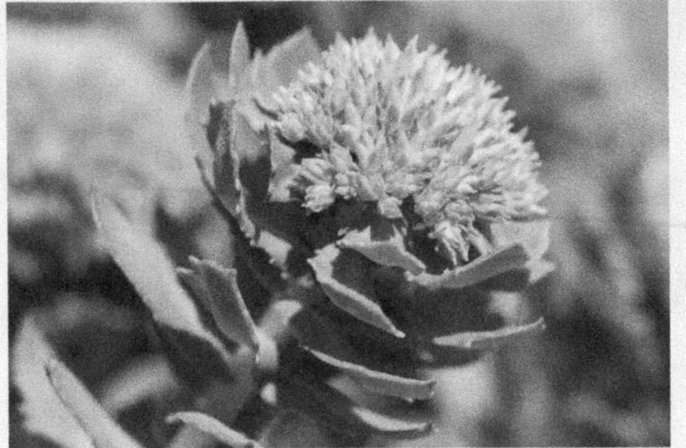

Extracts from the plant *Rhodiola rosea* increase human mental and memory capacity, which is thought to be due to inhibition of acetylcholine esterase (AChE). University of British Columbia (UBC) scientists report that the alcohol extract of *Rhodiola rosea* inhibits AChE activity by approximately 42%, with no indication of toxicity. They believe that this plant holds promise for the treatment of memory-impairing disorders, such as Alzheimer's disease.

Source: Hillhouse, B., D.S. Ming, C. French, and G.H. Towers. 2004. "Acetylcholine Esterase Inhibitors in *Rhodiola rosea*." *Pharmaceutical Biology* 42(1): 68–72.

restore the function of acetylcholine (see Figure 4.11). Of the five available treatment medications, all but one enhance the function of acetylcholine.

Norepinephrine Pathways arising from the locus ceruleus in the brain stem have numerous branches and project both up and down in the brain, releasing norepinephrine and influencing the level of arousal and attentiveness. It is perhaps through these pathways that stimulant drugs induce wakefulness. Norepinephrine pathways play an important role in the initiation of food intake, although other transmitter systems are also involved in the very important and therefore very complex processes of controlling energy balance and body weight.

Figure 4.10 Nigrostriatal Dopamine Pathway

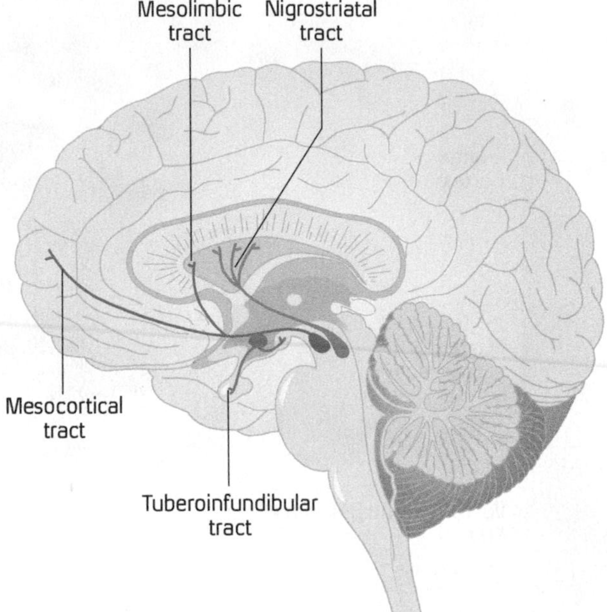

Source: Used with permission. http://thebrain.mcgill.ca/flash/a/a_03/a_03_cl/a_03_cl_que/a_03_cl_que.html

Serotonin Pathways containing **serotonin** arise from the brain-stem raphe nuclei and have projections both upward into the brain and downward into the spinal cord. Animal research has suggested one or more roles for serotonin in the complex control of food intake and the regulation of body weight. The diet drug Sibutramine causes its weight-reducing effects by blocking the reuptake of serotonin and norepinephrine.[16] Research on aggressiveness and impulsivity has also focused on serotonin. In studies with monkeys, low levels of serotonin metabolites in the blood have been associated with impulsive aggression, as well as with excessive alcohol consumption. Recent studies indicate a role for serotonin system dysfunction in individuals who commit suicide.[17] The use of selective serotonin reuptake inhibitors, such as Prozac, in treating major depressive disorder has also led to theories linking serotonin to depression. In all these cases (food intake and weight control, aggression and impulsivity, alcohol use, and depression), environmental influences play important roles, and other drugs that work through different neurotransmitter systems can also influence these behaviours. Therefore, it is much too simple to

serotonin: neurotransmitter found in the raphe nuclei; may be important for impulsivity, mood, and cognition, and plays a role in depression.

Figure 4.11 Acetylcholine

Acetylcholine esterase is an enzyme present within the synaptic cleft that hydrolyzes acetylcholine to choline and acetic acid, thereby inactivating it. Acetylcholine esterase inhibitors are used in the treatment of Alzheimer's disease.

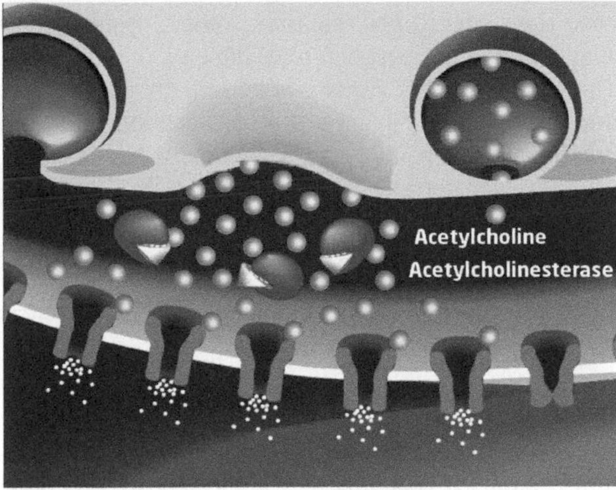

Source: Courtesy of Prof. Erik Jorgensen, Biology, Human Genetics, and Bioengineering, University of Utah.

attribute these behavioural problems to low serotonin levels alone. Hallucinogenic drugs, such as LSD, are believed to work by influencing serotonin pathways.

GABA (γ-amino butyric acid) **GABA** is one neurotransmitter that is not neatly organized into discrete pathways or bundles. GABA is found in most areas of the CNS and exerts generalized inhibitory functions. Many sedative drugs act by enhancing GABA inhibition (see Chapter 7). Etomidate (marketed as Amidate but available in Canada only through Health Canada's Special Access Program), a $GABA_A$ receptor agonist, is a short-acting intravenous anaesthetic agent used for the induction of general anaesthesia and for sedation. Etomidate has amnestic and sedative-hypnotic but not analgesic properties. At the University of Toronto Dr. Beverley A. Orser and colleagues demonstrated that deletion of a subunit of the $GABA_A$ receptor (alpha5 subunit) reduced the amnestic but not the sedative-hypnotic properties of etomidate. Thus the amnestic and sedative-hypnotic properties of etomidate can be dissociated on the basis of $GABA_A$ receptor pharmacology.[18]

Interfering with normal GABA inhibition, such as with the GABA-receptor-blocking drug strychnine, can lead to violent seizures resembling (but more severe than) convulsions seen in epilepsy.

Glutamate Like GABA, **glutamate** is found throughout the brain, and nearly all neurons have receptors that are activated by it. But, unlike GABA, stimulation of receptors that respond to glutamate makes cells more excitable. Thus, glutamate is often referred to as the brain's major excitatory neurotransmitter. Recently, increasing evidence indicates that specific glutamate pathways may be important for the expression of some psychoactive drug effects. For instance, abnormal glutamate transmission, caused by prolonged chronic cocaine

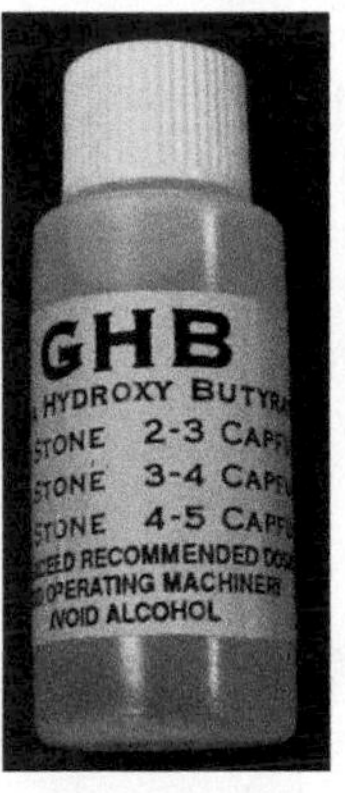

The club drug GHB (γ-hydroxy butyrate) is a close chemical relative of the neurotransmitter GABA.

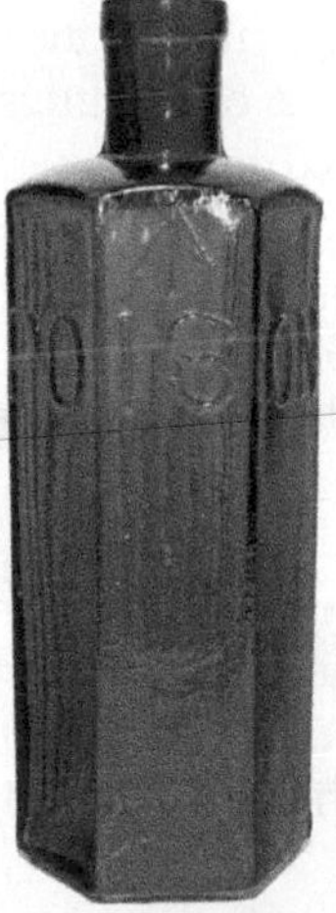

Antique pharmaceutical bottle used for storing poisonous substances. Distinctive shapes and textures helped those who couldn't read and people with visual impairments to distinguish poison bottles from other containers.

GABA: inhibitory neurotransmitter found in most regions of the brain.

glutamate: excitatory neurotransmitter found in most regions of the brain.

use, in the projection from the prefrontal cortex to the nucleus accumbens has been hypothesized to mediate relapse to cocaine use following a period of drug abstinence.[19] Researchers had long known that cocaine affects both dopamine and glutamate receptors on neurons, but the molecular details of those effects were unknown. Dr. Fang Liu at the University of Toronto, with a team of researchers led by Dr. John Q. Wang at the University of Missouri, Kansas City School of Medicine, has uncovered a connection between glutamate receptors in the brain and the euphoric effect of cocaine. The NMDA glutamate receptor is an important link for psychostimulants, such as cocaine, to modify excitability of striatal neurons and to stimulate behavioural activity in animal experiments. When rats were given cocaine, a specific subunit of dopamine receptors, called D2R, tended to attach to the NR2B subunit of the glutamate receptor and prevented its normal activation. The interaction between these receptors is direct and exists in a specific population of striatal neurons. The interaction can be increased by cocaine, producing a euphoric effect. If you block the interaction, then you block the cocaine effect.[20] Most of the data supporting this hypothesis have been obtained by using laboratory animals. Therefore, clinical implications of altered glutamate transmission in substance abuse remain unclear.

Endorphins Several chemicals in the brain produce effects similar to those of morphine and other drugs derived from opium. The term **endorphin** was coined in reference to endogenous (coming from within) morphine-like substances. Endorphins play a role in pain relief, but they are found in several places in the brain and circulating in the blood, and not all their functions are known. Although it is tempting to theorize about the role of endorphins in drug abuse or dependence, the actual evidence linking dependence to endorphins has not been strong, and other neurotransmitter systems (particularly dopamine and serotonin systems) have also been shown to influence behaviours related to dependence.

endorphin: opiate-like chemical that occurs naturally in the brain of humans and other animals.

agonist: a substance that facilitates or mimics the effects of a neurotransmitter on the postsynaptic cell.

antagonist: a substance that prevents the effects of a neurotransmitter on the postsynaptic cell.

precursors: chemicals that are acted on by enzymes to form neurotransmitters.

LO7 Drugs and the Brain

A drug is carried to the brain by the blood supply. How does each drug know where to go once it gets into the brain? The answer is that the drug goes everywhere. But because the drug molecules of LSD, for example, have their effect by acting on serotonin systems, LSD affects the brain systems that depend on serotonin. The way that LSD alters perceptions in the brain is unclear. Research suggests that LSD acts on serotonin receptors in two major parts of the brain. One area (the cerebral cortex) is involved in mood, cognition, and perception; the other area (the locus ceruleus) is described as the "novelty detector" because it receives sensory information from all parts of the body.[21] It was once thought that the LSD molecules that reach other types of receptors appear to have no particular effect. Seeman and colleagues at the University of Toronto have found that LSD affects dopamine D2 receptors, those same receptors that are involved in psychosis in schizophrenia, explaining why clinical **agonist** actions of LSD in eliciting psychotic symptoms are selectively treated in the hospital emergency room by haloperidol and other dopamine D2-selective **antagonists**.[22]

Because the brain is so well supplied with blood an equilibrium develops quickly for most drugs, so that the drug's concentration in the brain is about equal to that in the blood and the number of molecules leaving the blood is equal to the number leaving the brain to enter the blood. As the drug is removed from the blood (by the liver or kidneys) and the concentration in the blood decreases, more molecules leave the brain than enter it, and the brain levels begin to decrease.

We are able to explain the mechanisms by which many psychoactive drugs act on the brain. In most of these cases, the drug has its effects because the molecular structure of the drug is similar to the molecular structure of one of the neurotransmitter chemicals. Because of this structural similarity, the drug molecules interact with one or more of the stages in the life cycle of that neurotransmitter chemical. We can therefore understand some of the ways drugs act on the brain by looking at the life cycle of a typical neurotransmitter molecule.

Life Cycle of a Neurotransmitter

Neurotransmitter molecules are made inside the cell from which they are to be released. If they were just floating around everywhere in the brain, then the release of a tiny amount from a nerve ending wouldn't have much information value. However, the **precursors** from which the neurotransmitter is made circulate in the blood supply and generally in the brain. A cell that is going to make a particular neurotransmitter needs to bring in the right precursor in a greater concentration than exists outside the cell, so machinery is built into that cell's membrane for active **uptake** of the precursor. In this process, the cell expends energy to bring the precursor into the cell, even though the concentration inside the cell is already higher than that outside the cell. Obviously, this uptake mechanism must be selective and must recognize the precursor molecules as they float by. Many of the precursors are amino acids that are derived from proteins in the diet, and these amino acids are used in the body for many things besides making neurotransmitters. For example, the amino acid tyrosine is recognized by the norepinephrine neuron, which expends energy to take it in.

After the precursor molecule has been taken up into the neuron, it must be changed, through one or more chemical reactions, into the neurotransmitter molecule. This process is called **synthesis**. At each step in the synthetic chemical reactions, **enzymes** help the reactions along. These enzymes are themselves large molecules that recognize the precursor molecule, attach to it briefly, and hold it in such a way as to make the synthetic chemical reaction occur. Figure 4.12 provides a schematic representation of such a synthetic enzyme in action.

In our example diagram of the life cycle of the catecholamine neurotransmitters dopamine and norepinephrine (Figure 4.13), the precursor tyrosine is acted on first by one enzyme to make DOPA and then by another enzyme to make dopamine. In dopamine cells the process stops there, but in our norepinephrine neuron, a third enzyme is present to change dopamine into norepinephrine.

After the neurotransmitter molecules have been synthesized, they are stored in small vesicles near the terminal from which they will be released. This storage process also calls for recognizing the transmitter molecules and concentrating them inside the vesicles.

The arrival of the action potential in the presynaptic terminals causes calcium (Ca^{2+}) channels to open. Calcium enters the cells and assists the movement of the small vesicles filled with neurotransmitter toward the presynaptic terminal membrane so that the neurotransmitter is released into the **synapse**. Several thousand neurotransmitter molecules are released at once, and it takes only microseconds for these molecules to diffuse across the synapse. Once neurotransmitters are released into the synapse, they may bind with receptors on the membrane of the next neuron, sometimes referred to as the postsynaptic cell

Figure 4.12 Schematic Representation of the Action of a Synthetic Enzyme

A precursor molecule and another chemical fragment both bind to the enzyme. The fragment has a tendency to connect with the precursor, but the connection is made much more likely because of the way the enzyme lines up the two parts. After the connection is made, the new transmitter molecule separates from the enzyme.

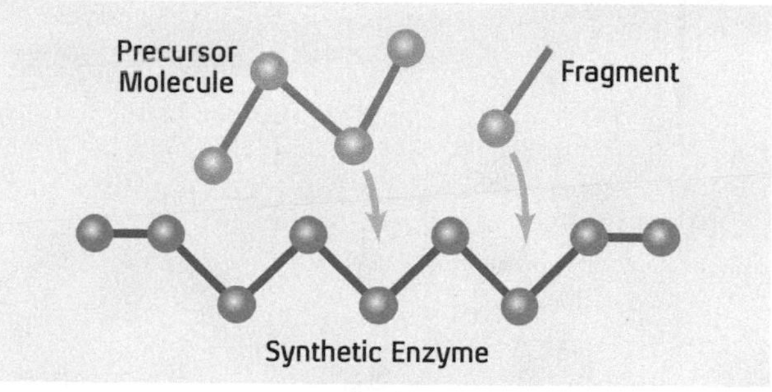

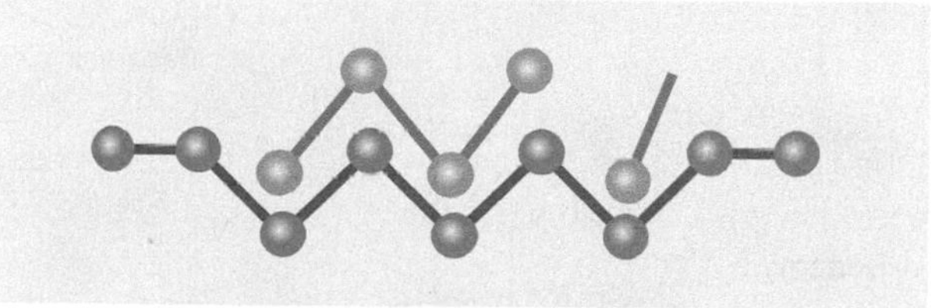

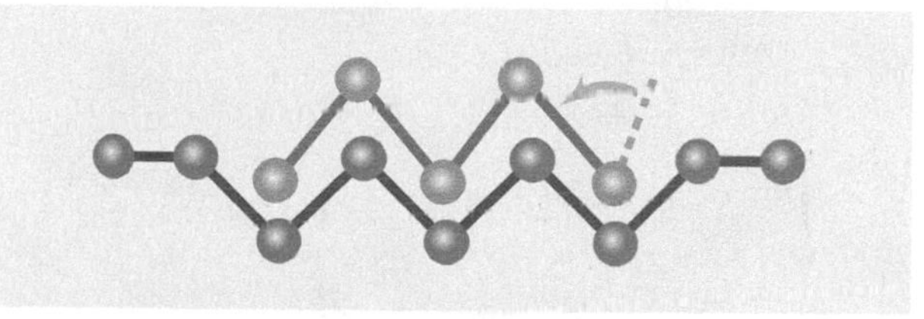

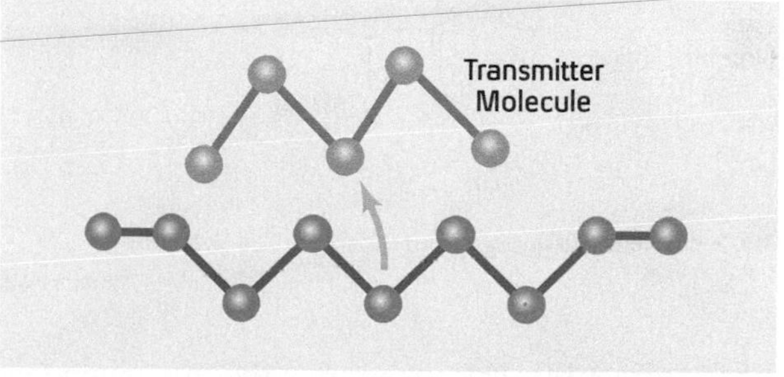

uptake: energy-requiring mechanism by which selected molecules are taken into cells.

synthesis: the forming of a neurotransmitter by the action of enzymes on precursors.

enzyme: large molecule that assists in either the synthesis or metabolism of another molecule.

synapse: the space between neurons.

Figure 4.13 Biosynthesis of the Catecholamines

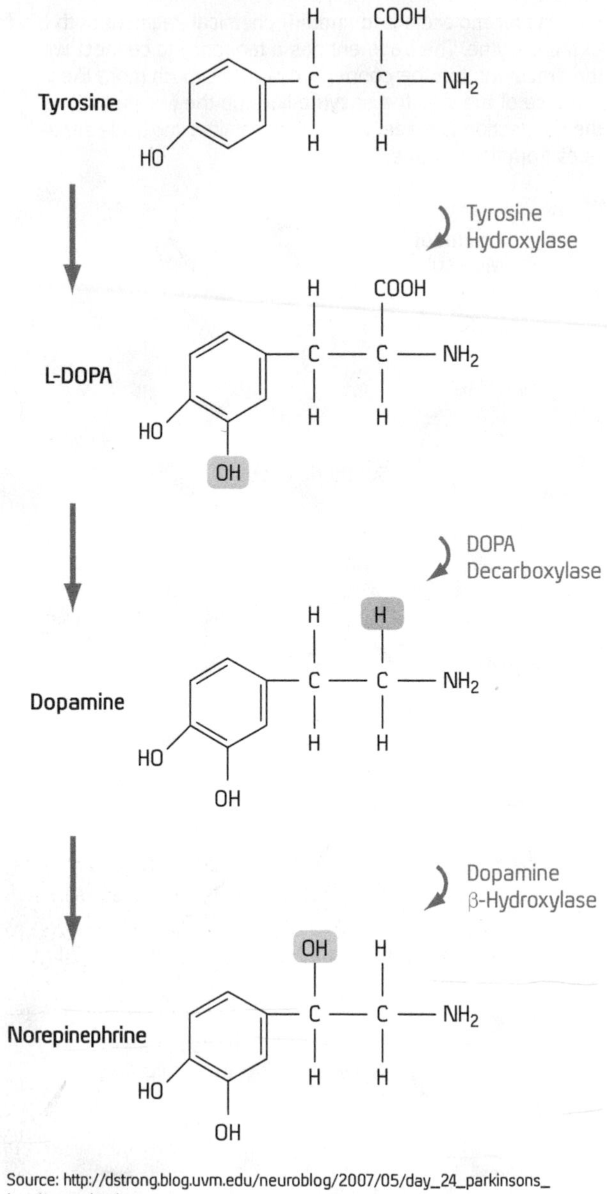

Tyrosine

H COOH
C — C — NH_2
HO H H

Tyrosine Hydroxylase

L-DOPA

H COOH
C — C — NH_2
HO OH H H

DOPA Decarboxylase

Dopamine

H H
C — C — NH_2
HO OH H H

Dopamine β-Hydroxylase

Norepinephrine

OH H
C — C — NH_2
HO OH H H

Source: http://dstrong.blog.uvm.edu/neuroblog/2007/05/day_24_parkinsons_huntingtons.html

(see Figure 4.14). This receptor is the most important recognition site in the entire process, and it is one of the most important places for drugs to interact with the natural neurotransmitter. In the process of binding, the neurotransmitter distorts the receptor, so that a tiny passage is opened through the membrane, allowing ions to move through the membrane. As a result, the postsynaptic cell can either become more or less excitable, and thus more or less likely to initiate an action potential.

Whether the effect of a neurotransmitter is excitatory or inhibitory depends on the type of receptor.

Figure 4.14 Neurotransmitter Release

Schematic representation of the release of neurotransmitter molecules from synaptic vesicles in the axon terminal of one neuron and the passage of those molecules across the synapse to receptors in the membrane of another neuron.

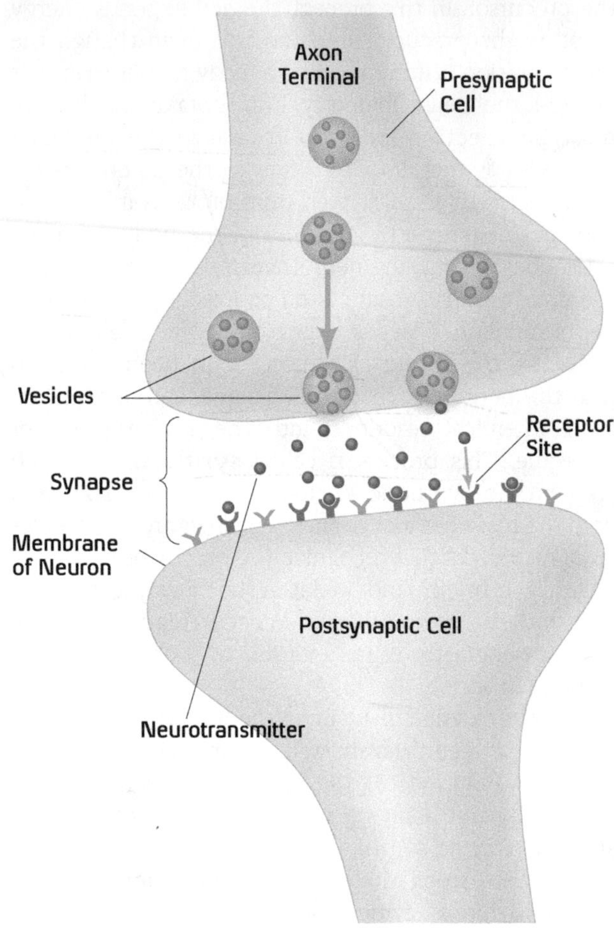

There are specific receptors for each neurotransmitter, and most neurotransmitters have more than one type of receptor in the brain. For example, the neurotransmitter GABA has at least three receptor types–$GABA_A$, $GABA_B$, and $GABA_C$–and stimulation of all seem to make the cell less excitable. Therefore, GABA is often called an inhibitory neurotransmitter (see Figure 4.15). Many of the sedative-like effects produced by drugs, such as barbiturates and benzodiazepines, are dependent on their binding to the $GABA_A$ receptors. Michael Poulter's group at the University of Western Ontario have discovered altered patterning of $GABA_A$ receptor subunits in the hippocampus and amygdala, two highly stressor-reactive regions of the mesolimbic system among people who committed suicide by hanging, drug overdose, or a jump from

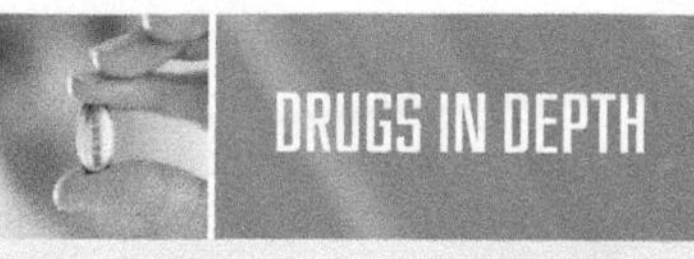

Endogenous Dopamine Release Mediates a Placebo Effect in People with Parkinson's Disease

At the Pacific Parkinson's Research Centre, University of British Columbia in Vancouver, researchers have demonstrated in a randomized control study that expectations play a central role in the mechanism of the placebo effect with release of endogenous dopamine in both nigrostriatal and mesolimbic projections. Thirty-five patients with mild to moderate Parkinson's disease undergoing levodopa treatment were told that they had a 75% or a 100% chance of receiving active medication and demonstrated significant dopamine release as measured by using [11C] raclopride positron emission tomography, accompanied by positive self-rated clinical responses. In truth, they had received a placebo.

This study by Stoessl and colleagues demonstrates the importance of salience over and above a patient's prior treatment response in regulating the placebo effect and has important implications for the interpretation and design of clinical trials.[23]

height. Poulter and colleagues' data support a role of regulation for $GABA_A$ subunit coordination across brain regions, which may have diverse implications for depression and suicide.[24] The function of GABA will be more fully explored in Chapter 7 in the discussion of psychotherapeutic agents for mental illness, including depression and anxiety.

Like GABA, acetylcholine also acts at multiple receptors in the brain: muscarinic and nicotinic (see Figure 4.16). At least five muscarinic receptors and at least 11 nicotinic receptors have been identified, and acetylcholine's action can be either excitatory or inhibitory, depending on the receptor stimulated. Of particular interest is acetylcholine's role in attentional processes in the human brain. Lambe and her research team at the University of Toronto have identified a specific subunit of the nicotinic acetylcholine receptor believed to play an important role in prefrontal cortical activity underlying attention. Published in the *Journal of Neuroscience*, Lambe and colleagues showed in mice that the rare genetic alpha5 subunit (a variant of the α subunit) of the nicotinic acetylcholine receptor powerfully enhances nicotinic neuroelectrical currents in

Figure 4.15 GABA Receptors

Binding of $GABA_A$ to its receptors opens a chloride channel, hyperpolarizing the membrane.

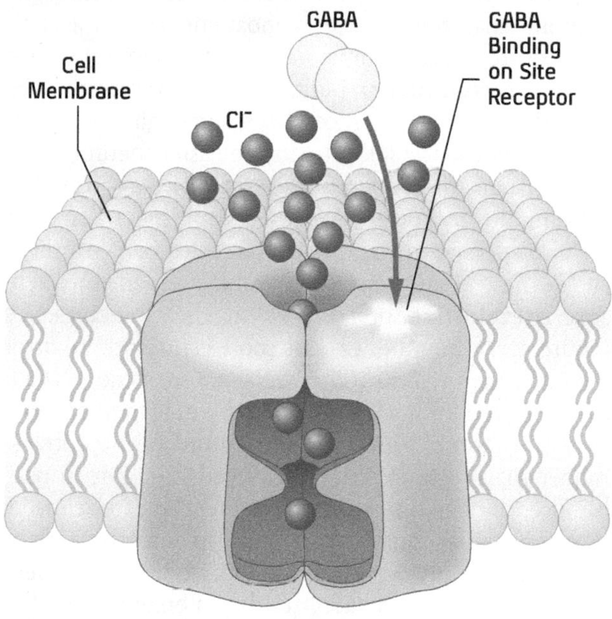

Figure 4.16 Acetylcholine Receptors

Binding of acetylcholine to its receptor opens a Na^+ channel, depolarizing the membrane.

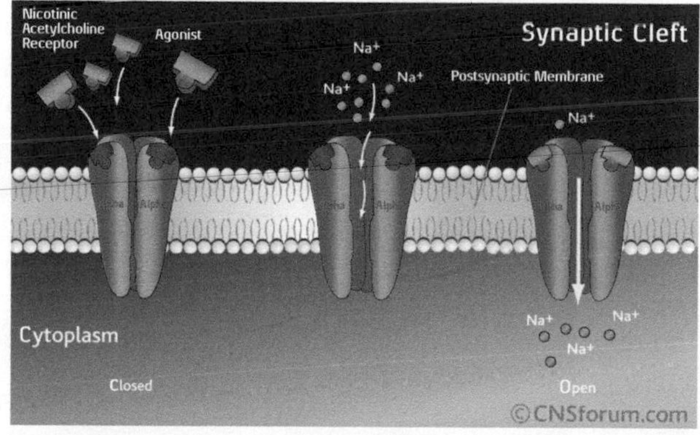

prefrontal cortical brain slices. In separate but related behavioural experiments, they show that the nicotinic receptor alpha5 subunit in adult brain circuitry is required for accurate performance by adult mice on challenging visual attention tasks. Together, these findings further demonstrate acetylcholine's complicated role in attentional performance.[25]

Because signalling in the nervous system occurs at a high rate, once a signal has been sent in the form of neurotransmitter release it is important to terminate that signal, so that the next signal can be transmitted. Thus, the thousands of neurotransmitter molecules released by a single action potential must be removed from the synapse. Two methods are used for this. The neurons that release the monoamine neurotransmitters serotonin, dopamine, and norepinephrine have specific **transporters** built into their terminals. The serotonin transporter recognizes serotonin molecules and brings them back into the releasing neuron, thus ending their interaction with serotonin receptors. The dopamine transporter and norepinephrine transporter are also specific to their neurotransmitters. With these and other neurotransmitters, enzymes in the synapse **metabolize**, or break down, the molecules (see Figure 4.17). In either case, as soon as neurotransmitter molecules are released into the synapse, some of them are removed or metabolized and never get to bind to the receptors on the other neuron. All neurotransmitter molecules might be removed in less than one-hundredth of a second from the time they are released; molecules are rapidly taken back up into the neuron from which they were released. Once inside the neuron, molecules are metabolized by an enzyme found in the cell.

Figure 4.17 Schematic Representation of the Action of a Metabolic Enzyme

The transmitter molecule binds to the enzyme in such a way that the transmitter molecule is distorted and "pulled apart." The fragments then separate from the enzyme.

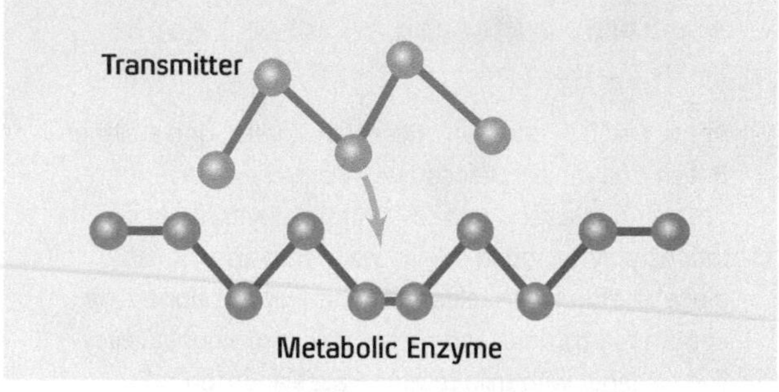

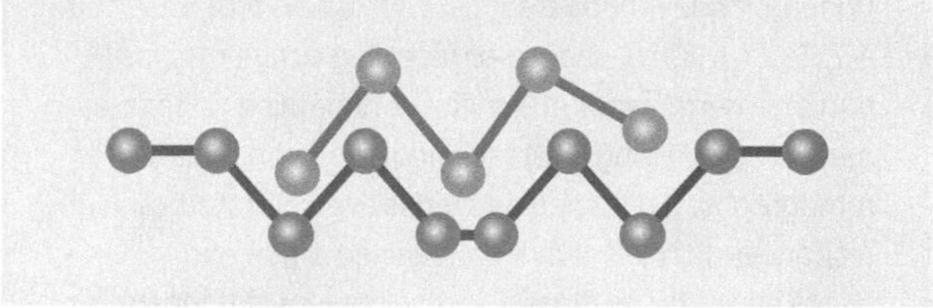

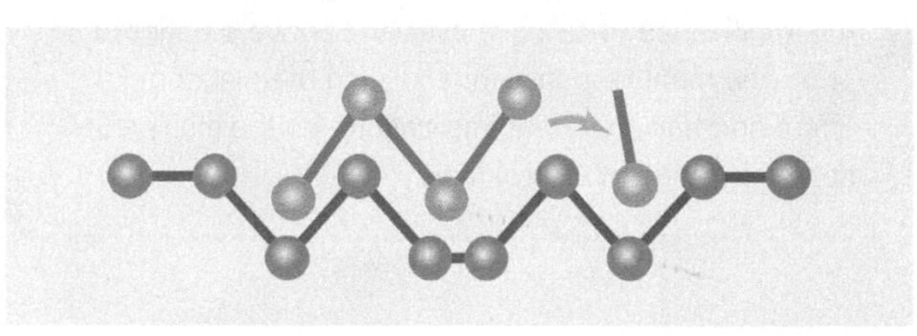

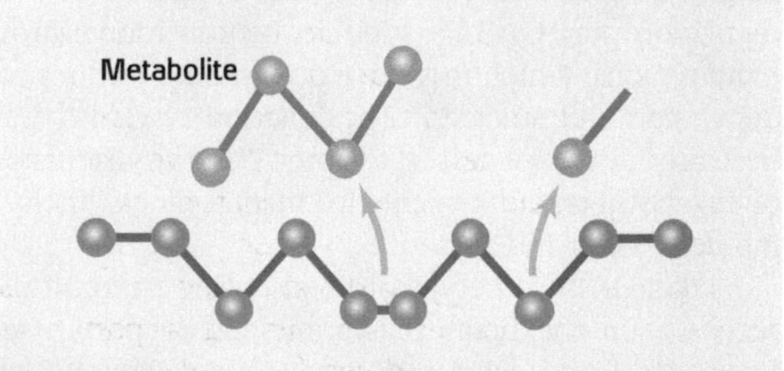

Examples of Drug Actions

It is possible to divide the actions of drugs on neurotransmitter systems into two main types. Through actions on synthesis, storage, release, reuptake, or metabolism, drugs can alter the availability of the neurotransmitter in the synapse. Either the amount of transmitter in the synapse, when it is released or how long it remains before being cleared from the synapse will be affected. The second main type of drug effect is directly on the receptors. A drug can act as an agonist by mimicking the action of the neurotransmitter and directly activating the receptor, or it can act as an antagonist by occupying the receptor and preventing the neurotransmitter from activating it.

Perhaps one of the most interesting mechanisms is interference with the transporters that clear neurotransmitters, such as norepinephrine, serotonin, and dopamine, from the synapse by bringing them back into the neuron from which they were just released. Both the stimulant drug cocaine and most of the antidepressant drugs block one or more of these transporters and cause the normally released neurotransmitter to remain in the synapse longer than normal. One of the most exciting research areas in the neurosciences is the search for greater understanding of how altering these reuptake processes can produce either cocaine-like or antidepressant effects, depending perhaps on the neurotransmitter systems affected and the time course of the drug's action.

transporter: mechanism in the nerve terminal membrane responsible for removing neurotransmitter molecules from the synapse by taking them back into the neuron.

metabolize: to break down or inactivate a neurotransmitter (or a drug) through enzymatic action.

Health Canada reports that although no best practice treatment guidelines exist for cocaine dependence, the use of several antidepressant drugs has shown promise in retaining users in the initial stages of treatment, particularly depressed people and those who snort cocaine. The most promising of these compounds is GBR 12909. Studies have shown that both cocaine and GBR 12909 inhibit the dopamine transporter, increasing the levels of dopamine in the synapse. This prolongs dopamine's pleasurable effects. GBR 12909 produces a much smaller dopamine spike but maintains levels for a longer time. In studies using monkeys, it was found that the injection of GBR 12909 greatly reduced cocaine self-administration.[26]

Drug Effects on Neurotransmitter Receptors

One method by which a drug can influence a receptor is by mimicking the action of the neurotransmitter (i.e., act as a receptor agonist). For example, heroin mimics the action of endorphins at opioid receptors. Nicotine has effects very similar to the effects of the neurotransmitter acetylcholine at some types of cholinergic receptors (they are called nicotinic acetylcholine receptors for this reason).

When the neurotransmitter binds to its receptor, in the process of matching up the structure of the transmitter molecule with the structure of the receptor, the receptor has to bend or stretch slightly, thus opening a small pore in the membrane. Suppose a drug molecule matched up so well with the receptor that the receptor didn't have to bend or stretch during the binding process. That drug molecule would fit the receptor better than the natural neurotransmitter. However, because the receptor doesn't have to change, there would be no effect on the electrical activity of the cell. Such agents are called antagonists, or "blockers," because by occupying the site they prevent the normal neurotransmitters from having a postsynaptic effect. Antipsychotic drugs (also called neuroleptic drugs or major tranquillizers), such as haloperidol (Haldol), block receptors for dopamine. When we refer to *blocking receptors,* only enough drug is given to block some of the receptors some of the time, so the net effect is to modulate, or alter, the activity in an ongoing system. Generally, if enough drug were given to block most of the receptors most of the time, the result would be highly toxic or even lethal.

What would happen if we tried to treat a psychotic patient who has Parkinson's disease with both L-dopa and haloperidol? The L-dopa is used to counteract damage to the dopamine systems in Parkinson's disease by making more dopamine available at the synapses. Haloperidol is used to control psychotic behaviour, and it acts by blocking dopamine receptors. Thus, the drugs seem to have opposing actions. In fact, haloperidol often produces side effects that resemble Parkinson's disease, and L-dopa often produces hallucinations in its users. The two drugs are not used in the same patient because each tends to reduce the effectiveness of the other.

LO8 Chemical Theories of Behaviour

Drugs that affect existing neurochemical processes in the brain often affect behaviour, and this has led to many attempts to explain normal (not drug-induced) variations in behaviour in terms of changes in brain chemistry. For example, differences in personality between two people might be explained by a difference in the chemical makeup of their brains, or changes in an individual's reactions from one day to the next might be explained in terms of shifting tides of chemicals. The ancient Greek physician Hippocrates believed that behaviour patterns reflected the relative balances of four humours: blood (hot and wet, resulting in a sanguine or passionate nature); phlegm (cold and wet, resulting in a phlegmatic or calm nature); yellow bile (hot and dry, resulting in a choleric, bilious, or bad-tempered nature); and black bile (cold and dry, resulting in a melancholic or gloomy nature). The Chinese made do with only two basic dispositions: *yin,* the moon, representing the cool, passive, "feminine" nature; and *yang,* the sun, representing the warm, active, "masculine" nature. Thus, any personality could be seen as a relative mixture of these two opposing forces.

Unfortunately, most of the chemical-balance theories that have been proposed based on relative influences of different neurotransmitters have not really been more sophisticated than these yin-yang and humoral notions of ancient times. For example, the major theory guiding the treatment of clinical depression proposes that too little activity of the **monoamine** neurotransmitters can cause depression and too much can cause a manic state. This proposition is known as the *monoamine theory of mood.* It

monoamine: a class of chemicals characterized by a single amine group; monoamine neurotransmitters include dopamine, norepinephrine, and serotonin.

is supported by evidence showing that monoamine-enhancing drugs, such as amphetamines and cocaine, elevate mood, and chronic use of large doses of these drugs can produce manic episodes. Furthermore, medications that augment the actions of monoamines by interfering with their uptake or metabolism have been used successfully to treat depression for more than 40 years. It should be noted that the antidepressant effects of these medications, however, are not apparent for at least seven to ten days, and sometimes not for weeks, following the initiation of treatment. The lag period occurs even though antidepressant medications increase the activity of monoamine neurotransmitters within minutes following drug administration. This suggests that although current antidepressant medications are useful, the underlying cause of depression is more complex than the simple proposed neurochemical imbalance. Nonetheless, because the rationale underlying the treatment of some psychopathologies–including depression, schizophrenia, and Alzheimer's disease–is based on correcting a neurochemical abnormality, it is tempting to speculate that depressed individuals differ from other people in terms of neurochemical levels or functioning. Two important points should be noted here. First, drug treatments for the vast majority of psychopathologies are not cures; they provide only relief from disease-related symptoms, indicating that much of the complexities associated with many psychopathologies have yet to be elucidated. Second, to date, no single neurochemical theory of depression has yet obtained sufficient experimental support to be considered an explanation.

LO9 Brain Imaging Techniques

Two techniques were developed during the 1980s for obtaining chemical maps of the brains of living humans. These techniques offer exciting possibilities for furthering our understanding of brain chemistry, abnormal behaviour, and drug effects.

One of the techniques is positron emission tomography (PET) (see Figure 4.18). In this technique, a radioactively labelled chemical is injected into the bloodstream, and a computerized scanning device then maps out the relative amounts of the chemical in various brain regions. Because all neurons in the brain rely on blood glucose for their energy, a labelled form of glucose can be used to see which parts of the brain are most active, and these vary depending on what the person is doing. The activity of the brain is colour-coded by the scientist. These false colour images represent the activity of different brain regions. The scientists may choose any colour to represent high activity versus low activity. In Figure 4.18, the scientists chose red to represent high activity relative to brain areas with reduced glucose metabolism, which is represented by blue. Similarly, blood flow to a particular brain region reflects the activity there, and labelled oxygen or other gases can map regional cerebral blood flow, which also changes depending on what the person is doing. More recently, labelled drugs that bind to dopamine, serotonin, or opiate receptors have been used, and it is therefore possible to see where the binding of those chemicals takes place in a living human brain.

Figure 4.18 PET Scan

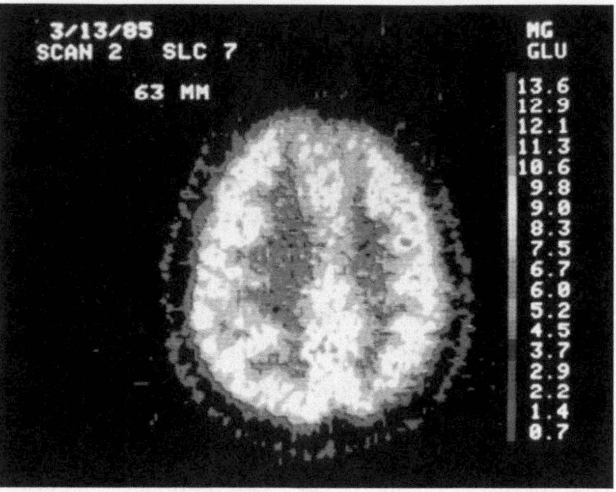

Source: National Cancer Institute Visuals Online (Dr. Giovanni Dichiro, Neuroimaging Section, National Institute of Neurological Disorders and Stroke).

Magnetic resonance imaging (MRI) is another brain imaging technique (see Figure 4.19). Rather than using radioactive labels, the technique relies on applying a strong magnetic field, measuring the energy released by various molecules. A radiofrequency (RF) pulse is produced from an emitter often attached to the subject–the RF field is turned on and off. The signals are complex, but with the aid of computers it is possible to detect certain chemical "fingerprints" in the signals. This technique gives a high-resolution image and does not require the administration of expensive radiochemicals; because it can provide much information not attainable with simple X-ray studies, it has been rapidly adopted by the medical community. A refinement of this technique (functional MRI, or fMRI), using different computational techniques, is beginning

Figure 4.19 MRI Scan

MRI scans can be used to view the structures of the brain. Functional MRI scans can be used to see the activity of specific brain regions following drug use.

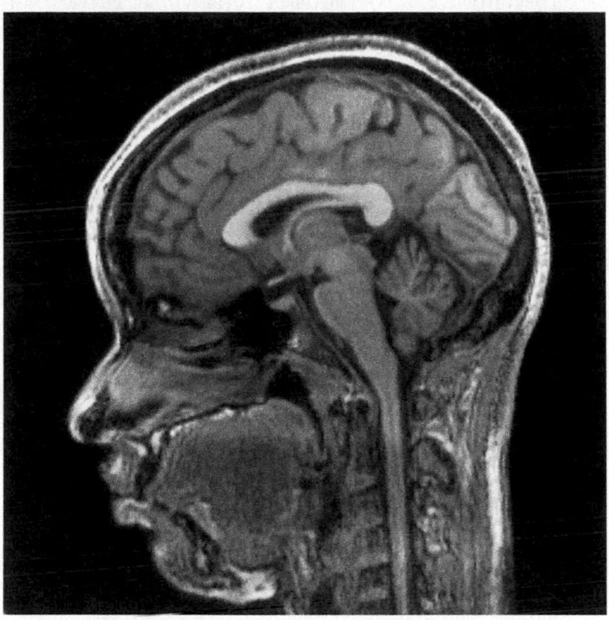

Source: Guy Croft SciTech/Alamy

to be used to study apparent changes in metabolic activity in specific brain regions. Also fMRI and MRI can be done on the same machines; the major difference between MRI and fMRI is the software used for analysis.

Although brain imaging (fMRI and PET) is an exciting technological advance that offers a glimpse into the working of the human brain, it is not without limitations. For example the production of a brain image involves many assumptions and complicated statistical analyses, which are often not standardized from one laboratory or hospital to the next. In addition, colour coding ("false colour" images and not pictures of the in vivo brain) of various amounts of brain activity can be arbitrary (e.g., some researchers may use a colour scheme that gives an illusion of enormous differences when only small differences actually exist). These limitations make it difficult, if not impossible, to compare brain scans collected in one laboratory with those from another in any meaningful manner. The analysis of brain imaging experiments has many problems, so much so that we might question whether or not every brain imaging study to date should be thrown out (except for the rare few that used rigorous statistical tools).

Summary

- Chemical signals in the body are important for maintaining homeostasis. Neurotransmitters are one type of chemical signal.
- The action potential is an electrical signal that initiates a chain of events that allows one neuron to communicate with another through the release of neurotransmitters.
- Neurotransmitters act over brief periods and very small distances because they are released into the synapse between neurons and are then rapidly cleared from the synapse.
- Receptors are specialized structures that recognize neurotransmitter molecules and, when activated, cause a change in the electrical activity of the neuron.
- The nervous system can be roughly divided into the central nervous system and the peripheral nervous system. The peripheral nervous system is composed of the somatic system and the autonomic system.
- The autonomic system, with its sympathetic and parasympathetic branches, is important because so many psychoactive drugs also have autonomic influences on heart rate, blood pressure, and so on.
- Specialized chemical pathways contain the important neurotransmitters dopamine, acetylcholine, norepinephrine, and serotonin.
- Key brain structures and chemical pathways include dopamine and the nigrostriatal and mesolimbic dopamine systems.
- The nigrostriatal dopamine system is damaged in Parkinson's disease, leading to muscular rigidity and tremors.
- The mesolimbic dopamine system is thought by many to be a critical pathway for the dependence produced by many drugs.
- Other important neurotransmitters are GABA and glutamate. The neurotransmitter GABA is inhibitory and the neurotransmitter glutamate is excitatory; both are found in most parts of the brain.
- Receptor types determine the action of a neurotransmitter at a particular site in the brain.

- Acetylcholine's action can be either excitatory or inhibitory, depending on the receptor it stimulates. Acetylcholine esterase inhibitors are drugs that alter the availability of the neurotransmitter acetylcholine.
- Haloperidol is a dopamine D2-selective antagonist that blocks the dopamine receptor.
- The life cycle of a typical neurotransmitter involves uptake of precursors, synthesis of the transmitter, storage in vesicles, release into the synapse, interaction with the receptor, reuptake into the releasing neuron, and metabolism by enzymes.
- Psychoactive drugs act either by altering the availability of a neurotransmitter at the synapse or by interacting with a neurotransmitter receptor.

Review Questions

1. What are some examples of homeostasis in the human body?
2. What are the similarities and differences between glia and neurons?
3. Describe the process of neurotransmitter release and receptor interaction.
4. Give some examples of the opposing actions of the sympathetic and parasympathetic branches of the autonomic nervous system. What is the neurotransmitter for each branch?
5. What is the function of the basal ganglia, and which neurotransmitter is involved?
6. What is the proposed role of the mesolimbic dopamine system in drug dependence?
7. Alzheimer's disease produces a loss of which neurotransmitter affecting primarily which brain structures?
8. What neurotransmitter seems to have only inhibitory receptors?
9. After a neurotransmitter is synthesized, where is it stored while awaiting release?
10. What are the two main ways in which drugs can interact with neurotransmitter systems?
11. PET and MRI are two examples of what technology?

CHAPTER 5

THE ACTIONS OF DRUGS

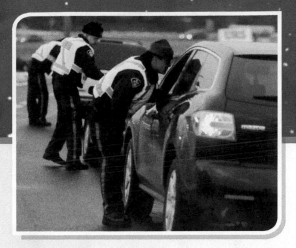

OBJECTIVES

When you have finished this chapter, you should be able to

- **LO1** Explain why plants are the source of many of the chemicals we use as drugs.
- **LO2** Distinguish among generic, brand, and chemical names for a drug.
- **LO3** Name the major drug categories.
- **LO4** Define pharmacodynamic factors including drug receptor interactions, the dose–response relationship, ED_{50}, LD_{50}, and the therapeutic index.
- **LO5** Describe drug action and specific and nonspecific drug effects, including placebo effects, therapeutic effects, and side effects.
- **LO6** Explain why pharmacological potency is not synonymous with effectiveness.
- **LO7** Explain the pharmacokinetic factors that determine drug action, including routes of drug absorption, distribution, metabolism, and excretion.
- **LO8** Discuss routes of administration and the importance of the blood–brain barrier.
- **LO9** List the mechanisms of drug actions.
- **LO10** Explain how drugs are metabolized and excreted.
- **LO11** Know the types of tolerance related to physical dependence.

LO1, LO2 Sources and Names of Drugs

Most of the drugs in use 50 years ago originally came from plants. Even now, most of our drugs either come from plants or are chemically derived from plant substances. Why do the plants of this world produce so many drugs? Suppose a genetic mutation occurred in a plant so that one of its normal biochemical processes was changed and a new chemical was produced. If that new chemical had an effect on an animal's biochemistry, when the animal ate the plant, the animal might become ill or die. In either case, that plant would be less likely to be eaten and more likely to reproduce others of its own kind. Such a selection process must have occurred many thousands of times in various places all over Earth. Many of those plant-produced chemicals have effects on the intestines or muscles; others alter brain biochemistry. In large doses the effect is virtually always unpleasant or dangerous, but in controlled doses those chemicals might alter the biochemistry just enough to produce interesting or even useful effects. In primitive cultures, the people who learned about these plants and how to use them safely were important figures in their communities. Those medicine men and women were the forerunners of today's pharmacists and physicians, as well as being important religious figures in their tribes.

Today the legal pharmaceutical industry is one of the largest and most profitable industries in North America, with sales exceeding $160 billion a year.[1] Canada and the United States generally show similar drug consumption rates, especially for cardiovascular, cholesterol, and psychotherapeutic medications. Canada ranks 36th in the world in terms of population, yet the Canadian pharmaceutical market is the eighth largest in the world, accounting for about 2% of the world market by sales[2,3] (see Figure 5.1). The Canadian pharmaceutical market has experienced strong growth and is the fourth fastest growing pharmaceutical industry after China, the United States, and Spain (see Figure 5.2). Generic drugs are more popular in the Canadian pharmaceutical industry than are brand names. The leading pharmaceutical company in Canada is Pfizer, while Apotex is the fifth largest pharmaceutical manufacturer but the leading generic producer.[4]

Figure 5.1 The Canadian Pharmaceutical Trade

The pharmaceutical trade has shown exceptional growth and vitality in the past ten years. Although exports regressed in value for the first time in 2008, this chart illustrates the spectacular growth of this industry in Canada.

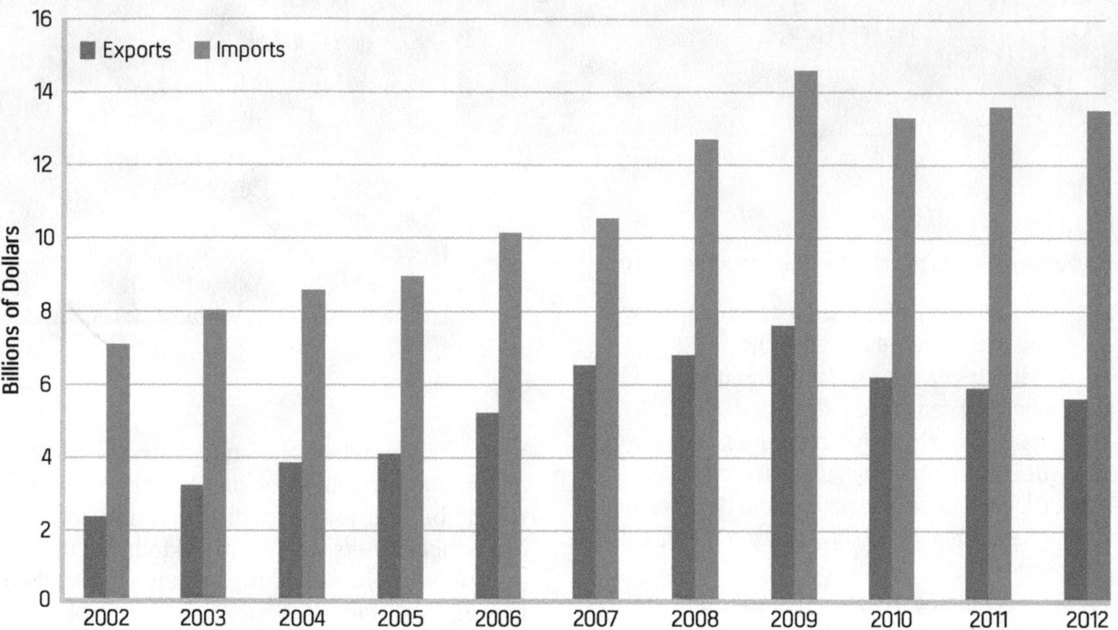

Source: Adapted from Industry Canada. Report 1: Canadian Total Exports of Pharmaceutical and Medicine Manufacturing for Latest Ten Years, Report 2: Canadian Total Imports of Pharmaceutical and Medicine Manufacturing for Latest Ten Years. 2008. Retrieved October 28, 2013.

For many of the largest-selling, still-patented drugs, Canadian pharmacy prices are often much lower than those of companies in the United States. In Canada, the lower prices are due to the increased regulation of pharmaceutical prices. The pervasive price control in Canada limits manufacturer's prices to the median price of seven reference nations.[5]

With such extensive sales, many people expect that billions of drugs are available. Not so. More than half of all prescriptions are filled with only 200 drugs.

Names of Drugs

Commercially available compounds have several kinds of names: brand, generic, and chemical. The **chemical name** of a compound gives a complete chemical description of the molecule and is derived from the rules of organic chemistry for naming any compound. Chemical names of drugs are rarely used except in a laboratory situation where biochemists or pharmacologists are developing and testing new drugs.

> **chemical name:** specifies the complete chemical description of a drug.
>
> **generic name:** specifies a particular chemical but not a particular brand.
>
> **brand name:** specifies a particular formulation and manufacturer of a drug.

Generic names are the official (i.e., legal) names of drugs and are listed in the *Compendium of Pharmaceuticals and Specialties* (CPS), Canada's leading source for drug information. Although a generic name refers to a specific chemical, it is usually shorter and simpler than the complete chemical name. Generic names are in the public domain, meaning they cannot be trademarked.

The **brand name** of a drug specifies a particular formulation and manufacturer, and the trademark belongs to that manufacturer. A brand name is usually quite simple and as meaningful (in terms of the indicated therapeutic use) as the company can make it. For example, the name Champix (Pfizer Canada) was chosen for the smoking cessation aid drug to indicate that it would mean victory over cigarette smoking. However, brand names are controlled by Health Canada, and overly suggestive ones are not approved. When a new chemical structure, a new way of manufacturing a chemical, or a new use for a chemical is discovered, it can be patented. Patent laws in Canada now protect drugs for 20 years (instead of the previous 17 years), and after that time the finding is available for use by anyone.[6] Having a patent means that for 20 years the company that has discovered and patented a drug can manufacture and sell it without direct competition. After that, other companies can apply to Health Canada to sell the "same" drug. Brand names, however, are copyrighted and protected by trademark laws. Therefore, the other companies have to use the drug's generic name or their own brand name. Health Canada requires these companies to submit samples to demonstrate that their version is chemically equivalent and to do studies to demonstrate that the tablets or capsules they are making will dissolve appropriately and result in blood levels similar to those of the original drug. When a drug "goes generic," the original manufacturer might reduce the price of the brand name product to remain competitive.

LO3 Categories of Drugs

A psychotropic substance or a psychoactive drug has an effect on the brain that results in temporary changes in thought processes, mood, and behaviour. Psychoactive drugs can be used recreationally to affect a person's consciousness (such as with alcohol), as an entheogen for spiritual purposes, and as medication (such as antidepressants for depression).

The classification of psychoactive drugs varies but most commonly depends on the effect of the drug on the brain. For example, amphetamine, cocaine, and nicotine are central nervous system (CNS) stimulants;

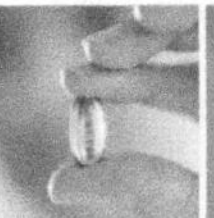

DRUGS IN DEPTH

Herbal Supplements

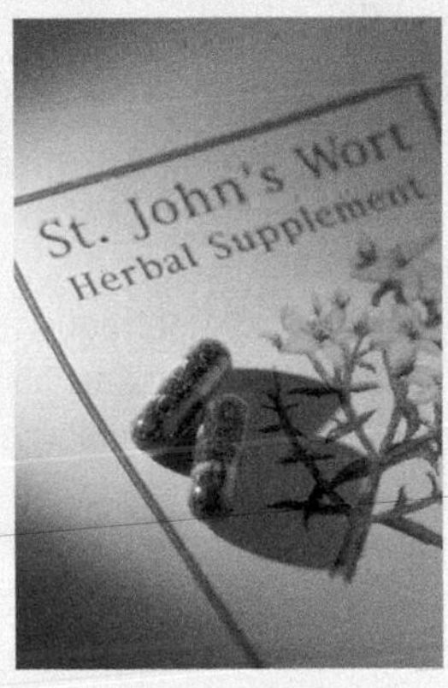

St. John's wort is used over the counter for depression but has many drug interactions.

St. John's wort, an herb that is believed to be helpful in relieving mild to moderate depression, should be taken only under a doctor's supervision. Health Canada's approval under the Natural Health Products Regulations is required for manufacturers of herbal supplements to sell their products. In a 2003 study looking at St. John's wort products bought in Canada and the United States, only a small fraction (2 out of 54) contained active ingredient; concentrations fell within 10% of what was claimed on the labels.[7] The Regulations, which came into effect at the beginning of 2004, helped to address the problem of quality, but St. John's wort does interact with other medications.

Foxglove is the common name for the *Digitalis purpurea* plant, from which the drug digitalis is obtained. The following quotation is taken from Earl Mindell's Herb Bible: "In 1775, English physician William Withering diagnosed a

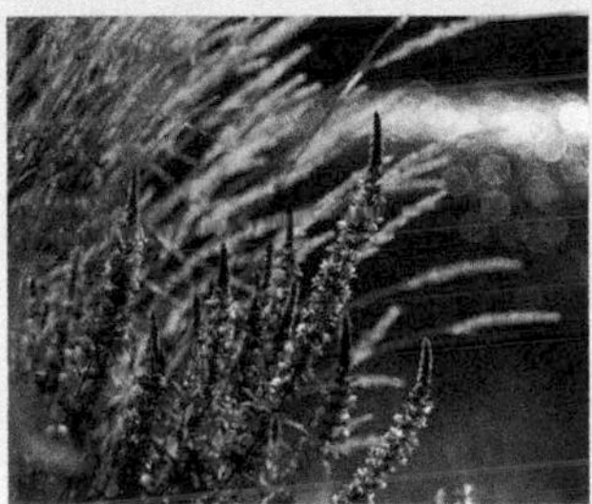

Digitalis purpurea

patient with congestive heart failure as hopeless and sent him home to die. A short time later, he learned that a local folk healer had cured his patient using a bunch of mysterious herbs. Amazed by the man's miraculous recovery, Withering investigated the herbs used by the healer and isolated foxglove (*Digitalis purpurea*) as the main ingredient. After performing several experiments, Withering discovered that this purple-flowered plant was a potent cardiotonic, that is, it improved the heart's pumping action, helping to rid the body of the excess fluid causing the congestion. Withering also learned that in wrong doses, foxglove could be lethal, triggering a fatal arrhythmia or irregularity in the heartbeat. For the next decade, Withering conducted numerous experiments to determine the precise amount of this drug needed to treat heart failure. He published his results in 1785, informing other physicians of this amazing new cure."[8] Digitalis is a highly efficacious treatment for heart failure. It does have unpredictable effects on the heart and must never be taken without a doctor's recommendation.[7]

Figure 5.2 Profitability by Gross Margin of Selected Industries in Canada, 2008

The pharmaceutical industry in Canada is one of the most profitable industry sectors after oil and gas extraction.

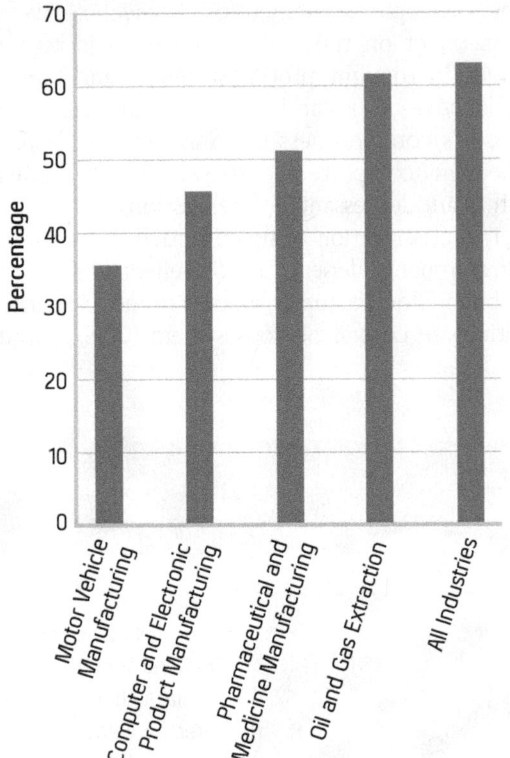

Source: Adapted from Industry Canada. Canadian Industry Statistics (CIS) (2011-11-28 [date modified]). Retrieved November 28, 2011, from http://www.ic.gc.ca/eic/site/cis-sic.nsf/eng/Home.

Figure 5.3 Most Commonly Used Injection Drugs in the Previous Three Months among Street Youth, 2003

Cocaine is the preferred injectable drug among Canadian street youth. ADHD experts report that in some rare occasions, the use of Ritalin to treat ADHD may increase a youth's propensity for cocaine and other stimulant addiction.

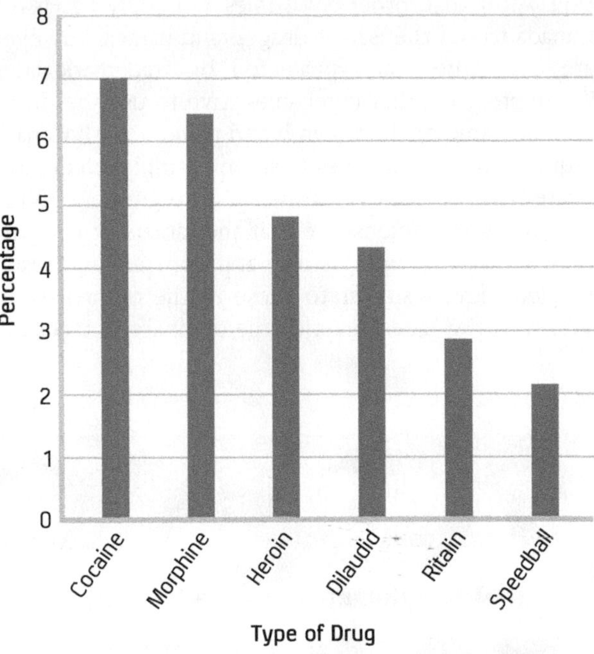

Source: Findings from Enhanced Surveillance of Canadian Street Youth, 1999–2003. Public Health Agency of Canada, 2007. Reproduced with permission from the Minister of Health, 2014.

barbiturates and alcohol are CNS depressants; morphine and codeine are analgesics (pain relievers); and LSD, ecstasy or MDMA, and PCP or angel dust are classified as hallucinogens or perception-altering agents (psychedelics).

Another class of drugs, psychotherapeutics, are used to treat psychological disorders (see Chapter 8). An example is Ritalin, an amphetamine-like prescription stimulant used to treat attention-deficit/hyperactivity disorder (ADHD). We are seeing an increase in Ritalin abuse by Canadian students[9] and street youth, who are attracted to its concentration-enhancing and stimulant effects. In the words of one user, "Coke's better. But Ritalin, it gives you the buzz and it gives you the—always you know, always want to do things, you know"[10] (see Figure 5.3 and the Drugs in the Media box).

The scheme presented in Figure 5.4 organizes the drugs according to their effects on the user, with first consideration given to the psychological effects. The figure gives the basic organization and examples of each type, but it is worthwhile to point out some of the defining characteristics of each major grouping.

At moderate doses, stimulant drugs produce wakefulness and a sense of energy and well-being. The more powerful stimulants, such as cocaine and amphetamines, can at high doses produce a manic state of excitement combined with paranoia and hallucinations. Conversely, withdrawal from chronic stimulant use can lead to decreased synaptic availability of the neurotransmitters dopamine (DA) and serotonin (5-HT), each associated with a constellation of symptoms (see Figure 5.5).

If you know about the behavioural effects of alcohol, then you know about the depressant drugs. At low doses they appear to depress inhibitory parts of the brain, leading to disinhibition or relaxation and talkativeness that can give way to recklessness. As the dose is increased, other neural functions become depressed, leading to slowed reaction times, uncoordinated movements, and unconsciousness. Stimulants and

DRUGS IN THE MEDIA

Prescription Amphetamine Abuse

Ritalin (methylphenidate), prescribed by doctors to treat attention-deficit/hyperactivity disorder (ADHD), stimulates the brain and body in a way similar to amphetamine and cocaine. It is not clear exactly how Ritalin works, but it helps people with ADHD reduce impulsive and hyperactive behaviour and pay attention to tasks. In school-age children, Ritalin has become a popular way to control difficult behaviours. Besides ADHD, Ritalin is also used to treat the sleep disorder known as narcolepsy, a condition that causes excessive sleepiness and the uncontrollable urge to sleep at inappropriate times. Unfortunately, Ritalin is abused by a small percentage of adults and youths who use it as a way to get high. How people who abuse Ritalin obtain the drug is a serious concern, with medications being stolen and, in some cases, children being bullied into giving up their medication. Abuse of Ritalin usually involves crushing pills into a powder so it can be snorted or dissolving them so it can be injected. Other similar medications such as Adderall (mixed amphetamine salts) are used by a small population of university and high school students to increase attention and prolong study hours. Flevated risks for prescription amphetamine abuse include highly competitive universities or private schools and its use has been referred to as "brain doping."[11] Use of prescription amphetamines by Canadian university students has been estimated at a high of 11%[12]; *Maclean's* magazine calls it "concentration for $5 a pill."[13]

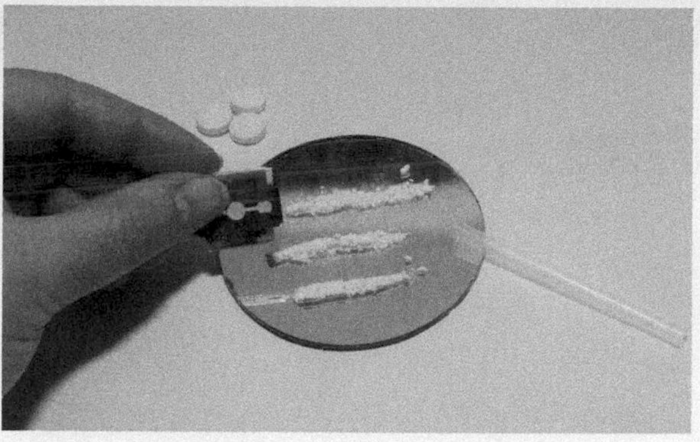

A small study conducted at the University of Toronto revealed that every student asked knew someone experimenting with Ritalin to help him or her either study or get high.

Some Canadian Statistics

- According to the Canadian Centre on Substance Abuse (CCSA), Canada is among the top 15 consumers of prescription amphetamines in the world[14]
- In a 2007 Newfoundland and Labrador study, 5.1% of students had used Ritalin without a prescription[15]
- In a 2011 study, 16 500 Ontario high school students reported using an ADHD drug for non-medical purposes[16]
- In a 2007 study, there was a significant drop among New Brunswick students using non-medical amphetamines and Ritalin (2.4% and 2%, down from 10.9% and 5.8%, respectively)[17]
- Health Canada estimates that 145 000 children are taking Ritalin in Canada. Purchasing pills from classmates, friends, and siblings with legitimate prescriptions is a major source for abusers[18]

Additional Sources: CBC Marketplace. *"Kiddie Coke": Using Ritalin to Get High.* 2003. Retrieved September 5, 2011, from http://www.cbc.ca/marketplace/pre-2007/files/health/ritalin/pageone.html; and Alberta Alcohol and Drug Commission. *ABCs of Ritalin (Methylphenidate).* 2003. Retrieved September 5, 2011, from http://www.adhdinfocentre.com/ritalin_2/abcs_ritalin.pdf.

depressants do not counteract each other. Although it may be possible to keep a drunk awake with cocaine, he or she would still be reckless, uncoordinated, and so on. Regular use of depressant drugs can lead to a **withdrawal syndrome** characterized by restlessness, shakiness, hallucinations, and sometimes convulsions when the intake of the drug is reduced.

Analgesics (pain relievers) include opioid drugs that produce a relaxed, dreamlike state; moderately high doses often induce sleep. Pharmacologically, this group is also known as the narcotics, and it is important to distinguish them from the "downers," or depressants. Opioids cause a clouding of consciousness without the reckless abandon, staggering, and slurred speech produced by alcohol and other depressants. Regular use of any of the opioids can lead to a withdrawal syndrome different from that of depressants and characterized by diarrhea, cramps, chills, and profuse sweating.

withdrawal syndrome: symptoms (e.g., muscle aches, anxiety attacks, sweating, nausea, convulsion, death) resulting from weaning of substance dependence.

Figure 5.4 Classification of Psychoactive Drugs

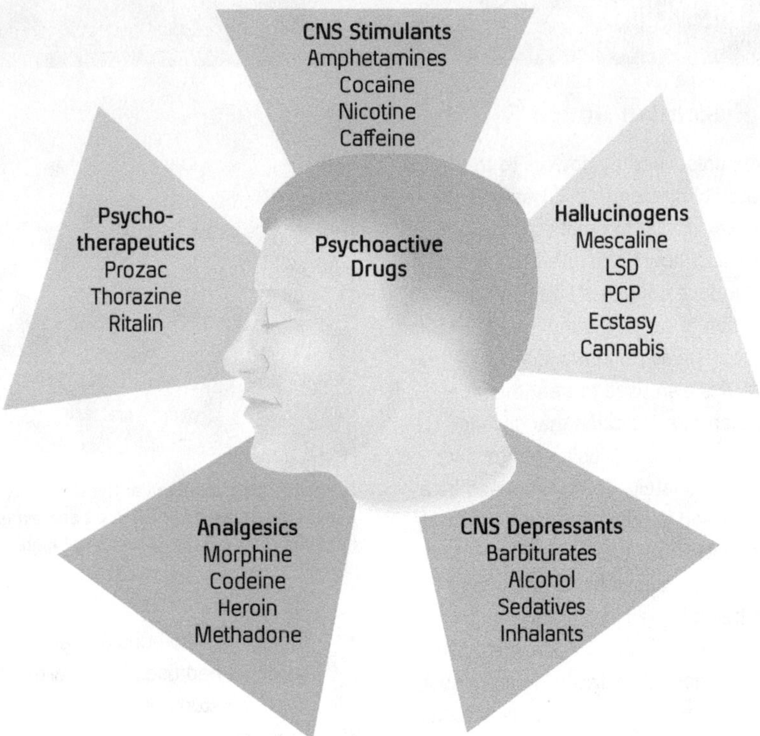

The hallucinogens produce altered perceptions, including unusual visual sensations and quite often changes in the perception of the person's own body.

The psychotherapeutic drugs include a variety of drugs prescribed by psychiatrists and other physicians for the control of mental health problems. The antipsychotics, such as haloperidol (Haldol), are also called neuroleptics. Chlorpromazine (Thorazine) was first synthesized in 1950 and became generally available for medical use in the mid-1950s (see Chapter 8). Neuroleptics can calm people experiencing psychosis and over time help them control hallucinations and illogical thoughts. The antidepressants, such as fluoxetine (Prozac), help some people recover more rapidly from seriously depressed mood states. Lithium is used to control manic episodes and to prevent mood swings in bipolar disorder.

As with any classification system, some things don't seem to fit into the classes. Nicotine and marijuana are two such drugs. Nicotine is often thought of as being a mild stimulant, but it also seems to have some of the relaxant properties of a low dose of a depressant. Marijuana is often thought of as a relaxant, depressive type of drug, but it doesn't share most of the features of that class. It is sometimes listed among the hallucinogens because at high doses it can produce altered perceptions, but that classification doesn't seem appropriate for the way most people use it.

LO4, LO5, LO6

Pharmacodynamics

Pharmacodynamics includes drug action and drug effects. Drug action refers to the interaction of the drug with its receptor; drug effects are the resulting behavioural, cognitive, and emotional changes that are produced following drug action.

Drug Effects

No matter what the drug or how much of it there is, it can't have an effect until it is taken. For there to be a drug effect, the drug must be brought together with a living organism. After a discussion of the basic concepts of drug movement in the body, you will be better able to understand such important issues as blood-alcohol concentration, the dependence potential of crack cocaine, and urine testing for marijuana use. What the drug does to the body is most often the reason we take the drug in the first place. We might like how it makes us feel whether we are sensation seeking or self-medicating to feel better.

Figure 5.5 The Dual-Deficit Model of Psychostimulant Addiction

According to the model, withdrawal from chronic stimulant use leads to decreased synaptic availability of dopamine (DA) and serotonin (5-HT) that, in turn, contributes to withdrawal symptoms, drug craving, and relapse. DA dysfunction underlies anhedonia (the inability to experience pleasure from what were enjoyable experiences) and psychomotor disturbances, whereas 5-HT dysfunction causes depressed mood, obsessive thoughts, and lack of impulse control. Protracted withdrawal phenomena are thought to contribute significantly to relapse. OCD is the abbreviation for obsessive-compulsive disorder.

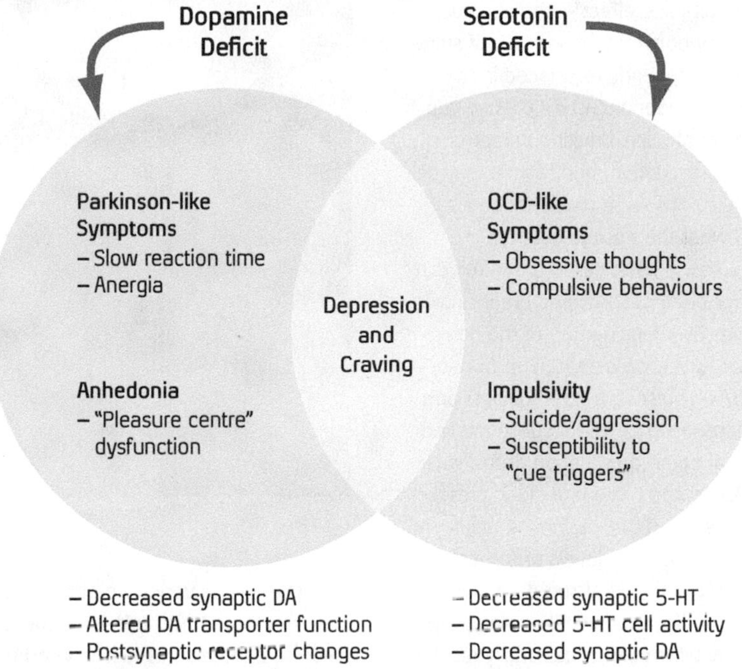

Source: Rothman, R. B., B. E. Blough, and M. H. Baumann. 2007. "Dual Dopamine/Serotonin Releasers as Potential Medications for Stimulant and Alcohol Addictions." *AAPS Journal* 9(1): E1–E10. Retrieved from http://www.aapsj.org/articles/aapsj0901/aapsj0901001/aapsj0901001.pdf.

Nonspecific (Placebo) Effects

The effects of a drug do not depend solely on chemical interactions with the body's tissues. With psychoactive drugs in particular, the influences of expectancy, experience, and setting are also important determinants of the drug's effect. For example, a good or bad "trip" on LSD seems to be more dependent on the experiences and mood of the user before taking the drug than on the amount or quality of drug taken. Even the effect of alcohol depends on what the user expects to experience. Nonspecific effects of a drug are those that derive from the user's unique background and particular perception of the world. In brief, the nonspecific effects include anything except the chemical activity of the drug and the direct effects of this activity. Nonspecific effects are also sometimes called placebo effects, because they can often be produced by a **placebo**, an inactive chemical that the user believes to be a drug.

The effects of a drug that depend on the presence of the chemical at certain concentrations in the target tissue are called specific effects. One important task for psychopharmacologists is to separate the specific effects of a drug from the nonspecific effects.

Suppose you design an experiment with two conditions. One group of people receives the drug you're interested in testing, in a dose that you have reason to believe should work. Each person in the second condition, or control group, receives a capsule that looks identical to the drug but contains no active drug molecules (a placebo). The people must be randomly assigned (random control trial or RCT) to the groups and be treated and evaluated identically except for the active drug molecules in the capsules for the experimental group. For this reason, tests for the effectiveness of a new drug must be done by using a **double-blind procedure**. Neither the participants nor the person

placebo: an inactive chemical or substance.

double-blind procedure: an experiment in which neither the researcher nor the participant knows whether the drug or a placebo is being used.

DRUGS IN THE MEDIA

The Grapefruit-Juice Effect

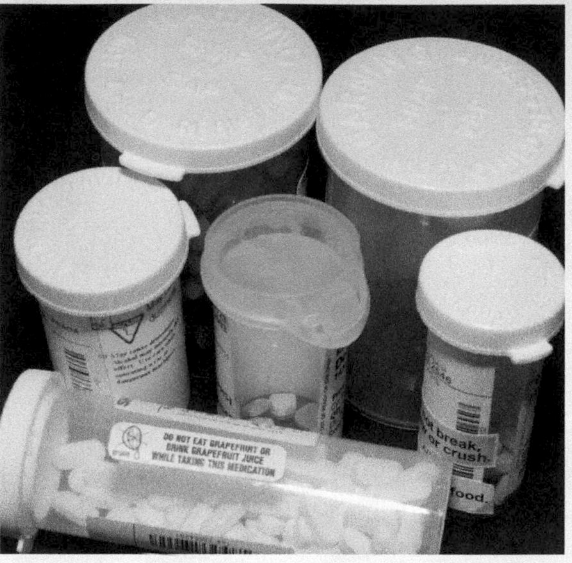

Reports about the "grapefruit-juice effect"—the observation that grapefruit juice may boost the absorption of some commonly prescribed drugs—recently resurfaced in the news, leaving some citrus fans wondering if it's OK to pop pills with their morning glass of juice. Drinking grapefruit juice to wash down some prescription medications may be dangerous because the juice can raise blood concentrations of the drug beyond what the dosage calls for.

Unlike other citrus juices, substances in grapefruit can interfere with the way your body absorbs and breaks down (metabolizes) certain drugs by inhibiting one of the body's intestinal enzyme systems "involving a specific isoform of cytochrome P450—CYP3A4—present in both the liver and the intestinal wall."[19] This interference can result in marked increases in serum levels of some prescription drugs, such as calcium-channel blockers used to control blood pressure and protease inhibitors given to treat HIV. An unknown chemical in grapefruit juice lowers the levels of a specific intestinal enzyme that normally breaks down drug molecules before they reach the bloodstream. This allows more of the drug to be absorbed, which can occasionally result in serious or life-threatening adverse reactions.

Although some drugs are prescribed with other drugs to enhance their effects, grapefruit juice should not be used for this purpose because its effects can be unpredictable and potentially dangerous. Only about one person in ten is affected, but in those who are, the juice can boost a drug's potency by as much as 40%.

As little as one glass of grapefruit juice (250 mL) can cause an increased blood drug level and the effects can last for three days or more. Therefore, even if you drink the juice in the morning and do not take your medication until bedtime, the level of the drug in your blood could still be affected.

The effects vary from one person to another, from one drug to another, and from one grapefruit juice preparation to another. This results in an unpredictable increase in blood drug level, which in some cases can cause serious effects.[20]

Although there has been considerable media focus on the grapefruit-juice effects, it is important to note that a number of other foods can alter the absorption or effects of some medications. For example, the absorption of tetracyclines, a class of antibiotics, is reduced by milk and dairy foods. This means that greater amounts of the antibiotic may be required to produce therapeutic effects. In Chapter 8, we discuss how some antidepressants can precipitate a hypertensive crisis when taken in combination with tyramine-containing foods (e.g., mature cheeses and soy sauce).

evaluating the drug's effect knows whether a particular individual is receiving a placebo or an experimental drug. Only after the experiment is over and the data have all been collected is the code broken so that the results can be analyzed.

Placebo effects have been shown to be especially important in two major kinds of therapeutic effects: treating pain (see Figure 5.6) and treating psychological depression. Therapeutic effects are the intended effects that treat a disease or an illness. The size of the placebo response in studies of depression has led to some recent controversy about just how effective antidepressants are. It has been known for the past 50 years that at least one-third of people who are psychologically depressed and are treated with placebos show improvement—in some published studies, the rates of placebo response have been even higher. One group of scientists reviewed all the data submitted to the U.S. Food and Drug Administration between 1987 and 2004 in support of new drug applications for 12

Figure 5.6 A Model Neuronal Network Explaining Placebo Analgesia-Related Activation of ACC Neurons

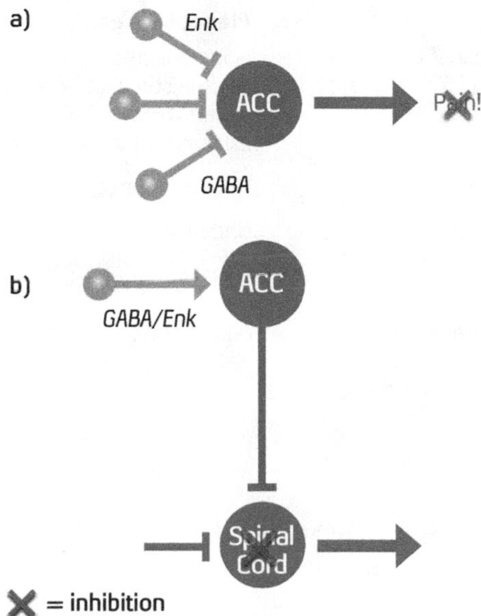

Source: A Model Neuronal Network Explaining Placebo Analgesia-Related Activation of ACC Neurons. Zhou, M. 2005. "Central Inhibition and Placebo Analgesia." *Molecular Pain* 1(21): 10.1186/1744-8069-1-21. Article retrieved from http://www.molecularpain.com/content/1/1/21.

of the most popular antidepressant medications on the U.S. market.[21] They concluded that about 80% of the effectiveness attributed to the antidepressant drugs could be obtained from a placebo.[22]

Placebos are substances with no active drug component that are often used in clinical trials where scientists want to show the effectiveness of their new drug on depression or pain. In both types of investigations scientists are finding that placebos (sometimes merely sugar pills) can relieve symptoms of depression and symptoms of pain. Does this mean the person is faking his or her symptoms? No, because if the experiment is designed correctly the person will not know (nor will the investigator) which pills (placebo or active drug) the person receives; this is called a double-blind study. So how can we explain the effects of these "sugar pills" on phenomena such as depression and pain? For pain, Zhou (2005) draws out a simple but elegant explanation (Figure 5.6). The use of a placebo leads to activation of inhibitory neurons within the anterior cingulate cortex (ACC), a structure that is part of the limbic system (see Chapter 4 for discussion of the limbic system). Inhibitory neurons mean that when these areas are activated they inhibit (or block) neural transmission, in this case for the perception of pain. These inhibitory neurons then release an inhibitory neurotransmitter: GABA. GABA is the major inhibitory neurotransmitter in the brain. In Figure 5.6(a), GABA acts on GABA receptors to inhibit ACC neurons that are involved in pain perception. In some neurons, another neurotransmitter, enkephalin (Enk), may also be released to produce similar inhibitory effects. How does the ACC inhibit pain? It is thought that GABA neurons may inhibit ACC neurons, as shown in Figure 5.6(b). If the ACC neurons are inhibited, so are the neural pathways in the spinal cord that transmit pain signals. Therefore, pain is reduced; this is referred to as an analgesic effect. For example, if you jam your finger in a car door, the pain signals from your finger are carried to an area of your brain that perceives pain. If the ACC inhibits the transmission of pain signals to the brain, you experience little or no pain.

Nonspecific effects are not caused by the chemicals in drugs, but they are still real effects that have a biological basis (see Table 5.1). A recent study of nonspecific drug effects used a technique known as quantitative electroencephalography, in which electrical activity was recorded from multiple electrodes placed on patients' heads. In a group of patients who were initially depressed, 38% of those treated with a placebo showed improved mood scores during the nine-week study. Those who showed improvement after placebo treatment were also likely to show changes in the electrical responses from the prefrontal cortex. Among the patients treated with either of two active antidepressant drugs 52% improved, and they showed a different pattern of electrical changes from the patients treated with a placebo.[23]

Dose–Response Relationships

Perhaps the strongest demonstration of the specific effects of a drug is obtained when the dose of the drug is varied and the size of the effect changes directly with the drug dose. A graph showing the relationship between the dose and the effect is called a **dose-response curve**. Typically, at very low doses no effect is seen. At some low dose, an effect on the response system being monitored is observed. This dose is the threshold, and as the dose of the drug is increased there are more molecular interactions and a greater effect on the response system. At the point where the system shows maximal response, further additions of the drug have no effect.

dose–response curve: a graph comparing the size of response to the amount of drug.

Table 5.1 Investigation of the Placebo Effect

Study Design	Groups	Objective	Placebo Effect
Standard two-group RCT*	Active drug and placebo	Study the efficacy of the active drug (with control for the placebo effect)	Not measured directly; comparison with baseline values gives inaccurate estimates of the placebo effect
Other two-group RCT	Placebo and untreated	Study the placebo effect	Underestimated
Standard three-group RCT	Active drug, placebo, and untreated	Study both the efficacy of the active drug (with control for the placebo effect) and the placebo effect	Underestimated
Multi-group RCT	Patients allocated to one of several doses of an active drug (or to one of several active drugs), to the placebo group, or to the untreated group	Study both the efficacy of the active drug (with control for the placebo effect) and the placebo effect	Potentially overestimated

*RCT (random control trial).

Source: De la Fuente-Fernández, R., M. Schulzer, and A. J. Stoessl. 2005. "The Placebo Effect in Neurological Disorders." *Lancet Neurology* 1: 85–91.

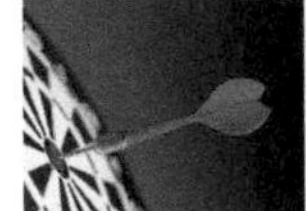

TARGETING PREVENTION

The Right Dose

One of the most important principles of pharmacology, and of much of research in general, is a concept called "dose–response" (see Figure 5.7). Just as the term implies, this notion refers to the relationship between some effect—let's say, lowering of blood pressure—and the amount of a drug. Scientists care a lot about dose–response data because these mathematical relationships signify that a medicine is working according to a specific interaction between different molecules in the body.

Sometimes it takes years to figure out exactly which molecules are working together, but when testing a potential medicine, researchers must first show that three things are true in an experiment. First, if the drug isn't there, you don't get any effect. In our example, that means no change in blood pressure. Second, adding more of the drug (up to a certain point) causes an incremental change in effect (lower blood pressure with more drug). Third, taking the drug away (or masking its action with a molecule that blocks the drug) means there is no effect.

Scientists most often plot data from dose–response experiments on a graph. A typical dose–response curve demonstrates the effects of what happens (the vertical Y-axis) when more and more drug is added to the experiment (the horizontal X-axis).

Source: The National Institutes of Health, "The Right Dose." http://publications.nigms.nih.gov/medbydesign/chapter1.html.

Figure 5.7 The Right Dose

Dose–response curves determine how much of a drug (X-axis) causes a particular effect, or a side effect, in the body (Y-axis).

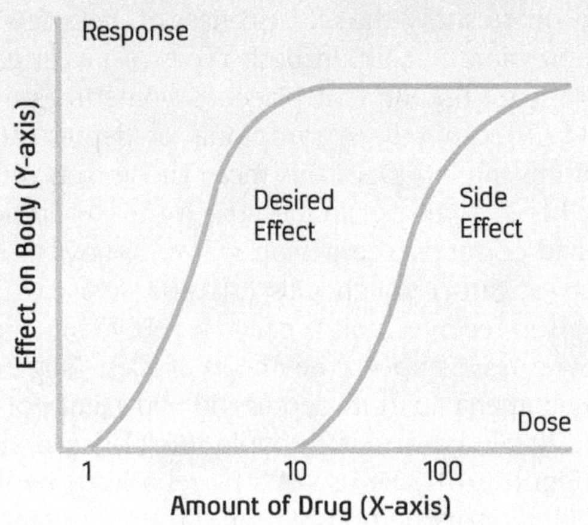

Source: Used with permission. http://publications.nigms.nih.gov/medbydesign/chapter1.html

Figure 5.8 Relationships between Alcohol Dose and Multiple Responses

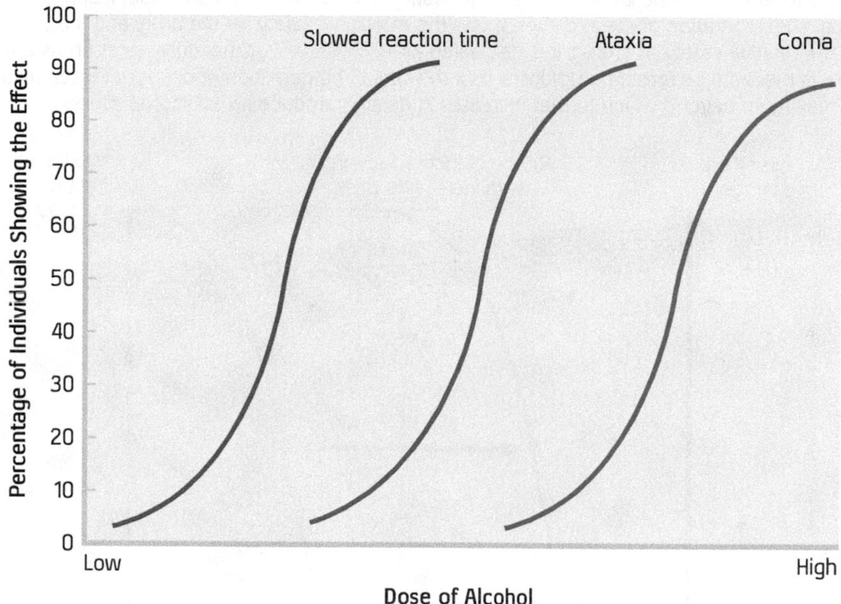

At higher drug dosages, increasing the dose does not increase a particular drug effect per se but will potentially increase other effects of the drug. Figure 5.8 shows a series of dose-response curves for three different effects of alcohol.

As the dose increases from the low end, an increasing number of people show a slowing of their reaction times. If we also have a test for **ataxia** (staggering or inability to walk straight), we see that, as the alcohol dose reaches the level at which most individuals are showing slowed reaction times, a few are also beginning to show ataxia. As the dose increases further, more people show ataxia, and some become **comatose** (they pass out and cannot be aroused). At the highest dose indicated, all the individuals would be comatose. We could draw curves for other effects of alcohol on such a figure; for example, at the high end we would begin to see some deaths from overdose, and a curve for lethality could be placed to the right of the coma curve. Figure 5.9 illustrates this concept by using the analgesic agent morphine.

In the rational use of drugs, four questions about drug dosage must be answered. First, what is the effective dose of the drug for a desired goal? For example, what dose of morphine is necessary to reduce pain? What amount of marijuana is necessary for an individual to feel euphoric? How much Aspirin will make the headache go away? The second question is what dose of the drug will be toxic to the individual? Combining those two, the third question is what the safety margin is–how different are the effective dose and the toxic dose? Finally, at the effective dose level, what other effects, particularly adverse reactions, might develop? Leaving aside for now this last question, a discussion of the first three deals with basic concepts necessary in understanding drug actions.

Estimating the safety margin is an important part of the preclinical (animal) testing that is done on any new drug before it is tried in humans. To determine an effective dose (ED), it is necessary to define an effect in animals that is meaningful in terms of the desired

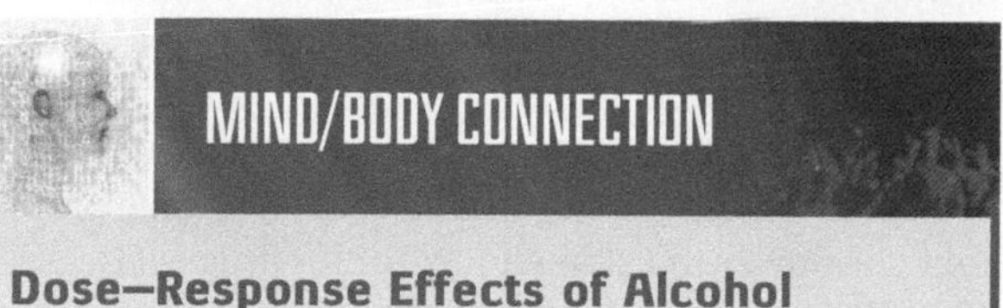

Dose–Response Effects of Alcohol

The first draught serveth for health, the second for pleasure, the third for shame, and the fourth for madness.

—Anacharsis

Source: http://www.brainyquote.com/quotes/quotes/a/anacharsis183134.html#HcuvO301A6UF8upM.99

ataxia: uncoordinated walking.

comatose: unconscious and unable to be aroused.

Figure 5.9 Dose–Response Curves for the Analgesic and Respiratory Depressant Effect of Morphine

The dose–response curve for the analgesic effects of a drug is usually quite distinct from the dose–response curve for the toxic effects of the same drug. The separation of these curves shows the margin of safety for the drug, and the therapeutic index (TI) is a quantitative index of the relative safety of a drug. It is calculated as $TI = TD_{50}/ED_{50}$; therefore, safer drugs tend to have larger TIs. Also shown in this figure is that with increasing drug doses past threshold (the detection of changes incited by the drug) there are increased effects, to a maximum beyond which further increases in dosage produce no additional effects.

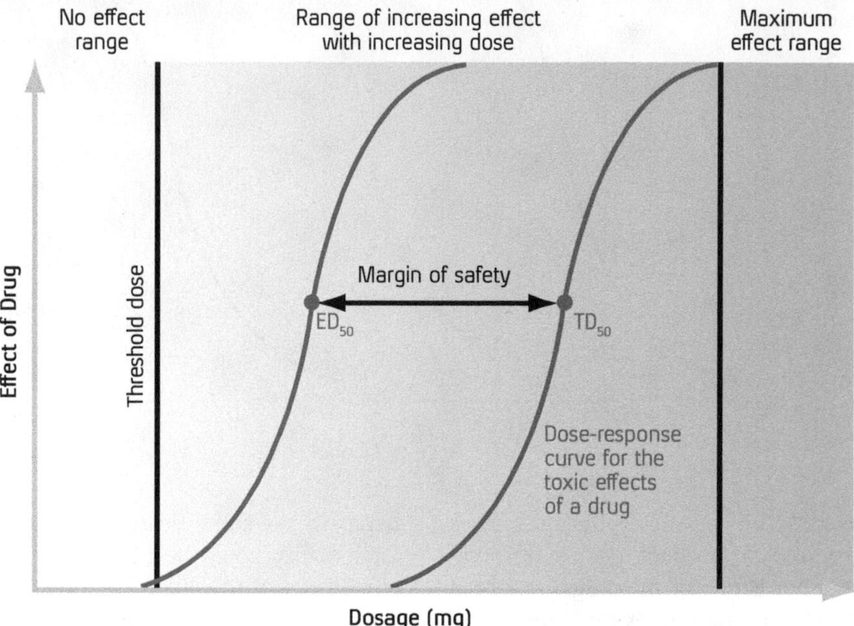

human use, although in some cases this is difficult. Say we will test a new sleeping pill (a hypnotic) on several groups of 20 mice each. Each group will receive a different dose, and an hour later we will check to see how many mice in each group are sleeping. Let us assume that at the lowest dose we tested, only 1 of the 20 mice was asleep, and at the highest doses all were asleep, with other values in between. By drawing a line through these points, we can estimate the dose required to put half of the mice to sleep (the **ED_{50}**, or the effective dose for 50% of the animals).

Toxicity is usually measured in at least one early animal study by determining how many mice die as a result of the drug. Let's say we check each cage the next day to see how many mice in each group died. From such a study we can estimate the **LD_{50}** (lethal dose for 50% of the mice). The **therapeutic index (TI)** is defined as LD_{50}/ED_{50}. Since the lethal dose should be larger than the effective dose, the TI should always be greater than 1. How large should the TI be if the company is going to go forward with expensive clinical trials? It depends partly on the TIs of the drugs already available for the same purpose. If the new drug has a greater TI than existing drugs, it is likely to be safer when given to humans.

This approach of estimating the dose to affect 50% of the mice is used in early animal tests because it is statistically more reliable to estimate the 50% point by using a small number of mice per group than it is to estimate the 1% or 99% points. However, with humans we don't do LD_{50} experiments but will take note of toxic or unwanted side effects of the drugs (TD_{50}). The TI in this case is defined as TD_{50}/ED_{50}. With some disorders, the best drugs available can help only half of the people. What we ultimately want is to estimate the dose that will produce a desired effect in the most people and without producing some unacceptable toxic reaction. The difference between these doses is called the **safety margin**.

ED_{50}: in animal drug trials, the effective dose for half of the animals tested.

LD_{50}: in animal drug trials, the lethal dose for half of the animals tested.

therapeutic index (TI): the ratio of LD_{50} to ED_{50}.

safety margin: the dosage difference between an acceptable level of effectiveness and the lowest toxic dose.

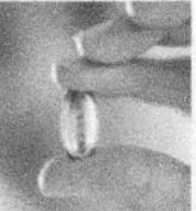

DRUGS IN DEPTH

The Placebo Effect

In a study conducted in 2005 at the University of Toronto, Zhuo investigated the neuronal mechanisms underlying placebo analgesia. Endogenous opioids in the CNS contribute to placebo analgesia and such effects are blocked if patients are given the opioid receptor antagonist naloxone. The anterior cingulate cortex (ACC) was previously identified, through human brain imaging, as being active during both placebo analgesia and opioid analgesia. The connections of the ACC to areas known to be involved in pain perception, such as midbrain periaqueductal grey (PAG), somehow activate the endogenous analgesia system originating from these areas, producing analgesic effects. Zhuo proposed a model neuronal network explaining placebo analgesia relating to the activation of the ACC (refer to Figure 5.6). These data support a role for neurotransmitter release in the nonspecific effects of placebos and challenge existing paradigms about placebo effects.[24]

Figure 5.10 Pet Scans

In these PET scans of a person with Parkinson's disease, the lower radioactivity observed in the striatum after placebo (saline injection; right) reflects increased occupancy of striatal D_2 receptors by dopamine (i.e., after placebo-induced dopamine release).

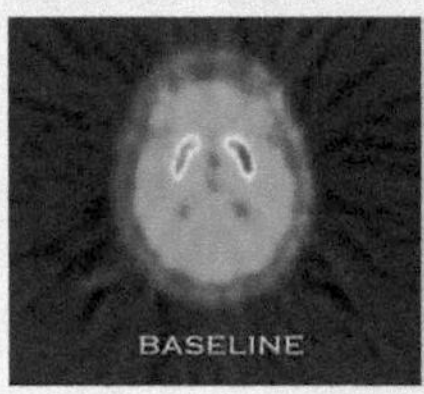

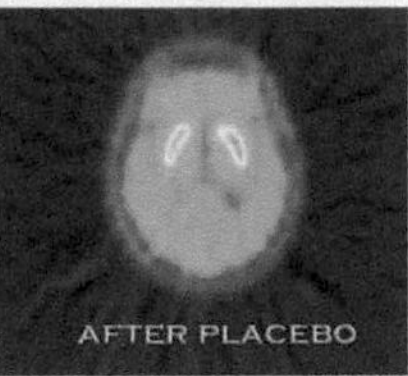

The placebo effect is not restricted to analgesia. At the University of British Columbia, Fuente-Fernández, Schulzer,

Figure 5.11 Theoretical Schematic of the Role of the Reward Circuitry in the Placebo Effect

Dopamine-producing neurons arising in the ventral midbrain (ventral tegmental area, VTA) that send projections to the ventral striatum (including the nucleus accumbens, NAcc) are activated by placebo-induced expectation of clinical benefit, which is a form of expectation of reward. This represents the permissive component of the placebo response (purple). Dopamine neurons in the prefrontal cortex (PFC) affect the activity of opioid, dopamine (DA), and serotonin (5-HT) transmission in other brain areas that control placebo responses, including a reduction in pain (placebo analgesia), improvement in motor performance in Parkinson's disease, and reduced depression. This pathway represents the cognitive component of the placebo effect (orange). The permissive component is common to all placebo effects, whereas the cognitive component is unique to the disease or condition of the patient. In this case, *placebo* refers to the actual placebo itself and to the environmental context in which the placebo is administered, which also may produce anticipatory effects as the result of conditioning.

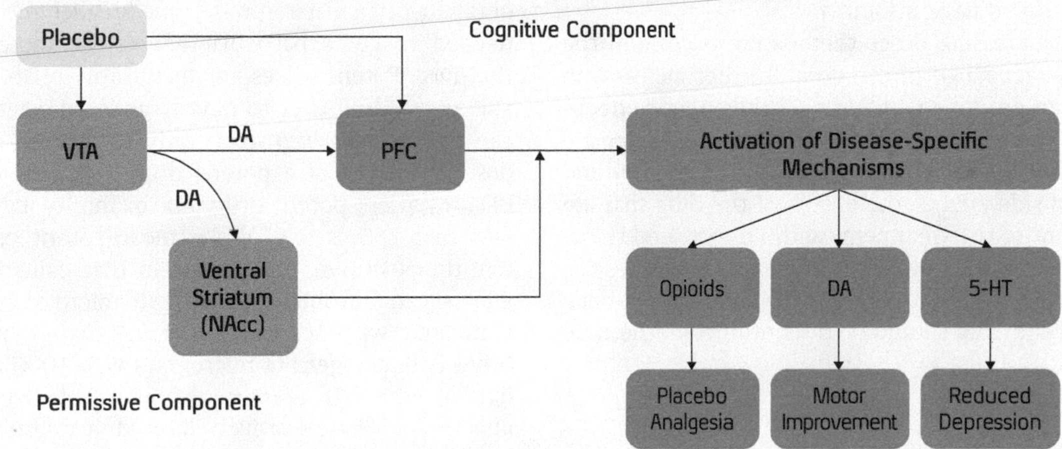

continued

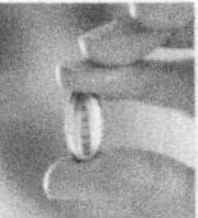

DRUGS IN DEPTH

The Placebo Effect

continued

and Stoessl proposed criteria for the investigation of the placebo effect with respect to Parkinson's disease, depression, and other neurological disorders.[25] In their paper published in *The Lancet*, they also discuss the evidence for the use of placebos in long-term substitution programs for the treatment of drug addiction (see Figure 5.10). The commonality of all these disorders is the involvement of the mesocorticolimbic and nigrostriatal dopaminergic system and the neural circuits involved in reward-related mechanisms.

Lidstone and colleagues at the Pacific Parkinson's Research Centre in Vancouver argue that while the placebo effect is mediated by the activation of the reward circuitry of the mesocorticolimbic dopamine system, patient expectation of a benefit plays a critical role (see Figure 5.11).[25] The suggestion of the use of placebos as a long-term strategy for the treatment of drug addiction is especially intriguing.

Sources: Levine J.D., N.C. Gordon, and H.L. Fields. 1978. "The Mechanism of Placebo Analgesia." *Lancet 2:* 654–657; Petrovic, P., E. Kalso, K.M. Petersson, and M. Ingvar. 2002. "Placebo and Opioid Analgesia—Imaging a Shared Neuronal Network." *Science 295:* 1737–1740; Wei, F., P. Li, and M. Zhuo. 1999. "Loss of Synaptic Depression in Mammalian Anterior Cingulate Cortex after Amputation." *Journal of Neuroscience 19:* 9346–9354; Tanaka, E. and R.A. North. 1994. "Opioid Actions on Rat Anterior Cingulate Cortex Neurons in Vitro." *Journal of Neuroscience 14:* 1106–1113; Basbaum, A.I. and H.L. Fields. 1984. "Endogenous Pain Control Systems: Brainstem Spinal Pathways and Endorphin Circuitry." *Annual Review of Neuroscience 7:* 309–338; Zhou, M. 2005. "Central Inhibition and Placebo Analgesia." *Molecular Pain 1*(21): doi 10.1186/1744-8069-1-21.

Most of the psychoactive compounds have an LD_1 (dosage required to kill 1% of the population) well above the ED_{95} (the dose of a drug that produces a desired effect in 95% of the population) level, so the practical limitation on whether or not, or at what dose, a drug is used is the occurrence of **side effects** (the effects of the drug that are not relevant to the treatment). It should be pointed out that side effects are not always bad things, even though this is the common perception. For example, medication that has the side effect of drowsiness may be beneficial at bedtime, especially if you have insomnia.

With increasing doses there is no increase in the maximal effect range of the drug. Further increases in drug dosing produce no additional therapeutic effects. Increased drug doses beyond maximum effect range are usually associated with an increase in the number and severity of side effects–the effects of the drug that are not relevant to the treatment, with no increased therapeutic effect. If the number of side effects becomes too great and the individual begins to suffer from them, the use of the drug should be discontinued or the dose lowered, even though the drug may be very effective in controlling the original symptoms. The selection of a drug for therapeutic use should be made on the basis of effectiveness in treating the symptoms with minimal side effects.

side effects: the unintended effects that accompany therapeutic effects.

potency: measured by the amount of drug (dose) required to produce an effect.

Potency

The **potency** of a drug is one of the most misunderstood concepts in the area of drug use. Potency refers only to the amount of drug that must be given to obtain a particular response. The smaller the amount needed to get a particular effect, the more potent the drug. Potency does not necessarily relate to how effective a drug is or to how large an effect the drug can produce. *Potency* refers only to relative effective dose; the ED_{50} of a potent drug is lower than the ED_{50} of a less potent drug. For example, it has been said that LSD is one of the most potent psychoactive drugs known. This is true in that hallucinogenic effects can be obtained with 50 micrograms (mcg), compared with several milligrams (mg) required of other hallucinogens (a microgram is 1/1000 of a milligram, which is 1/1000 of a gram). However, the effects of LSD are relatively limited–it doesn't lead to overdose deaths the way heroin and alcohol do. Alcohol has a greater variety of more powerful effects than LSD, even though in terms of the dose required to produce a psychological effect, LSD is thousands of times more potent.

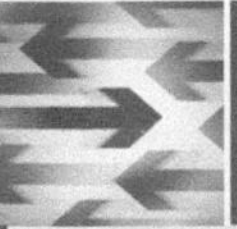

TAKING SIDES

Animal Toxicity Tests

Increasing interest in the welfare of laboratory animals has resulted in improved standards for housing, veterinary care, and anaesthesia. Some animal rights groups have suggested that most types of animal research should be stopped because the experiments are either unnecessary or misleading. The use of the LD_{50} test by drug companies, in which the researchers estimate the dose of a drug required to kill half the animals (usually mice), has been a particular target. The groups have claimed that these tests are outmoded and that toxicity could be predicted from computer models or work on isolated cell cultures.

A pamphlet published by People for the Ethical Treatment of Animals (PETA), a well-known animal rights group, claims on the one hand that the laboratory animals are sensitive beings with "distinct personalities, just like you and me," but on the other hand that toxicity tests on animals are not relevant to humans because of basic biological differences. In reality, most basic biological functions are quite similar among all mammals, whereas the greatest differences between laboratory mice and humans would probably be found in the areas of thoughts, emotions, and "personality."

A specific case cited by PETA was thalidomide testing, which it claims "passed animal safety tests with flying colors" and later caused thousands of human deformities. Some critical points in that argument were omitted, however. Thalidomide caused birth defects when taken during pregnancy. Otherwise, its human toxicity was quite low. Thalidomide was not tested on pregnant animals. If it had been, the birth defects would have been detected. And because of thalidomide, the laws were changed more than 30 years ago to require that drugs to be used by humans during pregnancy first undergo testing in pregnant animals.

Admittedly, giving drugs to pregnant animals to see if they produce birth defects or spontaneous abortions may seem cruel, but animal research is invaluable to the design of drugs safe for humans. Computer models have their uses, but they are limited in their predictive powers and are only as good as the physiological data that go into them. Would you volunteer to be the first living animal to take a new drug whose toxicity had been estimated by a computer model? Animal research saves lives.[26]

LO7 Pharmacokinetics of Drug Action

In addition to the chemical structures of drugs and whether they are designed as cardiogenic drugs, such as digitalis, or have mood-enhancing properties, such as St. John's wort, additional factors affect drug action and these include pharmacokinetic factors. Pharmacokinetics can be thought of as how drugs move through the body, and it includes **drug absorption**, **drug distribution**, **drug metabolism**, and **drug excretion** (ADME) (see Figure 5.12).

Time-Dependent Factors in Drug Actions

In the mouse experiment described earlier, we picked one hour after administering the drug to check for the sleeping effect. Obviously, we would have had to learn a bit about the **time course** of the drug's effect before picking one hour. Some very rapidly acting drug might have put the mice to sleep within 10 minutes and be wearing off by one hour, and we would pick a 20- or 30-minute time to check the effect of that drug. Absorption of a drug may be delayed in time-release preparations that are designed such that one dose of the drug will last the entire day or night.[27] The time course of a drug's action depends on many things, including how the drug is administered, how rapidly it is absorbed, and how it is eliminated from the body.

Figure 5.13 describes one type of relationship between administration of a drug and its effect over time. Between points A and B no effect is observed, although

drug absorption: the passage of a drug from the site of administration to the circulatory system.

drug distribution: the movement of drugs to and from the blood and various tissues of the body (for example, fat, muscle, and brain tissue).

drug metabolism: the process by which the body breaks down drugs.

drug excretion: the removal of drugs from the body.

time course: the timing of the onset, duration, and termination of a drug's effect.

Figure 5.12 Pharmacokinetics

Pharmacokinetics describes the absorption, distribution, metabolism, and excretion of drugs (ADME) in the body.

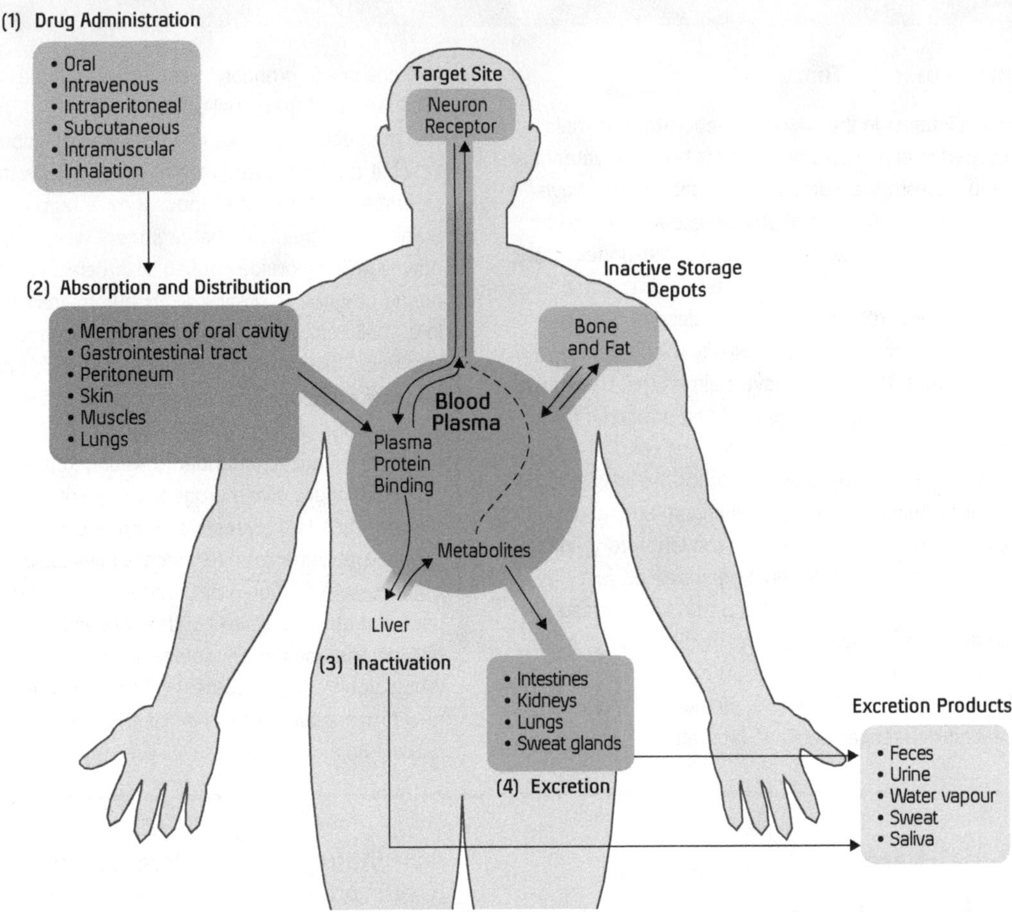

the concentration of drug in the blood is increasing. At point B the threshold concentration is reached, and from B to C the observed drug effect increases as drug concentration increases. At point C the maximal effect of the drug is reached, but its concentration continues increasing to point D. Although deactivation of the drug probably begins as soon as the drug enters the body, from A to D the rate of absorption is greater than the rate of deactivation. Beginning at point D the deactivation proceeds more rapidly than absorption, and the concentration of the drug decreases. When the amount of drug in the body reaches E, the maximal effect is over. The action diminishes from E to F, at which point the level of the drug is below the threshold for effect, although the drug is still in the body up to point G.

If the relationship described in Figure 5.13 is true for a particular drug, then increasing the dose of the drug will not increase the magnitude of its effect. Aspirin and other headache remedies are probably the most misused drugs in this respect–if two are good, four should be better, and six will really stop this headache. No way! When the maximum possible therapeutic effect has been reached, increasing the dose primarily adds to the number of side effects. The **efficacy** of a drug is its ability to produce a desired behavioural effect. Two Aspirins are efficacious in relieving a headache.

The usual way to obtain a prolonged effect is to take an additional dose at some time after the first dose has reached its maximum concentration and started to decline. The appropriate interval varies from one drug to another. If doses are taken too close together, the maximum blood level will increase with each dose and can result in **cumulative effects**.

efficacy: a drug's ability to produce a desired behavioural effect.

cumulative effects: the effects of giving multiple doses of the same drug.

Figure 5.13 Possible Relationships between Drug Concentration in the Body and Measured Effect of the Drug

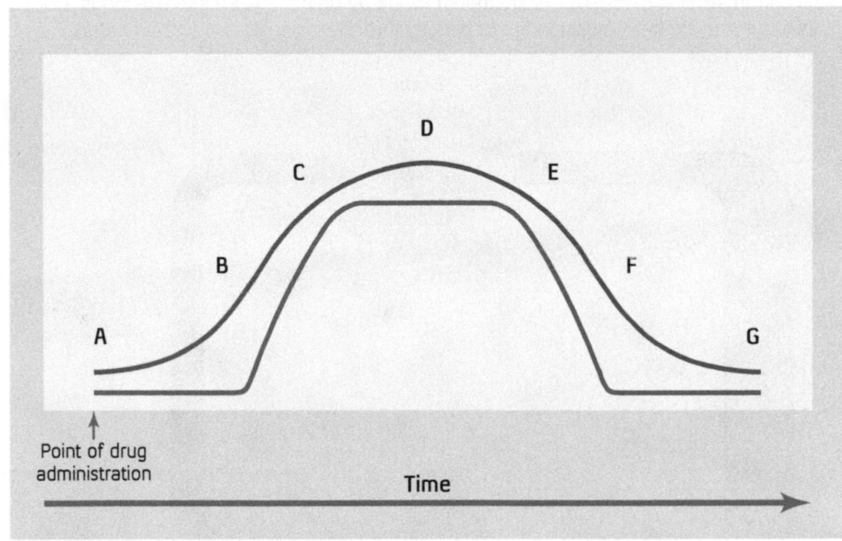

One of the important changes in the manufacture of drugs is the development of **controlled-release** preparations. These compounds are prepared so that after oral ingestion the active ingredient is released into the body over a six- to ten-hour period. With a preparation of this type, a large amount of the drug is initially made available for absorption, and then smaller amounts are released continually for a long period. The initial amount of the drug is expected to be adequate to obtain the response desired, and the gradual release thereafter is designed to maintain the same effective dose of the drug even though the drug is being continually deactivated. In terms of Figure 5.13, a time-release preparation would aim at eliminating the unnecessarily high drug level at C–D–E while lengthening the C–E time interval.

LO8 Mechanisms of Drug Action: Getting the Drug to the Brain

The chemistry of drug molecules determines whether drugs act quickly and slowly. The importance of lipid solubility will become clear as we see how molecules get into the brain.

A Little Chemistry

One of the most important considerations of whether a drug will get into the brain is the **lipid solubility** of the molecules. Shake up some salad oil with some water, let it stand, and the oil floats on top. When other chemicals are added, sometimes they "prefer" to be concentrated more in the water or in the oil. For example, if you put sodium chloride (table salt) in with the oil and water and shake it all up, most of the salt will stay with the water. If you crush a garlic clove and add it to the mix, most of the chemicals that give garlic its flavour will remain in the oil. The extent to which a chemical can be dissolved in oils and fats is called its lipid solubility. Most psychoactive drugs dissolve to some extent in either water or lipids, and in our oil-and-water experiment some fraction of the drug would be found in each.

Routes of Administration

We rarely put chemicals directly into our brains. All psychoactive drugs reach the brain tissue by way of the bloodstream. Most psychoactive drugs are taken by one of three basic routes: by mouth (enteral), injection (parenteral), or inhalation (topical) (see Figure 5.14).

Enteral Administration Enteral routes of drug administration involve the digestive tract and involve orally taking the drug or using a suppository (rectal/vaginal).

controlled release: a dosage form for drugs that are released or are activated over time.

lipid solubility: the tendency of a chemical to dissolve in fat, as opposed to in water.

Figure 5.14 Routes of Drug Administration and Distribution of Drugs through the Body

Drugs can enter the body through several mechanisms: by mouth (oral), by being inhaled into the lungs, or by being injected under the skin (subcutaneous), into the muscle (intramuscularly), or directly into the bloodstream (intravenous).

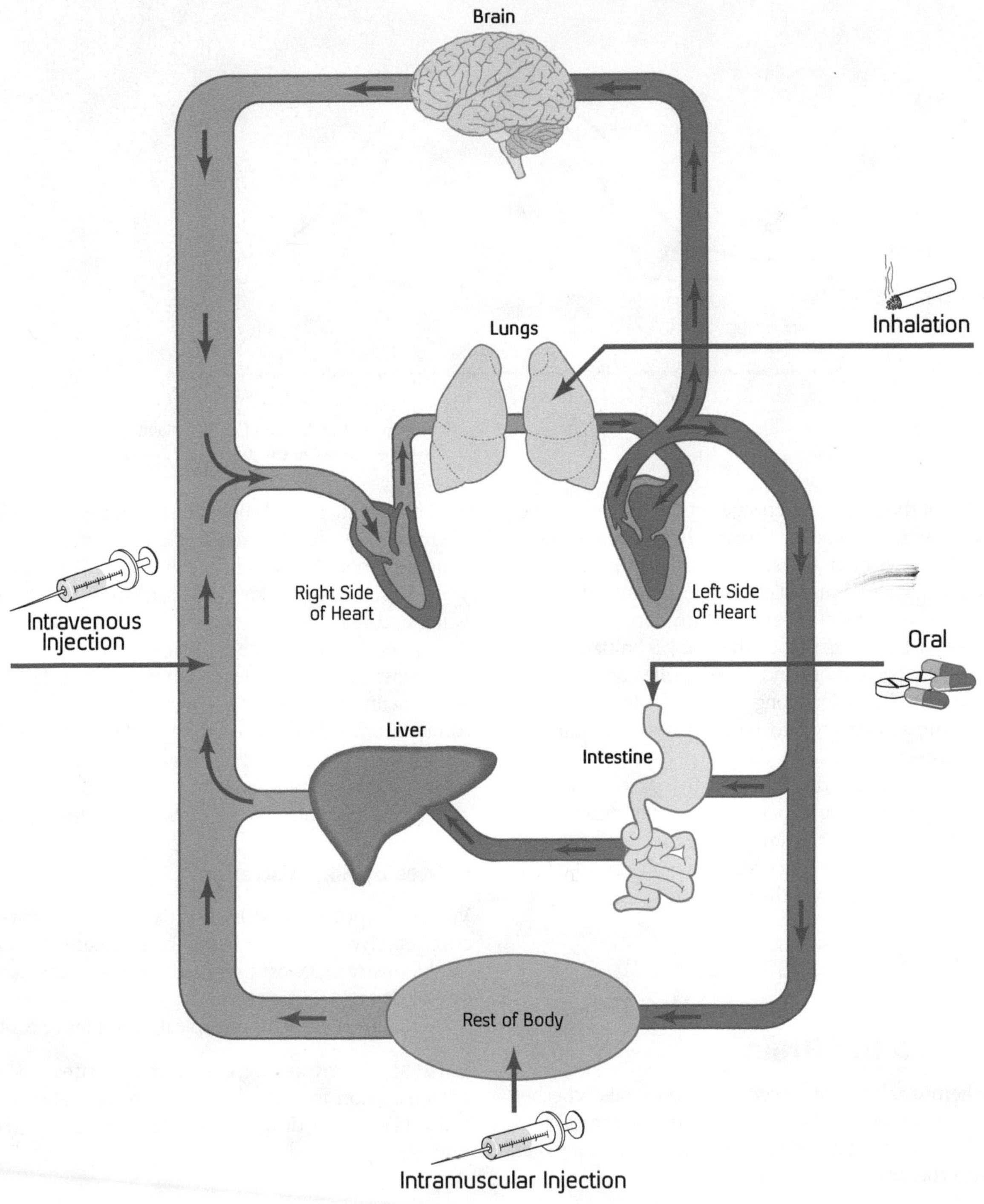

Oral Administration Most drugs begin their grand adventure in the body by entering through the mouth. Even though oral intake might be the simplest way to take a drug, absorption from the gastrointestinal tract is the most complicated way to enter the bloodstream. A chemical in the digestive tract must withstand the actions of stomach acid and digestive enzymes and not be deactivated by food before it is absorbed. The antibiotic tetracycline provides a good example of the dangers in the gut for a drug. This antibiotic readily combines with calcium ions to form a compound that is poorly absorbed. If tetracycline is taken with milk (calcium ions), blood levels will never be as high as if it were taken with a different beverage.

The drug molecules must next get through the cells lining the wall of the gastrointestinal tract and into the blood capillaries. If taken in capsule or tablet form, the drug must first dissolve and then, as a liquid, mix into the contents of the stomach and intestines. However, the more other material there is in the stomach, the greater the dilution of the drug and the slower it will be absorbed. The drug must be water soluble for the molecules to spread throughout the stomach. However, only lipid-soluble and very small water-soluble molecules are readily absorbed into the capillaries surrounding the small intestine, where most absorption into the bloodstream occurs.

Once in the bloodstream, the dangers of entering through the oral route are not over. The veins from the gut go first to the liver (see Figure 5.14). If the drug is the type that is metabolized rapidly by the liver (nicotine is one example), very little may get into the general circulation. Thus, nicotine is much more effective when inhaled than when swallowed.

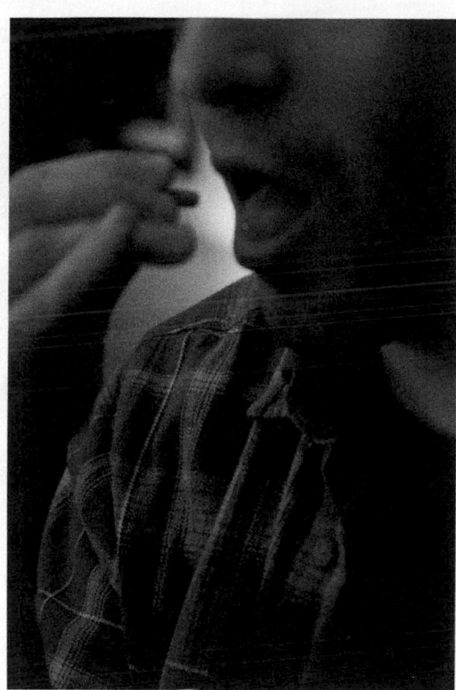

Absorption of a drug into the bloodstream through the gastrointestinal tract is a complicated process.

Rectal/Vaginal Administration Both rectal and vaginal suppositories take advantage of the characteristics of mucous membranes. Mucous membranes have a rich blood supply and drugs are absorbed directly into the bloodstream, avoiding the gastrointestinal tract. There are increased reports of adolescents administering alcohol using alcohol suppositories (called "booty bumping" or "butt bongs") and/or the insertion of "vodka soaked tampons in the vagina in girls or the rectum in guys" (see Huffington Post Canada). Blood alcohol levels can rise quickly into the death zone, with blood alcohol concentration (BAC) levels reported to exceed 0.20 g/100 mL. (For more information on BAC, see Chapter 9.)

Parenteral Administration Chemicals can be delivered by injection, with a hypodermic syringe directly into the bloodstream or deposited in a muscle mass or under the upper layers of skin. With the **intravenous (IV)** injection, the drug is put directly into the bloodstream, so the onset of action is much more rapid than with oral administration or with other means of injection. Another advantage is that irritating material can be injected this way, because blood vessel walls are relatively insensitive. Also, it is possible to deliver very high concentrations of drugs intravenously, which can be both an advantage and a danger. A major disadvantage of IV injections is that the vein wall loses some of its strength and elasticity in the area around the injection site. After many injections into a small segment of a vein, the wall of that vein eventually collapses, and blood no longer moves through it, necessitating the use of another injection site. The greatest concern about IV drug use is the danger of introducing infections directly into the bloodstream, either from bacteria picked up on the skin as the needle is being inserted or from contaminated needles and syringes containing traces of blood. This risk is especially great if syringes and needles are shared among users. This has been a significant means by which AIDS and other blood-borne diseases have been spread (see Chapter 2), and is one reason people advocate for harm reduction strategies for injection drug users (see Chapter 1).

Subcutaneous and **intramuscular** injections have similar characteristics, except that absorption is more rapid from intramuscular injection. Muscles have a better blood supply than the underlying layers of the

intravenous (IV): injection directly into a vein.

subcutaneous: injection under the skin.

intramuscular: injection into a muscle.

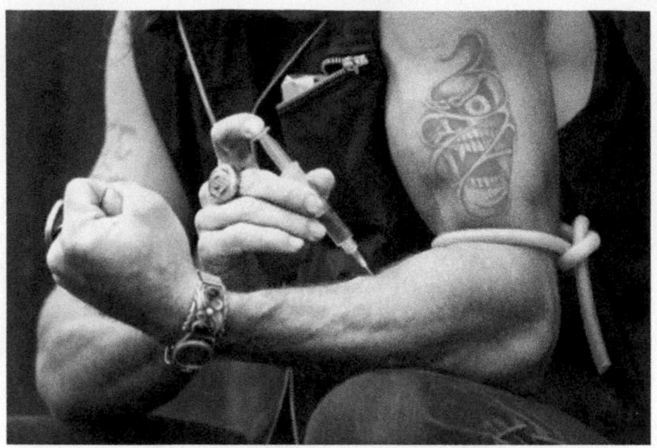

For many heroin users, the preferred route of administration is by intravenous injection.

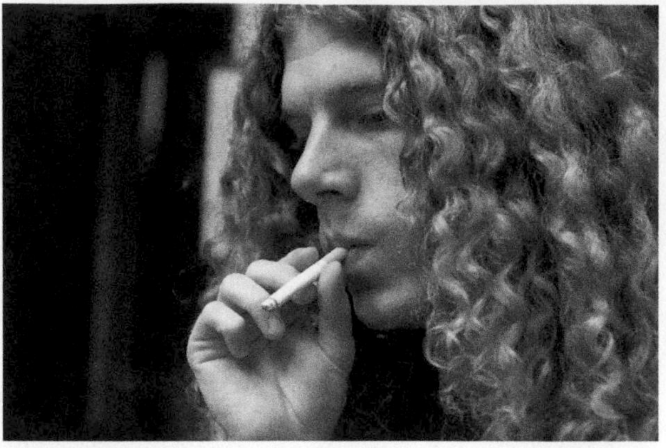

Inhalation is a very effective means of delivering a drug to the brain.

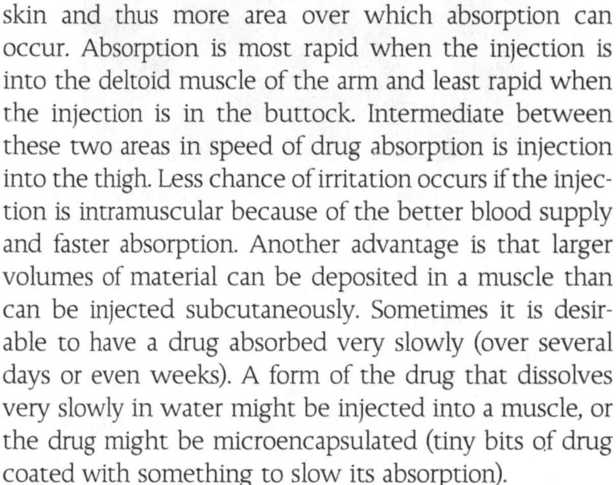

skin and thus more area over which absorption can occur. Absorption is most rapid when the injection is into the deltoid muscle of the arm and least rapid when the injection is in the buttock. Intermediate between these two areas in speed of drug absorption is injection into the thigh. Less chance of irritation occurs if the injection is intramuscular because of the better blood supply and faster absorption. Another advantage is that larger volumes of material can be deposited in a muscle than can be injected subcutaneously. Sometimes it is desirable to have a drug absorbed very slowly (over several days or even weeks). A form of the drug that dissolves very slowly in water might be injected into a muscle, or the drug might be microencapsulated (tiny bits of drug coated with something to slow its absorption).

One disadvantage of subcutaneous injection is that if the material injected is extremely irritating to the tissue, the skin around the site of injection might die and be shed. This method of injection is not very common in medical practice but has long been the kind of injection used by beginning opioid users. This is commonly called "skin popping."

Topical Administration **Topical administration** is a local effect where the drug is applied directly to the area where it is needed. When it comes to illicit drugs, this includes smoking (inhalation) and snorting.

Inhalation Inhalation is the drug delivery system used for smoking nicotine, marijuana, and crack cocaine, and for "huffing" gasoline, paints, and other inhalants; it is used medically with various anaesthetics. It is a very efficient way to deliver a drug. Onset of drug effects is quite rapid because the capillary walls are very accessible in the lungs, and the drug thus enters the blood quickly. For psychoactive drugs, inhalation can produce more rapid effects than even intravenous administration. This is because of the patterns of blood circulation in the body (refer to Figure 5.14). The blood leaving the lungs moves fairly directly to the brain, taking only five to eight seconds to do so. By contrast, blood from the veins in the arm must return to the heart and then be pumped through the lungs before moving on to the brain; this takes 10 to 15 seconds. Aerosol dispensers have been used to deliver some drugs via the lungs, but three considerations make inhalation of limited value for medical purposes. First, the material must not be irritating to the mucous membranes and lungs. Second, control of the dose is more difficult than with the other drug delivery systems. Last, and perhaps the prime advantage for some drugs and disadvantage for others, the drug is not stored in the body. This means the drug must be given as long as the effect is desired and that, when drug administration is stopped, the effect rapidly decreases.

Other Routes Topical application of a drug to the skin is not widely used because most drugs are not absorbed well through the skin. However, for some drugs this method can provide a slow, steady absorption over many hours. For example, a skin patch results in the slow absorption of nicotine over an entire day. This patch has been found to help prevent relapse in people who have quit smoking. Other applications include application to mucous membranes (e.g., nasal as well as oral mucosa), which results in more rapid absorption than through the skin because these

topical administration: application of a drug directly to the area where it is needed.

membranes are moist and have a rich blood supply. Most cocaine users, who snort or sniff cocaine powder into the nose, where it dissolves and is absorbed through the membranes, use the mucous membranes of the nose. Also, the mucosa of the oral cavity provide for the absorption of nicotine from chewing tobacco directly into the bloodstream without going through the stomach, intestines, and liver.

Drug Distribution and Transport in the Blood

When a drug enters the bloodstream its molecules often will attach to one of the protein molecules in the blood, albumin being the protein most commonly involved. The degree to which drug molecules bind to plasma proteins is important in determining drug effects. As long as a protein-drug complex exists, the drug is inactive and cannot leave the blood. In this condition, the drug is protected from inactivation by enzymes.

Equilibrium is established between the free (unbound) drug and the protein-bound forms of the drug in the bloodstream. As the unbound drug moves across capillary walls to sites of action, a release of protein-bound drug occurs to maintain the proportion of bound-to-free molecules. Considerable variation exists among drugs in the affinity that the drug molecules have for binding with plasma proteins. Alcohol has a low affinity and thus exists in the bloodstream primarily as the unbound form. In contrast, most of the molecules of THC, the active ingredient in marijuana, are bound to blood proteins, with only a small fraction free to enter the brain or other tissues. If two drugs were identical in every respect except protein binding, the one with greater affinity for blood proteins would require a higher dose to reach an effective tissue concentration. Conversely, the duration of that drug's effect would be longer because of the storage of molecules on blood proteins.

Because different drugs have different affinities for the plasma proteins, you might expect that drugs with high affinity would displace drugs with weak protein bonds, and they do. This fact is important because it forms the basis for one kind of drug interaction. When a high-affinity drug is added to blood in which there is a weak-affinity drug already largely bound to the plasma proteins, the weak-affinity drug is displaced and exists primarily in the unbound form. The increase in the unbound drug concentration helps move the drug out of the bloodstream to the sites of action faster and can be an important influence on the effect the drug has. At the very least, the duration of action is shortened.

More about the Blood–Brain Barrier

The brain is very different from other parts of the body in terms of drugs' ability to leave the blood and move to sites of action. As described in Chapter 4, the blood-brain barrier, a semipermeable structure between the blood and the fluid that surrounds neurons, keeps certain classes of compounds in the blood and away from brain cells. Thus, some drugs act only on neurons outside the central nervous system–that is, only on those in the peripheral nervous system–whereas others may affect all neurons.

The blood-brain barrier is not well developed in infants; it reaches complete development only after one or two years of age in humans. Although the nature of this barrier is not well understood, several factors are known to contribute to the blood-brain barrier. One is the makeup of the capillaries in the brain. They are different from other capillaries in the body, because they contain no pores. Even small water-soluble molecules cannot leave the capillaries in the brain; only lipid-soluble substances can pass the lipid capillary wall.

If a substance can move through the capillary wall, another barrier unique to the brain is met. About 85% of the capillaries are covered with glial cells; little extracellular space is left next to the blood vessel walls. With no pores and close contact between capillary walls and glial cells, almost certainly an active transport system is needed to move chemicals in and out of the brain. In fact, known transport systems exist for some naturally occurring agents (see Figure 5.15).

Small molecules (O_2, CO_2) are not ionized (positively or negatively charged), are therefore fat soluble, and pass straight through the capillary. Glucose, amino acids, and nutrients are actively transported by pumps across the blood-brain barrier. Ions do not cross it.

A final note on the mystery of the blood-brain barrier is that cerebral trauma can disrupt the barrier and permit agents to enter that normally would be excluded. Concussions and cerebral infections frequently cause enough trauma to impair the effectiveness of this screen, which normally permits only selected chemicals to enter the brain.

LO9 Mechanisms of Drug Actions

Many types of actions are suggested in Chapters 6 to 16 as ways in which specific drugs can affect physiochemical processes, neuron functioning, and, ultimately, thoughts, feelings, and other behaviours. It is

Figure 5.15 The Blood–Brain Barrier

The smallest and final branches of arteries (capillaries) are structurally different in the brain than they are in the body. In the body, gaps in endothelial cells permit the free flow of substances into and out of the blood. In the brain, these gaps are closed by tight junctions formed by astrocytes, which make the capillaries selectively permeable to things in the blood. Blood contents that cross the capillary wall must still cross a layer of astrocyte cells before becoming available to interneurons. The blood–brain barrier allows the brain to get what it needs (water, oxygen, and glucose) and protects the brain from foreign substances in the blood. In this figure, CSF means cerebrospinal fluid.

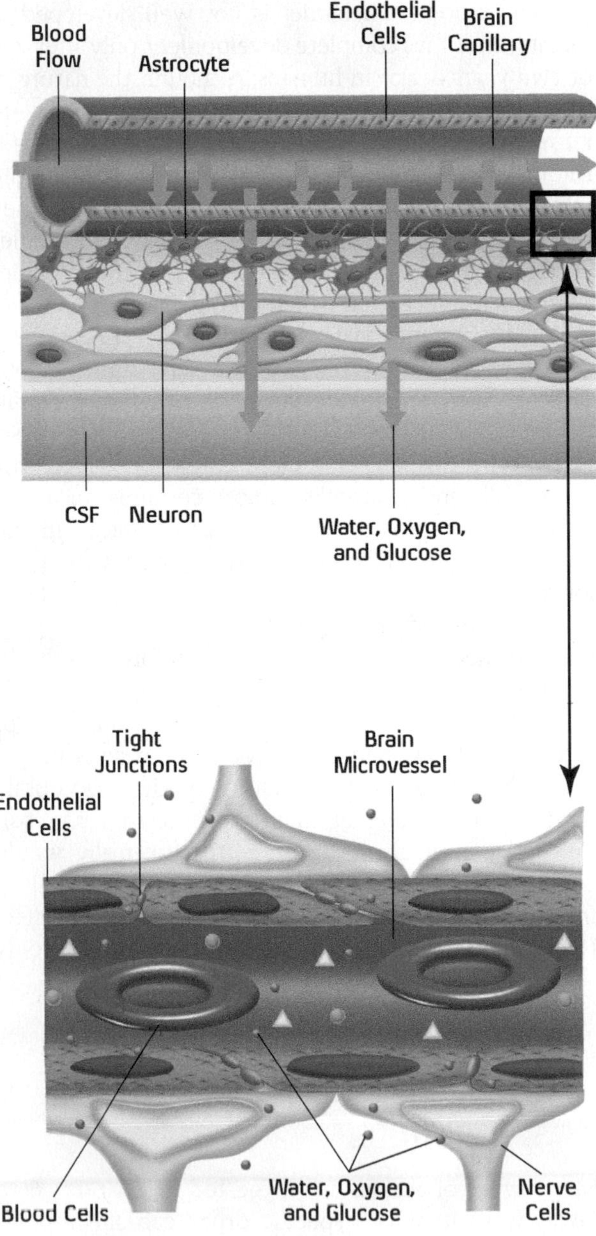

Source: © The McGraw-Hill Companies, Inc.

possible for drugs to affect all neurons, but many exert actions only on very specific presynaptic or postsynaptic processes.

Effects on All Neurons

Chemicals that have an effect on all neurons must do it by influencing some characteristic common to all neurons. One general characteristic of all neurons is the cell membrane. It is semipermeable, meaning that some agents can readily move in and out of the cell, but other chemicals are held inside or kept out under normal conditions. The semipermeable characteristic of the cell membrane is essential for the maintenance of an electric potential across the membrane. It is on this membrane that some drugs seem to act and, by influencing the permeability, alter the electrical characteristics of the neuron.

Most of the general anaesthetics have been thought to affect the central nervous system by a general influence on the cell membrane. The classical view of alcohol's action on the nervous system was that it has effects similar to the general anaesthetics through an influence on the neural membrane. However, evidence has pointed to more specific possible mechanisms for alcohol's effects (see Chapter 9), and even the gaseous anaesthetics might be more selective in their action than was previously thought.[28]

Effects on Specific Neurotransmitter Systems

The various types of psychoactive drugs (e.g., opioids, stimulants, depressants) produce different types of effects primarily because each type interacts in a different way with the various neurotransmitter systems in the brain. Chapter 4 pointed out that the brain's natural neurotransmitters are released from one neuron into a small space called a synapse, where they interact with receptors on the surface of another neuron. Psychoactive drugs can alter the availability of a neurotransmitter by increasing or decreasing the rate of synthesis, metabolism, release from storage vesicles, or reuptake into the releasing neuron. Drugs might also act directly on the receptor, either to activate it or to prevent the neurotransmitter chemical from activating it (see Figure 5.16).

With the existence of more than 50 known neurotransmitters, and considering that different drugs can interact with several of these in different combinations, and given the variety of mechanisms by which each drug can interact with the life cycle of a natural neurotransmitter, the potential exists for an endless variety

Figure 5.16 Receptors and Sites of Drug Action

Drug actions at a synapse. A drug can cause the neurotransmitter (NT) to leak out of a synaptic vesicle into the axon terminal, prevent release of NT into the synaptic cleft, promote release of NT into the synaptic cleft, prevent reuptake of NT by the presynaptic membrane, block the enzyme that causes breakdown of the NT, or bind to a receptor, mimicking the action of an NT.

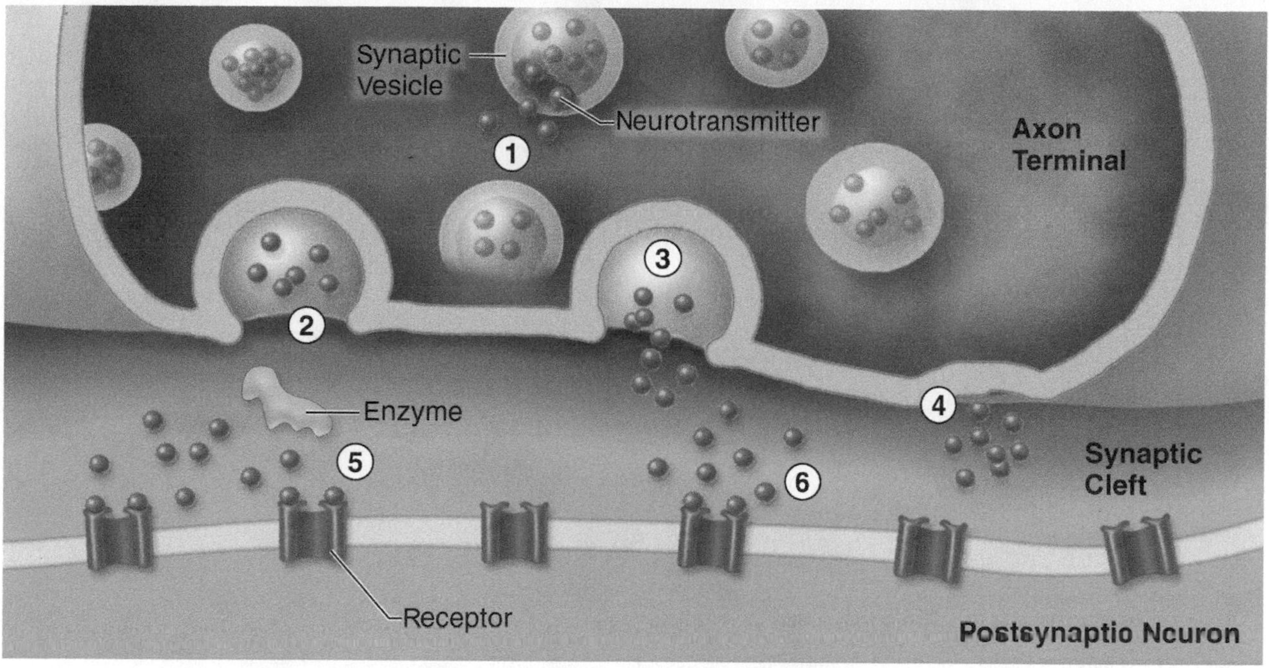

Source: Mader, Sylvia. 2011. *Inquiry into Life*, 13th ed. Boston: McGraw-Hill Higher Education. © The McGraw-Hill Companies, Inc.

of drugs with an endless variety of actions both presynaptically and postsynaptically (see Figure 5.17). However, all these actions are nothing more mysterious than a modification of the ongoing (and quite complex) functions of the brain.

LO10 Drug Metabolism and Deactivation

Before a drug can cease to have an effect, one of two things must happen to it. It may be excreted unchanged from the body (usually in the urine), or it must be chemically changed so that it no longer has the same effect on the body. Although different drugs vary in how they are deactivated, the most common way is for enzymes in the liver to act on the drug molecules to change their chemical structure. Drugs are being removed or metabolized by the body as soon as administered. Some substances are not easily removed (e.g., heavy metals) and accumulate in the body. This usually has two effects: (1) the **metabolite** no longer has the same action as the drug molecule, and (2) the metabolite is more likely to be excreted by the kidneys.

The kidneys operate in a two-stage process. In the first step, water and most of the small and water-soluble molecules are filtered out. Second, most of the water is reabsorbed, along with some of the dissolved chemicals. The more lipid-soluble molecules are more likely to be reabsorbed; so one way in which the liver enzymes can increase the elimination of a drug is by changing its molecules to a more water-soluble and less lipid-soluble form. All drugs are eliminated from the body in a chemically altered (metabolized) form or by excretion.

The most important drug-metabolizing enzymes found in the liver belong to a group known as the CYP450 family of enzymes. The CYP450 enzymes seem to be specialized for inactivating various general kinds of foreign chemicals that the organism might ingest. This is not like the immune system, in which foreign proteins stimulate the production of antibodies for that protein—the CYP450 enzymes

metabolite: a product of enzyme action on a drug.

Figure 5.17 Presynaptic and Postsynaptic Mechanisms

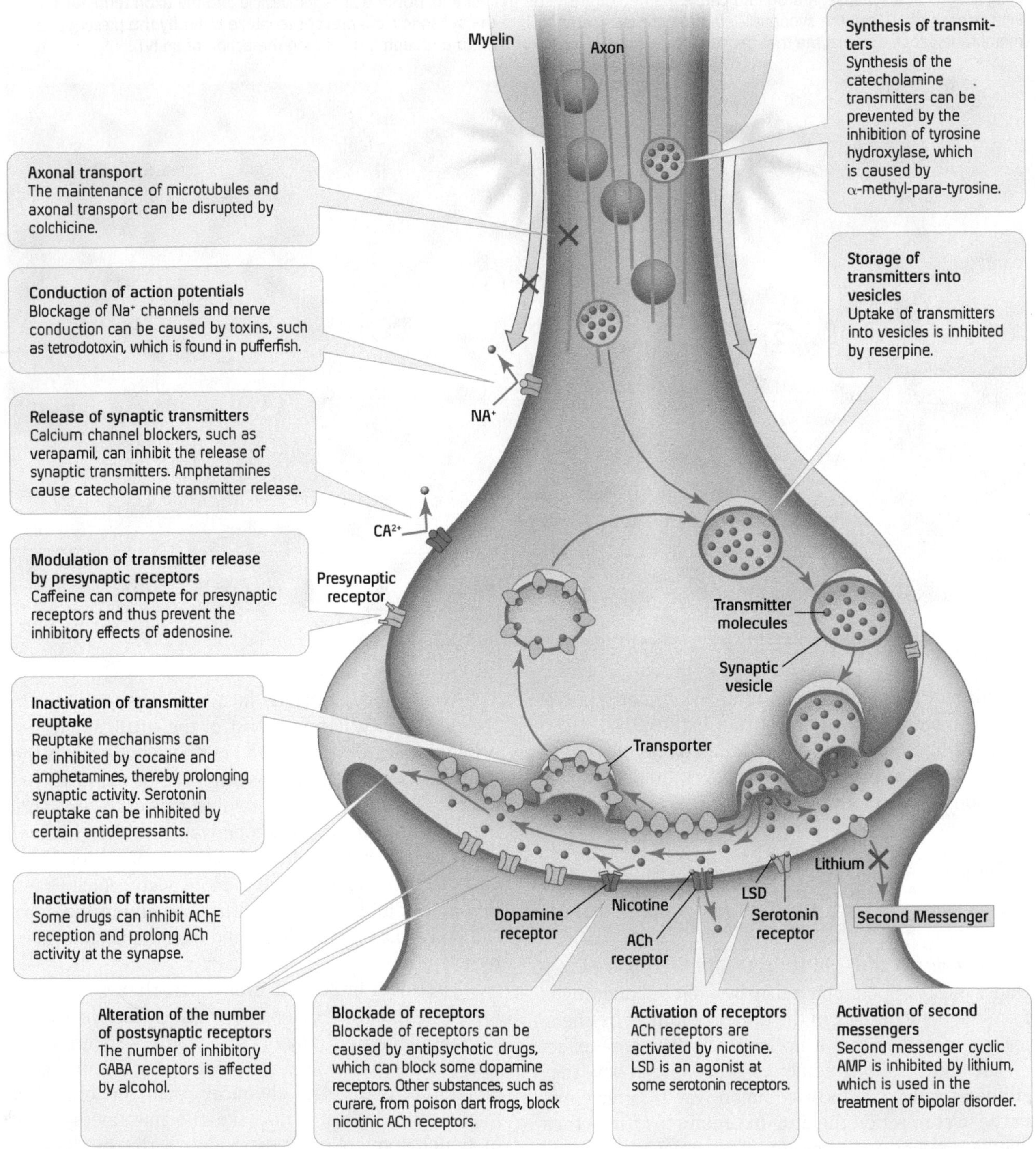
Myelin
Axon
Synthesis of transmitters
Synthesis of the catecholamine transmitters can be prevented by the inhibition of tyrosine hydroxylase, which is caused by α-methyl-para-tyrosine.
Axonal transport
The maintenance of microtubules and axonal transport can be disrupted by colchicine.
Storage of transmitters into vesicles
Uptake of transmitters into vesicles is inhibited by reserpine.
Conduction of action potentials
Blockage of Na+ channels and nerve conduction can be caused by toxins, such as tetrodotoxin, which is found in pufferfish.
NA+
Release of synaptic transmitters
Calcium channel blockers, such as verapamil, can inhibit the release of synaptic transmitters. Amphetamines cause catecholamine transmitter release.
CA2+
Modulation of transmitter release by presynaptic receptors
Caffeine can compete for presynaptic receptors and thus prevent the inhibitory effects of adenosine.
Presynaptic receptor
Transmitter molecules
Synaptic vesicle
Inactivation of transmitter reuptake
Reuptake mechanisms can be inhibited by cocaine and amphetamines, thereby prolonging synaptic activity. Serotonin reuptake can be inhibited by certain antidepressants.
Transporter
Lithium
Inactivation of transmitter
Some drugs can inhibit AChE reception and prolong ACh activity at the synapse.
Dopamine receptor
Nicotine
ACh receptor
LSD
Serotonin receptor
Second Messenger
Alteration of the number of postsynaptic receptors
The number of inhibitory GABA receptors is affected by alcohol.
Blockade of receptors
Blockade of receptors can be caused by antipsychotic drugs, which can block some dopamine receptors. Other substances, such as curare, from poison dart frogs, block nicotinic ACh receptors.
Activation of receptors
ACh receptors are activated by nicotine. LSD is an agonist at some serotonin receptors.
Activation of second messengers
Second messenger cyclic AMP is inhibited by lithium, which is used in the treatment of bipolar disorder.

already exist in the liver and are waiting for the introduction of certain types of chemicals. Various plants have evolved the ability to produce chemicals that do nothing directly for the plant but kill or make ill any animals that eat the plant. In defence, apparently many animals have evolved CYP450 enzymes for eliminating these toxic chemicals once they are eaten.

Although the CYP450 enzymes are always available in the liver, the introduction of drugs can alter their function. Many drugs, including alcohol and the barbiturates, have been shown to induce (increase) the activity of one or more of these drug-metabolizing enzymes. Once the body's cells detect the presence of these foreign molecules, they produce more of the enzyme that breaks down that molecule, in an effort to normalize the cell's chemistry (homeostasis–see Chapter 4). Enzyme induction has important potential not only for tolerance to that particular drug but also for interactions with other drugs that might be broken down by the same enzyme. The increased rate of metabolism could mean that a previously effective dose of an antibiotic or a heart medicine can no longer reach therapeutic levels. The enzyme activity typically returns to normal some time after the inducing drug is no longer being taken. For example, Health Canada has warned that St. John's wort can decrease blood concentrations of several drugs, presumably by inducing CYP450 enzymes.[29] Other drugs, including fluoxetine (Prozac) and other modern antidepressant drugs, have a high affinity for one of the CYP450 enzymes and "occupy" the enzyme molecules so that they effectively inhibit the enzyme's action on any other drug. Now a previously safe dose of blood-pressure medication or cough suppressant results in much higher blood levels that could be dangerous. Prescribing physicians have to be aware of the potential for these types of drug interactions, either to avoid using certain drugs together or to adjust doses upward or downward to compensate for enzyme induction or inhibition. Given the ethnic diversity of people who live in Canada, the influence of genetic variations in the cytochrome P-450 enzyme system on drug disposition and metabolism is a major focus of contemporary research in pharmacogenetics.[30]

Not all the metabolites of drugs are inactive. Both diazepam (Valium) and marijuana have **active metabolites** that produce effects similar to those of the original (parent) drug and prolong the effect considerably.

Drug Half-Life

A drug's **half-life** is the time it takes for half of the drug to lose its pharmacological or physiological effects and to be eliminated from the body (see Figure 5.18).

In fact, so-called **prodrugs** are being developed that are inactive in the original form and become active only after they are altered by the liver enzymes. Drugs that are metabolized into active particles have a longer half-life. The half-lives of some common drugs are presented in Table 5.2.

Figure 5.18 Drug Half-Life

The amount of drug remaining in blood plasma is decreased by half over equal time intervals. In this example the time is expressed in half-lives whereby each passing interval the drug is eliminated by 50%.

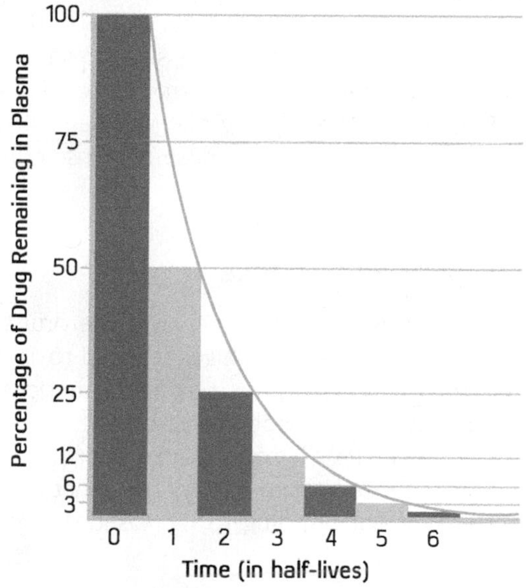

Table 5.2 Half-Life of Some Common Drugs

Drug	Trade or Street Name	Half-Life
Cocaine	Coke, big C, snow	1 hour
Morphine	Morphine	1.5–2 hours
Nicotine	Tobacco	2 hours
LSD	Acid	3 hours
Acetylsalicylic acid	Aspirin	3–4 hours
Ibuprofen	Advil	3–4 hours
Naproxen	Aleve	12 hours
THC	Marijuana	20–30 hours
Sertraline	Zoloft	2–3 days
Fluoxetine	Prozac	7–9 days

active metabolite: a metabolite that has drug actions of its own.

half-life: the time it takes for half of the drug to lose its pharmacological or physiological effects and to be eliminated from the body.

prodrugs: drugs that are inactive until acted on by enzymes in the body.

LO11 Mechanisms of Tolerance and Withdrawal Symptoms

The phenomena of tolerance and withdrawal symptoms have historically been associated with drug dependence. Tolerance refers to a situation in which repeated administration of the same dose of a drug results in gradually diminishing effects. Drug tolerance is associated with a shift of the dose-response curve to the right (see Figure 5.19).

Drug Disposition Tolerance

Sometimes the use of a drug increases the drug's rate of metabolism or excretion. This is referred to as **drug disposition tolerance**, or pharmacokinetic tolerance. For example, phenobarbital induces increased activity of the CYP450 enzymes that metabolize the drug. Increased metabolism reduces the effect of subsequent doses, perhaps leading to increased dosage. But additional amounts of the drug increase the activity of the enzymes even more, and the cycle continues. Another possible mechanism for increased elimination has to do with the pH (acidity) of the urine. Amphetamine is excreted unchanged in the urine, and making the urine more acidic can increase the rate of excretion. Both amphetamine itself and the decreased food intake that often accompanies heavy amphetamine use tend to make the urine more acidic. Amphetamine is excreted 20 times as rapidly in urine with a pH of 5 as in urine with a pH of 8.

Behavioural Tolerance

Particularly when the use of a drug interferes with normal behavioural functions, individuals may learn to adapt to the altered state of their nervous system and

drug disposition tolerance: tolerance caused by more rapid elimination of the drug.

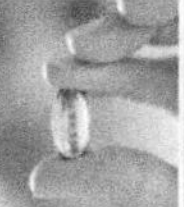

DRUGS IN DEPTH

Drug Interactions

Various drugs can interact with one another in many ways. They may have similar actions and thus have additive effects. One may displace another from protein binding, and thus one drug may enhance the effect of another even though they have different actions. One drug may stimulate liver enzymes and thus reduce the effect of another. Even restricting our discussion to psychoactive drugs, such a variety of interactions are possible that it would not make sense to try to catalogue them all here. Instead, a few of the most important interactions are described.

Respiratory Depression (Alcohol, Other Depressants, Opioids)

The single most important type of drug interaction for psychoactive drugs is the effect on respiration rate. All depressant drugs (sedatives, such as Valium and Xanax, barbiturates, sleeping pills), alcohol, and all narcotics tend to slow down the rate at which people breathe in and out, because of effects in the brain stem. Combining any of these drugs can produce effects that are additive and in some cases may be more than additive. Respiratory depression is the most common type of drug overdose death. People simply stop breathing.

Stimulants and Antidepressants

Although antidepressant drugs such as amitriptyline (Elavil) and Prozac are not in themselves stimulants, they can potentiate the effects of stimulant drugs, such as cocaine and amphetamine, possibly leading to manic overexcitement, irregular heartbeat, high blood pressure, or other effects.

Stimulants and Depressants

It might seem that the "uppers" and "downers" would counteract each other, but that's generally not the case when it comes to behaviour. Such drugs as Valium, Xanax, and alcohol may lead to disinhibition and recklessness. When combined with the effects of stimulants, explosive and dangerous behaviours are possible.

Cocaine + Alcohol = Cocaethylene

Although this may sound like a special case of combining a depressant and a stimulant (it is), there is another possible interaction in that cocaine can combine chemically with ethyl alcohol to produce a substance called cocaethylene—a potent stimulant that animal studies indicate may be more toxic than cocaine. The ramifications of this recent discovery are not yet clear.

Figure 5.19 Drug Tolerance

(a) The effect of a drug is proportional to its concentration at its site of action, increasing with increasing doses (blue line). Over time with repeated use, the drug effect does not reach the predicted effect based on dose, and the drug effects are decreased, which is indicative of tolerance. (b) A reduced drug response can come about through at least three mechanisms: drug disposition tolerance, behavioural tolerance, and pharmacodynamic tolerance. Through any of these, the dose–response curve is shifted to the right, resulting in the same dose having less effect (1) or a greater dose being required to produce the same effect (2).

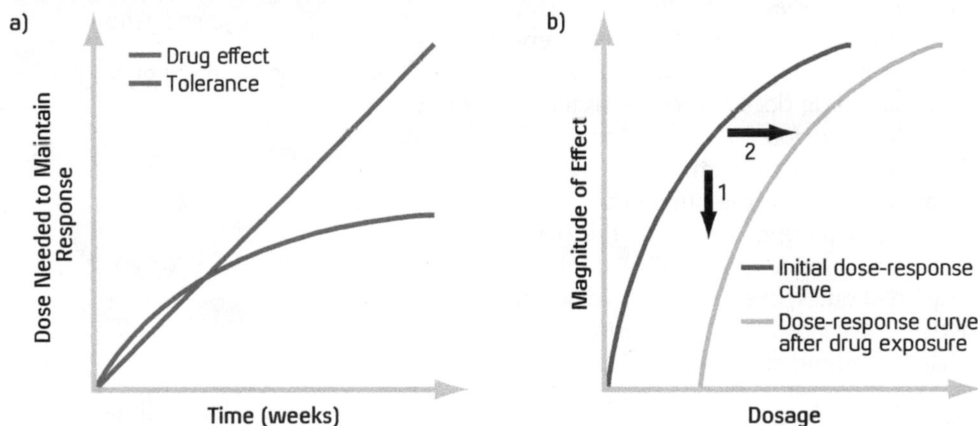

therefore compensate somewhat for the impairment. In some ways, this is analogous to a person who breaks a wrist and learns to write with the nonpreferred hand; the handwriting probably won't be as good that way, but with practice the disruptive effect on writing will be reduced. A person who regularly drives a car after drinking alcohol will never be as good a driver as he or she would be sober, but with experience the impairment may be reduced. In this type of tolerance, called **behavioural tolerance**, the drug may continue to have the same biochemical drug effect but with a reduced effect on behaviour.

Pharmacodynamic Tolerance

In many cases the amount of drug reaching the brain doesn't change, but the sensitivity of the neurons to the drug's effect does change. This is best viewed as an attempt by the brain to maintain its level of functioning within normal limits (an example of homeostatic set point; see Figure 5.20). There are many possible

behavioural tolerance: tolerance caused by learned adaptation to the drug.

Figure 5.20 Physical Dependence, Withdrawal, and Effect of Homeostatic and Compensatory Adaptations

With repeated drug administrations, the body adjusts its internal processes in an attempt to return to its initial level of functioning (homeostatic adaptations). The withdrawal that results once drug taking stops is closely linked to the development of physical tolerance. The body is still using compensatory adaptations but without the drug effects, and the results are opposite to the drug effects. As an example, alcohol is a CNS depressant and withdrawal from alcohol can result in excitability that can lead to seizures and death.

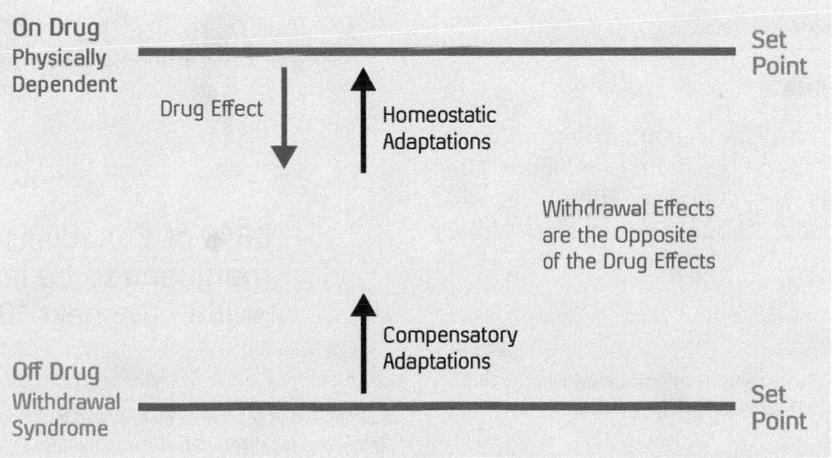

mechanisms for this. For example, if the central nervous system is constantly held in a depressed state through the regular use of alcohol or another depressant drug, the brain might compensate by reducing the amount of the inhibitory neurotransmitter GABA that is released, or by reducing the number of inhibitory GABA receptors (many studies show that the brain does regulate the numbers of specific types of receptors). This adjustment might take several days, and after it occurs the depressant drug doesn't produce as much CNS depression as it did before. If more of the drug is taken, the homeostatic mechanisms might further decrease the release of GABA or the number of GABA receptors. If the drug is abruptly stopped, the brain now does not have the proper level of GABA inhibition, and the CNS becomes overexcited, leading to wakefulness, nervousness, possibly hallucinations, and the sensation that something is crawling on the skin. In severe cases, brain activity becomes uncontrolled and seizures can occur. These withdrawal symptoms are the defining characteristic of physical dependence.

Dr. Shepard Siegel at McMaster University has found that some drug withdrawal symptoms are conditional responses elicited by stimuli paired with the drug effect. Treatment would involve having addicts consume a small dose of a drug and wait out the subsequent withdrawal symptoms. If this is done often enough the compensatory response to environmental cues would grow weaker.[31] Thus, **pharmacodynamic tolerance** leads not only to a reduced effectiveness of the drug but also to these withdrawal reactions. After several days the compensating homeostatic mechanisms return to a normal state, the withdrawal symptoms cease, and the individual is no longer as tolerant to the drug's effect. Cross-tolerance may also occur in which tolerance that develops to one substance in a class of drug will transfer to other substances in that same class, such as barbiturates and alcohol.

Drug Classifications

Psychoactive drugs may be classified depending on their behaviour effects on the brain (see Figure 5.21). Psychoactive drugs are chemical substances that serve to alter mood, thought processes, and/or behaviour. Drugs that stimulate neuronal activity are

pharmacodynamic tolerance: tolerance caused by altered nervous system sensitivity.

Cannabis is in a class of its own and includes marijuana and hashish. Marijuana legalization is a social debate.

Figure 5.21 Drug Effects by Classification

DRUG EFFECTS BY CLASSIFICATION

CLASSIFICATION AND EXAMPLES	EFFECTS (CAN HAVE AT LEAST ONE OF THESE EFFECTS)	HARMS/DANGERS (RISKS OF USING A DRUG CAN INCLUDE ONE OR MORE OF THESE)
CENTRAL NERVOUS SYSTEM DEPRESSANTS		
• Alcohol • Benzodiazepines: minor tranquillizers (Valium, Ativan), sleeping medications (Halcion, Imovane) • Barbiturates (Tuinal)	• decreased inhibitions • increased confidence • relaxation • intoxication • poor judgment • slurred speech • impaired memory/thinking • decreased motor skills	• respiratory depression • seizures • liver disease • heart disease • increased risk of cancer • fetal alcohol spectrum disorder • breathing problems • brain damage
OPIATES		
• Prescription pain relievers • Morphine • Codeine • Heroin	• pain relief (analgesia) • drowsiness • intoxication followed by euphoria • constipation • decreased breathing rate • pinpoint pupils	• hepatitis (from sharing needles) • HIV/AIDS (from sharing needles) • increased risk of some cancers • brain damage • pulmonary problems
CENTRAL NERVOUS SYSTEM STIMULANTS		
• Cocaine (incl. crack) • Methylphenidate (Ritalin) • Amphetamines • Nicotine • Caffeine • Methylenedioxymethamphetamine* (MDMA-ecstasy)	• euphoria • increased energy • increased heart rate, blood pressure • decreased appetite • feelings of enhanced sociability, sexuality, confidence	• paranoid psychosis • depression • HIV/AIDS (from sharing needles) • insomnia • sexual disinterest • dilated pupils • seizures • heart attacks/stroke • extreme anxiety, panic states • hallucinations
HALLUCINOGENS		
• Lysergic acid diethylamide (LSD) • Mescaline • Psilocybin ("magic mushrooms") • Phencydidine (PCP, "angel dust")	• visual and auditory distortions • hallucinations • altered body image • feelings of enhanced mental capacity • muscle twitches • dizziress, nausea, vomiting • out of touch with reality • distorted body image	• panic reactions • psychosis • flashbacks • poor judgment leading to serious injuries or death • anxiety and depression • memory and thinking problems

* A stimulart with hallucinogenic properties.

Source: 2008 NS Dept. of Health Promotion and Protection http://www.druged.ednet.ns.ca/Supplement/Appendices/IRE/Effects/Effects.html

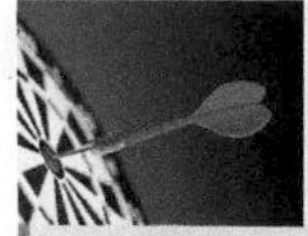

TARGETING PREVENTION

Avoiding Withdrawal Symptoms

Withdrawal symptoms may appear after ceasing the use of many psychoactive drugs, if the user has been taking high doses for a prolonged period. When a hospital patient needs to be treated with an opioid (analgesia) for pain control, how can the drug be given in such a way as to reduce the chances of developing physical dependence, as evidenced by withdrawal symptoms? Obviously, keeping doses as low as possible and giving the drug for as short a time as possible are two important keys. One way to keep the dose low while still obtaining adequate pain control is through the use of a PCA (patient-controlled anaesthesia or analgesia) pump. Within limits, each patient is allowed to administer just the amount of narcotic needed to control his or her pain. This prevents two problems: (1) giving more of the drug than is necessary just to make sure the pain is controlled, and (2) not giving quite enough of the drug so that the patient experiences pain and has to request and wait for more of the drug before the pain is relieved. Dependence may be less of a problem when the patient is allowed to take the drug as needed.

called CNS stimulants; examples are amphetamine, cocaine, and nicotine. Drugs that reduce neuronal activity are called CNS depressants; these include barbiturates and alcohol. Drugs that are given to relieve pain are called analgesics, and include morphine and codeine. Hallucinogens or perception-altering agents are often referred to as "psychedelics" and include drugs such as LSD, ecstasy or MDMA, and PCP or angel dust.

The solvents and inhalants classification includes chemical vapours or gases that produce a high when they are breathed in (inhalants). Volatile solvents, including gasoline, cleaning fluids, paint thinners, and hobby glue, among others, are the most commonly abused type of inhalants.

Another class of drugs is called psychotherapeutics. Some people have disorders that are caused by an imbalance in the chemical neurotransmitters in the brain. These powerful drugs correct the imbalance and allow those who need them to function normally. Psychotherapeutics or drugs for mental disease include neuroleptics (e.g., chlorpromazine), drugs used to treat schizophrenia, and drugs used to treat depression, such as Prozac. The different drug classifications will be examined in more detail in later chapters of this book.

Summary

- Most drugs are derived directly or indirectly from the hundreds of chemical substances found in plants.
- The legal pharmaceutical industry is one of the largest and most profitable industries in Canada.
- Brand names belong to one company; the generic name for a chemical may be used by any company. A chemical name is derived from the rules of organic chemistry for naming any compound. Chemical names are used in laboratories.
- Most psychoactive drugs can be categorized as stimulants, depressants, opioids, hallucinogens, or psychotherapeutic agents.
- Pharmacodynamics includes drug action and drug effects. Drug action refers to the interaction of the drug with its receptor; drug effects are the resulting behavioural, cognitive, and emotional changes that are produced following drug action.
- Specific drug effects are related to the concentration of the chemical; nonspecific effects are also called placebo effects, because they can often be produced by an inactive chemical (placebo) that the user believes to be a drug. A drug's therapeutic effects are the intended effects that treat a disease or an illness. Side effects are the unintended effects that accompany therapeutic effects.
- Double-blind procedures are important in determining the effects of drugs on behaviour. The expectation that a drug will have an effect is called a placebo effect; while this can produce changes in the brain, they are not necessarily related to the active chemical properties of a drug.
- Most psychoactive drugs are taken by one of three basic routes: by mouth, injection, or inhalation. Other less frequently used routes include topical application of a drug to the skin and application to mucous membranes.
- Drug absorption is the passage of a drug from the site of administration to the circulatory system. Drug metabolism is the process by which the body breaks down drugs. Drug distribution occurs when the drug moves to and from the blood and various tissues of the body (for example, fat, muscle, and brain tissue). In drug excretion, drugs are removed from the body.

- When a drug enters the bloodstream, its molecules usually attach to protein molecules in the blood. The degree to which drug molecules bind to plasma proteins is important in determining drug effects.
- Because each drug is capable of producing many effects, many dose-response relationships can be studied for any given drug. Typically, at very low doses no effect is seen. At increasing doses, an effect on the response system being monitored is observed.
- The ED_{50} is the effective dose for half of the animals tested. The LD_{50} is the lethal dose for 50% of the animals tested. The ratio of LD_{50} to ED_{50} is called the therapeutic index and is one indication of the relative safety of a drug for a particular use or effect.
- The potency of a drug is the amount needed to produce an effect, not how effective the drug is or how large an effect it can produce.
- The liver microsomal enzyme system is important for drug deactivation and for some types of drug interactions.
- Drug tolerance can result from changes in distribution and elimination, from behavioural adaptations, or from changes in the responsiveness of the nervous system caused by compensatory (homeostatic) mechanisms. Physical dependence (withdrawal) can be a consequence of this last type of tolerance.
- Virtually all psychoactive drugs have relatively specific pharmacodynamic effects on one neurotransmitter system or more, either through altering availability of the transmitter or by interacting with its receptor.
- The blood–brain barrier, a semipermeable structure between the blood and the fluid that surrounds neurons, protects the brain by keeping certain classes of compounds in the blood and away from brain cells. For a drug to be psychoactive, its molecules must be capable of passing through the blood–brain barrier.

Review Questions

1. Morton's makes table salt, also known as sodium chloride. What is the chemical name, what is the generic name, and what is the brand name?
2. Into which major category does each of these drugs fall: heroin, cocaine, alcohol, LSD, Prozac?
3. How does the administration of a placebo produce specific alterations of neurotransmitter system in the brain?
4. Why should LD_{50} always be greater than ED_{50}?
5. Why do people say that LSD is one of the most potent psychoactive drugs?
6. Which route of administration gets a drug to the brain most quickly?
7. If an older adult has less protein in the blood than a younger person, how would you adjust the dose of a drug that has high protein binding?
8. How might two drugs interact with each other through actions on the CYP450 enzyme system?
9. Which type of tolerance is related to physical dependence, and why?

SECTION

3

CHAPTER 6

Stimulants

How do the stimulant drugs cocaine and amphetamines act on the body?

CHAPTER 7

Other Depressants and Inhalants

How do the depressants work as sedatives and hypnotics?

CHAPTER 8

Psychotherapeutic Drugs: Medication for Mental Disorders

Which drugs are used in treatment of depression, schizophrenia, and other mental disorders?

UPPERS AND DOWNERS

In Section 3 we start by studying two categories of drugs that have straightforward actions on behaviour. Stimulants generally excite the central nervous system, while depressants generally inhibit it. In Chapter 8, we see that most drugs used to treat mental disorders have more complicated actions. Antidepressant drugs, used to treat depression, are not stimulants. When taken for several weeks, they can help raise a depressed mood into the normal range, but they don't produce the effects stimulants do. Likewise, the tranquillizers used to treat psychotic behaviour are not depressants and do not always produce the drowsiness that sedatives and sleeping pills do.

CHAPTER 6

STIMULANTS

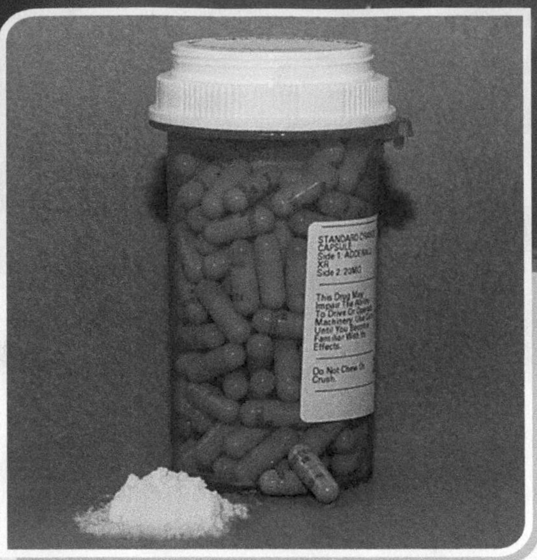

OBJECTIVES

When you have finished this chapter, you should be able to

- **LO1** Discuss the history of cocaine and amphetamines.
- **LO2** Describe early psychiatric uses of cocaine.
- **LO3** Describe how cocaine hydrochloride and crack cocaine are processed from coca.
- **LO4** Compare and contrast the illicit supply sources for cocaine and methamphetamine in Canada.
- **LO5** Compare and contrast the mechanism of action and route of administration of cocaine and amphetamines.
- **LO6** Compare and contrast acute and chronic toxicity concerns associated with cocaine and amphetamines.
- **LO7** Compare the chemical structure of amphetamine to the catecholamine neurotransmitters and to ephedrine.

Stimulants are the drugs that can keep you going, both mentally and physically, when you should be tired. There have been many claims about the other things these drugs can do for (and to) people. Do they really make you smarter, faster, or stronger? Can they sober you up? Improve your sex life? Do they produce dependence?

We can divide the stimulants somewhat arbitrarily: The readily available stimulants nicotine and caffeine are discussed in Chapters 10 and 11, and the restricted stimulants cocaine and the amphetamines are covered in this chapter. Since the widespread introduction of cocaine into Western Europe and North America in the nineteenth century, some people have always been committed to the regular recreational use of the stimulants, but neither cocaine nor the amphetamines have ever achieved widespread social acceptance as recreational drugs.

coca: a bush that grows in the Andes and produces cocaine.

cocaine: the active chemical in the coca plant.

LO1, LO2, LO3, LO4, LO5, LO6

Cocaine

Cocaine is a powerful central nervous system (CNS) stimulant that creates intense feelings of pleasure, increases alertness, and decreases appetite and the need for sleep.

History

The origin of the earliest civilization in the Americas, beginning around 5000 BCE of what was to become the Inca Empire in Peru, has been traced to the use of **coca**. Natives of the Andes Mountains in Bolivia and Peru still use coca today as their ancestors did: chewing the leaves and holding a ball of coca leaf almost continually in the mouth. The freedom from fatigue provided by the drug is legendary in allowing these natives to run or to carry large bundles great distances over high mountain trails. The psychoactive effects can be made stronger by adding some calcified lime to raise the alkalinity inside the mouth–this increases the extraction of **cocaine** and allows greater absorption into the blood supplying the inside of the mouth. It appears that humans in the Andes first settled down and formed communities around places where this calcified lime could be mined.[1] Eventually they took up the planting and harvesting of crops in the nearby fields–and one of those important crops was, of course, coca.

The terrain of the Andes in Bolivia and Peru is poorly suited for growing almost everything. *Erythroxylon coca,* however, seems to thrive at elevations of 600 to 2400 metres on the Amazon slope of the mountains, where more than 254 centimetres of rain fall annually. The shrub is pruned to prevent it from reaching the normal height of two to three metres, so that the picking, which is done three or four times a year, is easier to accomplish. The shrubs are grown in small, one-hectare patches called *cocals,* some of which are known to have been under cultivation for more than 800 years.

Before the sixteenth-century invasion by Pizarro, the Incas had built a well-developed civilization in Peru. The coca leaf was an important part of the culture, and although earlier use was primarily in religious ceremonies, coca was treated as money by the time the conquistadors arrived. The Spanish adopted this custom and paid coca leaves to the native labourers for mining and transporting gold and silver. Even then the coca leaf was recognized as increasing strength and endurance while decreasing the need for food.

Early European chroniclers of the Incan civilization reported on the unique qualities of this plant, but it never interested Europeans until the last half of the nineteenth century. At that time the coca leaf contributed to the economic well-being and fame of three individuals. They, in turn, brought the Peruvian shrub to the notice of the world.

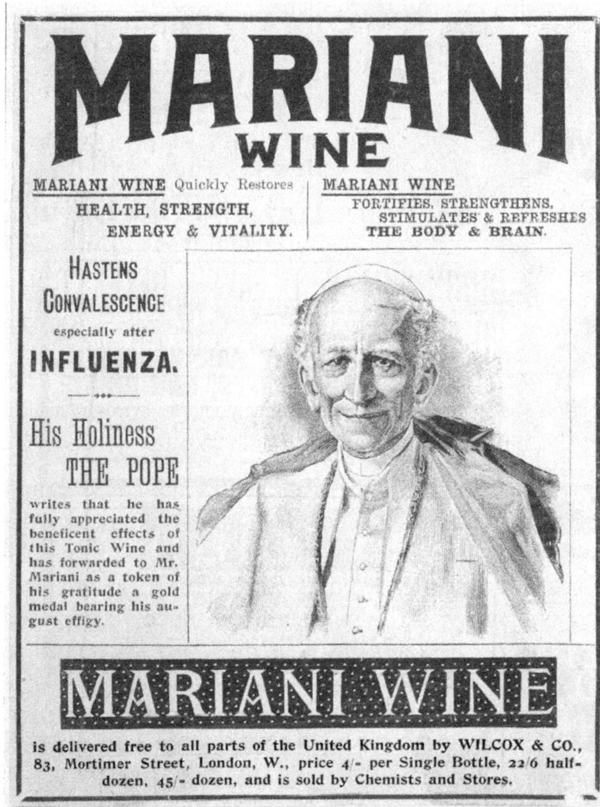

Vin Mariani was a tonic wine and patent medicine containing coca leaf extract created circa 1863 by French chemist Angelo Mariani.

Coca Wine

The first of the individuals was Angelo Mariani, a French chemist. His contribution was to introduce the coca leaf indirectly to the general public. Mariani imported metric tons of coca leaves and used an extract from them in many products. You could suck on a coca lozenge, drink coca tea, or obtain the coca leaf extract in any of a large number of other products. It was Mariani's coca wine, though, that made him rich and famous. Assuredly, it had to be the coca leaf extract in the wine that prompted the pope to present a medal of appreciation to Mariani. Not only the pope but also royalty and the general public benefited from the Andean plant. For them, as it had for the Incas for a thousand years and was to do for Americans who drank early versions of Coca-Cola (see Chapter 11), the extract of the coca leaf lifted their spirits, freed them from fatigue, and gave them a generally good feeling.

Local Anaesthesia

The second famous individual was Karl Koller, an Austrian ophthalmologist born in 1857 who was the first to introduce cocaine as a local anaesthetic for eye surgery. Before this discovery, he had tested such solutions as chloral hydrate and morphine as anaesthetics in the eyes of laboratory animals without success. Sigmund Freud was already fully aware of the pain-killing properties of cocaine, but Koller recognized its tissue-numbing capabilities. In 1884, Koller established cocaine's potential as a local anaesthetic to the medical community, revolutionizing eye surgery. Before the introduction of cocaine for eye surgery, it was complicated to execute because of the involuntary reflex motions of the eye to respond to the slightest stimuli. Later, cocaine was also used as a local anaesthetic in other medical fields, such as dentistry.

Early Psychiatric Uses

The third famous individual to encourage cocaine use was a young Viennese physician named Sigmund Freud, who studied the drug for its potential as a treatment medication in a variety of ailments, including depression and morphine dependence. In 1884, Freud wrote to his fiancée that he had been experimenting with "a magical

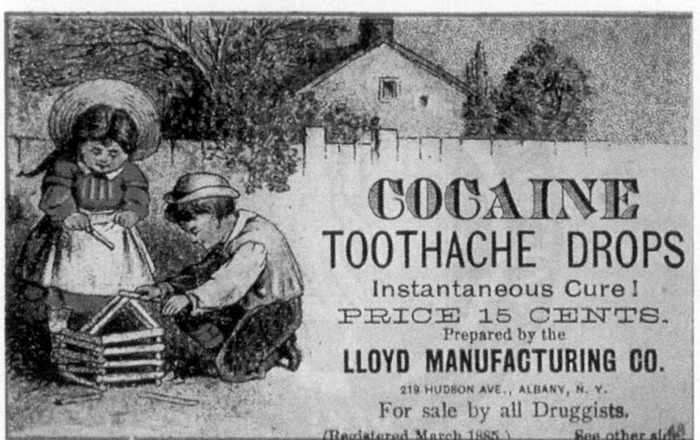

Cocaine was an ingredient in many patent medicines in North America.

drug." He wrote, "If it goes well I will write an essay on it and I expect it will win its place in therapeutics by the side of morphium, and superior to it. . . . I take very small doses of it regularly against depression and against indigestion, and with the most brilliant success." He urged his fiancée, his sisters, his colleagues, and his friends to try it, extolling the drug as a safe exhilarant, which he himself used and recommended as a treatment for morphine dependence. For emphasis he wrote in italics, "*inebriate asylums can be entirely dispensed with.*"[2]

In an 1885 lecture before a group of psychiatrists, Freud commented on the use of cocaine as a stimulant, saying, "On the whole it must be said that the value of cocaine in psychiatric practice remains to be demonstrated, and it will probably be worthwhile to make a thorough trial as soon as the currently exorbitant price of the drug becomes more reasonable"—the first of the consumer advocates!

Freud was more convinced about another use of the drug, however, and in the same lecture said,

> We can speak more definitely about another use of cocaine by the psychiatrist. It was first discovered in America that cocaine is capable of alleviating the serious withdrawal symptoms observed in subjects who are abstaining from morphine and of suppressing their craving for morphine. . . . On the basis of my experiences with the effects of cocaine, I have no hesitation in recommending the administration of cocaine for such withdrawal cures in subcutaneous injections of 0.03–0.05 g per dose, without any fear of increasing the dose. On several occasions, I have even seen cocaine quickly eliminate the manifestations of intolerance that appeared after a rather large dose of morphine, as if it had a specific ability to counteract morphine.[3]

Even great people make mistakes. The realities of life were harshly brought home to Freud when he used cocaine to treat a close friend, Fleischl, to remove his dependence on morphine. Increasingly larger doses were needed, and eventually Freud spent a frightful night nursing Fleischl through an episode of cocaine psychosis. After that experience, Freud generally opposed the use of drugs in the treatment of psychological problems.

Besides Mariani, Koller, and Freud, one well-known fictional character revealed that the psychological effects of cocaine, both the initial stimulation and the later depression, had been well appreciated by 1890:

> Sherlock Holmes took his bottle from the corner of the mantelpiece, and his hypodermic syringe from its neat morocco case. With his long, white nervous fingers, he adjusted the delicate needle and rolled back his left shirtcuff. For some little time his eyes rested thoughtfully upon the sinewy forearm and wrist, all dotted and scarred with innumerable puncture-marks. Finally, he thrust the sharp point home, pressed down the tiny piston, and sank back into the velvet-lined armchair with a long sigh of satisfaction.
>
> Three times a day for many months I had witnessed this performance, but custom had not reconciled my mind to it. . . .
>
> "Which is it today," I asked, "Morphine or cocaine?"
>
> He raised his eyes languidly from the old black-letter volume which he had opened.
>
> "It is cocaine," he said, "a seven-per-cent solution. Would you care to try it?"
>
> "No, indeed," I answered brusquely. "My constitution has not got over the Afghan campaign yet. I cannot afford to throw any extra strain upon it."
>
> He smiled at my vehemence. "Perhaps you are right, Watson," he said. "I suppose that its influence is physically a bad one. I find it, however, so transcendently stimulating and clarifying to the mind that its secondary action is a matter of small moment."[4]

Although physicians were well aware of the dangers of using cocaine regularly, non-medical and quasimedical use of cocaine was widespread at the start of the twentieth century. It was one of the secret ingredients in many patent medicines and elixirs but was also openly advertised as having beneficial effects. The Parke-Davis Pharmaceutical Company noted in 1885 that cocaine "can supply the place of food, make the coward brave, and silent eloquent" and called it a "wonder drug."[5]

Legal Controls on Cocaine

In North America, little concern was given to cocaine until the end of the 1960s, when amphetamines became harder to obtain, and cocaine use again began to increase. As had occurred nearly a century before, the virtues of cocaine were now being touted by a number of individuals, ranging from physicians to celebrities. North America's second era of flirtation with cocaine was under way. In 1974, psychiatrist Peter Bourne, who would soon become President Jimmy Carter's chief drug adviser, wrote, "Cocaine . . . is probably the most benign of illicit drugs currently in widespread use. At least as strong a case could be made for legalizing it as for legalizing marijuana."[6] A respected psychiatrist, writing in a premier psychiatric text echoed the above remarks: "Used no more than two or three times a week, cocaine creates no serious problems. . . . Chronic cocaine abuse does not usually appear as a medical problem."[7] These endorsements bore a striking resemblance to those of Sigmund Freud in 1884, who wrote in his famous essay titled "Über Coca," "Opinion is unanimous that the euphoria induced by coca is not followed by any feeling of lassitude or other state of depression. . . . It seems probable . . . that coca, if used protractedly but in moderation, is not detrimental to the body."[8] Had we forgotten our experience with cocaine a century earlier? If so, it wouldn't take long for people to become alarmed.

Cocaine use before 1985 in North America had come to symbolize wealth and fame, in part because street sales of the drug were mainly in the hydrochloride form in quantities that made the price relatively expensive. As a result, most consumers were affluent. Because a convenient method for smoking cocaine was not yet widely available, the majority of users snorted the drug. The abuse potential of snorted cocaine is lower than that of smoked or intravenous cocaine. The infrequent use of smoked cocaine changed in the mid- to late-1980s, when enterprising dealers began selling smokeable cocaine in the form of crack (it makes a cracking sound when burned/smoked). The cocaine experience was now available to anyone with $5 to $10, a lighter, a glass pipe, and access to a dealer. With the availability of a seemingly cheaper form of cocaine, use increased among some groups. Because the majority of crack cocaine sold by street-level dealers is considerably adulterated, it is actually more expensive than powder cocaine.

In Canada, drug regulations are covered by the Controlled Drugs and Substances Act and the Food and Drug Act. The Controlled Drugs and Substances Act was passed in 1996, repealing the Narcotic Control Act and Parts III and IV of the Food and Drug Act (parts dealing with the advertisement of controlled substances). This Act classified drugs into schedules from I to VIII. In Canada, cocaine is classified into Schedule I. Unlawful possession is subject to fines up to $1000 or imprisonment for up to six months or both for a first offence. Penalties are greater for possession of larger amounts or subsequent offences (i.e., conviction for trafficking can bring life imprisonment).

Supplies of Illicit Cocaine in Canada

According to the United Nations Office on Drugs and Crime *World Drug Report 2009*, Colombia remained the world's largest cultivator of coca bush, with 81 000 hectares, followed by Peru (56 100 hectares), and Bolivia (30 500 hectares).[9] In 2008 estimated global cocaine production decreased by 15% over 2007 (845 metric tons in 2008 and 994 metric tons in 2007). This decrease was attributable to a strong reduction in cocaine production in Colombia (28%), which was not offset by increases in Bolivia and Peru. Colombia remains the primary source country for powder cocaine destined for the Canadian market; however, in 2007 cocaine originating from Peru increased significantly in comparison to previous years.

In all of these countries, attempts to control production are complex: U.S. Drug Enforcement Administration (DEA) agents assist local police, who may be in conflict with army units fighting against local guerrillas. Often the price and availability of coca in these countries are determined more by local politics than by the DEA's eradication and interdiction efforts. Although we might pay some farmers to grow alternative crops, the high profits from growing illicit cocaine draw others to plant new fields. An economic analysis of the impact of eradication efforts indicates that even the most successful projects result in at best only temporary shortages.[10]

Mexico's role as a transit country for cocaine destined for Canada has increased not only by way of the Mexico-U.S.-Canada highway corridor but also by direct shipments via air and marine modes. In spite of the increased smuggling activity originating in Mexico in 2007, the United States remained the primary transit country for cocaine destined for Canada.[11] The largest proportion of cocaine smuggled into Canada continues to be concentrated at major ports of entry located in British Columbia, Ontario, and Quebec. Before 2006, the largest quantities of cocaine seized arrived via the air mode; recently, the land mode was ranked as the primary smuggling method.

An increasing trend noted at Canadian international airports was the smuggling of cocaine in liquid form. Canada Border Services Agency reported seizing 83.52 kilograms of liquid cocaine in 2007, of which the majority originated in Peru. By transforming cocaine from powder form into liquid, drug traffickers are attempting to further avoid detection by port authorities. The liquid cocaine was concealed by air passengers in their luggage within bottles of alcohol or in hygiene and health products. The most frequent point of seizure was at Toronto's Pearson International Airport.

Once smuggled into Canada, cocaine is trafficked from the Pacific region to other Western provinces, while the central provinces of Quebec and Ontario have been identified as supplying the user population in the Maritimes. Although various transportation methods, such as the use of domestic flights, courier companies, and passenger coaches (buses), have been well documented in the delivery of cocaine to various locations within Canada, there has been a noted increase along major highways in the use of passenger vehicles and commercial transportation trucks with false compartments.

Pharmacology of Cocaine

Science has led us to a much better understanding of the mechanisms responsible for cocaine's ability to produce its pleasurable effects, the regions of the brain activated by both chemical forms of cocaine (hydrochloride and freebase), and the neurotransmitters responsible for its effects.

Source Coca (*Erythroxylum coca*) is a plant in the family Erythroxylaceae, native to north-western South America. The plant plays a significant role in traditional Andean culture, as noted at the beginning of the chapter. Coca is best known throughout the world because of its alkaloids, which include cocaine, a powerful stimulant. The plant resembles a blackthorn bush and grows to a height of two to three metres. The branches are straight, and the leaves, which have a green tint, are thin, opaque, and oval, and taper at the extremities. A marked characteristic of the leaf is an areolated portion bounded by two longitudinal curved lines, one line on each side of the midrib, and more conspicuous on the underside of the leaf.

coca paste: a crude extract containing cocaine in a smokeable form.

cocaine hydrochloride: the most common form of pure cocaine, it is stable and water soluble.

freebase: a method of preparing cocaine as a chemical base so that it can be smoked.

The flowers are small and disposed in little clusters on short stalks; the corolla is composed of five yellowish-white petals, the anthers are heart-shaped, and the pistil consists of three carpels united to form a three-chambered ovary. The flowers mature into red berries. Coca leaves contain, besides the oils that give them flavour, the active chemical cocaine (up to almost 2%). Cocaine was isolated before 1860, but there is still debate over who did it first and exactly when. Simple and inexpensive processing of 500 kilograms of coca leaves yields 1 kilogram of cocaine. An available supply of pure cocaine and the newly developed hypodermic syringe improved the drug delivery system, and in the 1880s physicians began to experiment with the drug.

Chemical Structure The chemical structure of cocaine is shown in Figure 6.1. This is a fairly complicated molecule, which doesn't resemble any of the known neurotransmitters in an obvious way. In fact, the structure of cocaine doesn't give us much help at all in understanding how the drug works in the brain.

Forms of Cocaine

As was pointed out in Chapter 1, it is important to understand how a drug is taken when determining the potential effects of that drug. As a part of the process of making illicit cocaine, the coca leaves are mixed with an organic solvent, such as kerosene or gasoline. After thorough soaking, mixing, and mashing, the excess liquid is filtered out to form a substance known as **coca paste**. In South America, this paste is often mixed with tobacco and smoked.

The paste can also be made into **cocaine hydrochloride**, a salt that mixes easily in water and is so stable that it cannot be heated to form vapours for inhalation. Recreational users of this form of cocaine either snort (sniff) or inject the drug intravenously. Some users who wanted to smoke cocaine used to convert it into **freebase** by extracting it into a

Figure 6.1 Cocaine

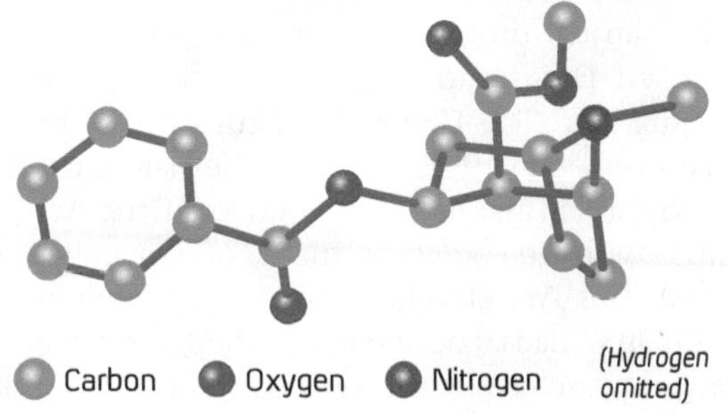

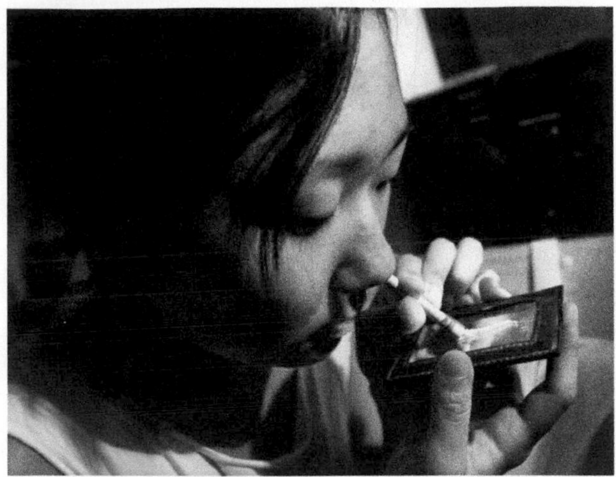

Users of cocaine hydrochloride, the most common form of pure cocaine, either snort the drug or inject it intravenously.

volatile organic solvent, such as ether. The freebase can be heated and the vapours inhaled. This method of smoking cocaine can be very dangerous because the combination of fire and ether fumes is extremely explosive. The popularity of this form of freebasing began to decline in the early 1980s, when it was discovered that mixing cocaine with simple household chemicals, including baking soda and water, and then drying it resulted in a lump of smokeable cocaine (**crack** or **rock**).

Mechanism of Action

The more we learn about cocaine's effects on the brain, the more complex the drug's actions seem. Figure 6.2 illustrates, using a rat's brain, the reward pathways responsible for the reinforcing effects of drugs of abuse

crack: a street name for a simple and stable preparation of cocaine base for smoking.

rock: another name for crack.

Figure 6.2 Neural Reward Circuits Important in the Reinforcing Effects of Drugs of Abuse

As shown in the rat brain, mesocorticolimbic dopamine (DA) systems originating in the ventral tegmental area include projections from cell bodies of the ventral tegmental area to the nucleus accumbens, amygdala, and prefrontal cortex; glutamatergic (GLU) projections from the prefrontal cortex to the nucleus accumbens and the ventral tegmental area; and projections from the gamma-aminobutyric acid (GABA) neurons of the nucleus accumbens to the prefrontal cortex. Opioid interneurons modulate the GABA-inhibitory action on the ventral tegmental area and influence the firing of norepinephrine (NE) neurons in the locus ceruleus. Serotonergic (5-HT) projections from the raphe nucleus extend to the ventral tegmental area and the nucleus accumbens. The figure shows the proposed sites of action of the various drugs of abuse in these circuits.

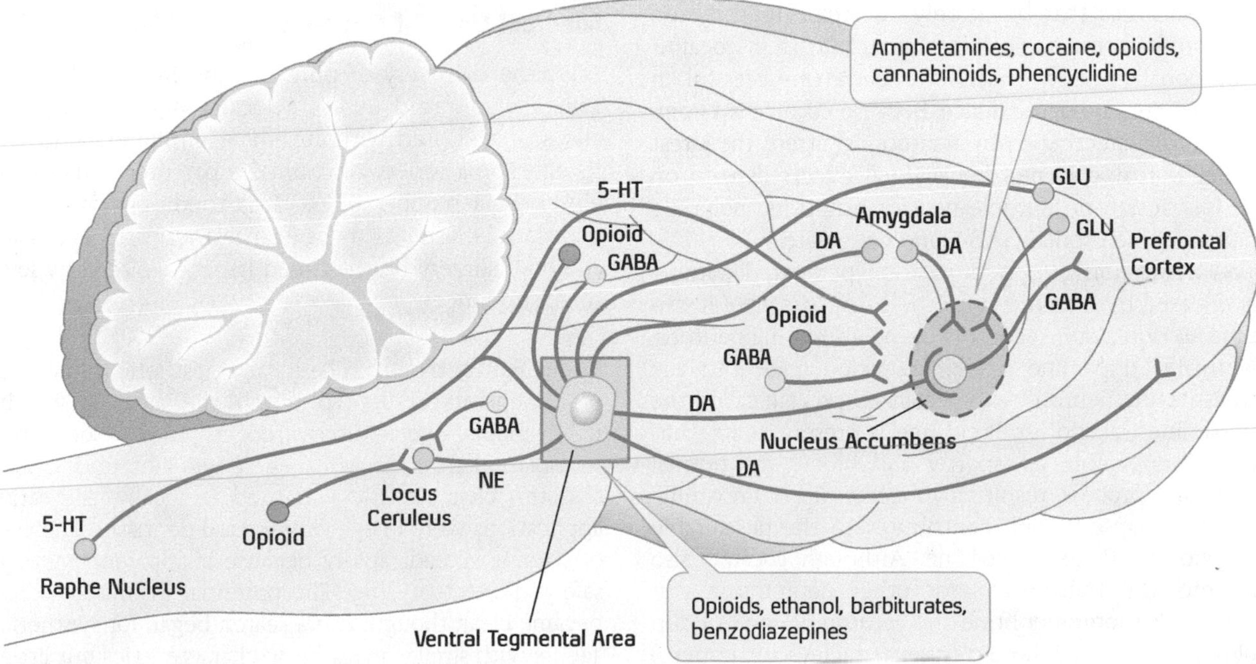

Source: Camí, J., and M. Farré. 2003. "Drug Addiction." *New England Journal of Medicine* 349(10): 975–86.

Figure 6.3 Cocaine's Effect on Dopamine in the Brain

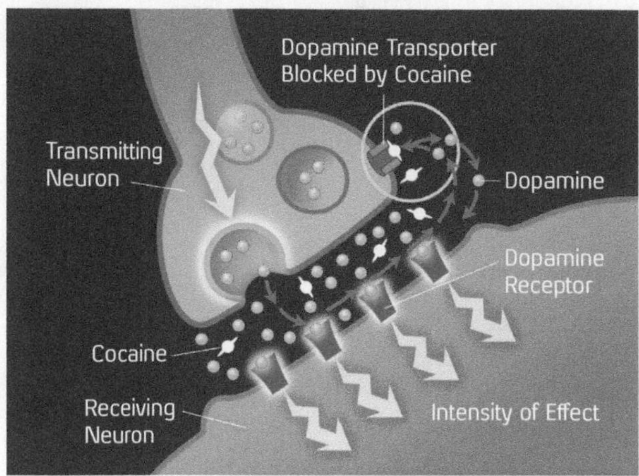

Source: National Institute on Drug Abuse. *Cocaine: Research and Addiction* (Research Report Series, NIH Publication Number 10-4166). 2010. Retrieved March 20, 2011, from http://drugabuse.gov/ResearchReports/Cocaine/cocaine.html.

and shows the proposed sites of action of various drugs.[12] Cocaine blocks the reuptake of dopamine, norepinephrine, and serotonin, causing a prolonged effect of these neurotransmitters (see Figure 6.3). The observation that the blockage of dopamine receptors or the destruction of dopamine-containing neurons lessened the amount of cocaine that laboratory animals self-administered led many cocaine researchers to focus on dopamine neurons. After several years of intense scientific research, enthusiasm regarding dopamine's exclusive role in cocaine-related behaviours has been tempered, in part, because drugs that block only dopamine reuptake do not produce the same behavioural effects as cocaine. Additionally, these drugs have been unsuccessful in treating cocaine dependence. Because cocaine is a complex drug, affecting many neurotransmitters, the latest belief is that cocaine's behavioural effects depend on an interaction of multiple neurotransmitters, including dopamine, serotonin, GABA, and glutamate.[12]

In the normal communication process, dopamine is released by a neuron into the synapse, where it can bind to dopamine receptors on neighbouring neurons. Normally, dopamine is then recycled back into the transmitting neuron by a specialized protein called the dopamine transporter. If cocaine is present, it attaches to the dopamine transporter and blocks the normal recycling process, resulting in a buildup of dopamine in the synapse, which contributes to the pleasurable (euphoric) effects of cocaine. Although cocaine also inhibits the transporters for other neurotransmitter chemicals (norepinephrine and serotonin), the buildup of dopamine in the limbic system (nucleus accumbens) is thought to underlie its powerful pleasurable effect.

Absorption and Elimination

People can, and do, use cocaine in many ways. Chewing and sucking the leaves allows the cocaine to be absorbed slowly through the mucous membranes. This results in a slower onset of effects and much lower blood levels than are usually obtained via snorting, the most common route by which the drug is used recreationally. In snorting, the intent is to get the very fine cocaine hydrochloride powder into the nasal passages—right on the nasal mucosa. From there it is absorbed quite rapidly and, through circulatory mechanisms that are not completely understood, reaches the brain rather quickly.

The intravenous use of cocaine delivers a very high concentration to the brain, producing a rapid and brief effect. For that reason, intravenous cocaine used to be a favourite among compulsive users, many of whom switched from intranasal to intravenous use. However, the smoking of crack is now preferred by most compulsive users because this route is less invasive (no needles) and the onset of its effects is just as fast.

The cocaine molecules are metabolized by enzymes in the blood and liver, and the activity of these enzymes is variable from one person to another. In any case, cocaine itself is rapidly removed, with a half-life of about one hour. The major metabolites, which are the basis of urine screening tests, have a longer half-life of about eight hours.

Medical Uses of Cocaine

After the discovery of pure cocaine in the 1860s, it gained widespread use as a local anaesthetic. It was also sold and used without any scientific evidence of its effect in a variety of countless patented tonics and elixirs for a number of medical conditions. It is still occasionally used as a local anaesthetic for eye, ear, and nose surgery but has been largely replaced by less toxic substances.

Local Anaesthesia The local anaesthetic properties of cocaine—its ability to numb the area to which it is applied—were discovered in 1860 soon after its isolation from coca leaves. It was not until 1884 that this characteristic was used medically; the early applications were in eye surgery and dentistry. The use of cocaine spread rapidly because it apparently was a safe and effective drug. The potential for misuse soon became clear, though, and a search began for synthetic agents with similar anaesthetic characteristics but little or no potential for misuse. This work was rewarded in

1905 with the discovery of procaine (Novocain), which is still in wide use.

Many drugs have been synthesized since 1905 that have local anaesthetic properties similar to those of cocaine but have little or no ability to produce CNS stimulation. Those drugs have largely replaced cocaine for medical use. However, because cocaine is absorbed so well into mucous membranes, it remains in use for surgery in the nasal, laryngeal, and esophageal regions.

Other Claimed Benefits Because cocaine produces a feeling of increased energy and well-being, it enjoyed an important status among achievers of the 1980s who self-prescribed it to overcome fatigue. Many athletes and entertainers felt that they could not consistently perform at their peak without the assistance of cocaine, and this resulted in increased cocaine use among these groups. Cocaine has not been used medically for its CNS effects for many years, in part because its effects are brief, but mostly because of concern about the development of dependence.

Causes for Concern

No evidence exists that occasional use of small amounts of cocaine is a threat to the individual's health. However, many people have increased the amount they use to the point of toxicity.

Acute Toxicity Acute cocaine poisoning leads to profound CNS stimulation, progressing to convulsions, which can lead to respiratory or cardiac arrest. This is in some ways similar to amphetamine overdose, with the exception that there is much greater individual variation in the uptake and metabolism of cocaine, so that a lethal dose is much more difficult to estimate. In addition, there are very rare, severe, and unpredictable toxic reactions to cocaine and other local anaesthetics, in which individuals die rapidly, apparently from cardiac failure. Cocaine can trigger the chaotic heart rhythm called ventricular fibrillation by preventing the vagus nerve from controlling the heartbeat.[13] Intravenous cocaine users might also experience an allergic reaction either to the drug or to some additive in street cocaine. The lungs fill rapidly with fluid, and death can occur.

It was reported in 1992 that the combination of cocaine and alcohol (ethanol) in the body could result in the formation of a chemical called **cocaethylene**, which was subsequently shown in mice to be more toxic than cocaine. However, studies in humans have shown that cocaethylene is less potent than cocaine with respect to its cardiovascular and subjective effects.[14]

Chronic Toxicity Regularly snorting cocaine, and particularly cocaine that has been "cut" with other things, can irritate the nasal septum, leading to a chronically inflamed, runny nose. Because of the high temperatures required for smoking crack, the unsafe quality of the paraphernalia used (makeshift devices, such as pop cans, inhalers, or other metal or glass implements), and repeated inhalation because of its short duration of effect, users often have persistent cuts, burns, and open sores or wounds on their lips, gums, and inner mouth lining.[15] Use of cocaine in a binge, during which the drug is taken repeatedly and at increasingly high doses, can lead to a state of increasing irritability, restlessness, and paranoia. In severe cases, this can result in a full-blown paranoid psychosis, in which the individual loses touch with reality and experiences auditory hallucinations.[16] This experience is disruptive and quite frightening. However, most individuals seem to recover from the psychosis as the drug leaves the system.

There has been concern for several years about the effects of chronic cocaine use on the heart muscle. It appears that, in some users, frequent, brief disruption of the heart's function can damage the heart muscle itself.[17] It is not clear how often such damage occurs.

Dependence Potential Cocaine can produce dependence in some users, particularly among those who inject it or inhale the vapours of smokeable cocaine. Each year, cocaine accounts for one of the largest proportions of admission for drug treatment.[18] Additionally, in laboratory experiments, human research volunteers will perform rigorous tasks to receive a dose of cocaine.[19] Virtually every species of laboratory animal, when given the opportunity, will readily self-administer cocaine and if given unlimited access to cocaine they will self-administer the drug until their eventual death.[20] Thus, it appears that cocaine can be a powerfully reinforcing drug: Take it and it will make you want to take it again.

Throughout the 1970s, the importance of this dependence potential went unrecognized, partly because cocaine was expensive and in short supply and largely because the common method of using

cocaethylene: a chemical formed when ethanol and cocaine are co-administered.

cocaine during this time was snorting it. The 1980s saw an increase in freebasing and then of the more convenient form of smokeable cocaine: crack or rock. As relatively large numbers of people began to smoke cocaine in the mid-1980s, the dependence potential of this form of use became clear to the public and to the users themselves.

Because at one time drug dependence was linked to the presence of physical withdrawal symptoms (when the abused substance was removed), a number of experiments have studied whether physical withdrawal symptoms appear on abrupt cessation after repeated cocaine use. After prolonged daily cocaine administration in animals, there were no obvious withdrawal signs (for example, no diarrhea or convulsions), and many scientists concluded that cocaine produced no physical dependence and was therefore not a dependence-producing drug. More recent experience has led to a different way of looking at this issue. Abuse potential of a drug is no longer defined solely by the presence of physical withdrawal symptoms during drug abstinence. As was discussed in Chapter 2, a person may be diagnosed with a stimulant (cocaine) use disorder if he or she exhibits a set of maladaptive behaviours listed in the DSM-5, which may or may not include physical withdrawal symptoms. Following several days of cocaine use (a binge), a constellation of withdrawal symptoms may be present, including cocaine craving, irritability, anxiety, depressed mood, increased appetite, and exhaustion. The severity of withdrawal symptoms from cocaine are related to the dosage and purity of cocaine administered, frequency of use, chronicity of use, route of administration, extent of other drug use (i.e., alcohol, benzodiazepine, opioid), and the extent and severity of drug-related medical and psychiatric complications.

Reproductive Effects Early reports of babies being born under the influence of cocaine resulted in lurid media accounts of the "crack baby" phenomenon, which unfortunately overstated both the number of such children and the expected long-term effects. However, more recent data from well-controlled human studies indicate that, among children six years old and younger, there are no consistent negative associations between prenatal cocaine exposure and several developmental measures, including physical growth, test scores, and language.[21] The long-term effects of prenatal cocaine exposure on older children are less well known because limited data are available. Nevertheless, the use of cocaine during pregnancy is not recommended because of more immediate problems associated with cocaine use during pregnancy—the risk increases for both spontaneous abortions (miscarriages) and a torn placenta. It should be noted that of all the drugs used during pregnancy the one most associated with birth defects and cognitive behavioural problems is the legal drug alcohol.

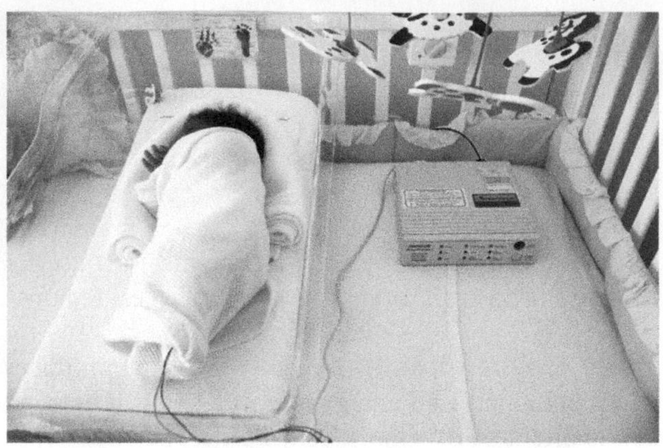

Cocaine use during pregnancy increases the risk of serious complications. Although the early negative effects of prenatal exposure have been overstated in media accounts, the long-term effects on exposed children aren't well known.

Current Patterns of Cocaine Use

The United Nations Office on Drugs and Crime *World Drug Report 2009* estimates that the annual prevalence of cocaine use worldwide ranges from 15.6 million to 20.8 million people in 2007. In Canada, the *Canadian Alcohol and Drug Use Monitoring Survey* (CADUMS) is an ongoing general population survey of alcohol and illicit drug use among Canadians ages 15 years and older, designed to provide detailed national and provincial estimates of alcohol and drug-related behaviours and outcomes. The results for the 2009 survey were based on telephone interviews with 13 082 respondents, across all ten provinces, representing 25 957 435 Canadian residents. Table 6.1 shows changes in cocaine use between the *Canadian Addiction Survey* (CAS 2004) and the CADUMS surveys (2008 and 2009) by age and gender.

The *Northwest Territories Addiction Survey 2006* is based on the core components of the questionnaire used in the CAS 2004. A total of 845 residents 15 years of age or older completed the survey. It was estimated that 11.6% of respondents had used cocaine or crack over their lifetime, with males reporting higher rates than females (15.7% for males versus 7.2% for females). It was also reported that 1.8% of residents had used cocaine or crack in the past 12 months, but the report emphasizes caution in interpretation because of high

Table 6.1 Cocaine Use in Canada, CAS 2004 and CADUMS 2008 and 2009

	Cocaine/Crack Use in the Past Year by Age					
	Age 15–24			Age 25+		
	CAS 2004	CADUMS 2008	CADUMS 2009	CAS 2004	CADUMS 2008	CADUMS 2009
Sample size	2 085	1 443	955	11 519	15 197	15 197
Users of cocaine/crack	5.5 (4.0–7.4)	5.9 (3.9–0.9)	3.0* (1.6–5.3)	1.2 (0.9–1.6)	0.8 (0.6–1.1)	0.9 (0.5–1.5)
	Cocaine/Crack Use in the Past Year by Gender					
	Male			**Female**		
	CAS 2004	**CADUMS 2008**	**CADUMS 2009**	**CAS 2004**	**CADUMS 2008**	**CADUMS 2009**
Sample size	5 721	6 583	5 260	8 188	10 057	7 823
Users of cocaine/crack	2.7 (2.1–3.5)	2.3 (1.7–3.3)	1.5 (0.9–2.6)	1.1 (0.8–1.6)	0.9 (0.6–1.6)	0.9 (0.5–1.6)

*Estimate is qualified because of high sampling variability; interpret with caution.

Source: Adapted from Health Canada. *Canadian Alcohol and Drug Use Monitoring Survey 2009*, Tables 4 and 5. 2010. Retrieved September 26, 2011, from http://www.hc-sc.gc.ca/hc-ps/drugs-drogues/stat/_2009/tables-tableaux-eng.php.

sampling variability.[22] Even though cocaine's source countries are in Mexico and South America, it would appear that its availability and past-year use rates are comparable to the national past-year use rates shown in Table 6.1. No longer can cocaine be considered a drug of the affluent in Canada as it was in the 1970s.

The *Student Drug Use Survey in the Atlantic Provinces* (SDUSAP) *2007: Atlantic Technical Report* surveyed 17 545 students in Nova Scotia, Prince Edward Island, Newfoundland and Labrador, and New Brunswick in grades 7, 9, 10, and 12. Less than 5% of the students reported having used cocaine or crack in the last year. Students in grades 7-12 would typically be between 13 and 19 years of age (teenagers). This rate is comparable to the national past-year cocaine/crack use in 15-24-year-olds (teenagers and young adults) shown in Table 6.1. Additionally, less than 5% reported having used amphetamine or methylphenidate in the past year without a doctor's prescription, and less than 2% reported having used crystal methamphetamine.[23]

Cocaine's Future

In attempting to predict the future, we can learn from two writers who have made successful predictions about cocaine use in the past. The first, writing in the early 1970s, pointed out that historically, as cocaine use declined, amphetamine use increased. Looking at the decline in amphetamine use in the late 1960s, he predicted the increased use of cocaine that we saw in the 1970s and early 1980s.[24] The other writer[5] pointed out that at the height of cocaine use in 1986, we were

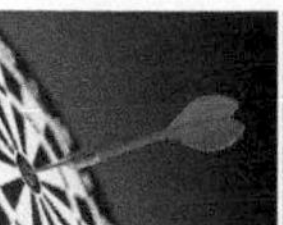

TARGETING PREVENTION

Cocaine and Friendship

Imagine you have a good friend, Terri, who has been using cocaine off and on for a year. However, in the past couple of months it seems that Terri's use has become more frequent. You have had to stop lending her money because she never pays it back. When you hinted that her cocaine use might be getting out of hand, she did not respond. When you tried direct confrontation, she angrily denied that she had a problem. You are still good friends. You certainly don't want to turn Terri in to the police, but you are getting pretty worried. What do you think you should do?

There are multiple answers to this problem. It might be interesting to discuss this hypothetical situation with a group of friends to find out how they would want to be treated under the circumstances.

reliving an earlier cycle of cocaine use that occurred around the start of the twentieth century.

When cocaine was introduced in the 1880s, the experts had mostly positive opinions about its effects, and it was regarded as a fairly benign substance. In the second stage (1890s), more people used cocaine, and its dangers and side effects became well known. In the third stage, in the early 1900s, society turned against cocaine and passed laws to control it. After many years with little cocaine use, in the early 1970s the drug again had the reputation of being fairly benign and not capable of producing "real" dependence. In the 1980s, we were again in the second stage, in which increasing use eventually made us all aware of the potential dangers. This comparison led to the prediction that Canadians would again turn away from cocaine and would pass increased legal restrictions on it. This prediction came true during the late 1980s. Cocaine use has increased slightly since then, but the more interesting story has been the re-emergence of another illicit stimulant drug, amphetamine (and in particular, methamphetamine). Once again, it seems that as use of cocaine decreased, the market shifted somewhat toward amphetamines.

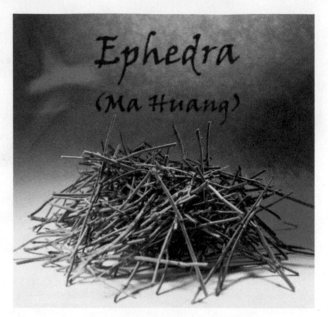

The active ingredient in the herb *ma huang* is ephedrine, which is chemically similar to amphetamine.

LO7 Amphetamines

Like cocaine, the amphetamines are powerful CNS stimulants. They produce a number of effects, including increased energy, wakefulness, alertness, reduced hunger, and feelings of wellness.

History

For centuries the Chinese have made a medicinal tea from herbs they call *ma huang,* which North American scientists classify in the genus *Ephedra*. The active ingredient in these herbs is called **ephedrine**, and it is used to dilate the bronchial passages in asthma patients. Bronchial dilation can be achieved by stimulating the sympathetic branch of the autonomic nervous system, and that is exactly what ephedrine does (it is referred to as a **sympathomimetic** drug). This drug also has other effects related to its sympathetic nervous system stimulation, such as elevating blood pressure. In the late 1920s, researchers synthesized and studied the effects of a new chemical that was similar in structure to ephedrine: **Amphetamine** was patented in 1932.

All major effects of amphetamine were discovered in the 1930s, although some of the uses were developed later. Amphetamine's first use was as a replacement for ephedrine in the treatment of asthma. Quite early it was shown that amphetamine was a potent dilator of the nasal and bronchial passages and could be efficiently delivered through inhalation. The Benzedrine (brand name) inhaler was introduced as an over-the-counter (OTC) product in 1932 for treating the stuffy noses caused by colds.

Some of the early work with amphetamine showed that the drug would awaken anaesthetized dogs. As one writer put it, amphetamine is the drug that won't let sleeping dogs lie! This led to the testing of amphetamine for the treatment of **narcolepsy** in 1935. Narcolepsy is a condition in which the individual spontaneously falls asleep as many as 50 times a day. Amphetamine enables these patients to remain awake and function almost normally. In 1938, however, two narcolepsy patients treated with amphetamine developed acute paranoid psychotic reactions. The paranoid reaction to amphetamine has reappeared regularly and has been studied (discussed later in this chapter).

ephedrine: a sympathomimetic drug used in treating asthma.

sympathomimetic: a drug that stimulates the sympathetic branch of the autonomic nervous system.

amphetamine: a synthetic CNS stimulant and sympathomimetic.

narcolepsy: a disease that causes people to fall asleep suddenly.

In 1937, amphetamine became available as a prescription tablet, and a report appeared in the literature suggesting that amphetamine, a stimulant, was effective in reducing activity in hyperactive children. Two years later, in 1939, notice was taken of a report by amphetamine-treated narcolepsy patients that they were not hungry when taking the drug. This appetite-depressant effect became the major clinical use of amphetamine. A group of psychology students at the University of Minnesota began experimenting with various drugs in 1937 and found that amphetamine was ideal for "cramming," because it allowed them to stay awake for long periods. Truck drivers also noted this effect, and they used "bennies" to stay awake during long hauls.

Wartime Uses In 1939, amphetamine went to war. There were many reports that Germany was using amphetamines to increase the efficiency of its soldiers. Such statements provided the basis for other countries to evaluate the utility of amphetamines. A 1944 report in the *Air Surgeon's Bulletin,* titled "Benzedrine Alert," stated, "This drug is the most satisfactory of any available in temporarily postponing sleep when desire to sleep endangers the security of a mission."[25] Some early studies were reported, including one in which

> 100 Marines were kept active continuously for 60 hours in range firing, a 25-mile forced march, a field problem, calisthenics, close-order drill, games, fatigue detail and bivouac alerts. Fifty men received seven 10-milligram tablets of benzedrine at six hour intervals following the first day's activity. Meanwhile, the other 50 were given placebo (milk sugar) tablets. None knew what he was receiving. Participating officers concluded that the benzedrine definitely "pepped up" the subjects, improved their morale, reduced sleepiness and increased confidence in shooting ability. . . . It was observed that men receiving benzedrine tended to lead the march, tolerate their sore feet and blisters more cheerfully, and remain wide awake during "breaks," whereas members of the control group had to be shaken to keep them from sleeping.

In addition to Germany's use of amphetamines during World War II, Canadian, U.S., and Japanese soldiers were issued amphetamines by military personnel to help them stay alert and to reduce fatigue. However, the German high command was disturbed by the side effects associated with amphetamines and they became prohibited after Russians captured elite Waffen SS troops who were equipped with guns but no bullets. It was later revealed that this fighting unit, in a fit of paranoia after amphetamine use, had wasted all of their ammunition firing at imaginary enemies the night before.[26]

Amphetamines were widely used in Japan during World War II to maintain production on the home front and to keep the fighting men going. To reduce large stockpiles of methamphetamine after the war, the drug was sold without prescription, and the drug companies advertised them for "elimination of drowsiness and repletion of the spirit." Such widespread use was accompanied by considerable overuse and abuse. In 1948 and again in 1955, strict amphetamine controls were enacted, along with treatment and education programs. Although the Japanese government claimed to have "eliminated" the amphetamine-abuse problem before 1960, there were smaller Japanese "epidemics" of methamphetamine use in the 1970s and 1980s.

The "Speed Scene" of the 1960s Amphetamine use in North America peaked between the 1950s and early 1970s. Most of the misuse of amphetamines was through the legally manufactured and legally purchased oral preparation. Truck drivers, students, and athletes were groups that abused amphetamines in Canada during that time because they were easily available in this country. It is difficult to pinpoint exactly when intravenous (IV) abuse of amphetamines began in North America, but it was probably among IV users of heroin and cocaine. In the 1920s and 1930s, when IV use of those drugs was spreading among the drug subculture, the combination of heroin and cocaine injected together was known as the **speedball**, presumably because the cocaine rush or flash occurs rapidly after injection, thus speeding up the high. So, on the streets, one name for cocaine was "speed." When the amphetamines became so widely available after World War II, some of these enterprising individuals discovered that they could get an effect similar to that of cocaine if they injected amphetamine along with the heroin. Thus, amphetamines came to be known as **speed** by that small drug underground that used heroin intravenously. By the 1960s, amphetamines had become so widely available at such a low price that more IV drug users were using them, either in combination with heroin or alone. Currently, levels of amphetamine abuse have decreased in North America, presumably because of a greater awareness of their abuse potential and limited therapeutic benefits, which

speedball: the combination of heroin and cocaine injected together.

speed: a street name for cocaine, and then later amphetamine.

have resulted in regulations governing their prescribing in Canada. Amphetamines are a Schedule I drug in Canada's Controlled Drugs and Substances Act.

The most desired drug on the streets was methamphetamine, which was available in liquid form in ampoules for injection. Hospital emergency rooms sometimes used this drug to stimulate respiration in patients suffering from overdoses of sleeping pills (no longer considered an appropriate treatment), and physicians also used injectable amphetamines intramuscularly to treat obesity. In the San Francisco Bay area, reports appeared in the early 1960s of "fat doctors" who had large numbers of patients coming in regularly for no treatment other than an injection of methamphetamine.

Because some heroin users would inject amphetamines alone when they could not obtain heroin, some physicians also felt that methamphetamine could serve as a legal substitute for heroin and thus be a form of treatment. In those days, amphetamines were not considered to produce dependency, so these physicians were quite free with their prescriptions.[24] Reports of those abuses led to federal regulation of amphetamines within the new concept of dangerous drugs in the 1965 U.S law. Unfortunately, the publicity associated with these revelations and the ensuing legislation caught the attention of young people whose identity as a generation was defined largely by experimentation with drugs their parents and government told them were dangerous. To the Haight-Ashbury district of San Francisco came the flower children, to sit in Golden Gate Park, smoke marijuana, take LSD, and discuss peace, love, and the brotherhood of humanity. They moved in next door to the old, established drug subculture, in which IV drug use was endemic. That mixture resulted in the speed scene and young people who became dependent on IV amphetamines. Although in historical perspective the speed scene of the late 1960s was relatively short-lived and only a small number of people were directly involved, it was the focus of a great deal of national concern, and it helped change the way the medical profession and society at large viewed these drugs, which had been so widely accepted.

As the abuse of amphetamines began to be recognized, physicians prescribed less of the drugs. Their new legal status as dangerous drugs put restrictions on prescriptions and refills, and in the 1970s the total amount of these drugs that could be manufactured was limited. Thus, within less than a decade, amphetamines went from being widely used and accepted pharmaceuticals to being less widely used, tightly restricted drugs associated in the public mind with drug-abusing hippies.

As controls tightened on legally manufactured amphetamines, at least three reactions continued to affect the drug scene. The first reaction was that a market began to develop for "look-alike" pills: legal, milder stimulants (usually caffeine or ephedrine) packaged in tablets and capsules that were virtually identical in colour, shape, and markings to prescription amphetamines. Later the makers of look-alikes began to expand the variety of shapes and sizes to attract a wider market. Because these pills contained legally available, OTC ingredients, their sellers could not be prosecuted. By the early 1980s, the odds were good that if someone bought "speed" pills from a street dealer they were actually getting look-alikes. The U.S. national high school survey had to apply a correction factor to its data to account for these look-alikes and get a more accurate measure of actual amphetamine use. The U.S. FDA began to crack down on manufacturers and distributors of pills containing large amounts of caffeine or mixtures of caffeine and other legal stimulants, and passed regulations making it illegal to distribute any substance that is misrepresented to be a controlled substance. The section on "Supplies of

(a)

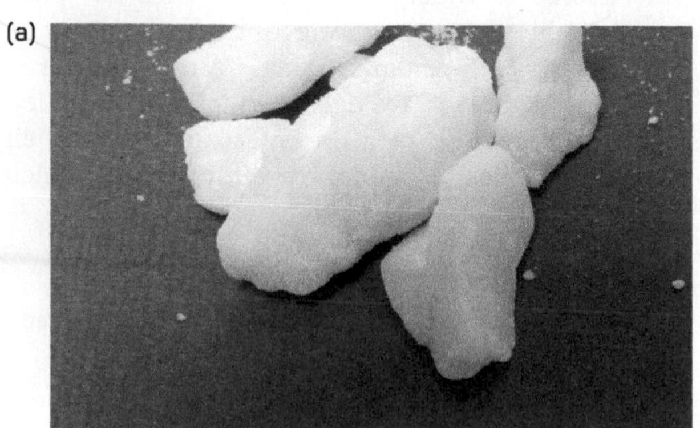

(b)

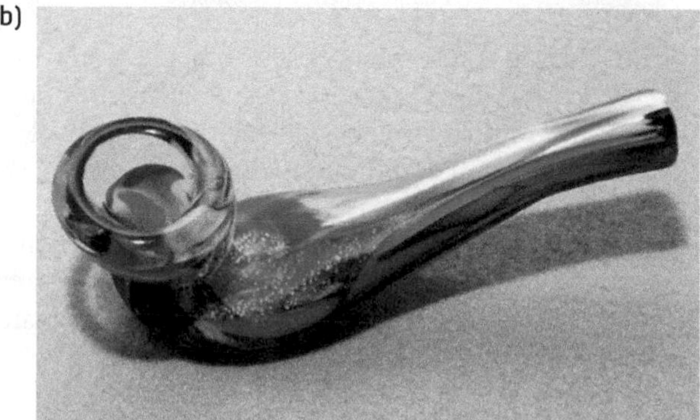

Ice is a smokeable form of methamphetamine (a) crystals, (b) pipe.

Illicit Methamphetamine in Canada" below describes the regulations enacted by Canada to decrease export of precursors and essential chemicals to produce methamphetamine.

The reduced availability of legally manufactured amphetamines had a second important effect. As the price went up and the quality of the available speed became more questionable, the drug subculture began, slowly and without fanfare, to rekindle its interest in a more "natural," reportedly less dangerous stimulant–cocaine. In 1970, federal agents in Miami reported that "the traffic in cocaine is growing by leaps and bounds."[24] And as we now know, they were seeing only the small beginnings of a cocaine trade that would swell to much greater size by the mid-1980s.

The Return of Methamphetamine The third reaction to limited amphetamine availability was an increase in the number of illicit laboratories making methamphetamine, which acquired the name **crank**. Most illicit methamphetamine is produced in small "stovetop laboratories," which might exist for only a few days in a remote area before moving on. The process for making methamphetamine has been on the streets since the 1960s, and illicit laboratories have been raided every year. By the late 1990s, however, the number of illicit methamphetamine laboratories confiscated by the authorities had increased more than eight-fold, a clear indication that methamphetamine was the next drug fad. A major concern with clandestine methamphetamine laboratories is that fumes and residue associated with these laboratories are dangerous.[27]

In 1989, the media began warning of the next drug epidemic: the "smoking" of methamphetamine hydrochloride crystals, also known by the street names **ice, crystal meth**, chalk, crank, fire, speed, gak, glass, Tina, and yaba. Although many media accounts regarding methamphetamine-related effects and its dependence-producing potential were exaggerated, methamphetamine abuse rose dramatically during the 1990s. By 1999, more than 9 million Americans had used methamphetamine at least once. Five years earlier this number was less than 4 million. In recent history, methamphetamine abuse has been viewed as a western phenomenon; methamphetamine is the most common primary drug of abuse cited for treatment admissions in Honolulu and San Diego. Other indicators of increased methamphetamine use include data from DAWN, which show methamphetamine-associated emergency department admissions and deaths have remained considerably higher than for any other "club drug," a term derived from the association of certain drugs with dance clubs, for more than a decade.[28,29] The drug of the 1960s urban hippie has now become associated with other subgroups including biker gangs, rural Canadians, and urban gay communities. Although methamphetamine use has received a lot of media attention recently, its use in Canada is relatively low compared with other drugs of abuse. Table 6.2 shows

crank: a street name for illicitly manufactured methamphetamine.

ice, crystal meth: street names for crystals of methamphetamine hydrochloride.

Table 6.2 Past-Year and Lifetime Use of Methamphetamine

	Overall	Males	Females	15–24-Year-Olds	25+ Year-Olds
N	13 082	5 260	7 822	955	15 197
Past-Year Methamphetamine Use					
	0.1% (0.0%–0.3%)	NR	NR	NR	NR
Lifetime Methamphetamine Use					
	0.9% (0.6%–1.4%)	1.4% (0.9%–2.3%)	0.5% (0.2%–0.9%)	1.8%* (0.9%–3.7%)	0.8% (0.5%–1.2%)

NR = not reported because of high sampling variability

*Estimate is qualified because of high sampling variability; interpret with caution.

Source: Adapted from Health Canada. *Canadian Alcohol and Drug Use Monitoring Survey: Summary of Results for 2010.* 2011. Retrieved September 13, 2011, from http://www.hc-sc.gc.ca/hc-ps/drugs-drogues/stat/_2010/summary-sommaire-eng.php.

the prevalence rate and 95% confidence interval for past-year and lifetime use of methamphetamine by age and gender from the 2009 CADUMS.

Supplies of Illicit Methamphetamine in Canada

According to the Royal Canadian Mounted Police *Drug Situation in Canada 2007 Report*, demand for methamphetamine in Canada is not broad-based but rather originates from those segments of the community where the drug is associated with certain lifestyles.[30] In core production regions, such as British Columbia, Ontario, and Quebec, availability is high and prices are relatively stable. In British Columbia, where an estimated 75% of all meth lab seizures occurred in 2007, the bulk of operations were economic-based labs run by organized crime groups. The average price range across Canada is estimated at between $80 and $150 per gram, but a gram of meth can go for as low as $50 in high-density production areas, such as Vancouver and mainland British Columbia.

While powder and crystal methamphetamine are readily available, consumption of the drug in tablet form is on the rise. In a continuing trend, consumers in Quebec prefer methamphetamine in tablets. Patterns in 2007 showed Canadian meth labs to have advanced levels of production capacity and capabilities to provide a flourishing supply beyond the demands of domestic trade. The Asia-Pacific region continued to grow as a consumer region for powder methamphetamine manufactured and transported directly from Canada.

Canada has earned a reputation as an important methamphetamine source country. The Canadian and U.S. governments have legislated several regulations designed to suppress methamphetamine production and purity by limiting access to the precursor chemicals (ephedrine and pseudoephedrine) typically used in its production. Following the 1997 pseudoephedrine regulation in the United States, many large-scale producers turned to precursor chemicals from Canada, as these chemicals were not yet regulated here.[31] Partly because of this and because of concerns about its own methamphetamine problems, Canada implemented three precursor chemical regulations anticipated to impact large-scale producers.[32,33]

The first two Canadian regulations addressed precursor chemicals, which by definition are used in the preparation of a drug and become part of its molecular structure; the third regulation addressed essential chemicals, which are used in the preparation of a drug but do not become part of its molecular structure.[34] Canada's essential chemical regulation has affected primarily producers of lower-quality methamphetamine, leaving higher-purity methamphetamine on the market by default in the United States.[35]

Pharmacology of Amphetamines

Research has led to a better understanding of the mechanisms responsible for amphetamine's ability to produce its pleasurable effects, the regions of the brain activated, and the neurotransmitters responsible for its effects.

Source Amphetamines are produced through chemical synthesis by pharmaceutical companies or in illicit laboratories on the street.

Chemical Structure Figure 6.4 illustrates some similarities in the structures of amphetamines and related drugs. First, note the likeness between the molecular structures of the catecholamine neurotransmitters (dopamine and norepinephrine) and the basic amphetamine molecule. It appears that amphetamine produces its effects because it is recognized as one of these catecholamines at many sites in both the central and the peripheral nervous systems. The amphetamine molecule has both "left-handed" and "right-handed" forms (l and d forms). The original Benzedrine was an equal mixture of both forms. The d form is several times as potent in its CNS effects, however, and in 1945 d-amphetamine was first marketed as Dexedrine for use as an appetite suppressant.

Next, look at the methamphetamine molecule, which simply has a methyl group added to the basic amphetamine structure. This methyl group seems to make the molecule cross the blood-brain barrier more readily and thus further increase the CNS potency. (If more of the molecules get into the brain, then fewer total molecules have to be given.) However, the behavioural significance of this in humans has yet to be determined, as studies directly comparing the two compounds report no difference on many measures, including subjective drug-effect ratings and heart rate. Notice the structures for ephedrine, the old Chinese remedy that is still used to treat asthma, and for phenylpropanolamine (PPA). Before 2000, PPA was an ingredient in OTC weight-control preparations (see Chapter 12) and in many of the look-alikes. Both of these molecules have a structural addition that makes them not cross the blood-brain barrier as well; therefore, they produce peripheral effects without as much CNS effectiveness.

Figure 6.4 Molecular Structures of Stimulants

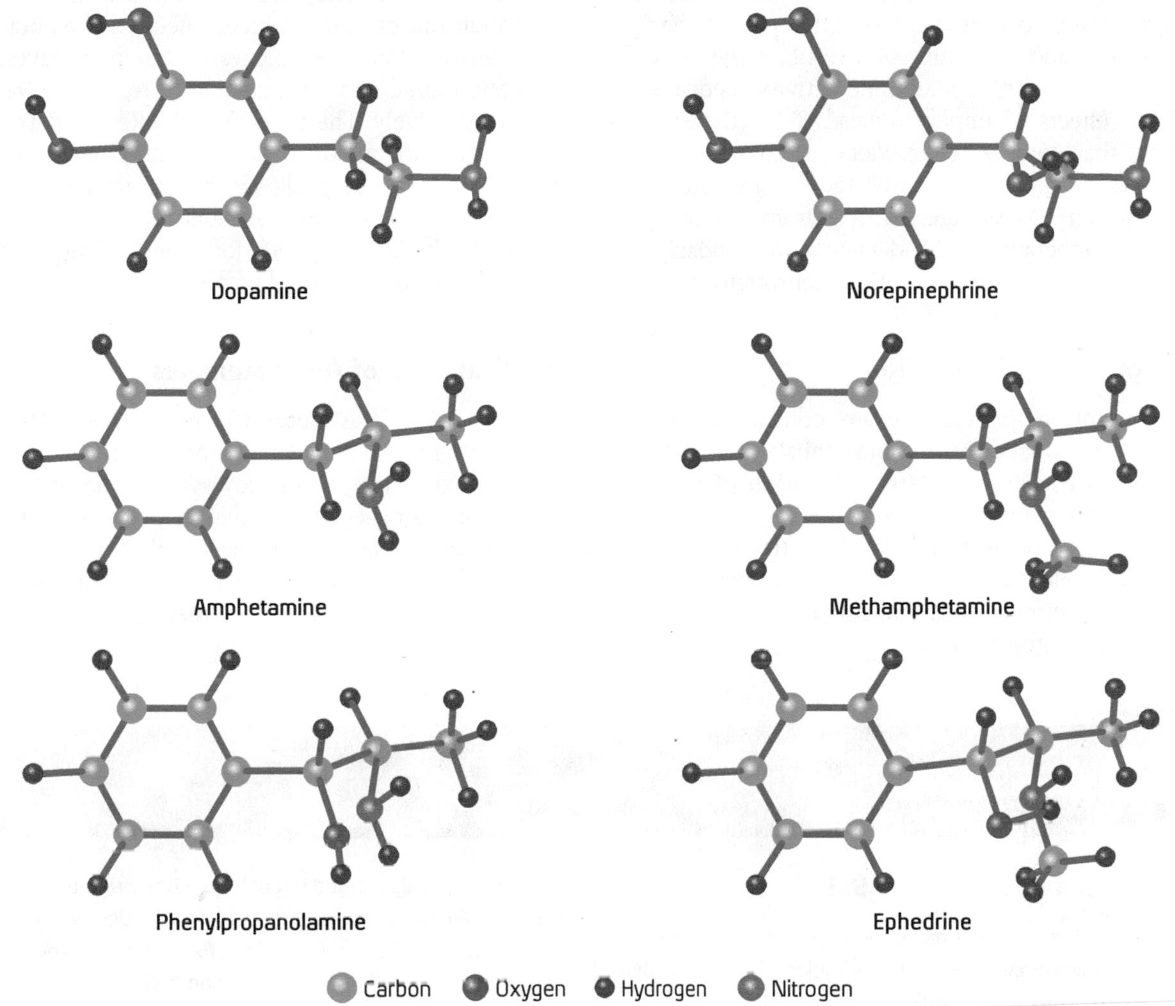

Mechanism of Action

Amphetamines increase the release of dopamine, norepinephrine, and serotonin from their storage vesicles, resulting in an increased concentration of these monoamines in the synapse.[36] In addition, amphetamines also block the reuptake of dopamine, norepinephrine, and serotonin. Typically, neurons recycle monoamines by taking the released neurotransmitters back up into the terminal through a process of reuptake. Therefore, the effects of the monoamines are much more powerful when the reuptake process is blocked. Whereas cocaine has a similar affinity for transporters of all three monoamines, amphetamines have negligible binding to the serotonin transporter and are five to nine times as potent at the norepinephrine transporter as at the dopamine transporter.[37,38] Amphetamine attenuates monoamine metabolism by inhibiting monoamine oxidase.[39] While there is a relatively low potency of amphetamines at monoamine oxidase, we cannot discount a contribution from MAO inhibition to its spectrum of physiological activity.

Findings from studies of laboratory animals strongly implicate dopamine in mediating amphetamine-related reinforcement. For example, researchers have reported that amphetamines produce substantial increases in dopamine levels in the nucleus accumbens, a brain region thought to be important for drug-related reinforcement. In humans, while amphetamine-induced euphoria and brain dopamine elevations have been positively correlated, dopamine antagonists do not block the euphoria produced by amphetamine.[40] These observations suggest that exclusive focus on dopamine might be overly simplistic. Recent evidence shows that amphetamines are more potent releasers of norepinephrine than of dopamine and serotonin. As a result, some researchers speculate that norepinephrine activity mediates the euphoric effects of amphetamines.[41] Nevertheless, it is unlikely that complex drug effects, such as subjective effects and drug taking, are mediated via one neurotransmitter system. As we are learning from our study of cocaine, amphetamine-related effects are probably the result of interactions with multiple neurotransmitters.

Absorption and Elimination

Like cocaine, amphetamines are consumed through a variety of routes: intravenous, inhalation, oral, and intranasal. Virtually complete elimination of the drug occurs within two days of the last dose.

With high doses a tachyphylaxis (rapid tolerance) may be seen. Because amphetamine produces its effects largely by displacing the monoamine transmitters from their storage sites, with large doses the monoamines might be sufficiently depleted, so that another dose within a few hours may not be able to displace as much neurotransmitter, and a reduced effect will be obtained.

Methamphetamine bioavailability of intravenous, inhalation, oral, and intranasal is 100%, 90%, 67%, and 79%, respectively. The time to peak effect is fastest for intravenous, followed by smoking and oral administration, while time to peak effect of intranasal administration is unknown. The authors refer the reader to Cruickshank and Dyer, 2009 for review of clinical pharmacokinetics of methamphetamine.

Medical Uses of Amphetamines

In the 1930s, the potential medical usefulness of amphetamines was recognized for both their stimulant and anorexiant properties. However, by the late 1940s, the enthusiasm began to diminish because of reports that amphetamines were being widely abused. Despite the high dependence potential of amphetamines, they are still used for a variety of medical conditions, as described below.

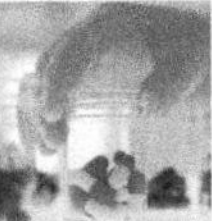

DRUGS IN THE MEDIA

Canadian Use of "Bath Salts"

"Bath salts" is the street name for a synthetic cathinone that contains amphetamine-type stimulants such as methylenedioxypyrovalerone (MDPV), mephedrone, or methylone.[42,44,45,46,47,48,50] The drug is commonly snorted or taken orally, but can also be injected and smoked.[42,44,46,50] The term "bath salts" is due to its resemblance to hygiene products that are added to bath water for cleansing.[44,45,47,48,49,50] The desired effects of the drug are increased energy, alertness, sociability, and libido, but the negative effects include hallucinations, decreased appetite, chest pain (due to heart palpations, hypertension, and tachycardia), hyperthermia or increased body temperature, agitation, and paranoia which can lead to violent behaviour.[42,44,45,47,48,49,50] Withdrawal effects may include depression, anergia or lack of energy, amnesia, inability to concentrate, and cravings.[42,44] Chronic use is associated with mood swings, insomnia, kidney failure, and muscle breakdown.[44]

Bath salts are relatively new and the statistics for Canadian consumption are limited. Possession and trafficking of bath salts is a concern in the Atlantic provinces; import to this area is mainly through the U.S. state of Maine, and the drug is distributed through New Brunswick then into the other Atlantic provinces.[42,45,46,47,48,50] From October 2012 through January 2013, persons from Pictou County, Nova Scotia were arrested for possession and trafficking bath salts,[43] with the largest drug seizures of bath salts in Canada thus far.[51,52,53] See Table 6.3 for a breakdown of bath salt activity across the country, ordered from west to east based on local reports between May 3 and May 22, 2012.

Mephedrone and methylone, the active ingredients in bath salts, are controlled substances in Canada. Recently, MDPV was made illegal because it was placed in the same category as heroin and cocaine.[42,45,47,48] Possession, trafficking, importing, exporting, and production of MDPV, mephedrone, and methylone is illegal and may result in fines, a criminal record, or a prison sentence.[44,47,48,50] Since bath salts are relatively new and there is limited information and statistics about the drug, Health Canada is currently working with law-enforcement agencies, such as the Royal Canadian Mounted Police, to determine new strategies to address risks to public health and safety and to communities related to the use of bath salts.[48,50]

continued

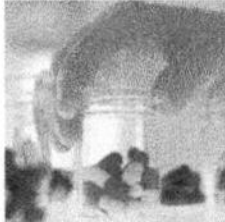

DRUGS IN THE MEDIA

Canadian Use of "Bath Salts"

continued

Table 6.3 Level of Concern Regarding the Use of Bath Salts among Canadian Municipalities

Low ◯ ◯ ◯ ◯ ◯ High

Level of Concern	City	Notes
◯	Vancouver	No reports
◯	Edmonton	No reports
◯	Prince Albert	Two cases of self-disclosed use of bath salts in the fall of 2011. Detox and outpatient facilities report people talking about bath salts, but no confirmed use.
◯	Winnipeg	Report of a few individuals claiming to have used bath salts irregularly when they were unable to obtain other drugs; however, nothing has been confirmed.
◯	Toronto	There is little to report in Toronto specific to MDPV. It is one of many "research chemicals" used among youth in Toronto's club and party scene. Use of these drugs is still limited, although growing. Data about local use of research chemicals are non-existent and reports are anecdotal. The most complete information comes from the TRIP Project, a harm reduction program working with youth in the club and party scene. TRIP has begun using test kits to see what pills actually contain. A TRIP staff member, who is also a member of Toronto's Research Group on Drug Use, noted that "the last pressed E pill tested by a volunteer came out positive for cathinones and piperazines." For more information, see TRIP's website: http://www.tripproject.ca/trip/?q=node/2005. At the provincial level, the 2011 Ontario student survey (OSDUHS) assessed the reported use of mephedrone or bath salts among students in grades 7 to 12. However, the estimates were suppressed because they were too low to estimate with the sample of 9,000. The Centre for Addiction and Mental Health (CAMH) has concluded that there is no evidence that mephedrone had measurably diffused to the student population.
◯	Ottawa	Neither treatment providers nor the police report encountering "bath salts." However, there is an expectation among some that areas of the Ottawa Valley could be seeing bath salts in the near future. This expectation is due to a seizure of bath salts by the Ontario Provincial Police in the neighbouring community of Arnprior.
◯	Montreal	No reports
◑	New Glasgow, NS	In April New Glasgow police reported a few cases of individuals acting erratically and posing a danger to themselves as a result of using bath salts. Local health authorities have reported at least fourteen (14) incidents related to bath salts in the past few months. These include cases reported by hospital emergency departments in New Glasgow and Truro, where individuals ingesting bath salts required emergency care. These incidences also include calls and admissions to local withdrawal management centres. Local authorities have found bath salts mixed with other drugs such as cannabis, so there is great concern that users may be unaware they are ingesting the substance. The Pictou County Health Authority has been meeting with local law enforcement to discuss the emergence of bath salts and discuss demand reduction and supply reduction strategies.

Source: CCENDU Drug Alert: "Bath Salts." Canadian Centre on Substance Abuse, Canadian Community Epidemiology Network on Drug Use Alerts and Bulletins. Published June 5, 2012. http://www.ccsa.ca/Resource%20Library/CCSA-CCENDU-Drug-Alert-Bath-Salts-2012-en.pdf. Reproduced with permission from the Canadian Centre on Substance Abuse.

The authors thank Danielle Bouthillier for article contribution.

Figure 6.5 Mood Changes over Time

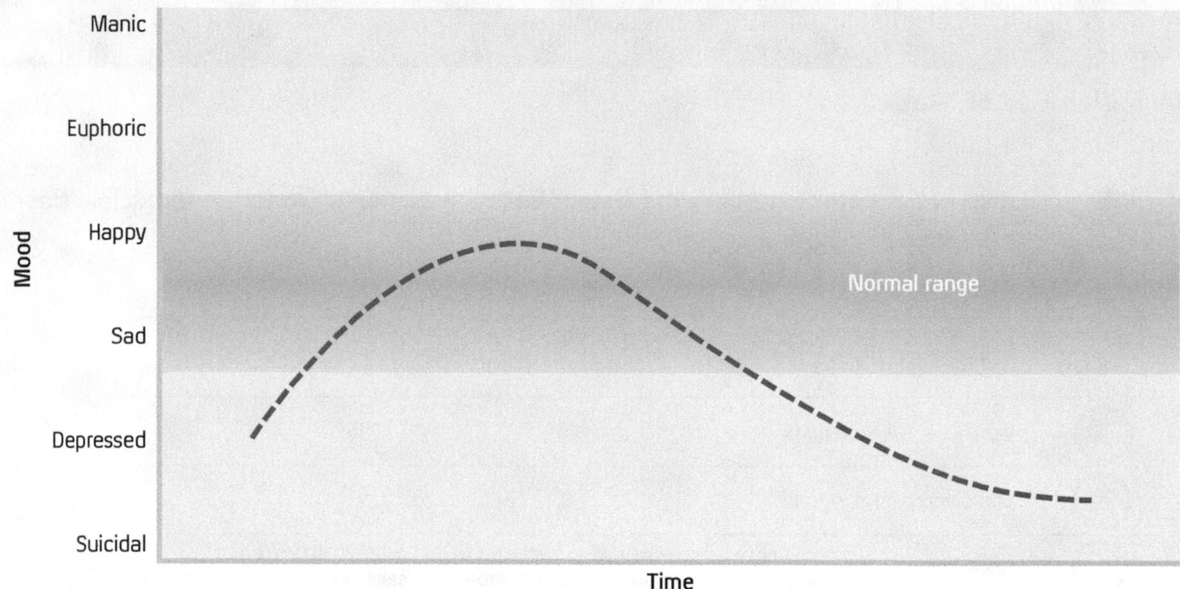

Previous Use for Depression During the 1950s and early 1960s, amphetamines were prescribed for depression and feelings of fatigue. If we look at an individual's mood as potentially ranging from very depressed, up through sadness into a normal range, and then into euphoria and finally the excited, manic range (Figure 6.5), we can better understand amphetamine's effects on mood. The person who is seriously depressed is not just sad; he or she feels helpless and hopeless with no energy and might think of suicide. Amphetamines are capable of temporarily moving the mood up the scale, so that a depressed person might, for a few hours, move into a normal range. But when the drug wears off, that person doesn't stay "up." The mood drops, often below the predrug level. To keep the mood up, the person needs to keep taking amphetamine. Amphetamine does interfere with sleep, so some physicians prescribed sleeping pills for nighttime. These patients often went for a daily "ride" on an emotional roller coaster, waking up depressed and taking a pill to get going in the morning, and either coming off the drug or taking a "downer" at night. As we will see in Chapter 8, other treatments are now used for depression, and amphetamines are rarely used for this purpose.

Weight Control Probably the most common medical use for amphetamines through the mid-1960s was for weight control. Studies show that amphetamine use reduces food intake and body weight. According to the 2004 *Canadian Community Health Survey: Nutrition*, 23.1% of Canadians aged 18 or older–an estimated 5.5 million adults–were obese.[54] This was significantly higher than estimates derived from self-reported data collected in 2003, which yielded an obesity rate of 15.2%. Another 8.6 million, or 36.1%, were overweight. With 33% of Americans overweight as well, the market is vast for a pill that would help us lose weight. For years the common medical response was some form of amphetamine or related sympathomimetic stimulant. Physicians dispensed prescriptions for pills and some gave injections, and a number of people did lose weight. But in the 1960s, when people began to view the amphetamines with greater concern, it was also clear that some people who took these stimulants regularly were still overweight.

To understand the role of stimulant drugs in weight control, let's imagine a typical experiment to test the value of amphetamine in treating obesity. Patients who meet some criterion for being overweight are recruited for the study. All are brought to a hospital or clinic, where they are weighed, interviewed, examined, and given a diet to follow. Half are given amphetamine and half a placebo in a double-blind design. Each week the patients return to the hospital, where they are interviewed, weighed, and given their supply of drug for the next week. After two months the drug code is broken and the amount of weight loss in each group is calculated. This type of study virtually always finds that both groups lose weight, mostly in the first two or three weeks. After that, the weight loss is much slower. This initial weight loss by both groups probably is a result of beginning a new diet and being involved in a medical study in which they know they will be weighed each week. Over the first two or three weeks the amphetamine group will lose a little more weight than the placebo group. The difference between the two groups after two or three weeks might be about one kilogram, which is statistically significant but probably not medically or cosmetically important. As the study continues, the gap stays about the same. In other words, in such studies the amphetamine effect is real but small and limited in duration. Even with moderate dose increases, four to six weeks seems to be the limit before tolerance occurs. Increasing to high doses might produce some further effect, but these experiments don't allow that, and it would be foolhardy as a treatment approach. The use of amphetamines for weight reduction came under attack from various sources, and the FDA in 1970 restricted the legal use of amphetamines to three types of conditions: narcolepsy, hyperkinetic (hyperactive) behaviour, and "short-term" weight-reduction programs.

Amphetamine and several related stimulant drugs are still used for weight control. Methamphetamine is available by prescription for short-term weight loss, as are the other sympathomimetics diethylpropion, phentermine, phenmetrazine, phendimetrazine, and some related but slightly different drugs, fenfluramine and mazindol. The FDA allows the sale of all these drugs even though experts point out that the drugs make a clinically trivial contribution to the overall weight reduction seen in the experiments. The package insert for each of these drugs includes the following FDA mandated statements:

> The natural history of obesity is measured in years, whereas most studies cited are restricted to a few weeks duration; thus, the total impact of drug induced weight loss over that of diet alone must be considered clinically limited. . . . [Drug name] is indicated in the management of exogenous obesity as a short-term (a few weeks) adjunct in a regimen of weight reduction based on caloric restriction. The limited usefulness of agents of this class must be weighed against possible risk factors inherent in their use.[55]

In November 1997, another new weight-control drug, sibutramine (Meridia), was introduced. Intended for use only in those who were extremely overweight, this drug was believed to act by blocking reuptake of both norepinephrine and serotonin. In October 2010, Abbott Laboratories voluntarily withdrew Meridia from the Canadian market.[56] The company's decision was based on data from the *Sibutramine Cardiovascular Outcomes Trial,* which demonstrated an increased risk of serious cardiovascular events associated with Meridia use in patients at high risk of cardiovascular events.

Narcolepsy Narcolepsy is a sleep disorder in which individuals do not sleep normally at night and in the daytime experience uncontrollable episodes of muscular weakness and falling asleep. Although interest has increased in sleep disorders in general, and sleep-disorder clinics are now associated with almost every major medical centre in Canada, the best available treatment for a long time was to keep the patient awake during the day with amphetamine or methylphenidate, a related stimulant. Recently, Health Canada approved modafinil (Alertec) to promote wakefulness in patients with narcolepsy. Modafinil's mechanism of action is complex and not completely understood, but increasing evidence indicates that its therapeutic effects depend on increasing the activity of glutamate and the catecholamine neurotransmitters norepinephrine and dopamine. Unlike amphetamines and other stimulants, modafinil appears to have low abuse potential[57] and has been demonstrated to be effective in the treatment of narcolepsy and excessive daytime sleepiness for up to 40 weeks, suggesting a lack of tolerance development.[58]

Hyperactive Children Even though it has been more than 50 years since the first report that amphetamine could reduce activity levels in hyperactive children, and even though hundreds of thousands of children are currently being treated with stimulant drugs for this problem, we still have controversy over the nature of the disorder being treated, we still don't understand what the drugs are doing to reduce hyperactivity, and we still don't have a widely accepted solution to the apparent paradox: Why does a stimulant drug appear to produce a calming effect?

The disorder itself was referred to as childhood hyperactivity for many years, and the children who received that label were the ones who seemed absolutely incapable of sitting still and paying attention in class. Many of these children had normal or even above-average IQ scores yet were failing to learn. During the 1960s, lead toxicity or early oxygen deprivation were proposed as the possible cause of a small amount of brain damage. Pointing out that many of these children exhibit "soft" neurological signs (impairments in coordination or other tests that are not localizable to a particular brain area), the term minimal brain dysfunction (MBD) became popular. By 1980, there was a belief that there had been too much focus on activity levels and that the basic disorder was a deficit in attention, which usually, but not always, was accompanied by hyperactivity. Thus, the *Diagnostic and Statistical Manual of Mental Disorders* (DSM) of the American Psychiatric Association used the term attention deficit disorder. However, *DSM-IV-TR* recognized the strong relationship between attention deficit and hyperactive behaviour by using the term attention deficit hyperactivity disorder.[59] The definition of **attention-deficit/hyperactivity disorder (ADHD)** has been updated in the fifth edition of the *Diagnostic and Statistical Manual of Mental Disorders* (DSM-5) to more accurately characterize the experience of affected adults. This revision is based on nearly two decades of research showing that ADHD, although a disorder that begins in childhood, can continue through adulthood for some people. Previous editions of the DSM did not provide appropriate guidance to clinicians in diagnosing adults with the condition. ADHD was also moved within the manual and can now be found in the "Neurodevelopmental Disorders" chapter to reflect brain developmental correlates with ADHD. The same primary 18 symptoms for ADHD that are used in the DSM-IV are used in the DSM-5 to diagnose ADHD. They continue to be divided into two major symptom domains: inattention and hyperactivity/impulsivity. And, like in the DSM-IV, at least six symptoms in one domain are required for an ADHD diagnosis. The criteria used to diagnose this disorder are listed in the box on the next page.

The cause or causes of ADHD are not well understood. The fact that it is at least three times more common in boys than in girls hasn't helped us understand its cause. Also, in many cases the problems seem to lessen once the child reaches puberty. It was once thought that this was an absolute developmental change, but now we recognize that as many as one-third of the children continue to have hyperactivity problems into adulthood.

Some progress has been made toward a better understanding of the etiology of the disorder. Data from twin studies, for example, indicate that genetic factors contribute substantially to the expression of ADHD. Findings from other studies suggest the disorder is associated with prefrontal cortex deficits, especially in catecholamine-rich regions.[60] The clear evidence demonstrating the beneficial effects of amphetamines and **methylphenidate (Ritalin)** in the treatment of ADHD bolsters this latter finding. These medications increase brain catecholamine activity, which would, in theory, reverse catecholamine-associated deficits. Although this theory is plausible, there are other theories and none has yet been widely accepted. Table 6.4 lists some side effects of methylphenidate.

Table 6.4 Methylphenidate Side Effects

Headache
Drowsiness
Dizziness
Nose and throat irritation
Sleeplessness
Involuntary movement (tic)
Aggression
Feeling anxious
Unexpected changes in mood
Cough
Abnormal heart beat
Fast or irregular heart beats/heart rate (palpitations/tachycardia)
Stomach pains or discomfort
Feeling sick or being sick

Source: http://drugs.webmd.boots.com/drugs/drug-304-Methylphenidate.aspx

One concern is that treatment with stimulant medications will lead to substance abuse, even though findings from controlled studies show that stimulant therapy is protective against substance abuse (i.e., the occurrence of substance-use disorders is actually decreased). Despite this, an increasing number of non-stimulant medications are being assessed for utility. Atomoxetine (Strattera) has been shown to be efficacious in the treatment of ADHD.[61] Atomoxetine's ability to increase catecholamines in the prefrontal cortex has been hypothesized to be the basis for these effects. Unlike stimulant therapies used to treat ADHD, atomoxetine does not increase dopamine transmission in the nucleus accumbens and does not appear to have abuse potential.

One of the more disturbing side effects of stimulant therapy is a suppression of height and weight increases during drug treatment. Amphetamine produces a slightly greater effect in most studies than methylphenidate. If drug treatment is stopped over the summer vacation, a growth spurt makes up for most of the suppressed height and weight gain. Even more disturbing is the possible

ADHD: attention-deficit/hyperactivity disorder.

methylphenidate (Ritalin): a stimulant used in treating ADHD.

DSM-5

Diagnostic Criteria for Attention-Deficit/Hyperactivity Disorder

A. A persistent pattern of inattention and/or hyperactivity-impulsivity that interferes with functioning or development as characterized by either (1) or (2) or both:

(1) Six (or more) for children and five (or more) for older adolescents and adults (over age 17 years) of the following symptoms of inattention have persisted for at least six months to a degree that is maladaptive and inconsistent with developmental level:

Inattention

a. Often fails to give close attention to details or makes careless mistakes
b. Often has difficulty sustaining attention in tasks or play
c. Often does not seem to listen when spoken to directly
d. Often does not follow through on instructions and fails to finish schoolwork, chores, or duties
e. Often has difficulty organizing tasks and activities
f. Often avoids, dislikes or is reluctant to engage in activities that require sustained mental effort
g. Often loses things necessary for tasks or activities
h. Is often easily distracted by extraneous stimuli
i. Is often forgetful in daily activities

(2) Six (or more) for children and five (or more) for older adolescents and adults (over age 17 years) of the following symptoms of hyperactivity-impulsivity have persisted for at least six months to a degree that is maladaptive and inconsistent with developmental level:

Hyperactivity and impulsivity

a. Often fidgets with hands or feet or squirms in seat
b. Often leaves seat in classroom or in other situations in which remaining seated is expected
c. Often runs about or climbs excessively in situations in which it is inappropriate
d. Often has difficulty playing or engaging in leisure activities quietly
e. Is often "on the go" or often acts as if "driven by a motor"
f. Often talks excessively

Impulsivity

g. Often blurts out answers before questions have been completed
h. Often has difficulty awaiting turn
i. Often interrupts or intrudes on others

B. Several inattentive or hyperactive-impulsive or inattentive symptoms that caused impairment were present before age 12 years.

C. Some impairment from the symptoms is present in two or more settings.

D. There must be clear evidence of clinically significant impairment in social, academic, or occupational functioning.

E. The symptoms do not occur exclusively during the course of a Pervasive Developmental Disorder or other disorder and are not better accounted for by another mental disorder.

Source: Reprinted with permission from the Diagnostic and Statistical Manual of Mental Disorders, Fourth Edition (Copyright © 2000) and the Diagnostic and Statistical Manual of Mental Disorders, Fifth Edition (Copyright © 2013). American Psychiatric Association.

misdiagnosis of ADHD and subsequent treatment with stimulant mediation in children who do not require it.

The seemingly indiscriminate but medically prescribed use of stimulant drugs to influence the behaviour of school-aged children has evoked much social protest and commentary. (See the Black Box warning on the following page.)

"Smart Pills" A number of studies in the 1960s seemed to show that rats learned faster and performed better if they were given amphetamine or some other stimulant. Abbott Laboratories obtained a patent for the stimulant it named Cylert, which it was testing as a "smart pill." Much animal and human research has since been done on the role of stimulants in improving mental performance. One way to represent the effects of stimulants can be seen in Figure 6.6, which schematically relates degree of mental performance to the arousal level of the CNS. At low levels of arousal, such as when the individual is sleepy, performance suffers. Increasing the arousal level into the normal range with a stimulant can then improve performance. At the very high end of the arousal scale, the person is so maniacal or so involved in repetitive, stereotyped behaviour that performance suffers, even on the simplest of tasks. The region of the graph

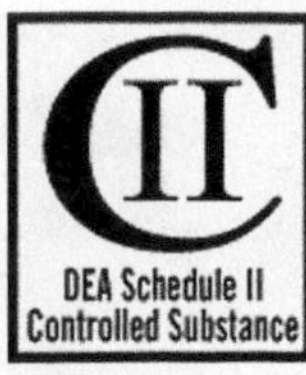

FDA "Black Box" Warning Label

The Food and Drug Administration (FDA) requires the following "black box" warning on all methylphenidate drugs, including Ritalin, which means that medical studies indicate Ritalin carries a significant risk of serious, or even life-threatening, adverse effects.

WARNING

RITALIN-SR IS A FEDERALLY CONTROLLED SUBSTANCE (CII) BECAUSE IT CAN BE ABUSED OR LEAD TO DEPENDENCE. KEEP RITALIN-SR IN A SAFE PLACE TO PREVENT MISUSE AND ABUSE. SELLING OR GIVING AWAY RITALIN-SR MAY HARM OTHERS, AND IS AGAINST THE LAW.

TELL YOUR DOCTOR IF YOU OR YOUR CHILD HAVE (OR HAVE A FAMILY HISTORY OF) EVER ABUSED OR BEEN DEPENDENT ON ALCOHOL, PRESCRIPTION MEDICINES OR STREET DRUGS.

Used with permission of Medicalopedia. Retrieved from http://www.medicalopedia.org/1908/ritalin-abuse-among-students-is-increasing-alarmingly/

Figure 6.6 Effects of Stimulants on Performance

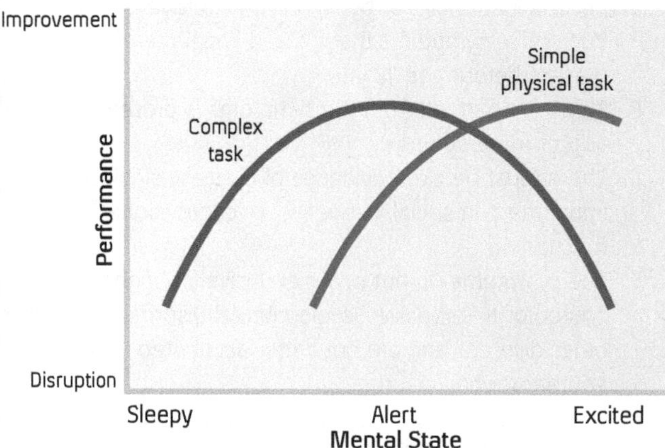

labelled "Excited" shows that some simple tasks can be improved above normal levels, but complex or difficult tasks are disrupted because of difficulty in concentrating, controlling attention, and making careful decisions. Cylert never made it to the market as a smart pill, but the company later introduced it as an alternative to Ritalin in the treatment of ADHD.

Figure 6.6 reveals that anyone trying to improve his or her mental performance level with amphetamines or other stimulants is taking a chance. Depending on the type of task, predrug performance level, and dose, a person might obtain improvement or disruption. A small dose could be beneficial to a tired person driving alone at night on a deserted highway but would probably only add to the confusion of a school bus driver trying to negotiate the King's Highway 401 (which is known simply as the 401 in Ontario and is the busiest highway in North America) at 7:30 a.m. with a load of noisy students. As for the students, a small dose of a stimulant might help keep them awake to study when they should be sleeping, but a larger dose? An old piece of folklore recounts something that probably never happened but has the ring of possible truth to it. It involves a student who stayed awake for days studying with the help of amphetamines, went into a final exam "wired up," wrote feverishly and eloquently for two hours, and only later when she received her exam back with an F saw that she had written the entire answer on one line, using the line over and over, so that it was solid black and the rest of the paper was blank.

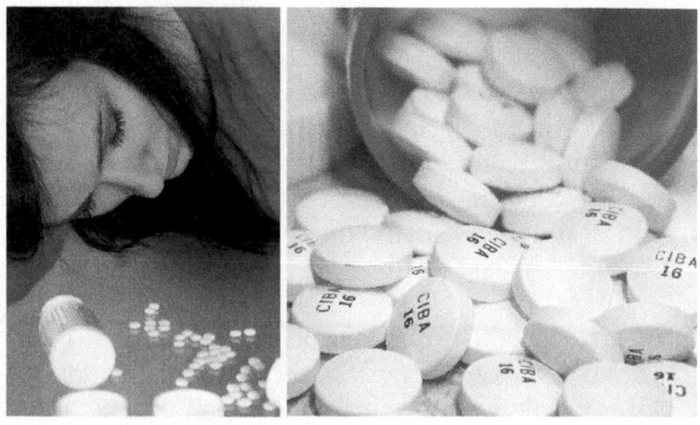

Stimulants such as Ritalin are used as a study aid by some postsecondary students.

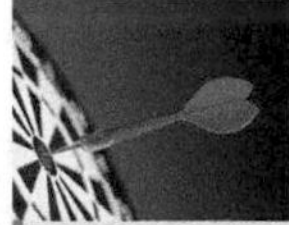

TARGETING PREVENTION

Overdiagnosis of Attention-Deficit/Hyperactivity Disorder (ADHD) in Children

Attention-deficit/hyperactivity disorder (ADHD) is a common disorder in school-aged children. There are many theories as to what causes ADHD; diet, prenatal and birth complications, and genes are among the factors suggested. It is the most common diagnosed neurobiological disorder in children (Morrow et al., 2012).

After analyzing the school systems in the United States, Morrow et al. (2012) designed a cohort study in Canada to see whether birth month had any effect on ADHD diagnosis. This study was done in British Columbia, where the cut-off date for entry into primary school was December 31. They hypothesized that because children born in December would be the youngest in their grade, they would show more behavioural problems associated with ADHD symptoms than any of the other months. Results showed that boys born in December were 30% more likely to be diagnosed and girls born in December were 70% more likely to be diagnosed (Morrow et al., 2012). These results are shown in Figure 6.7.

The authors thank Sarah Coughlin for article contribution.

Source: Morrow, R. L., J. Garland, J. M. Wright, M. Maclure, S. Taylor, and C. R. Dormuth. 2012. "Influence of Relative Age on Diagnosis and Treatment of Attention-Deficit/Hyperactivity Disorder in Children," *Canadian Medical Association Journal* 184(7): 755–762. doi:10.1503/cmaj.111619

Figure 6.7 Number of Children Receiving Treatment for ADHD

This figure depicts the number of children receiving treatment for ADHD by percentage according to month of birth. The graph accounts for sex of the child as well as the children combined (Morrow et al., 2012).

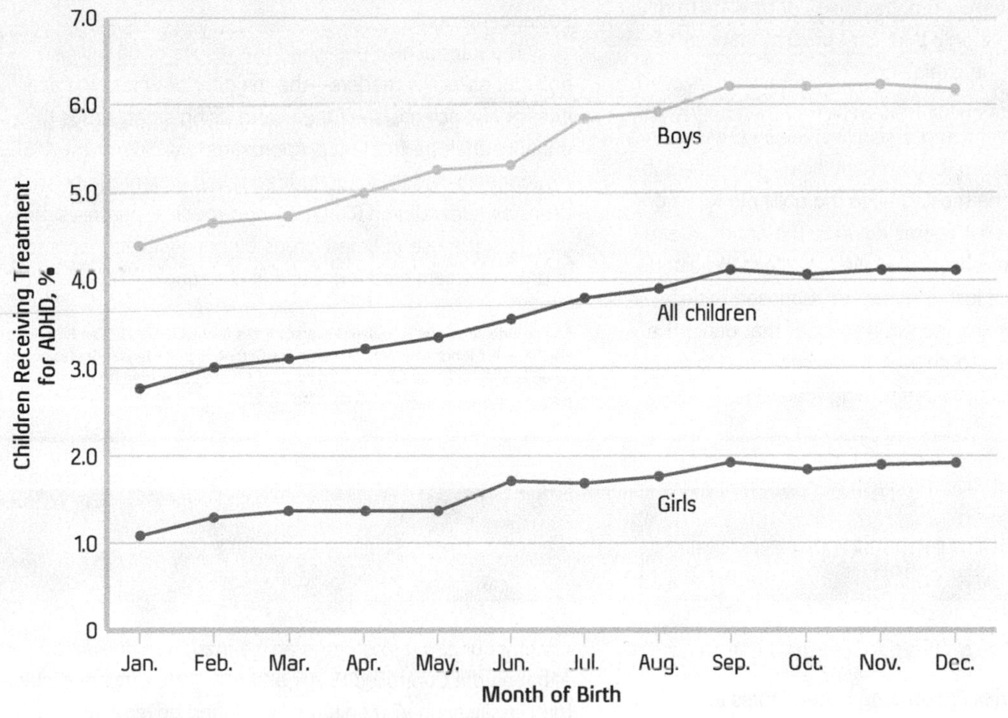

Source: Used with permission of The Canadian Medical Association Journal. Access Copyright.

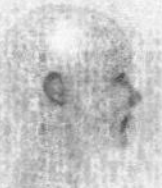

MIND/BODY CONNECTION

Can Pills Make You Smarter?

Surveys are finding an increasing number of students are turning to cognitive-enhancing drugs, such as Ritalin, modafinil, Adderall, and even speed, to improve their academic performance. These substances are often referred to as "smart drugs"—or things that are used to enhance mental performance. Some popular smart drugs, such as coffee, are easily available while others, such as the ADHD drug Ritalin, are available only through prescriptions. One survey, conducted in 2008, indicated that on some campuses as many as one in four students uses these kinds of drugs for non-medical purposes.

Mike Gorgal (name has been changed), a second-year history student at the University of Ottawa, acquires Ritalin from a friend whose father is a doctor. He began taking the drug during a particularly stressful time this semester. He said the Ritalin helps him focus on his work for hours, but has tried to not become dependent on the drug. "I make it a point not to do it very often, because I don't want to rely on it too much and I'd only take it if I procrastinate something way too long," he explained.

He has never tried any other cognitive-enhancing substances, other than coffee, but said that Ritalin puts him in a "trance" in which he can focus on anything—even the subjects that bore him the most. "I have the ability to focus on my own; it's just when it comes down to the grind . . . and I need to get the work done . . . I take the Ritalin to help me focus and to help me just do what I'm supposed to do."

While it's becoming increasingly clear that under the pressure of university, to do well, to succeed, and to maintain scholarships, students are turning toward both legal and illegal substances. What isn't clear is whether or not their actions are considered ethical in society.

Some see the use of these drugs as cheating, because not every student has access to them. Others say their use is no different from using coffee. Gorgal doesn't think using smart drugs is problematic.

Commentary on the responsible use of cognitive-enhancing drugs published in 2008 in the journal *Nature* argues that taking Ritalin or other cognitive-enhancing drugs is not significantly different from eating well, taking advantage of a tutor, or getting sleep before an exam. "Drugs may seem distinctive among enhancements in that they bring about their effects by altering brain function, but in reality so does any intervention that enhances cognition," stated the article. "Recent research has identified beneficial neural changes engendered by exercise, nutrition, and sleep, as well as instruction and reading. In short, cognitive-enhancing drugs seem morally equivalent to other, more familiar, enhancements."

The journal also published the results of an online poll that asked its readers—the majority of whom are academics and scientists—if they were using smart drugs to enhance their performance. Approximately 20% of the 1400 respondents said they had indeed taken advantage of such drugs as Adderall and Ritalin for non-medical purposes. Do you think the use of smart drugs by university students to improve academic performance is cheating?

Source: Adapted from Canadian University Press Newswire. 2001. "Can Pills Make You Smarter? More and More Students Are Getting High for Higher Grades," by Amanda Shendruk, *The Fulcrum* (University of Ottawa). Retrieved from http://newswire.cup.ca/articles/39571 on June 22, 2011.

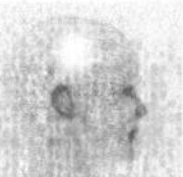

MIND/BODY CONNECTION

Drug Prescription Monitoring in Canada

In 2011, Canadian prescription drug expenditures totalled approximately $27.7 billion nationwide.[62] However, some of these prescriptions were more stringently monitored and controlled than others. In general, monitored drugs include any controlled drug that is listed in the schedules of the Controlled Drugs and Substances Act, with the exception of compounded testosterone and benzodiazepines.[63] Although the Controlled Drugs and Substances Act describes the classification of monitored drugs and governs the distribution and possession of these drugs and their precursors, it does not directly govern the monitoring of drug *prescriptions* in Canada.[64]

Currently, there is no surveillance system in place to monitor drug prescriptions at the national level.[64] Having

continued

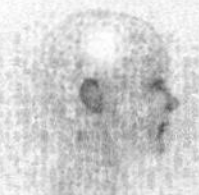

MIND/BODY CONNECTION

Drug Prescription Monitoring in Canada

continued

recognized the growing need for prescription monitoring, most provinces, including Nova Scotia, have designed and implemented their own prescription monitoring programs.[64,66] While the provincial programs each share the common goal of monitoring and reducing the inappropriate use of controlled drugs,[64] there is considerable variation in the organizations by which they are administered, the process of how they obtain their data, and in some cases, even the drugs that are determined to require monitoring.[64] As a result, there is an unfortunate disconnect between the various prescription monitoring systems across Canada.

The Nova Scotia Prescription Monitoring Program is widely believed to be the most advanced surveillance system in Canada.[65] Initially, prescription monitoring in Nova Scotia relied on the use of a triplicate prescription pad.[66] Under this system, physicians and pharmacists were required to each retain a copy of the prescription, with the third copy being mailed to the Prescription Monitoring Association of Nova Scotia for the manual collection of data.[66] However, an online system was later implemented that allowed for the immediate collection and analysis of prescription information, causing the triplicate prescription pad to be replaced by the duplicate prescription pad.[66] Under this new system, pharmacists are now able to enter monitored drug prescriptions into the online system while the drug is being dispensed, allowing them to access the most up to date patient and prescription information.[67] Upon submission, they are alerted of any potential drug misuse, including if the patient frequently obtains monitored drug prescriptions from several prescribers, if the prescription has been stolen, or if the prescription has previously been filled at another pharmacy.[60]

In March 2013, the Canadian Centre on Substance Abuse released a report titled *First Do No Harm: Responding to Canada's Prescription Drug Crisis*, outlining the development of a 10-year nationwide strategy against prescription drug abuse.[69] Understanding that prescription drug abuse is a national issue, the National Advisory Council on Prescription Drug Misuse took a collaborative approach in the development of this strategy. This was done through the incorporation of concerns and expertise from various stakeholders, including the government, health care professionals, and patients themselves.[69] With the overall goal of reducing the harm associated with the misuse of prescription drugs in Canada,[69] the strategy places considerable attention on the development of a comprehensive national surveillance system.

According to the report, the system would allow for information regarding monitored drug prescriptions to be collected and analyzed at the national level,[69] facilitating open communication between health care providers across the country. With the current system of individual provinces governing their own prescription monitoring programs, health care providers in one province generally do not have access to information regarding drug prescriptions from other provinces. This disconnect gives patients who purposely misuse prescription drugs, such as opioids and stimulants, the opportunity to obtain them from several provinces without being caught, thus undermining the purpose of the provincial prescription monitoring program. As a short-term goal, the report suggests establishing prescription monitoring programs in every Canadian province and territory by 2015.[69] Furthermore, it goes on to suggest that key aspects of prescription monitoring programs, including how data are collected and reported, should be standardized by 2017[69] to allow for more effective patient-centred care.

The Non-Insured Health Benefits (NHIB) Program provides health care coverage for First Nations and Inuit persons in Canada.[70] In addition, the NHIB program also has an established Prescription Monitoring Program (NHIB-PMP) that aims to reduce the misuse of prescription medications, including opioids and stimulants.[70] As a part of the NHIB program, patient drug profiles are randomly reviewed by a health care professional.[70] If at any point potential misuse is suspected, the patient will be placed directly into the monitoring program.[70] Patients are then required to obtain their prescriptions for opioids, stimulants, and benzodiazepines from a single prescriber, and must also have them all dispensed at the same pharmacy.[70] The Non-Insured Health Benefits Program also places limits on how much medication can be dispensed at any given time, as another means of control.[71] For example, pharmacists are presently only permitted to dispense a maximum 30-day supply of opioids for pain relief.[71]

The need for a national surveillance system to monitor prescription drugs has intensified in recent years in part

continued

MIND/BODY CONNECTION

Drug Prescription Monitoring in Canada

continued

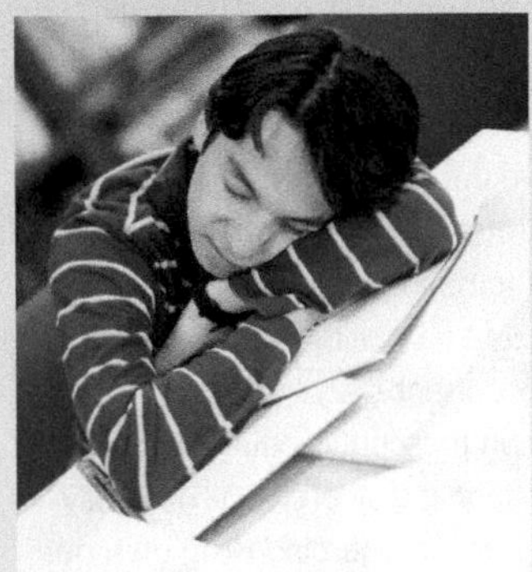

Students are feeling the pressure to achieve great academic success. As a result, many are turning to Ritalin for a quick solution.

due to an increase in the incidence of Ritalin abuse among university students.[72] Ritalin is a stimulant medication that is commonly prescribed to people suffering from attention-deficit/hyperactivity disorder (ADHD).[72] For overwhelmed university students, the drug has become quite appealing due to its ability to increase attention, alertness, and wakefulness.[73] In the pharmacy setting, Ritalin is highly secured through its storage in a locked area, along with other controlled substances. Currently, there are restrictions on the amount of Ritalin a patient can be prescribed to take on a daily basis. For children, the maximum dose is 60 mg per day; for adults, the maximum dose is 100 mg per day.[74] Furthermore, although there is no definite limit, the medication is generally dispensed in low quantities, providing the patient with enough pills for one to three months.

Unfortunately, more and more university students are turning to the Schedule III drug,[75] without a prescription, to achieve greater academic success.[72] In some cases, students visit several doctors complaining of symptoms that would warrant them a prescription for the drug. In other cases, students with legitimate prescriptions are selling their

Figure 6.8 Statistics on Teen Abuse of Prescription Drugs

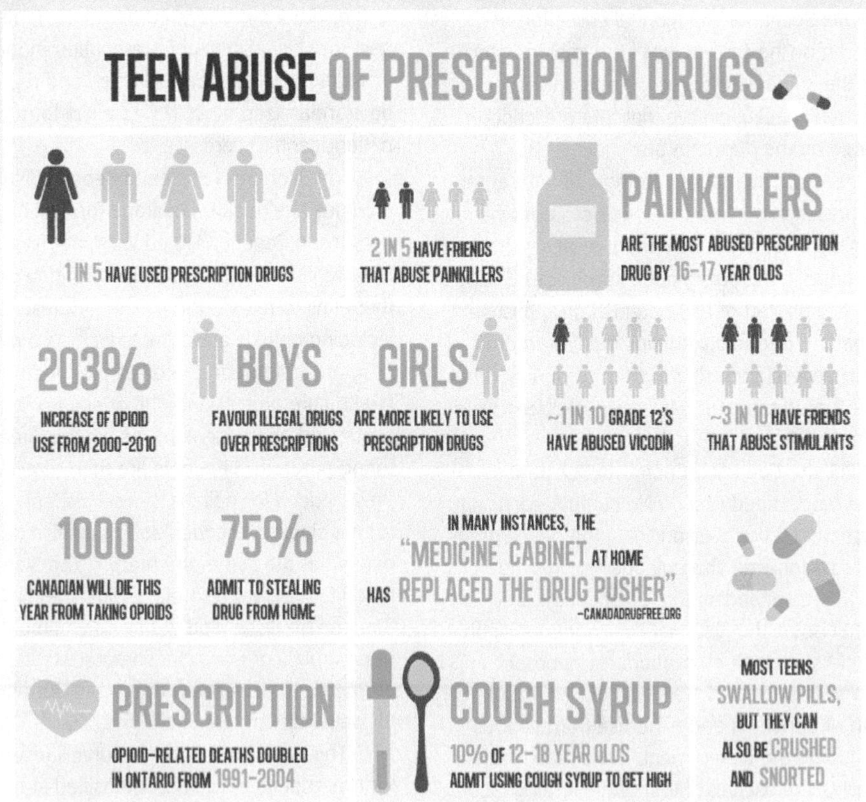
TEEN ABUSE OF PRESCRIPTION DRUGS
1 IN 5 HAVE USED PRESCRIPTION DRUGS
2 IN 5 HAVE FRIENDS THAT ABUSE PAINKILLERS
PAINKILLERS
ARE THE MOST ABUSED PRESCRIPTION DRUG BY 16–17 YEAR OLDS
203%
INCREASE OF OPIOID USE FROM 2000–2010
BOYS
FAVOUR ILLEGAL DRUGS OVER PRESCRIPTIONS
GIRLS
ARE MORE LIKELY TO USE PRESCRIPTION DRUGS
~1 IN 10 GRADE 12'S HAVE ABUSED VICODIN
~3 IN 10 HAVE FRIENDS THAT ABUSE STIMULANTS
1000
CANADIAN WILL DIE THIS YEAR FROM TAKING OPIOIDS
75%
ADMIT TO STEALING DRUG FROM HOME
IN MANY INSTANCES, THE "MEDICINE CABINET AT HOME HAS REPLACED THE DRUG PUSHER"
-CANADADRUGFREE.ORG
PRESCRIPTION
OPIOID-RELATED DEATHS DOUBLED IN ONTARIO FROM 1991–2004
COUGH SYRUP
10% OF 12–18 YEAR OLDS ADMIT USING COUGH SYRUP TO GET HIGH
MOST TEENS SWALLOW PILLS, BUT THEY CAN ALSO BE CRUSHED AND SNORTED

Source: *Used with permission of Health Canada.*

continued

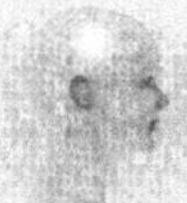

MIND/BODY CONNECTION

Drug Prescription Monitoring in Canada

continued

Ritalin medication to make a profit. Finally, many Ritalin abusers are turning to online pharmacies to gain access to the prescription drug. Figure 6.8 provides some statistics on teen abuse of prescription drugs in Canada.

The idea of purchasing medication online may seem somewhat bizarre, but the trend is becoming increasingly common. In Canada, several pharmacies have legitimate Web sites that offer online access to pharmaceutical services.[76] As with in-store pharmacies, legitimate online pharmacies must ensure that their services operate in accordance with established standards of practice, as well as all federal and provincial legislation.[77] On its homepage, a Canadian online pharmacy must clearly show that it is duly licensed and accredited, and must also indicate the location and contact information of the in-store pharmacy.[77] Furthermore, it must ensure that proper assessments of need are conducted and that prescription counselling is provided.[77] Although there is strict legislation in place to regulate online pharmacies in Canada, it does not appear to be very effective.[78] A quick Google search will yield several online pharmacies, including some alleging to be Canadian, that are still operating despite being illegal. Although purchasing prescriptions online has many advantages, including easier access to a pharmacist and generally lower medication costs,[79] there are disadvantages as well. Many online pharmacies are illegal and employ cyber-doctors who, after a quick online consultation, prescribe medications to patients.[79] According to Health Canada, patients who use illegal online pharmacies must exercise great caution.[76] Many illegal online pharmacies sell medications that are considered harmful in Canada and generally require monitoring.[76] In the absence of careful monitoring by health care professionals, patients who obtain medications online may be at risk of adverse drug interactions.[76] Furthermore, many online pharmacies are simply scams aimed at gathering users' personal and financial information.[80] As a piece of advice, Health Canada suggests that any concerns about the legitimacy of an online pharmacy should be directed toward the pharmacy licensing body in that province.[76]

The authors thank Sarah Leblanc for article contribution.

Athletics Under some conditions the use of amphetamines or other stimulants at an appropriate dose can produce slight improvements in athletic performance. The effects are so small as to be meaningless for most athletes, but at the highest levels of competition even a 1% improvement can mean the difference between winning a medal and coming in sixth. The temptation has been strong for athletes to use amphetamines and other stimulants to enhance their performances, and this topic is discussed in more detail in Chapter 16.

Causes for Concern

The abuse potential of amphetamines and methamphetamines is considered to be very high because of their ability to produce extreme feelings of euphoria. Additionally, these drugs can be administered in a variety of ways, including injection and inhalation, resulting in extremely high dosages being administered when users become tolerant to the pleasurable effects. This combination of effects leads to a variety of problems in the short and long term.

Acute Toxicity During the period of amphetamine intoxication with above-normal doses, the altered behaviour patterns (acute behavioural toxicity) can cause some dangers. As we have seen, even at moderate doses complex decision making can be temporarily impaired. At higher doses, especially administered for extended periods, the user tends to be easily panicked and to become suspicious to the point of paranoia. Combine this with increased feelings of power and capability, and there is concern that incidents of violence may increase.

There were multiple reports of the association of amphetamine use and violence and aggression in the late 1960s and early 1970s. Those reports returned along with increased amphetamine use in the 1990s. But violence is a lifestyle characteristic of many methamphetamine users, and a causal relationship between violent behaviour and methamphetamine use is not well established. Although evidence that amphetamine use is related to increased levels of aggression continues to grow, the underlying processes or mechanisms remain somewhat elusive. Recent findings suggest that amphetamine users may have an impaired capacity to control or inhibit aggressive impulses. Amphetamine use is also associated with increased positive symptoms of psychosis (particularly paranoia) that contribute to a perception of the environment as a hostile, threatening place. Additionally, high levels of impulsivity related to amphetamine use may also play a role. Each of these three factors independently may lead to an increase in aggression with increased use of amphetamine. However, the interactive or synergistic effects of these three factors may be particularly problematic.[81] In addition, the amount of demonstrated violence because of methamphetamine use is considerably lower than that resulting from alcohol use.

At one time there was concern that large doses of amphetamines would push the blood pressure so high that small strokes would occur and cause slight brain damage, which would be cumulative for repeated high-dose users. However, no direct evidence has been obtained indicating this to be a problem.

It has been shown in rats that high doses of methamphetamine result in the production in the brain of a chemical that selectively destroys catecholamine neurons.[82] The possible long-term behavioural consequences for humans are unclear because the dosing regimens used in animal studies have been excessive and do not mimic the use of amphetamines by humans. What is clear, however, is that contaminants formed during the manufacturing of illicit methamphetamine have been shown to produce toxic effects on brain cells.[83]

Chronic Toxicity The development of a paranoid psychosis has long been known to be one of the effects of sustained cocaine use. The first amphetamine psychosis was described in 1938, but little attention was given to this syndrome until the late 1950s. Possible reasons for the psychosis included that heavy methamphetamine users have schizoid personalities or that the psychosis is really caused by sleep deprivation, particularly dream-sleep deprivation. The question of the basis for amphetamine psychosis was resolved by the demonstration that it could be elicited in the laboratory in individuals who clearly were not prepsychotic and who did not experience great sleep deprivation. The paranoid psychosis after high-dose IV use of amphetamine is primarily the result of the drug and not the personality predisposition of the user. Evidence shows that the paranoid psychosis results from dopaminergic stimulation, probably in the mesolimbic system. In some cases in which paranoid psychoses have been produced by amphetamines, the paranoid thinking and loss of touch with reality have been slow to return to normal, persisting for days or even weeks after the drug has left the system. There is no good evidence for permanent behavioural or personality disruption.

Another behaviour induced by high doses of amphetamine is compulsive and repetitive actions. The behaviour might be acceptable (the individual might compulsively clean a room over and over) or it might be bizarre (one student spent a night counting corn flakes). There is a precedent for this stereotyped behaviour in animal studies using high doses of amphetamine; it probably results from an effect of amphetamine on dopaminergic systems in the basal ganglia.

Dependence Potential Theories about the abuse potential of amphetamines parallel the history of such theories regarding cocaine. For years, experts argued about whether the amphetamines were truly addicting. Because abrupt cessation of amphetamine use didn't produce the kind of obvious physical withdrawal symptoms seen with barbiturate or heroin withdrawal, most people decided amphetamines did not produce real dependence. By today's standards, as defined by the DSM-5,[84] amphetamine-like compounds are capable of producing dependence, although the empirical evidence demonstrating a withdrawal syndrome (the "crash") in humans on cessation of amphetamine use is limited. Anecdotally, amphetamine-related withdrawal has been described to be analogous to cocaine-related withdrawal. Symptoms may include craving, lethargy, depressed mood, and so on.

It has been known for years that amphetamines could be habit forming—that is, they could produce psychological dependence. Until a few years ago, that was not considered important. Amphetamines were even considered by some to be a so-called soft drug. They were available by prescription, and most users did not develop psychological dependence. The idea seemed to be that, although it could be habit forming in some individuals, its potential for abuse was limited. Now we realize that important factors, such as dose and route of administration, were not being considered. Small doses (5 or 10 milligrams) taken orally by people acting under their physician's orders for some purpose other than achieving a high rarely result in dependence. A larger dose injected intravenously for the purpose of getting high can result in a rapid development of dependence. Taken in this way, amphetamine is as potent a reinforcer as any known drug. Data from studies of laboratory animals reveal that rats and monkeys will quickly learn to press a lever that produces IV injections of amphetamine. If required to do so, an animal will press hundreds of times for a single injection.[85]

Summary

- Before the sixteenth century, the Incas used the coca leaf primarily in religious ceremonies and as currency. Early European explorers reported on the unique qualities of the coca plant, but it never really interested Europeans until the last half of the nineteenth century.
- Viennese physician Sigmund Freud studied cocaine for its potential treatment for a variety of ailments, including depression and morphine dependence. At a lecture in 1885 before a group of psychiatrists, Freud commented on the use of cocaine as a stimulant.
- In manufacturing illicit cocaine, coca leaves are mixed with an organic solvent. After thorough soaking, mixing, and mashing, excess liquid is filtered leaving coca paste. The paste can be made into cocaine hydrochloride, a salt that dissolves easily in water and can be snorted or injected.
- Cocaine hydrochloride can be converted into the smokeable freebase form of cocaine (crack or rock) by extracting it into a volatile organic solvent, such as ether. The freebase can be heated and the vapours inhaled.
- Cocaine blocks the reuptake of dopamine, norepinephrine, and serotonin, resulting in prolonged effects of these neurotransmitters at their receptors.
- Colombia remains the world's largest cultivator of coca bush, followed by Peru and Bolivia. Mexico's role as a transit country for cocaine destined for Canada has increased not only by way of the Mexico-U.S.-Canada highway corridor but also by shipments by air or marine modes.
- Cocaine is a complicated molecule structurally and doesn't resemble any of the known neurotransmitters in an obvious way. The structure of cocaine doesn't give science much help in understanding how the drug works on the brain.
- Acute cocaine poisoning leads to profound CNS stimulation, which can progress to convulsions and respiratory or cardiac arrest. Snorting cocaine irritates the nasal septum, leading to a chronically inflamed, runny nose.
- Because of the high temperatures required for smoking crack, the unsafe quality of the paraphernalia used, and repeated inhalation, users often have persistent cuts, burns, and open sores or wounds on the lips, gums, and inner mouth lining.
- For centuries the Chinese have made medicinal tea from herbs they call *ma huang*, classified in the genus *Ephedra*. The active ingredient in these herbs is called *ephedrine*, which dilates the bronchial passages in people with asthma.
- In the late 1920s, researchers synthesized and studied the effects of a new chemical that was similar in structure to ephedrine: Amphetamine was patented in 1932. The major effects of amphetamine were discovered in the 1930s, although some of the uses were developed later. Amphetamine's first use was as a replacement for ephedrine in the treatment of asthma.
- Amphetamines increase the release of dopamine, norepinephrine, and serotonin from their storage vesicles, resulting in an increased concentration of them in the synapse. In addition, amphetamines can also block the reuptake of dopamine, norepinephrine, and serotonin.
- Demand for methamphetamine in Canada is not broad-based but originates from specific segments of the community. In core production regions, such as British Columbia, Ontario, and Quebec, availability is high and prices relatively stable. In British Columbia, where an estimated 75% of all meth lab seizures in 2007 occurred, the bulk of operations were economic-based labs run by organized crime groups. The Asia-Pacific region continued to grow as a consumer region for powder methamphetamine manufactured and transported directly from Canada.
- Amphetamines are structurally similar to catecholamine neurotransmitters (dopamine and norepinephrine). Amphetamines seem to produce their effects because they are recognized as one of these catecholamines at many sites in both the central and the peripheral nervous systems.
- The methamphetamine molecule simply has a methyl group added to the basic amphetamine structure. This addition of a methyl group to the base amphetamine molecule seems to let it cross the blood–brain barrier more readily than amphetamines, increasing its CNS potency.
- Even at moderate doses of amphetamines, complex decision making can be temporarily impaired. At higher doses and with extended use, people may easily panic and become suspicious to the point of paranoia. The first amphetamine psychosis was described in 1938, but little attention was given to this syndrome until the late 1950s.

Review Questions

1. At about what periods in history did cocaine reach its first and second peaks of popularity, and when was amphetamine's popularity at its highest?
2. How did Mariani, Freud, and Koller popularize the use of cocaine?
3. How are coca paste, freebase, crack, and ice similar?
4. What similarities and what differences are there in the toxic effects of cocaine and amphetamine?
5. Contrast the typical "speed freak" of the 1960s with the typical cocaine user of the early 1980s and with our stereotype of a modern crack smoker.
6. How does the chemical difference between methamphetamine and amphetamine relate to the behavioural effects of the two drugs?
7. Compare the dependence potential of cocaine with that of amphetamine.

CHAPTER 7

OTHER DEPRESSANTS AND INHALANTS

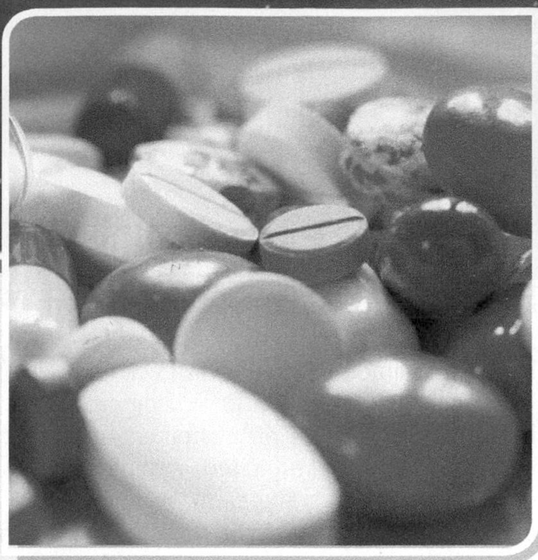

OBJECTIVES

When you have finished this chapter, you should be able to

- **LO1** List the depressant drugs and describe their general set of common behavioural effects.
- **LO2** Explain how concerns about barbiturate use led to acceptance of newer classes of sedative-hypnotics.
- **LO3** Describe the mechanism of action for benzodiazepines.
- **LO4** Describe differences in appropriate dose and duration of action for daytime anxiolytic effects as opposed to hypnotic effects of prescription depressants.
- **LO5** Explain why it is not recommended that people use sleeping pills for more than a few days in a row.
- **LO6** Describe how the time of onset of a depressant drug relates to abuse potential and how duration of action relates to the risk of withdrawal symptoms.
- **LO7** List several types of substances that are abused as inhalants.
- **LO8** Discuss issues related to depressant and inhalant use in vulnerable populations.
- **LO9** Describe gamma-hydroxybutyrate's typical dose range and behavioural effects and its effects when combined with alcohol.

Downers, depressants, sedatives, hypnotics, anxiolytics–known by many names, these prescription drugs all have a widespread effect in the brain that can be summed up as decreased CNS activity. What are the behavioural effects? The depressant drugs discussed in this chapter (barbiturates, benzodiazepines, nonbenzodiazepine hypnotics, and drugs used to facilitate sexual assault) share many characteristics with the major CNS depressant, alcohol, which will be discussed in detail in Chapter 9. Most people have a good idea of the effects of alcohol, and these drugs have effects that are generally similar: depending on the dose and the situation, people may experience relaxation, exhilaration, inebriation, drowsiness, or become stuporous and uncoordinated. We consider these CNS **depressants** as a class because of those common effects. Alcohol is such an important substance that it has its own chapter (Chapter 9). Beginning with the introduction of the **barbiturates** in the early 1900s, there has been a series of prescription drugs marketed for two medical purposes. Many people have used low doses of these drugs to reduce anxiety, to keep them calm and relaxed. When prescription drugs are used in that way, we will refer to them as **sedatives**. Current examples of popular sedatives include Xanax and Ativan, both members of the chemical class **benzodiazepines**. The other common medical use for the CNS depressants is to induce sleep. When these medications are used as sleeping pills we refer to them as **hypnotics**. Current examples of popular sleep medications include Ambien and Lunesta, both examples of the newest type of nonbenzodiazepine hypnotics. In this chapter we also discuss the non-medical use of various **inhalants** (e.g., glue, paint, solvents), because the typical effects of inhaling the fumes from these products also fall into the category of

depressants: drugs that slow activity in the CNS.

barbiturates: a chemical group of sedative-hypnotics.

sedatives: drugs used to relax, calm, or tranquillize.

benzodiazepines: a chemical grouping of sedative-hypnotics.

hypnotics: drugs used to induce sleep.

inhalants: volatile solvents inhaled for intoxicating purposes.

CNS depressant effects. Also included is the depressant drug **GHB**, which has attained notoriety as a date-rape drug.

LO1, LO2 History and Pharmacology

Before Barbiturates

Chloral Hydrate In the early 1900s a Chicago bartender named Mickey Finn became briefly famous when he was prosecuted for adding chloral hydrate to the drinks of some of his customers, after which they would become incapacitated and be robbed by one of his "house girls." The term "Mickey Finn" entered our language as slang for a drug added to someone's drink without his knowledge. This technique was used in several movie scripts, where it was referred to as "slipping" someone a "mickey." First synthesized in 1832, chloral hydrate was not used clinically until about 1870. It is rapidly metabolized to trichloroethanol, which is the active hypnotic agent. When taken orally, chloral hydrate has a short onset period (30 minutes), and one to two grams will induce sleep in less than an hour.

In 1869, Dr. Benjamin Richardson introduced chloral hydrate to Great Britain. Ten years later he called it "in one sense a beneficent, and in another sense a maleficent substance, I almost feel a regret that I took any part whatever in the introduction of the agent into the practice of healing."[1] He had learned that what humankind can use, some will abuse. Chloral hydrate abuse is a tough way to go; it is a gastric irritant, and repeated use causes considerable stomach upset.

Chloral hydrate is available in Canada as a 500 mg capsule or as a 100 mg/mL syrup. Indications for the use of chloral hydrate are outlined by Health Canada. These include short-term use as a hypnotic/sedative or hypnotic to either reduce anxiety or induce sleep prior to surgical or medical procedures. While the mechanism of action of chloral hydrate is not well understood, it is reported that the drug's active metabolite trichloroethanol underlies its CNS depressive effect. Like many drugs, tolerance occurs. It is documented that tolerance to the sedating effects of the drug can develop within 5 days to 2 weeks of continued use. Pharmacokinetically, chloral hydrate is rapidly absorbed through oral and rectal passages. Sleep onset with hypnotic doses is observed within 30 to 60 minutes following administration, with the duration of drug action lasting 4 to 8 hours. Benzodiazapines, as well as a variety of other agents, have become first-line therapy and chloral hydrate is not used as regularly as in past decades.[2]

GHB: gamma-hydroxybutyrate; chemically related to GABA and used recreationally as a depressant.

duration of action: the length of time a drug is effective; how long a drug's effects last.

Paraldehyde Paraldehyde was synthesized in 1829 and introduced clinically in 1882. Paraldehyde would probably be in great use today because of its effectiveness as a CNS depressant with little respiratory depression and a wide safety margin, except for one characteristic: It has an extremely noxious taste and an odour that permeates the breath of the user. Its safety margin and its ability to sedate patients led to widespread use in mental hospitals before the 1950s. Anyone who worked in, was a patient in, or even visited one of the large state mental hospitals during that era remembered the odour of paraldehyde.

Bromides Bromide salts were used so widely in patent medicines to induce sleep in the nineteenth century that the word *bromide* entered our language as a reference to a story that was tiresome and boring. Bromides accumulate in the body, and the depression they cause builds up over several days of regular use. Serious toxic effects follow repeated hypnotic doses of these agents. Dermatitis and constipation are minor accompaniments; with increased intake, motor disturbances, delirium, and psychosis can develop. Very low (ineffective) doses of bromides remained in some OTC medicines until the 1960s.

Barbiturates

Although the barbiturates have largely been replaced by more modern drugs, they were the first CNS depressant prescription medications to be widely used and abused. First introduced in 1903, the barbiturates became so important that eventually over 2500 different examples of this chemical class were synthesized, and quite a few were marketed. Examples of once-popular barbiturates include phenobarbital, amobarbital, and secobarbital. The barbiturates are grouped according to their **duration of action** (how long the drug's effects last), which also happens to correspond to how quickly they act after being taken by mouth (time of onset). The short-acting barbiturates begin to produce effects in as little as 15 minutes and have effects lasting only 2 or 3 hours, whereas the long-acting drugs may take an hour to produce effects, but they may last for 8 hours or more.

When these drugs were used during the daytime to reduce nervousness and anxiety, low doses (30–50 mg) of a long-acting barbiturate like phenobarbital were widely prescribed as sedatives. If, on the other hand, we were using these drugs as sleeping pills, these would have been higher doses (100–200 mg) of a shorter-acting drug like secobarbital.

Although the majority of people who took these medications did so without harm, the barbiturates were associated with overdose deaths, both accidental and intentional. As with other CNS depressants, the cause of death is typically respiratory depression (breathing slows and eventually stops) and in a great many cases this is due to the combined effects of alcohol and a depressant drug. Also, if we remember that these drugs produce effects similar to alcohol, it should not surprise us that sometimes people took barbiturates to get high. Regular use of high doses, either for sleeping or intoxication, resulted in tolerance, and some people then increased the dose to several hundred milligrams per day. With these high daily doses, dangerous withdrawal symptoms could result if the person stopped the drug use abruptly (physical dependence).

Now let's consider the importance of duration of action for abuse and dependence. As we saw in previous chapters, when people decide on their own to take a drug to produce a change in the way they feel, the drug's effect may be seen as *reinforcing* the behaviour of taking the drug. We know from many years of research that reinforcement is strongest when it is immediate. Therefore, the short-acting drugs with rapid onset are more likely to lead to psychological dependence ("compulsive" drug use). Physical dependence (withdrawal symptoms) are more likely to occur when a drug leaves the body quickly, as opposed to declining slowly over a longer time. So, the short-acting drugs are more likely to produce withdrawal symptoms. During the heyday of barbiturate prescribing, neither overdose deaths nor dependence were big concerns among those being treated with sedatives (low doses of longer-acting drugs). The problems typically resulted from the prescriptions for sleeping pills (higher doses of shorter-acting drugs). However, concerns about overdoses, psychological dependence, and physical dependence led to a bad reputation for all barbiturates, and by the 1950s the door was wide open for a safer substitute.

Table 7.1 lists some of the barbiturates available in Canada. Pharmacokinetics refers to what the body does to the drug: absorption, distribution, metabolism, and excretion. These pharmacokinetic properties are affected by the route of administration and dose of the drug taken and are reflected in the drug's onset of action, half-life, and duration of drug effects. The drugs with the shortest time of onset are highly lipid-soluble, absorbing and entering the brain rapidly, while those with the shortest duration of action tend to be more rapidly metabolized and leave the brain quickly. These unique pharmacokinetic properties of specific agents are reflected in their varying time courses and are important to understand the different uses of these drugs and their likelihood for dependence.

Meprobamate

Meprobamate (Miltown) was patented in 1952, and was believed to be a new and unique type of CNS depressant. The U.S. FDA approved its use in 1955 and it quickly became widely prescribed, based partly on a successful publicity campaign and partly on physicians' concerns about prescribing barbiturates.

Under Canada's Controlled Drugs and Substances Act (CDSA), meprobamate is listed as a Schedule III drug. It is sold as a combination product called 282-MEP, which contains meprobamate in combination with acetylsalicylic acid (ASA), caffeine, and codeine, and is prescribed for muscle pain. It was pulled from the Canadian market in 2013 due to safety concerns.[3]

It gradually became clear that meprobamate, like the barbiturates, can also produce both psychological and physical dependence. Physical dependence can result from taking a bit more than twice a normal daily dose. In 1970, meprobamate became a Schedule IV

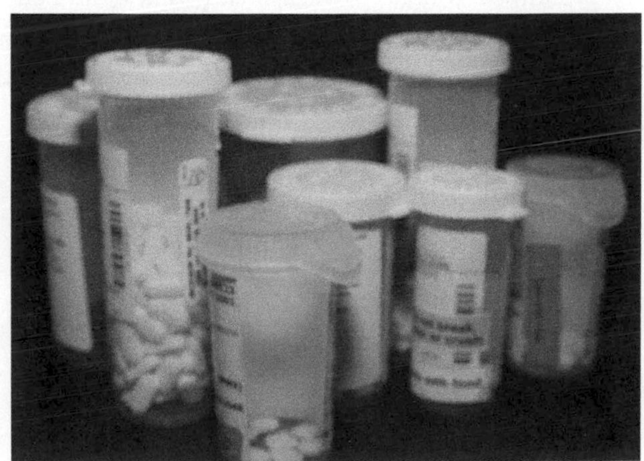

The risk of dependence on prescription sedatives depends on the timing of their effects and on the dose.

Table 7.1 Pharmacokinetic Properties of Barbiturates

Generic Name	Route of Administration	Onset of Action (minutes)	Dosage Form Strengths (mg)	Half-Life (hours)	Duration of Action
Butalbital	Oral	15–60	Tablet 50 mg in combination with 330 mg ASA and 40 mg caffeine	35	4–6 h
	Oral		Capsule 50 mg in combination with 300 mg ASA, 40 mg caffeine and 15 or 30 mg codeine		
Pentobarbital	IM, IV	1	IM, IV injection 50 mg/mL	35–50	15 min
Phenobarbital	IM, IV	1	Solution 30 mg/mL; 120 mg/mL	80–120	10–12 h
Phenobarbital	Oral		Tablet 15, 30, 60, and 100 mg		
	Oral		Elixir 5 mg/mL		
	Oral		Tablet 40 mg in combination with 0.2 mg belladonna and 0.6 mg ergotamine		
Primidone	Oral	n/a	Tablets 1.5, 3, 6 mg	10–12	10–12 h
Thiopental	IV	1	Tablet 10 mg	8–10	10–30 min

Abbreviations: ASA = acetylsalicylic acid; IM = intramuscular; IV = intravenous

Source: Adapted from the *Compendium of Pharmaceuticals and Specialties, 2009* (44th ed.). Ottawa: Canadian Pharmacists Association, 2009.

controlled substance, and although it is still available for prescriptions under several brand names, the benzodiazepines have largely replaced it.

In retrospect, it seems ironic that the medical community so readily accepted meprobamate as being safer than barbiturates. By deciding that the "barbiturates" were dangerous, the focus was on the chemical class, rather than on the dose and the manner in which the drug was used. Thus, a new, "safer" chemical was accepted without considering that its safety was not being judged under the same conditions. This mistake has occurred frequently with psychoactive drugs. It occurred again with methaqualone.

Methaqualone

With continued reports of overdoses and physical dependence associated with secobarbital and amobarbital sleeping pills, in the 1960s the market was wide open for a hypnotic that would be less dangerous. Maybe it was too wide open.

Methaqualone was synthesized in India and found to have sedative properties. Germany introduced methaqualone as an over-the-counter (nonprescription) drug in 1960, had its first reported methaqualone suicide in 1962, and discovered that 10 to 20% of the drug overdoses in the early 1960s resulted from misuse of methaqualone. Germany changed the drug to prescription-only status in 1963. From 1960 to 1964, Japan also had a problem with methaqualone abuse, which was the culprit in more than 40% of drug overdoses in that country. Japan placed very strict restrictions on the prescribing of methaqualone, which reduced the number of subsequent overdoses.

Apparently no one in North America was paying much attention to these problems in other countries, because in 1965, after three years of testing, Quaalude and Sopor, brand names for methaqualone, were introduced in the United States as prescription drugs with a package insert that read "Addiction potential not established."

Was methaqualone really very different from the barbiturates? For a while, physicians thought it was safer. Street users referred to it as the "love drug" (one of many drugs to have been called this) or "heroin for lovers," implying an aphrodisiac effect. In reality the effect is probably not different from the disinhibition produced by alcohol or other depressants. Methaqualone causes the same kind of motor incoordination as alcohol and the barbiturates. Both psychological and physical dependence can develop to methaqualone as easily and rapidly as with the barbiturates, and for a few years methaqualone was also near the top of the charts for drug-related deaths. If it was different, it wasn't much different.

Oral administration of methaqualone results in a rapid sense of euphoria. Tolerance to the hypnotic and euphoric effects of methaqualone occurs quickly, prompting users to increase the dose. Repeated administration of high doses of methaqualone can produce physical dependence, severe withdrawal-related psychotic symptoms, and life-threatening seizure activity. Methaqualone is no longer available as a prescription drug in North America.

Benzodiazepines

The first of the benzodiazepines was chlordiazepoxide, which was marketed under the trade name Librium (possibly because it "liberates" one from anxieties) in the United States and Librax in Canada.[4]

Librium was marketed in 1960 as a more selective "anti-anxiety" agent that produced less drowsiness than

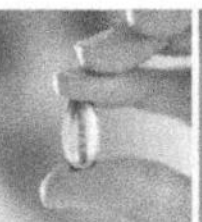

DRUGS IN DEPTH

Sodium Pentathol

Sodium pentathol, also known as thiopental sodium, is an ultra-short-acting barbiturate that has had a variety of interesting uses different from the other barbiturates discussed in this chapter. Sodium pentathol is administered intravenously, and has a very rapid onset. When used as an anaesthetic for brief surgical procedures, unconsciousness can occur in less than a minute. Because this drug is very lipid soluble, it moves rapidly into the brain. In fact, after one minute more than half of the drug can be found in the brain itself, a testament both to the enormous amount of blood that flows through the brain and to the high lipid content of brain tissue. At this point, if no further drug is administered, the thiopental molecules redistribute to other tissues in the body, and the person will regain consciousness in 4 to 5 minutes.

Sodium pentathol has also been used in lower doses to make people relaxed and more talkative. This effect has historically been used both in psychotherapy (in attempts to break through defence mechanisms and/or reveal suppressed memories), and in interrogations, as a so-called "truth serum." Fortunately or unfortunately, the effectiveness of this technique is questionable (to say nothing of the ethical and legal issues). The mechanisms of action and effects are similar to alcohol, so consider whether the old Latin phrase "*in vino veritas*" (in wine there is truth) is valid in your own experience. When people are slightly intoxicated, they are certainly more talkative and less inhibited. But are they more truthful? Whether in psychotherapy or in an interrogation, one should certainly question the validity of anything said during a state of intoxication, just as you would if the person had been drinking.

Also of current importance is the use of thiopental for lethal injections when carrying out sentences of death in most states in the U.S. Although consciousness may be lost quickly with thiopental, it takes several minutes for the person to stop breathing and die. Therefore, other drugs are typically used to produce death more rapidly. In the typical three-drug procedure for lethal injection, thiopental is first administered to induce unconsciousness. Second, a curare-like drug is given that paralyzes the muscles, including respiratory muscles. Third, a drug is given that stops the heart. In 2008, the U.S. Supreme Court issued an opinion that did uphold the use of this procedure. At issue was the fact that these injections are often not administered by trained medical personnel, and if for some reason the convict is not unconscious, he or she could experience what amounts to a very painful heart attack, possibly while conscious but paralyzed and unable to move. The Court's conclusion was that not enough evidence was presented to establish the likelihood of this botched procedure, so they upheld the Kentucky law that provides for its use in the death penalty.

the barbiturates and had a much larger safety margin before overdose death occurred in animals. Clinical practice bore this out: Physical dependence was almost unheard of, and overdose seemed not to occur except in combination with alcohol or other depressant drugs. Even strong psychological dependence seemed rare with this drug. The conclusion was reached that the benzodiazepines were as effective as the barbiturates and much safer. Librium became not only the leading psychoactive drug in sales but also the leading prescription drug of all. It was supplanted in the early 1970s by diazepam (Valium), a more potent (lower-dose) agent made by the same company. From 1972 until 1978, Valium was the leading seller among all prescription drugs. Since then no single benzodiazepine has so dominated the market, but alprazolam (Xanax) is currently the most widely prescribed among this class of drugs.

As these drugs became widely used, reports again appeared of psychological dependence, occasional physical dependence, and overdose deaths. Diazepam was one of the most frequently mentioned drugs in the DAWN system coroners' reports, although almost always in combination with alcohol or other depressants. What happened to the big difference between the barbiturates and the benzodiazepines? One possibility is that it might not be the chemical class of drugs that makes the big difference but the dose and time course of the individual drugs. *Overdose* deaths are more likely when a drug is sold in higher doses, such as those prescribed for hypnotic effects. *Psychological dependence* develops most rapidly when the drug hits the brain quickly, which is why intravenous use of heroin produces more dependence than oral use, and why smoking crack produces more dependence than chewing coca leaves. *Physical dependence* occurs when the drug leaves the system more rapidly than the body can adapt—one way to reduce the severity of withdrawal symptoms is to reduce the dose of a drug slowly over time. Drugs with a shorter duration of action leave the system quickly and are much more likely to produce withdrawal symptoms than are longer-acting drugs.

Chlordiazepoxide was sold in low doses for daytime use and has a slow onset of action and an even longer duration of action than phenobarbital. Chlordiazepoxide produced few problems with either compulsive use or withdrawal symptoms, and overdoses were almost unheard of. Diazepam has a more rapid onset than chlordiazepoxide, but because of slow metabolism and the presence of active metabolites, it also has a long duration of action (see Table 7.2). We might expect a drug with these characteristics to produce more psychological dependence than chlordiazepoxide but only rarely to produce withdrawal symptoms. This is exactly what happened.

Benzodiazepines are reportedly the most frequently prescribed psychotropic medication. Among adults in Canada and the United States, 3% to 4% are using benzodiazepines,[5] with approximately 100 million prescriptions written each year.[6] Benzodiazepines are indicated for a variety of psychiatric and medical conditions, including anxiety disorders, sleep disorders, seizure disorders, movement disorders, and muscle spasticity. They are used in anaesthesiology and for the symptomatic treatment of agitation associated with other psychiatric and neurological disorders, including psychotic, mood, and cognitive disorders. In emergencies, they are the preferred treatment of withdrawal from alcohol and sedative-hypnotics, as well as for agitation from stimulants and seizures. The clinical efficacy of the benzodiazepines is similar, but these drugs differ in their pharmacokinetic properties, such as potency, onset of action, and other pharmacokinetic parameters.[7]

Figure 7.1 illustrates the time course of depressant actions of drugs found in this drug classification. Secobarbital, a short-acting barbiturate, has a relatively rapid onset, entering the brain quickly with increased potential for psychological dependence. Its duration of action is relatively short, which underlies severe withdrawal symptoms for the chronic user. As its primary use was to induce sleep, large doses were often prescribed. Secobarbital was associated with overdose and both physical and psychological dependence. In comparison, phenobarbital had a slower onset but longer duration of action and was less likely to produce psychological dependence and withdrawal symptoms. It was rarely associated with overdose. Table 7.3 shows the half-life of some popular sedative-hypnotics.

As if to underscore the basic similarity that exists among all the depressant drugs, in the 1990s a new version of the "Mickey Finn" was popularized. **Rohypnol** (flunitrazepam), a benzodiazepine sold as a hypnotic in many countries around the world but not in the United States, hit the news when reports surfaced of its being put into the drinks of unsuspecting women by their dates. The combination of Rohypnol and alcohol was reputed to produce a profound intoxication, during which the woman would be highly suggestible and unable to remember what had happened to her. In reality, Rohypnol effects are not much different

Rohypnol: a benzodiazepine; the "date-rape drug."

Table 7.2 Pharmacokinetic Properties of Benzodiazepines

Generic Name	Brand Name	Onset of Action*	Dosage Form Strengths (mg)	Approximate Equivalent Oral Dose (mg)†	Active Metabolites
			Short Acting		
Midazolam	Versed	–	–	–	Yes
Triazolam	Halcion	F	Tablets 0.125, 0.25 mg	0.25	No
			Intermediate Acting		
Alprazolam	Xanax	I	Tablets 0.25, 0.5, 1, 2 mg	0.5	Yes
Bromazepam	Lectopam	I	Tablets 1.5, 3, 6 mg	3	Yes
Clobazam	Frisium	I	Tablet 10 mg	10	Yes
Clonazepam	Rivotril	I	Tablets 0.5, 2 mg	0.25	No
Lorazepam	Ativan	I	Tablets‡ 0.5, 1, 2 mg	1	No
Nitrazepam	Mogadon	I	Tablets 5, 10 mg	5	No
Oxazepam	Serax	S	Tablets 10, 15, 30 mg	15	No
Temazepam	Restoril	I	Capsules 15, 30 mg	15	No
			Long Acting		
Chlordiazepoxide	Librium	I	Capsules 5, 10, 25 mg	10	Yes
Clorazepate	Tranxene	F	Capsules 3.75, 7.5, 15 mg	7.5	Yes
Diazepam	Valium	F	Tablets‡ 2, 5, 10 mg	5	Yes
Flurazepam	Dalmane	F	Capsules 5, 10 mg	15	Yes

*F = fast (<1 h), I = intermediate (1–3 h), S = slow (>3 h)

†Approximate equivalent dosages: There is no agreed upon equivalency table for the benzodiazepines. The above equivalencies may vary slightly for each individual.

‡Other forms available.

Source: Adapted from the *Compendium of Pharmaceuticals and Specialties 2009* (44th ed.). Ottawa: Canadian Pharmacists Association, 2009.

Figure 7.1 Schematic Diagram of the Relative Time Courses of Two Barbiturates and Two Benzodiazepines after Oral Administration

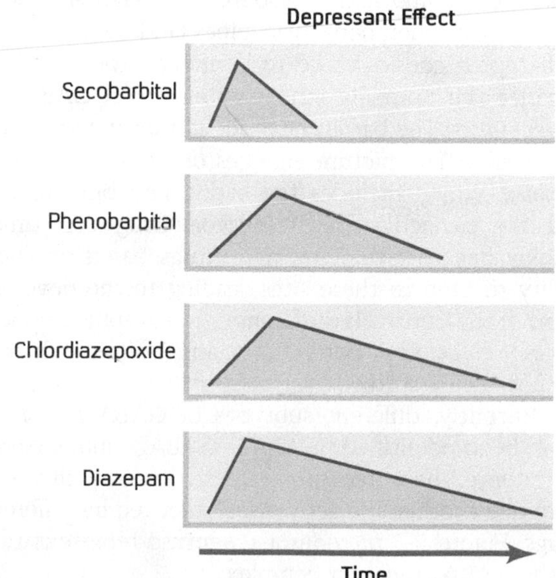

from the effects of other benzodiazepines (or any of the CNS depressants) when combined with alcohol, but popular folklore quickly established it as a date-rape drug. In 1997, the drug's manufacturer changed

Table 7.3 Some Popular Sedative-Hypnotics

Type	Half-Life (hours)
Anxiolytics	
Alprazolam (Xanax)	6 to 20
Chlordiazepoxide (Librax)	5 to 30
Clonazepam (Klonopin)	30 to 40
Diazepam (Valium)	20 to 100
Lorazepam (Ativan)	10 to 20
Hypnotics	
Temazepam (Restoril)	5 to 25
Zolpidem (Ambien)	1
Eszopiclone (Lunesta)	6

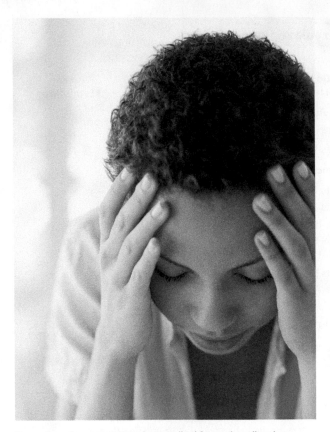

Benzodiazepines are commonly prescribed for anxiety disorders.

the formulation of the pill so that when it dissolves in a drink it produces a characteristic colour.

Nonbenzodiazepine Hypnotics

The most recent additions to the class of depressant drugs do not have the chemical structure of the benzodiazepines, but they have similar effects. Zolpidem (Ambien) was introduced in 1993, followed later by zaleplon (Sonata) and eszopiclone (Lunesta).

Zopiclone, a close relative of eszopiclone, is available in Canada and the United Kingdom, but not in the United States. Because the generic names of these drugs are hard to pronounce, but all begin with the same letter, they are often informally referred to as the "Z-drugs." In general, they are very similar to the benzodiazepines, but are called "nonbenzodiazepine" because they have a different chemical structure.

Zolpidem (Ambien) quickly became the most widely prescribed hypnotic drug on the market. It has a rapid onset and short duration of action, similar to the short-acting barbiturates that were once so popular. It has been shown to help induce sleep, but because of its short duration users didn't always remain asleep for 7 or 8 hours. This rapid, short action led to the introduction of an extended-release version (Ambien CR) to maintain longer sleep. However, taking advantage of the rapid onset, in 2011 the FDA approved a sublingual tablet (Intermezzo) to be taken when people awaken in the middle of the night. (Sublingual tablets are placed under the tongue, dissolve in the mouth, and often act more quickly than when swallowed.)

GABA: an inhibitory neurotransmitter.

Although many initially hoped that the nonbenzodiazepines would be more specific and avoid some of the problems of earlier drugs, there have been reports of withdrawal reactions and other complications with them as well. They are listed, along with the benzodiazepines, in Schedule IV, one step below the Schedule III classification of the barbiturates.

LO3 Mechanism of Action of Benzodiazepines

An important key to understanding the effects of these sedative-hypnotic agents was found in 1977 when it was reported that diazepam molecules had a high affinity for specific receptor sites in brain tissue. Other benzodiazepine types of sedatives also bound to these receptors, and the binding affinities of these various drugs correlated with their behavioural potencies in humans and other animals. It was soon noticed that the benzodiazepine receptors were always near receptors for the amino acid neurotransmitter **GABA**. It now appears that when benzodiazepines (and their nonbenzodiazepine cousins) bind to their receptor site, they enhance the normally inhibitory effects of GABA on its receptors. The barbiturates act at a separate binding site nearby. The picture emerges of a GABA receptor *complex*, which includes the barbiturate binding site and the benzodiazepine receptor. Drug companies quickly began developing new drugs based on their ability to bind to these sites, leading to the development of the entire class of nonbenzodiazepine hypnotics, as well as other potentially useful compounds that are now being studied.[8]

Recently, different subtypes of GABA receptors have been identified ($GABA_A$, $GABA_B$, and $GABA_C$ receptors). These receptors are structurally different from one another and activated or blocked by different drugs. Figure 7.2 provides a schematic representation of the $GABA_A$ receptor complex.

Figure 7.2 Schematic Drawing of the Gamma-Aminobutyric Acid ($GABA_A$) Benzodiazepine Receptor Complex

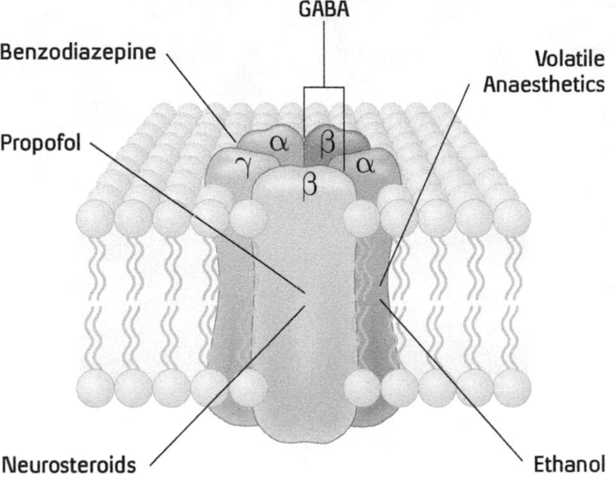

Source: Lovinger, David M. National Institute of Health, National Institute on Alcohol and Alcohol Abuse. *Communication Networks in the Brain*, Figure 4. 2008. Retrieved June 22, 2011, from http://pubs.niaaa.nih.gov/publications/arh313/196-214.htm.

Figure 7.3 $GABA_A$ Receptor

A schematic of the $GABA_A$ receptor protein $[(\alpha1)_2(\beta2)_2(\gamma2)]$. Illustrated are the five combined subunits that form the protein. These five subunits include a chloride (Cl^-) ion channel pore, two GABA active binding sites at the α1 and β2 interfaces, and at the α1 and γ2 interface a benzodiazepine (BDZ) allosteric binding site.

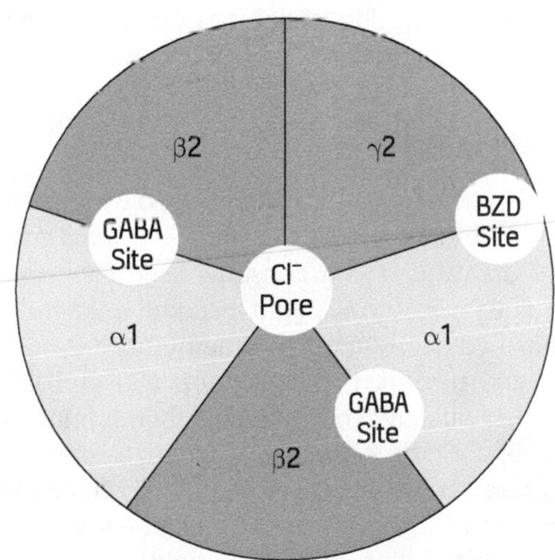

Source: Wikipedia, The Free Encyclopedia. "The $GABA_A$ Receptor." Retrieved November 9, 2011, from http://en.wikipedia.org/wiki/GABA$_A$_receptor.

The $GABA_A$ receptor is comprised of five subunits. The α type comprises two, the β type comprises two, and the γ type comprises one of the subunits. GABA-benzodiazepine receptor complex activation results in an increased chloride ion influx (see Figure 7.3), resulting in hyperpolarization of the neuronal membrane inhibiting the neuron and any resultant action potential.

It should be noted that benzodiazepines do not independently activate the flow of chloride ions into the neuron. Rather, benzodiazepines facilitate the action of GABA and resultant influx of chloride ions into the neuron. Other depressant drugs, including barbiturates, anaesthetic steroids, volatile solvents, and alcohol, also activate this receptor complex at slightly different sites. Regardless, the effect is the same. The inhibitory effects of GABA are enhanced.

LO4, LO5 Beneficial Uses of Depressants

As Anxiolytics

> Raze out the written troubles of the brain, and with some sweet oblivious antidote
> Cleanse the stuff'd bosom of that perilous stuff
> Which weighs upon the heart. . .

As these lines from Shakespeare's *Macbeth* reveal, humans have often sought a "sweet oblivious antidote" to the cares and woes of living. Alcohol has most frequently been used for that purpose, but the sedative drugs also play a major role in modern society.

In Canada in recent decades, the barbiturates, then meprobamate, and then the benzodiazepines have been among the most widely prescribed medications. Four benzodiazepines are listed among the top 100 most commonly prescribed medications: alprazolam (Xanax), lorazepam (Ativan), clonazepam (Klonopin), and diazepam (Valium). Table 7.4 shows the frequency of use of individual benzodiazepines in four cycles of the *National Population Health Survey* (NPHS) for those reporting use between 1994 and 2000. The NPHS cohort consisted of 17 276 household residents sampled from the general population. Lorazepam was reported as having the highest frequency of use. The frequency of use for clonazepam increased across the four cycles, whereas the frequency of use for alprazolam and diazepam decreased. These are all relatively long-lasting drugs used primarily as **anxiolytics** (to reduce anxiety).

The combined sales of these anxiolytics make them one of the most widely prescribed drug classes.

anxiolytics: drugs, such as Valium, used in the treatment of anxiety disorders; literally, "anxiety-dissolving."

Table 7.4 Frequency (%) of Use of Individual Benzodiazepines from Canada's *Longitudinal National Population Health Survey*, between 1994 and 2000

Benzodiazepine	1994–1995	1996–1997	1998–1999	2000–2001
Alprazolam	10.0	12.1	8.1	5.6
Bromazepam	4.7	3.5	3.9	4.2
Clonazepam	9.9	10.2	13.9	14.8
Diazepam	9.1	7.2	5.9	5.9
Flurazepam	5.7	3.2	3.7	NP
Lorazepam	35.1	35.3	39.9	38.3
Oxazepam	10.6	NP	8.9	8.1
Temazepam	9.1	9.0	7.3	7.2

NP = data were not provided in the table from the source.

Source: Kassam, A., and S. B. Patten. 2006. "Canadian Trends in Benzodiazepine and Zopiclone Use." *Canadian Journal of Clinical Pharmacology* 13(1): 121–27.

Most physicians used to accept the widely held view that various types of dysfunctional behaviour (e.g., phobias, panic attacks, obsessive-compulsive disorders, psychosomatic problems) result from various forms of psychological stress that can be lumped under the general classification of "anxieties." So if anxieties produce dysfunctional behaviour and these drugs can reduce anxieties, then the drugs will be useful in reducing the dysfunctional behaviour. Although this approach seems logical, in reality not all of these conditions respond well to antianxiety drugs. For specific phobias (e.g., fear of spiders), behaviour therapy is a more effective treatment. And for obsessive-compulsive disorder and most of the official "anxiety disorders" (Chapter 8), certain antidepressant drugs seem to be most effective. Most of the prescriptions for anti-anxiety medications are not written by psychiatrists, nor are they written for patients with clearly defined anxiety disorders. In addition, many patients take the drugs daily for long periods. Galen, a second-century Greek physician, estimated that about 60% of the patients he saw had emotional and psychological, as opposed to physical, illness. It is currently estimated that for a typical general practitioner, about half of the patients have no treatable physical ailment. Many of these patients who complain of nervousness, distress, or vague aches and pains will be given a prescription for an anxiolytic, such as Xanax. One way to look at this is that the patients may be suffering from a low-level generalized anxiety disorder, and the sedative is reducing the anxiety. A more cynical way of looking at it is that some patients are asking to be protected from the cares and woes of daily living. The physician prescribes something that can make the patient feel better in a general way. The patient doesn't complain as much and comes back for more pills, so everyone is happy.

Although most physicians would agree that the benzodiazepines are probably overprescribed, in any individual case it may be impossible to know whether the patient just enjoys getting a "feel-good pill" or feels better because of a specific anti-anxiety effect. Whatever the reason for each person, based on history, the market for prescription anxiolytics will continue to be very large and profitable.

As Sleeping Pills

Although one or two beers might relax a person and reduce inhibitions a bit, the effect of larger amounts is more dramatic. If you consume several beers at an active, noisy party, you might become wild and reckless. But if you consume the same number of beers, go to bed, and turn off the lights, you will probably fall asleep fairly quickly. This is essentially the principle on which hypnotic drug therapy is based: a large enough dose is taken to help you get to sleep more quickly.

Insomnia is the term used to include several symptoms: trouble falling asleep, trouble staying asleep, or waking up too early. In a recent analysis of a large national health survey in the United States, among adults aged 20–39, almost 17% of women and about 9% of men reported one or more of these concerns (rates of insomnia are greater in older populations). In this sample of over 5000 people, once the differences between men and women in rates of depression (Chapter 8) were accounted for, there was no longer

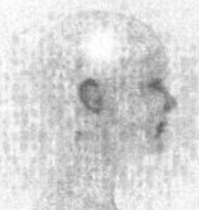

MIND/BODY CONNECTION

Learning to Relax

Most people shouldn't need pills to relax or to sleep. Here's a procedure you can use to relax before you study or as a refreshing study break. You can also use it to help you go to sleep at night.

Sit in a comfortable chair in a quiet room. Tense or contract each muscle group for a slow count of ten, then relax slowly for a count of ten. For each group, notice the difference between the feeling of tension and the warm, soft feeling of relaxation. Go from tension to relaxation slowly. Think of a balloon slowly leaking air and collapsing, or of a flower bud opening and folding back.

1. Tense and slowly relax your fists and forearms.
2. Bend your elbows and tense and relax your biceps.
3. Straighten your arms and tense and relax your triceps.
4. Wrinkle up and relax your forehead.
5. Clench and relax your jaw.
6. Shrug and relax your shoulders.
7. Fill your lungs and let air out slowly.
8. Pull in and relax your stomach.
9. Push down your feet to tense and relax your thighs.
10. Tip up your toes to tense and relax your shins.
11. Raise your heels to tense and relax your calves.

The whole procedure should take about 20 minutes the first time; it will take much less time later. Eventually, you will be able to put your body in a state of complete relaxation almost at will.

a significant gender difference for insomnia.[9] What this means is that people who visit their doctors complaining of insomnia should probably be evaluated for depression. This could be especially important, because in controlled trials comparing placebo to the new nonbenzodiazepine hypnotics, there was a doubling of the risk of depression for the group given the active drug. So, taking these sleeping pills can worsen depression in some people.[10]

Previous research has shown that most people who are concerned about insomnia do not take prescription hypnotic drugs, and there are effective nonmedical ways of dealing with insomnia. However, there is a large enough market for these drugs to encourage new drug development and quite a bit of television advertising.

After 1976, the benzodiazepines displaced the barbiturates in the sleeping-pill market. By the early 1990s, triazolam (Halcion) sales had reached $100 million per year in North America and $250 million worldwide. However, concerns were raised about the safety of the drug, and Upjohn, the drug's manufacturer, was sued by a woman who claimed the drug made her so agitated and paranoid that she had killed her own mother. That case was settled out of court, but it brought attention to the drug and to other claims that it produced an unusual number of adverse psychiatric reactions in patients. Halcion has been banned in five countries because of these side effects. It has survived

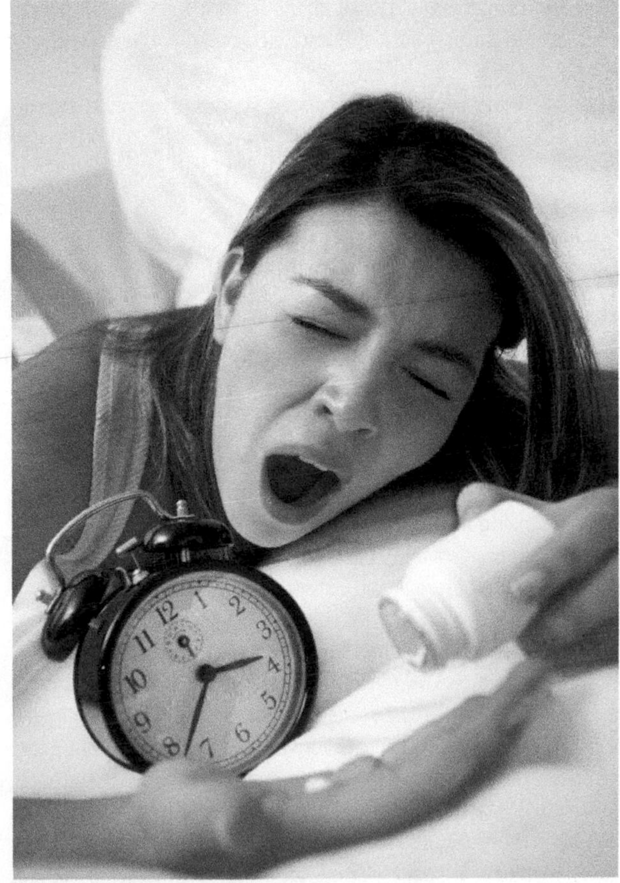

About one-third of adults report trouble sleeping.

two FDA reviews and remains on the market, but its sales have declined markedly.

The nonbenzodiazepine drug zolpidem (Ambien) binds selectively to the GABA-A receptor and has therefore been suggested to be a more specific hypnotic agent. Clinically it appears to be similar to Halcion, with rapid onset and short duration of action. Ambien has become the most-prescribed hypnotic drug in the United States, and several companies have been licensed to sell generic zolpidem as well. In spite of well-financed advertising campaigns by other nonbenzodiazepine competitors, zolpidem remains in the top spot. Concerns have been raised about sleepwalking, eating, and even driving while people are in a semi-waking state after taking these nonbenzodiazepine hypnotics. These concerns led the FDA to investigate such reports, and in 2008 all hypnotic drugs were required to attach a warning label about sleep-driving and other dangerous behaviours that might occur after taking these drugs.

We should be asking ourselves a few questions about the popularity of these new sleeping pills. Based on the history of hypnotic medications, every few years a new type of drug is marketed that promises to be safer than the old drugs. We then find out only after the new drugs have been widely accepted that they can produce the same old problems with overdose and dependence. This has happened with meprobamate, then methaqualone, and then the benzodiazepine hypnotics. Why should we be so ready to believe that these nonbenzodiazepine hypnotics will be different? This is particularly interesting when we realize that these Schedule IV controlled substances not only are widely advertised on television ("Ask your doctor!"), but also are being promoted with "free trial" offers. Should companies be allowed to offer free trials of a drug that has a reasonable potential for leading to dependence? And, although it doesn't show up on our list of the top 10 drugs in the DAWN system in Chapter 2, a special DAWN report released in 2013 found that zolpidem (Ambien)-related emergency room visits more than tripled between 2005 and 2010.[11] Because use of nonbenzodiazepine hypnotics is still increasing, we can expect to see higher rates of drug-related emergencies in the future.

If you or someone you know has trouble sleeping, before resorting to the use of medication it would be wise to follow the suggestions given in the Targeting Prevention box. These tactics will probably help most people deal with sleeplessness.

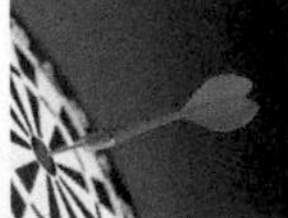

TARGETING PREVENTION

Falling Asleep without Pills

The following procedures are recommended ways of dealing with insomnia. If you occasionally have trouble sleeping, ask yourself which of these rules you typically follow, and which ones you often don't. Could you adopt some of these procedures?

- Establish and maintain a regular bedtime and a regular rising time. Try to wake up and get out of bed at the appointed time, even if you had trouble sleeping the night before. Avoid excessive sleep during holidays and weekends.
- When you get into bed, turn off the lights and relax. Avoid reviewing in your mind the day's stresses and tomorrow's challenges.
- Exercise regularly. Follow an exercise routine, but avoid heavy exercise late in the evening.
- Prepare a comfortable sleep environment. Too warm a room disturbs sleep; too cold a room does not solidify sleep. Occasional loud noises can disturb sleep without fully awakening you. Steady background noise, such as a fan, may be useful for masking a noisy environment.
- Watch what you eat and drink before bedtime. Hunger may disturb sleep, as may caffeine and alcohol. A light snack may promote sleep, but avoid heavy or spicy foods at bedtime.
- Avoid the use of tobacco.
- Do not lie awake in bed for long periods. If you cannot fall asleep within 30 minutes, get out of bed and do something relaxing before trying to fall asleep again. Repeat this as many times as necessary. The goal is to avoid developing a paired association between being in bed and restlessness.
- Do not nap during the day. A prolonged nap after a night of insomnia may disturb the next night's sleep.
- Avoid the chronic use of sleeping pills. Although sedative-hypnotics can be effective when used as part of a coordinated treatment plan for certain types of insomnia, chronic use is ineffective at best and can be detrimental to sound sleep.

As Anticonvulsants

A thorough description of seizure disorders (the **epilepsies**) is beyond the scope of this book. Both the barbiturates and the benzodiazepines are widely used for the control of epileptic seizures. Other antiepileptic drugs, such as valproic acid, carbamazepine, and lamotrigine, are usually prescribed in preference to benzodiazepines or barbiturates, but they may be used in combination. These other anticonvulsants are also widely used as mood stabilizers in psychiatric patients (Chapter 8).

Anticonvulsant medications are given chronically, so tolerance tends to develop. The dose should be kept high enough to control the seizures without producing undesirable drowsiness. Abrupt withdrawal of these drugs is likely to lead to seizures, so medication changes should be done carefully. Despite these problems, the sedative drugs are currently a necessary and useful treatment for epilepsy.

LO6 Causes for Concern

Dependence Liability

Psychological Dependence Most people who have used either barbiturates or benzodiazepines have not developed habitual use patterns. However, it was clear with the barbiturates that some individuals do become daily users of intoxicating amounts. Again, the short-acting barbiturates seemed to be the culprits. When Librium, the first benzodiazepine, was in its heyday, relatively little habitual use was reported. As Librium was displaced by the newer, more potent Valium, we saw increasing reports of habitual Valium use, perhaps because its onset, although slower than that of the short-acting barbiturates, is more rapid than that of Librium. Then Xanax, another rapid-acting benzodiazepine, became the most widely prescribed sedative, and reports of Xanax dependence appeared.

Animals given the opportunity to press a lever that delivers intravenous barbiturates will do so, and the short-acting barbiturates work best for this. Animals will also self-inject several of the benzodiazepines, but at lower rates than with the short-acting barbiturates. When human drug abusers were allowed an opportunity to work for oral doses of barbiturates or benzodiazepines on a hospital ward, they developed regular patterns of working for the drugs. When given a choice between pentobarbital and diazepam, the subjects generally chose pentobarbital.[12] These experiments indicate that these sedative drugs can serve as reinforcers of behaviour, but that the short-acting barbiturates are probably more likely to lead to dependence than are any of the benzodiazepines currently on the market.

Physical Dependence A characteristic withdrawal syndrome can occur after chronic use of large enough doses of any of the sedative-hypnotic drugs. This syndrome is different from the narcotic withdrawal syndrome and quite similar to the alcohol withdrawal syndrome. After chronic use of benzodiazepines, common side effects include anxiety, impaired concentration and memory, insomnia, nightmares, muscle cramps, increased sensitivity to touch and to light, and many others. More severe withdrawal symptoms occur after abrupt withdrawal from chronic use of larger doses, and may include delirium tremens, delusions, convulsions (may lead to death), and severe depression.[13]

This syndrome is nearly identical to the alcohol withdrawal syndrome and different in character from the narcotic withdrawal syndrome, longer lasting, and probably more unpleasant. In addition, withdrawal from the sedative-hypnotics or alcohol is potentially life-threatening, with death occurring in as many as 5% of those who withdraw abruptly after taking large doses.

Although it is said that withdrawal symptoms are less common after abrupt cessation of the newer non-benzodiazepine hypnotics, there is at least one case report of a woman experiencing seizures during withdrawal after extended use of zolpidem.[14]

Because there is a cross-dependence among the barbiturates, the benzodiazepines, and alcohol, it is theoretically possible to use any of these drugs to halt the withdrawal symptoms from any other depressant. Drug treatment is often used, and a general rule is to use a long-acting drug, given in divided doses until the withdrawal symptoms are controlled. Typically, one of the benzodiazepines is used during detoxification from any of the CNS depressants, although one of the specific anticonvulsants may also be used effectively.[15]

Toxicity

The major areas of concern with these depressant drugs are the behavioural and physiological problems encountered when high doses of the drug are present in the body (acute toxicity). Behaviourally, all these drugs are capable of producing alcohol-like intoxication

epilepsies: disorders characterized by uncontrolled movements (seizures).

with impaired judgment and incoordination. Obviously, such an impaired state vastly multiplies the dangers involved in driving and other activities, and the effects of these drugs combined with alcohol are additive, so that the danger is further increased. On the physiological side, the major concern is the tendency of these drugs to depress the respiration rate. With large enough doses, as in accidental or intentional overdose, breathing ceases. Again, the combination of these depressants and alcohol is quite dangerous. Although benzodiazepines are usually quite high on the list of drugs associated with deaths in the DAWN coroners' reports, in almost every case the culprit is the drug in combination with alcohol or another drug, rather than the benzodiazepine alone (see Chapter 2).

Patterns of Abuse

Almost all of the abuse of the sedative-hypnotic agents has historically involved the oral use of legally manufactured products. Two characteristic types of abusers have been associated with barbiturate use, and these two major types probably still characterize a large fraction of sedative abusers. The first type of abuser is an older adult who obtains the drug on a prescription, either for daytime sedative use or as a sleeping pill. Through repeated use, tolerance develops and the dose is increased. Even though some of these individuals visit several physicians to obtain prescriptions for enough pills to maintain this level of use, many would vehemently deny that they are "drug abusers." This type of chronic use can lead to physical dependence.

The other major group tends to be younger and consists of people who obtain the drugs simply to get high. Sleeping pills might be taken from the home medicine cabinet, or the drugs might be purchased on the street. These younger abusers tend to take relatively large doses, to mix several drugs, or to drink alcohol with the drug, all for the purpose of becoming intoxicated. With this type of use, the possibility of acute toxicity is particularly high.

Benzodiazepine Use in First Nation and Inuit Populations

In Canada the federal government via Health Canada oversees drug benefit programs for First Nations and Inuit people, including the Non-Insured Health

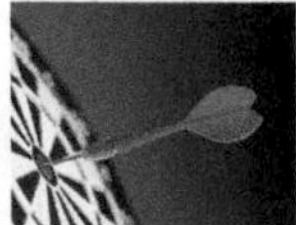

TARGETING PREVENTION

Combining Depressants with Alcohol or Opioids

All of the CNS depressant drugs covered in this chapter (anxiolytics, sleeping pills, anticonvulsants, inhalants, and GHB) can produce two kinds of dangerous effects. For one, in high enough doses they produce an intoxication similar to alcohol, and that intoxication increases the dangerousness of many kinds of activities, from driving to sex to just about any kind of active sport (see behavioural toxicity, Chapter 2).

The second danger lies in overdoses. As we saw in Chapter 2, each year there are several thousand deaths in Canada and the United States in which the use of benzodiazepine or nonbenzodiazepine drugs are mentioned. While it is theoretically possible to die from an overdose of any of these drugs alone, in practical terms this is very rare. In virtually every overdose death involving Valium, Xanax, or Ambien, some other substance is present. Most of the time it is alcohol. However, other combinations can be just as deadly, and as abuse has increased of such prescription opioids as hydrocodone and oxycodone, more opioid-sedative combination deaths are also occurring. For example, the Australian actor Heath Ledger's death in New York in 2008 was due to a combination of several benzodiazepines and opioids. No alcohol was reported in his case.

Clearly, some people must know that they are taking dangerous combinations of drugs. No single physician would have prescribed all the different medicines found in Mr. Ledger's blood, for example, and no pharmacist would have filled all of those prescriptions without warning of the dangers. But alcohol is such a common thing in some people's lives that they don't think about it when they also take a sleeping pill. Many might not know about the danger of combining medications. One should always take care when combining two drugs or any drug with alcohol, and read and pay attention to warnings provided with any prescription drug.

Benefits (NIHB) program. NIHB provides coverage for specific prescription drugs, dental care, vision care, medical supplies and equipment, and short-term crisis intervention mental health counselling. A Drug Use Evaluation Advisory Committee (DUEAC) was established in December 2003. This NIHB initiative provides recommendations to promote improvement in health outcomes of First Nations and Inuit people. A review of benzodiazepine use from April 1, 2002, until March 31, 2004 (24 months) of 80 495 individuals in the NIHB program revealed each had at least one claim for a benzodiazepine, resulting in more than 900 000 individual claims.[16] Females (63%) predominated, between the ages of 18 and 64 years (87%), who resided in Western regions (Figure 7.4). The percentage of persons with at least one prescription exceeding the equivalent of 40 milligrams diazepam per day is shown in Figure 7.5. Data presented in Figure 7.5 are not adjusted for age and are representative of all age groups. Among First Nations and Inuit peoples, the rate of overuse and potential misuse of benzodiazepines is consistent with the pattern of use of the general population in Canada.

Figure 7.4 Percentage of Total NIHB Eligible Population with at Least One Benzodiazepine Claim, by Region

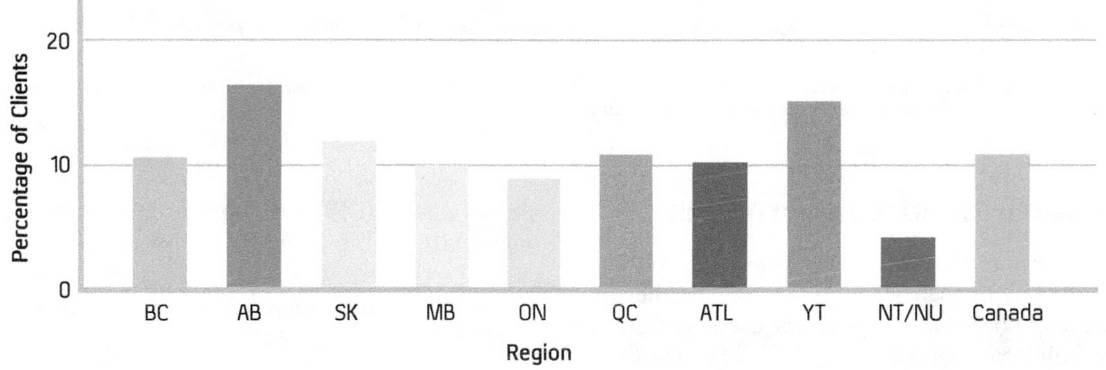

Source: *Drug Utilization Review of Benzodiazepine Use in First Nations and Inuit Populations.* Health Canada, 2005. Minister of Public Works and Government Services Canada, 2011.

Figure 7.5 Percentage of Clients with at Least One Prescription for More Than 40 Milligrams Diazepam Equivalents

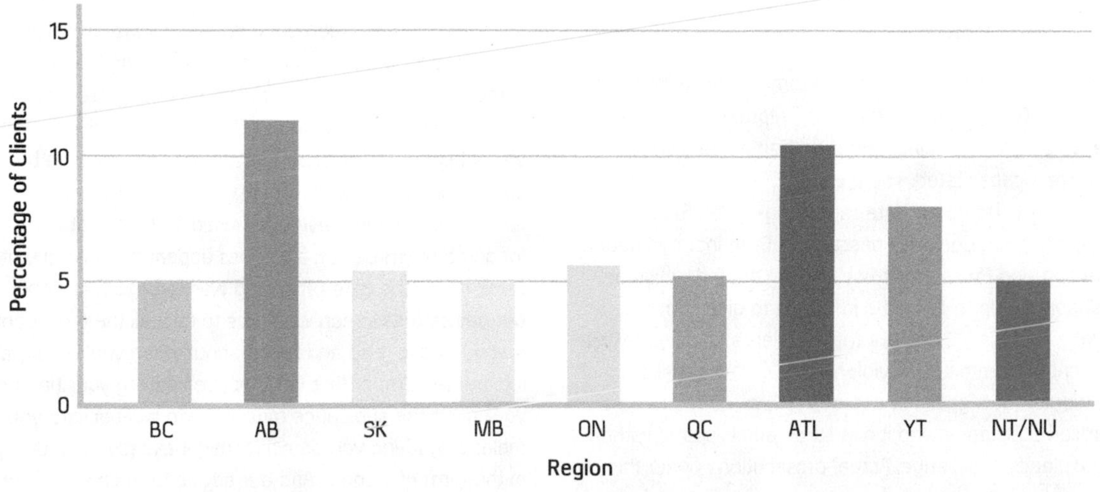

Source: *Drug Utilization Review of Benzodiazepine Use in First Nations and Inuit Populations.* Health Canada, 2005. Minister of Public Works and Government Services Canada, 2011.

Table 7.5 Summary of Hospital-reported Sexual Assault and Drug-facilitated Sexual Assault (DFSA) for Vancouver and Surrounding Communities, January 1993–May 2002*

Year of Assault	Total Number of Sexual Assaults	Number of DFSAs	Proportion of DFSAs (%) Among Total Sexual Assaults
1993	186	17	9.1
1994	147	12	8.2
1995	130	8	6.2
1996	164	14	8.5
1997	165	17	10.3
1998	162	16	9.9
1999	208	45	21.6
2000	156	40	25.6
2001	180	51	28.3
2002 (Jan–May)**	96	26	27.1

Notes:
*Excludes individuals presenting to the SAS who resided outside the SAS catchment area (Vancouver, Richmond, North Shore, Howe Sound)
**Data only available to May 31, 2002

Source: McGregor, M.J., J. Ericksen, L.A. Ronald, P.A. Janssen, A. Van Vliet, and M. Schulzer. 2004. "Rising Incidence of Hospital-reported Drug-facilitated Sexual Assault in a Large Urban Community in Canada: Retrospective Population-based Study." *Canadian Journal of Public Health* 95(6): 441–5.

Drugs Used to Facilitate Sexual Assault

Alcohol is the most frequent culprit in sexual assault.[17,18] However, for more than 20 years reports of other prescription and nonprescription drugs used to facilitate sexual assault have been escalating.[19, 20, 21] *Drug-facilitated sexual assault* (DFSA) is the use of substances to commit sexual assault. A Vancouver-based Canadian study of sexual assault victims presenting to the hospital emergency department showed an alarming increase since 1999 in the number of DFSA (Table 7.5).[22]

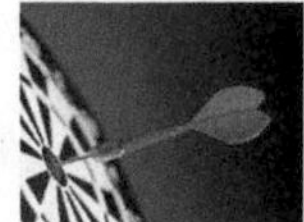

TARGETING PREVENTION

Date-Rape Drugs

You've all heard the stories about women having "roofies" (Rohypnol), GHB, or some other drug slipped into a drink while they weren't looking, and then being raped while they were incapacitated. There was a flurry of news and magazine articles about date-rape drugs in 1996, and in that year the U.S. Congress passed the Drug-Induced Rape Prevention and Punishment Act, making it a federal crime punishable by up to 20 years in prison to give someone a controlled substance without the recipient's knowledge, with the intent of committing a violent crime. Notice that alcohol itself would not trigger the use of this law—it has to be a controlled substance, and it has to be administered without the recipient's knowledge. Actual prosecutions under this law have been rare, partly because rape is usually charged under state laws.

Studies have been done in Canada, the United States, the United Kingdom, and Australia examining blood or urine samples from women who claimed that they were given a drug without their knowledge. The most common finding was a high blood alcohol content, and in more than half the cases in each study, no other drug was detected. In some cases a drug might have been used that was not detected for some reason, but it also does appear that in many of these cases the date-rape drug was too much alcohol.[23] So, our advice for women would be to take all the precautions that you have read and heard about when you're out partying, but remember that while you're keeping your hand over your glass the substance most likely to incapacitate you and make everything you do riskier might already be in that glass in the form of alcohol. And our advice for men is to remember that if she is incapable of giving her consent, it can be considered rape no matter how she became incapacitated.

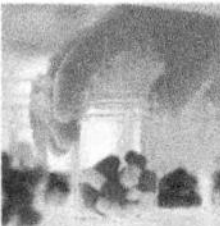

DRUGS IN THE MEDIA

Midazolam: A New Date-Rape Drug?

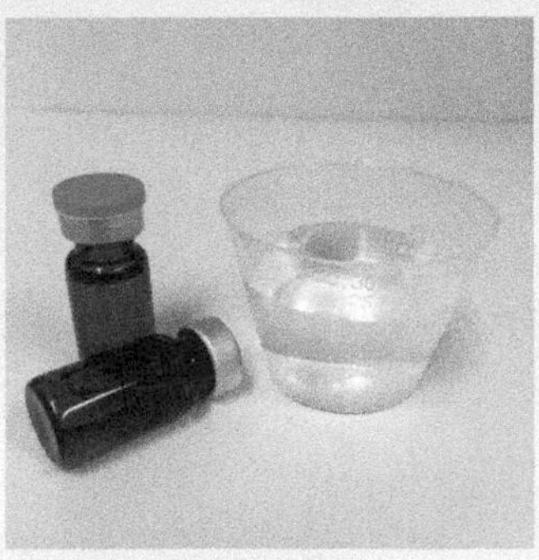

Benzodiazepines are a class of drugs that act as $GABA_A$-receptor agonists, and are prescribed in various clinical settings for their potent anxiolytic, hypnotic, antispasmodic, anticonvulsive, and amnesic effects.[24,25] Midazolam is a potent 1,4-benzodiazepine with an imidazole structure,[26] widely utilized in both adult and pediatric acute care settings because of its rapid onset and short half-life.[25] These characteristics facilitate safer dose titration, giving clinicians more control over achieving the desired clinical effect while minimizing adverse events.[24] Midazolam can be given via multiple routes, including but not limited to the oral, intramuscular, and intravenous routes.[24,25,27] It can be compounded as a colourless, water-soluble liquid[25] that is also odourless and tasteless. These physical characteristics, combined with the rapid pharmacokinetics and predictable clinical effects, give midazolam a dangerous potential for use as a date-rape drug.

In August 2014, at least 16 vials of midazolam were stolen from the Queen Elizabeth II Health Sciences Centre in Halifax. Each vial contained 5 mL of the drug, at a concentration of 1 mg/mL. The drugs were stolen from various resuscitation carts throughout the hospital, which are used in cardiac arrests and other serious emergencies. The vials were stored in sealed drug boxes, along with several other non-narcotic medications, but only the midazolam was found to be missing by hospital staff who perform daily inventory checks on the carts. The first thefts were noted by hospital staff on August 5. Security footage did not show any person(s) who may have stolen the drug, and initial investigations failed to reveal any suspects. The thefts continued, and on August 14 the police were notified. The public and local universities were quickly made aware of the risks of midazolam and its potential use in a sexual assault. Police urged the public to drink responsibly, to be wary of where their drinks came from, and to report any suspicious activity to bar staff and police officers.[28]

What if a sexual assault occurred, and the victim had no recollection of events after a certain point in the evening? One of the effects of midazolam is anterograde amnesia: forgetting events, or being unable to form memories after a point in time,[27,29] such as the moment of drug administration. Depending on the laboratory technology used, toxicological analysis of urine samples can reveal which substance(s) were delivered, but only if the recipient has not fully metabolized and excreted the target molecule to levels below the detection thresholds of the assay.[30] Using enzyme-multiplied immunoassay technique (EMIT), gas chromatography (GC), and mass spectroscopy (MS), Fraser et al. (1991)[26] analyzed forensic urine samples for midazolam and its metabolites. The authors confirmed the major metabolite, α-hydroxy midazolam, as the ubiquitous target molecule.

In a case of suspected benzodiazepine ingestion and subsequent sexual assault, a toxicologist may direct attention toward an analysis of urinary metabolites, as well as the parent drug, to confirm its presence in the victim's body. In Canada, midazolam is not available as an oral preparation outside of hospital or clinic settings.[31,32] Therefore, in a community setting, a sexual assault victim who tested positive for midazolam and/or its major metabolites should alert law enforcement to the possibility of a local sex offender who used the drug to facilitate rape.

The authors thank Ryan J. Mitchell, BScN, RN for article contribution.

A prospective study conducted by Du Mont and colleagues of women and men reporting sexual assault to seven hospital-based sexual assault treatment centres in Ontario revealed a cocktail of drugs used in sexual assault over a 22-month period.[33] Table 7.6 shows the types and percentages of CNS-active substances that were detected at collection. The column labelled Unexpected Drugs refers to ones for which the respondent reported not having actually consumed the drug but it was found by toxicological analysis.

LO7, LO8 Inhalants

Some people will do almost anything to escape reality. Gasoline, glue, paint, lighter fluid, spray cans of almost anything, nail polish, and Liquid Paper all contain

Table 7.6 Toxicological Results by Delay in Presentation and Unexpected Findings

Drugs Detected	Number and Percent of Total Cases (N = 178 (%*))	Time Delay ≤ 1 day (N = 142 (%))	Number and Percent of Unexpected Drugs (N = 87 (%))
Alcohol	55 (30.9)	53 (96.4)	1 (1.8)
Benzodiazepines			
Lorazepam	11 (6.2)	8 (72.7)	6 (54.5)
Diazepam	1 (0.6)	0 (0.0)	1 (100.0)
Clonazepam	2 (1.1)	2 (100.0)	0 (0.0)
Nitrazepam	1 (0.6)	1 (100.0)	1 (100.0)
Benzodiazepine metabolites	5 (2.8)	4 (80.0)	5 (100.0)
Opioids			
Codeine	8 (4.5)	7 (87.5)	6 (75.0)
Morphine	7 (3.9)	5 (71.4)	7 (100.0)
Oxycodone	6 (3.4)	5 (83.3)	5 (83.3)
Methadone	2 (1.1)	0 (0.0)	1 (50.0)
Hydromorphone	1 (0.6)	0 (0.0)	1 (100.0)
Antidepressants			
Citalopram	12 (6.7)	10 (83.3)	6 (50.0)
Venlafaxine	8 (4.5)	7 (87.5)	1 (12.5)
Fluoxetine	2 (1.1)	2 (100.0)	0 (0.0)
Mirtazapine	2 (1.1)	2 (100.0)	0 (0.0)
Other	5	3	2
Antipsychotics			
Quetiapine	5 (2.8)	3 (60.0)	1 (20.0)
Methotrimeprazine	1 (0.6)	1 (100.0)	0 (0.0)
Street drugs			
Cannabinoids	60 (33.7)	50 (83.3)	35 (58.3)
Cocaine	38 (21.4)	28 (73.7)	28 (73.7)
MDMA	13 (7.3)	12 (92.3)	8 (61.5)
Amphetamines	13 (7.3)	12 (92.3)	12 (92.3)
Ketamine	2 (1.1)	2 (100.0)	2 (100.0)
GHB	2 (1.1)	2 (100.0)	1 (50.0)
Other			
Diphenhydramine	8 (4.5)	7 (87.5)	7 (87.5)
Pseudoephedrine	7 (3.9)	7 (100.0)	6 (85.7)
Dimenhydrinate	6 (3.4)	5 (83.3)	4 (66.7)
Chlorpheniramine	5 (2.8)	4 (80.0)	5 (100.0)
Other	6	4	6

Notes:
Percentages do not total to 100 as more than one drug could be found in a sample.
*Toxicology results were available for 178 participants.

Source: Adapted from Du Mont, J., S. Macdonald, N. Rotbard, D. Bainbridge, E. Asllani, N. Smith, and M.M. Cohen. 2010. "Drug-facilitated Sexual Assault in Ontario, Canada: Toxicological and DNA Findings." *Journal of Forensic and Legal Medicine* 17(6): 333–8.

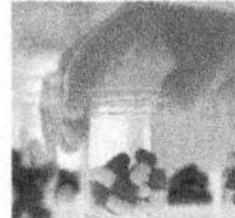

DRUGS IN THE MEDIA

Rape Victim Takes Story Public

First she says she was raped by two Florida men who slipped her GHB, and then by the justice system that let them off scot-free. But even after all this time, AJ Januszczak refuses to surrender and is one of the first known victims of the date-rape drug to warn others about GHB. It was Feb. 18, 1996, when few knew the bodybuilding drug GHB was being slipped into cocktails to incapacitate rape victims. Januszczak was spending the winter in Florida, paying her way by bartending at a strip club, and was out with her sister near Boca Raton. They noticed two beefy men they'd briefly met earlier at another club. One bought her a drink and kept bringing it to her on the dance floor. She recalls becoming dizzy and seeing a smirk cross his face. And then she remembers nothing at all. After a frantic search, her sister found her with the two men in a dark corner of the parking lot. Januszczak was unconscious, naked from the waist down and according to paramedics, just minutes from death.

Blood tests later found she'd been overdosed with more than 18 mg of GHB in her 90-pound body. A 200-pound bodybuilder usually uses 1.5 to 2 mg. Nicknamed the "leg spreader," two bottles of GHB were seized by police from the truck belonging to one of the men. A condom with the DNA of all three and an empty GHB bottle was found in the bushes.

Three months later, the two prominent bodybuilders were arrested. Both insisted the sexual intercourse was consensual. But a dozen women came forward claiming they, too, had been drugged and raped by them. A grand jury added kidnapping and conspiracy charges. And then, just days before the high-profile case was set for trial, the state attorney's office reluctantly withdrew the charges. The men had hired expensive lawyers, including the attorney who won the acquittal of alleged rapist William Kennedy Smith, and their tough probing had unravelled the case. Their client's truck had been searched illegally and so the GHB found there was inadmissible. Her torn clothes had never been taken into evidence. The GHB bottle found in the bushes had been mishandled by the sheriff's office. The two men walked free.

Januszczak remained determined to hold them accountable. So she followed the lead of O.J. Simpson's victims and filed a civil lawsuit. But she was only to be violated again. Januszczak claims she was tricked into signing an ultimately worthless agreement with her alleged attackers: By agreeing not to take them to court, they'd each pay her $500 000. But there was a catch—she'd have to sue their insurance company, State Farm Fire and Casualty, for the money.

"I didn't want money. I wanted a trial," she insists. The "novel" lawsuit was initially successful but reversed on appeal. By law, insurance companies can't be forced to pay for criminal acts. The supreme court of Florida refused to overturn the decision. Once again, she was left without the justice she had sought. Still, she refused to be a victim. Januszczak has never stopped trying to warn others about the date-rape drug: First telling her story on the *Geraldo* show in 1997 and in a [newspaper] column two years later. Her advocacy helped change the law in the U.S.—GHB, legal in Florida at the time of her attack—was made a controlled substance four years later.

Writing her "raw truth" has helped her find peace at last. "I just felt like I've been hanging on to the pain," she explains. "It meant coming to terms with it." And now she wants to reach other rape survivors with her message. "Never underestimate the power of your voice," Januszczak says fiercely. "Fight back and don't give up."

Source: *Adapted from Michele Mandel. "Rape Victim Takes Story Public," QMI Agency. Used with permission.*

volatile solvents that, when inhaled, can have effects that are similar in an overall way to the depressants. High-dose exposure to these fumes makes users intoxicated, often slurring their speech and causing them to have trouble walking a straight line, as if they were drunk on alcohol.

Although most people think first of the abuse of volatile solvents such as glues, paints, and gasoline, other types of substances can be abused through sniffing or inhaling in a similar manner (Table 7.7). Two major groups are the gaseous anaesthetics and the nitrites, as well as volatile solvents.

Gaseous Anaesthetics

Gaseous anaesthetics have been used in medicine and surgery for many years, and abuse of these anaesthetics occurs among physicians and others with access to

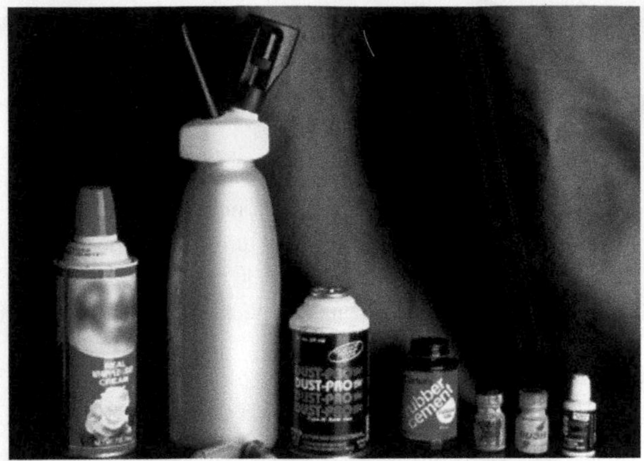

Chemicals abused by inhalation can be found in a variety of household products.

these gases. One of the oldest, nitrous oxide, was first used in the early 1800s and quite early acquired the popular name "laughing gas" because of the hilarity exhibited by some of its users. During the 1800s, travelling demonstrations of laughing gas enticed audience members to volunteer to become intoxicated for the amusement of others. Nitrous oxide is also one of the safest anaesthetics when used properly, but it is not possible to obtain good surgical anaesthesia unless the individual breathes almost pure nitrous oxide, which leads to suffocation through a lack of oxygen. Nitrous oxide is still used for light anaesthesia, especially by dentists. It is also often used in combination with one of the more effective inhaled anaesthetics, allowing the use of a lower concentration of the primary anaesthetic. Nitrous oxide is also found as a propellant in whipping-cream containers and is sold in small bottles ("whippets") for use in home whipping-cream dispensers. Recreational users have obtained nitrous oxide from both sources.

Nitrites

Amyl nitrite was first introduced into medicine in the mid-1800s as a treatment for chest pain. Inhaling the vapours of this drug relaxes blood vessels, including the coronary arteries. This increases blood flow, but also briefly lowers blood pressure. Amyl nitrite is still used in emergency medicine as a treatment for cyanide

Table 7.7 Some Chemicals Abused by Inhalation

Substances	Chemical Ingredients
Volatile Solvents	
Paint and paint thinners	Petroleum distillates, esters, acetone
Paint removers	Toluene, methylene chloride, methanol, acetone
Nail polish remover	Acetone, ethyl acetate
Correction fluid and thinner	Trichloroethylene, trichloroethane
Glues and cements	Toluene, ethyl acetate, hexane, methyl chloride, acetone, methyl ethyl ketone, methyl butyl ketone, trichloroethylene, tetrachloroethylene
Dry-cleaning agents	Tetrachloroethylene, trichloroethane
Spot removers	Xylene, petroleum distillates, chlorohydrocarbons
Aerosols, Propellants, Gases	
Spray paint	Butane, propane, toluene, hydrocarbons
Hair spray	Butane, propane
Lighters	Butane, isopropane
Fuel gas	Butane, propane
Whipped cream, "whippets"	Nitrous oxide
Air duster ("Dust-Off")	1,1 difluoroethane
Anaesthetics	
Current medical use	Nitrous oxide, halothane, enflurane
Former medical use	Ether, chloroform
Nitrites	
Locker Room, Rush, poppers	Isoamyl, isobutyl, isopropyl nitrite, butyl nitrite

poisoning. For much of the twentieth century amyl nitrite was sold in small glass vials that could be snapped in half or crushed to release the vapours under the nose. During the 1960s there was some recreational use of these "poppers." The increased blood flow created a sense of warmth, and increased blood flow to the sexual organs might have accounted for the street lore that nitrites can enhance sexual pleasure. At high doses there is also a brief sense of lightheadedness or faintness resulting from lower blood pressure. Although these glass vial "poppers" are much less available these days, the term "poppers" remains as the most common street name for illicitly sold nitrites. In addition to amyl nitrite, butyl, isopropyl, and isobutyl nitrite produce similar effects. These products have been used in various cleaning products, and some users have inhaled those products to achieve the same effect.

Nitrites have never been used by a significant percentage of people in the general population, but magazine and newspaper articles in the late 1970s reported their popularity among some urban men who have sex with men, and reports in the 1980s noted a statistical correlation with HIV infection within this group. Perhaps due to this concern, the 1988 Anti-Drug Abuse Act listed several nitrites as controlled substances and called for manufacturers to limit their use in commercial products.

Volatile Solvents

The modern era of solvent abuse, or at least of widely publicized solvent abuse, can be traced to a 1959 investigative article in the Sunday supplement of a Denver, Colorado, newspaper. This article reported that young people in a nearby city had been caught spreading plastic model glue on their palms, cupping their hands over their mouths, and inhaling the vapours to get high. The article warned about the dangers of accidental exposure to solvent fumes, and an accompanying photograph showed a young man demonstrating another way to inhale glue vapours—by putting the glue on a handkerchief and holding it over the mouth and nose. The article described the effects as similar to being drunk. That article both notified the police, who presumably began looking for such behaviour, and advertised and described the practice to young people: Within the next six months, the city of Denver went from no previously reported cases of "glue-sniffing" to 50 cases. More publicity and warnings followed, and by the end of 1961 the juvenile authorities in Denver were seeing about "30 boys a month." The problem expanded further in Denver over the next several years, while similar patterns of publicity, increased use, and more publicity followed in other cities. In 1962, the magazines *Time* and *Newsweek* both carried articles describing how to sniff model glue and warning about its dangers, and the Hobby Industry Association of America produced a film for civic groups that warned about glue sniffing and recommended that communities make it illegal to sniff any substance with an intoxicating effect. Sales of model glue continued to rise as the publicity went nationwide.[34]

Since 1962, recreational use of various solvents by young people has occurred mostly as more localized fads. One group of kids in one area might start using cooking sprays, the practice will grow and then decline over a couple of years, and meanwhile in another area the kids might be inhaling a specific brand and even colour of spray paint.

Although some "huffers" are adults (e.g., alcoholics without the funds to buy alcohol), most are young. The ready availability and low price of these solvents make them attractive to children. In the high school senior class of 2012, 3% of the students reported having used some type of inhalant in the past year, whereas 6% of the eighth-graders reported using an inhalant within the past year.[35] Inhalant use has traditionally been more common among marginalized populations.[36]

Because so many different solvents are involved, it is impossible to characterize the potential harm produced by abuse of glues, paints, correction fluids, and so on. Several of the solvents have been linked to kidney damage, brain damage, and peripheral nerve damage, and many of them produce irritation of the respiratory tract and result in severe headaches. However, several users of various inhalants have simply suffocated. Although most of the children who inhale solvents do so only occasionally and give it up as they grow older and have more access to alcohol, some become dependent and a few will die.

Laws to limit sales of these household solvents to minors or to make it illegal to use them to become intoxicated have been passed in some areas, but typically they have little effect. Too many products are simply too readily available. Look around your own home or on the shelves of a supermarket or discount store—how many products have a warning about using them in an enclosed place? That warning is used by some people to indicate an inhalant to try! This is one type of substance abuse that families and communities should attack with awareness, information, and direct social intervention.

Table 7.8 Annual Prevalence of Inhalant Use in the Atlantic Provinces by Students in Grades 7, 9, 10, and 12 (1996–2008)

Year	Nova Scotia		New Brunswick		Newfoundland and Labrador		Prince Edward Island	
	%	99% ci	%	99% ci	%	99% ci	%	99% ci
1996	7.2	±1.2	5.9	±1.2	8.0	±1.4	7.2	±1.4
1998	7.0	±1.2	5.3	±1.2	7.2	±1.3	6.7	±1.3
2002	4.8	±1.0	5.2	±1.0	5.6	±1.8	5.8	±1.4
2008	4.4	±1.0	2.6	±0.6	4.4	±1.0	3.6	±1.1

ci = confidence interval

Source: Adapted from Table 5: Trends in the annual prevalence of substance use, 1996-2007. PAGE 11 IN Poulin, C & Elliot, D (2007). *Student Drug Use Survey in the Atlantic Provinces-2007: Atlantic Technical Report.* Retrieved from http://www.health.gov.nl.ca/health/publications/atl_tech_report_2007_web_cover.pdf.

Rates of Volatile Solvent Abuse in Canada

In the 2004 *Canadian Addiction Survey*, 1.9% of males 15 years and older and 0.7% of females reported use of an inhalant in their lifetime. This was an increase of 1.2% and 0.3%, respectively, from 1994.[37] Table 7.8 depicts the annual prevalence of inhalant use in the Atlantic provinces among students in grades 7, 9, 10, and 12, from 1996 to 2008. Alarmingly, inhalant use is prevalent in the younger children.[37]

Research and clinical practice have detected increased rates of volatile solvent abuse among vulnerable youth including street youth, inner city youth, and some First Nations and Inuit youth living in select rural and remote areas of the country. In Toronto, 10% of street youth had reported inhaling solvents within the past month.[38] A 2003 report from Pauingassi First Nation in Manitoba concluded that half of children under 18 years of age and living on the reserve reported solvent use.[39]

Factors surrounding the abuse of volatile solvents among First Nations and Inuit youth in select communities include high rates of poverty, boredom, loss of self-respect, unemployment, family breakdown, and poor social and economic structures.[40] It would be naïve to discount the historic impact of residential schooling, systemic racism and discrimination, and multigenerational losses of land, language, and culture as contributing factors. Although depicted as higher in comparison to the rest of Canada, the current rate of volatile solvent abuse among Canada's Aboriginal youth is not known. The media portrayal of Inuit youth in Davis Inlet, Newfoundland, getting high on gasoline has been well-publicized.

Recognizing the problem, Health Canada established the National Youth Solvent Abuse Program (NYSAP) and in October 1993 opened ten youth solvent addiction centres across the country to provide treatment programs for youth ages 12–25 years. A national committee of solvent abuse treatment centre representatives oversees NYSAP to ensure coordination of treatment services comprised of pretreatment, treatment, and posttreatment care in which families and youth are active participants.

To date, the possession and use of volatile solvents is not an offence under Canadian federal law. Governing provincial/territorial and municipal laws are not consistent across the country. The Alberta Public Health Act, the Saskatchewan Safer Communities and Neighbourhoods Act, and Manitoba Safer Communities and Neighbourhoods prohibit provision and use of inhalants, while the Manitoba Minors Intoxicating Substance Control Act makes it unlawful for anyone to provide a person under 18 with a substance that could be abused in this manner.[41] It is not clear what effects these programs have had on deterring solvent abuse.

LO9 GHB (Gamma-Hydroxybutyric Acid)

Gamma-hydroxybutyrate (GHB) occurs naturally in the brain as well as in other parts of the body. Its structure is fairly close to the inhibitory neurotransmitter GABA. GHB has been known for some time to be a CNS depressant, and has been used in other countries as an anaesthetic. Because it appears to play a role in general cellular metabolism, for a time it was sold as a dietary supplement and taken (mostly in fairly low doses) by athletes and bodybuilders hoping to stimulate muscle growth. There is no good evidence that

GHB is effective for this use, but its widespread availability in the 1980s led some to "rediscover" its powerful CNS depressant effects. Taking larger quantities of GHB alone, or combining GHB with alcohol, produces a combined depressant effect similar to what would be produced by combining alcohol with any of the other depressants discussed in this chapter, from chloral hydrate to the benzodiazepines.

The usual recreational dose of GHB taken alone ranges from 1 to 5 grams (1000 to 5000 mg). It has a fairly short half-life of about one hour. The behavioural effects are similar to alcohol, and higher doses produce muscular incoordination and slurring of speech. Increasing recreational use led the FDA to ban the inclusion of GHB in dietary supplements in 1990. The use of GHB and alcohol as a date-rape combination led in 2000 to action directing that it be listed as a Schedule I controlled substance. Evidence from the Monitoring the Future survey indicated that in 2012 only about 1.4% of high school seniors reported using GHB in the past year, down from about 2% in 2000, the first year GHB use was studied.[42]

Summary

- The barbiturates, benzodiazepines, inhalants, and other depressant drugs all have many effects in common with each other and with alcohol.
- Depressants may be prescribed in low doses for their sedative effect or in higher doses as sleeping pills (hypnotics).
- Over the past 40 years, the barbiturates have been mostly displaced by the benzodiazepines.
- The barbiturates and benzodiazepines both increase the inhibitory neural effects of the neurotransmitter GABA.
- Drugs that have a rapid onset are more likely to produce psychological dependence.
- Drugs that have a short duration of action are more likely to produce withdrawal symptoms.
- Overdoses of these depressant drugs can cause death by inhibiting respiration, particularly if the drug is taken in combination with alcohol.
- The abused inhalants include gaseous anaesthetics, certain nitrites, and volatile solvents.
- Abuse of inhalants, especially of the volatile solvents, can lead to organ damage, including neurological damage, more readily than with alcohol or other psychoactive substances.

Review Questions

1. What was the foul-smelling drug that was so widely used in mental hospitals before the 1950s?
2. Which use of a benzodiazepine (sedative vs. hypnotic) calls for a higher dose?
3. What is the relationship between psychological dependence and the time course of a drug's action?
4. The barbiturates and benzodiazepines act at which neurotransmitter receptor?
5. Why should hypnotic drugs usually be prescribed only for a few nights at a time?
6. What is zolpidem (Ambien)?
7. What are the characteristics of the sedative-hypnotic withdrawal syndrome?
8. What happens to a person who takes an overdose of a sedative-hypnotic?
9. How are the effects of the nitrites different from the effects of inhaled solvent fumes?
10. What are the effects of combining GHB with alcohol?

CHAPTER 8

PSYCHOTHERAPEUTIC DRUGS: MEDICATION FOR MENTAL DISORDERS

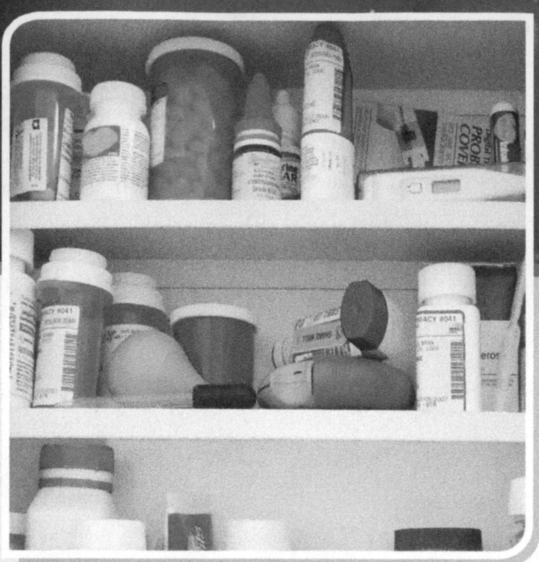

OBJECTIVES

When you have finished this chapter, you should be able to

- **LO1** Discuss what is meant by concurrent disorders and why we are seeing an increase in Canada.
- **LO2** Discuss why many professionals oppose the medical model of mental disorders.
- **LO3** Describe the classification of anxiety disorders and phobias, psychosis, and mood and depressive disorders.
- **LO4** Explain how the model by Hebb characterizes the progression of panic disorder and its implications for pharmacotherapy.
- **LO5** Explain the historical context and the importance of the discovery of the phenothiazine antipsychotics.
- **LO6** List several currently available antipsychotic drugs, distinguishing between typical and atypical antipsychotics.
- **LO7** Discuss theories of antipsychotic drug action, and explain how evidence-based practice guides antipsychotic use.
- **LO8** Explain how the sales trend of antidepressants has changed since Health Canada issued black-box warnings.
- **LO9** Explain why it is simplistic to say that antidepressant drugs work by restoring serotonin activity to normal.
- **LO10** Describe how lithium is used in treating bipolar disorder.
- **LO11** Discuss the consequences of drug treatments for mental illness.

For many individuals diagnosed with psychological disorders, the primary mode of treatment is drug therapy. Psychotherapeutic drugs are powerful psychoactive medications that help control psychotic behaviour, depression, and mania in thousands of people, reducing human suffering and health care costs, yet these drugs are far from cures, and many have undesirable side effects. Psychotherapeutics is the drug category classification of medications prescribed for the treatment of mental disorders. Should mental disorders be approached with chemical treatments? Do these treatments work? How do they work? What can these drugs tell us about the causes of mental illness? Although we don't yet have complete answers for any of these questions, we do have partial answers for all of them.

LO1, LO2, LO3, LO4

Mental Illness

Mental illnesses, also often referred to as psychological disorders, are characterized by alterations in thinking, mood, or behaviour (or some combination thereof) and can be associated with significant distress and impaired functioning. The symptoms of mental illness can vary from mild to severe, depending on the type of mental illness, the individual, the family, and the socioeconomic environment. Mental illness is the second leading cause of human disability and premature death in Canada.[1,2] Depression, for example, is much more than simple unhappiness. Clinical depression, sometimes called major depression, is a mood disorder that is a significant mental health problem. Major depression occurs in 10-25% of women–almost twice the rate in men.[3]

Research shows that more than 50% of those seeking help for an addiction also have a mental illness, and

Figure 8.1 Links between Substance Abuse and Mental Health

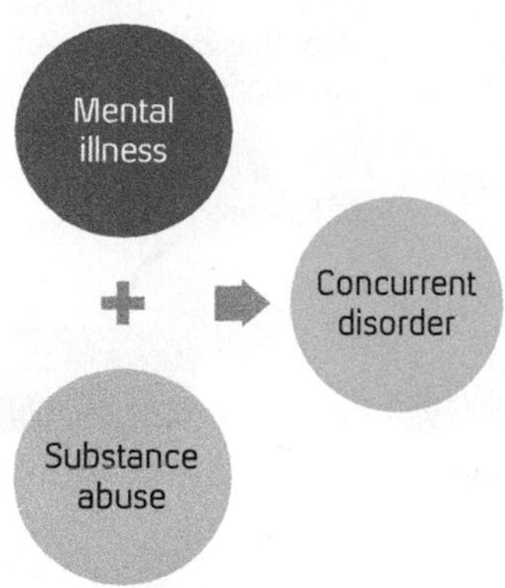

Source: Canadian Centre on Substance Abuse. When Mental Health and Substance Abuse Problems Collide. 2013. Reproduced with permission from the Canadian Centre on Substance Abuse.

15–20% of those seeking help from mental health services are also living with an addiction.[4] (Figure 8.1 provides an illustration of links between substance abuse and mental health.) The Centre for Addiction and Mental Health (CAMH) is Canada's largest addiction and mental health teaching hospital. CAMH combines education, research, clinical care, policy development, and health promotion to help transform the lives of people affected by mental health and addiction issues.[5] Concurrent disorders present a challenge for treatment: 70% of mental illnesses appear before the age of 25, and the rates of concurrent disorders are significantly higher among adolescents.[6] Drug and alcohol abuse disorders are linked to high rates of treatment nonadherence (i.e., not following a treatment plan, including not taking medications as prescribed) and to lower rates of recovery, increased risk of aggression and violence, increased attempted and completed suicide rates, and a less favourable response to conventional treatments.[4,7]

Concurrent Disorders

Mental disorders, like substance-abuse disorders, tend to be chronic, relapsing illnesses.[8] In schizophrenia, and to a lesser extent other psychological disorders, substance abuse is particularly prevalent.[9] In fact, in people with mental disorders, the risk of substance abuse is two to four times as high as in the general population.[4,8,10,11] Tobacco and cannabis tend to be the two most abused drugs. In people with schizophrenia the prevalence of cigarette smoking is two- to three-fold higher (58–88%) than in the general population. Cannabis follows tobacco as the most-used substance by people with co-occurring psychotic disorders. It has been suggested that cannabis use can trigger psychosis and schizophrenia. A study from Sweden that followed people for 15 years found that the risk of schizophrenia in adulthood was six times as high in frequent users of cannabis (those who used cannabis on more than 50 occasions in early adolescence) as in nonusers.[4] Two proposed models of increased substance abuse among individuals with mental disorders are presented in Figure 8.2. The self-medication hypothesis suggests that people choose a particular drug that is effective in combatting symptoms of psychosis. The symptoms are lessened with the drug, which provides **negative reinforcement**. The primary addiction hypothesis suggests that the neurobiology of psychosis and the brain areas involved increase a person's vulnerability to substance abuse. Increased vulnerability may produce increased pleasure with use, which provides **positive reinforcement**. Both hypotheses are supported in Canadian research.[4]

The Medical Model

Before the nineteenth century, attempts to understand or explain mental illnesses involved either magical or religious explanations, such as demon possession, or biophysical explanations.[12] Increasing focus on mental illness as an illness with neurobiological causes and underpinnings had beneficial results. It has helped promote the development of new treatments, reduced the stigma that may arise as a result of magical or religiously determined theories of mental illness, and encouraged investment in research, treatment, and care. Indeed, concern about stigma and its impact on people with mental illness has been increasingly addressed through public education campaigns that equate mental illness

negative reinforcement: the reinforcing of a response by giving an aversive stimulus when the response is not made and omitting the aversive stimulus when the response is made.

positive reinforcement: the offering of desirable effects or consequences for a behaviour with the intention of increasing the chance of that behaviour being repeated in the future.

Figure 8.2 Two Models to Explain Co-occurring Psychotic and Substance Use Disorders

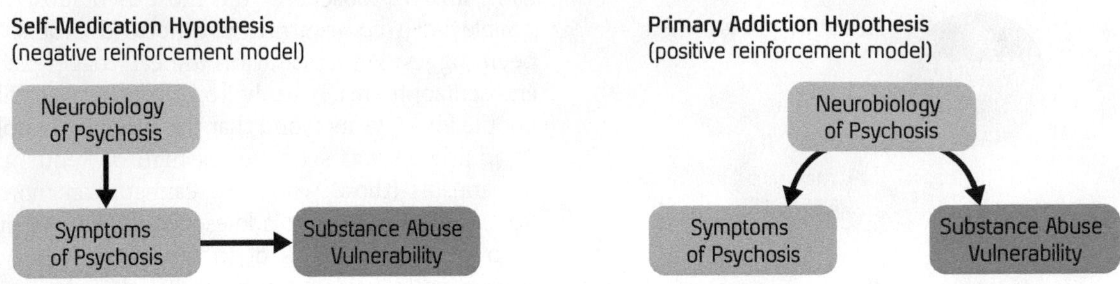

Source: Canadian Centre on Substance Abuse. *Substance Abuse in Canada: Concurrent Disorders*. Ottawa: Author, 2009.

with any other illness of the body.[13] The problem is that the use of the term *mental illness* seems to imply a particular model for behavioural disorders or dysfunctions. The medical model has been attacked by both psychiatrists (who are medical doctors) and psychologists (who generally hold nonmedical doctorates, such as a Ph.D. or Psy.D.).

According to this model, the *patient* appears with a set of *symptoms*, and on the basis of these symptoms a *diagnosis* is made as to which *disease* the patient has. Once the disease is known, its *cause* can be determined and the patient provided with a *cure*. In general terms the arguments for and against a medical model of mental illness are similar to those for and against a medical model of dependence, presented in Chapter 2. For an infectious disease, such as tuberculosis or syphilis, a set of symptoms suggests a particular disorder, but a specific diagnostic test for the presence of certain bacteria or antibodies is used to confirm the diagnosis, identify the cause, and clarify the treatment approach. Once the infection is cleared up, the disorder is cured.

For mental disorders a set of behavioural symptoms is about all we have to define and diagnose the disorder. A person might be inactive, not sleeping or eating, and quiet, and what little is said might be quite negative. This behaviour might lead us to call the person depressed. Does that mean the person has a disease called depression, with a physical cause and a potential cure? Or does it really only give a description of how he or she is acting, in the same way as we might call someone *crabby*, *friendly*, or *nerdy*?

Mental illness affects thinking, mood, or behaviour and can be associated with distress and impairment of functioning. The symptoms can vary from mild to severe[14] and may require hospitalization (see Figure 8.3). The prevalence of perceived distress, which may precede clinical diagnosis, among Canadian university students was assessed by the 2004 *Canadian Campus Survey*. About 33% of undergraduate students self-reported four or more symptoms indicative of elevated distress. Elevated distress was higher among women than men (33.5% versus 23.9%), higher among those attending university in British Columbia (30.7%) or Ontario (32.8%) than nationally (29.2%), and lowest among recreationally oriented students (21%) compared with others. The most common symptoms of distress were more often reported by women than by men and included feeling constantly under strain (reported by 47% of all students, 53% of women, and 41% of men), losing sleep over worry (38% of women and 25% of men), and feeling unhappy or depressed (36% of women and 28% of men). Examination of the trends between 1998 and 2004 revealed that the overall prevalence of elevated psychological distress (29.8% for women and 29.2% for men) remained stable during this period.[15]

A similar study conducted in people ages 55 and older in New Brunswick living in private households reported the following use of prescription medication: 17% used medication to assist sleep; 9.5% to treat depression; and 9.4% to reduce anxiety or panic attacks. Comparatively, senior women are more likely than their male counterparts to report the use of any prescription medication. However, there was no significant difference for gender in the tendency to have used any of the specific types of pharmaceutical drugs prescribed for sleep, anxiety, or depression. Stress is reported to be a primary contributing factor.[16]

The behaviours that we refer to as indicating depression are varied and probably have many

Figure 8.3 The Proportion of All Hospitalizations That Are Due to One of Seven Mental Illnesses*; in General Hospitals by Age and Sex, Canada, 1999–2000

Mental disorders accounted for 3.8% of all general hospital admissions in 1999. The rates were much higher (more than 10%) for both men and women ages 15–44 years.

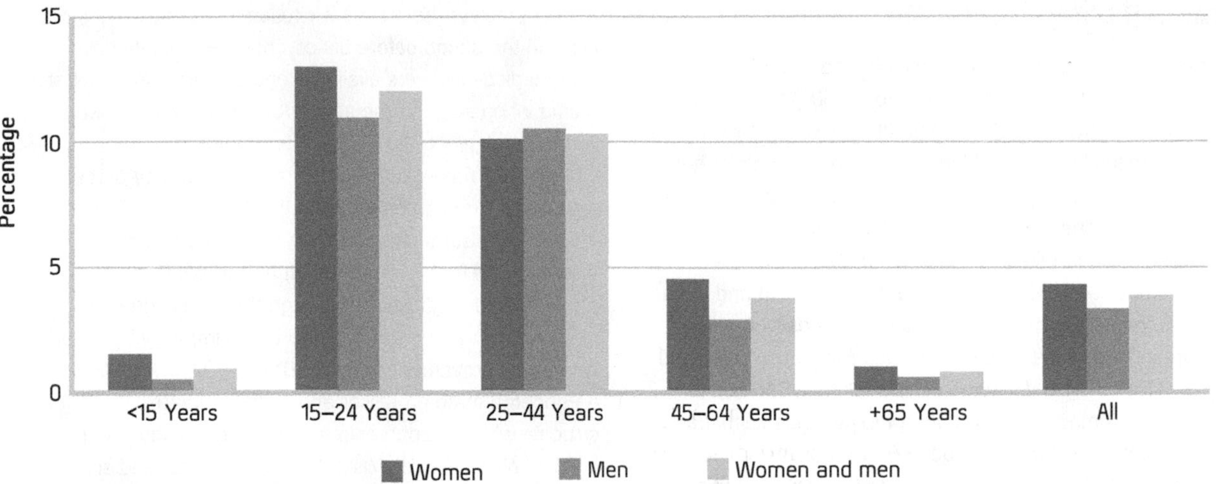

* Most responsible diagnosis is one of anxiety disorders, bipolar disorders, schizophrenia, major depression, personality disorders, eating disorders, and attempted suicide.

Source: Health Canada. *A Report on Mental Illnesses in Canada.* Ottawa, Ontario, Canada, 2002. © Health Canada Editorial Board Mental Illnesses in Canada. Canadian Cataloguing in Publication data: ISBN H39-643/2002E; 0-662-32817-5.

different causes, most of them not known. We are far from being able to prescribe a cure for depression that will be generally successful in eliminating these symptoms.

Despite these attacks on the medical model, it still seems to guide much of the current thinking about behavioural disorders. The fact that psychoactive drugs can be effective in controlling symptoms, if not in curing disorders, has lent strength to supporters of the medical model. If chemicals can help normalize an individual's behaviour, a natural assumption might be that the original problem resulted from a chemical imbalance in the brain–and that measurements of chemicals in urine, blood, or cerebrospinal fluid could provide more specific and accurate diagnoses and give direction to efforts at drug therapy. This kind of thinking gives scientists great hope, and many experiments have attempted to find the chemical imbalances, so far with very little success.

Classification of Mental Disorders

Because human behaviour is so variable and because we do not know the causes of most mental disorders, classification of people with mental illnesses into diagnostic categories is difficult. Nevertheless, some basic divisions are widely used and important for understanding the uses of **psychotherapeutic drugs**. In 2013, the American Psychiatric Association (APA) published the fifth edition of its *Diagnostic and Statistical Manual of Mental Disorders* (referred to as the DSM-5).[17] This manual provides criteria for classifying mental disorders into hundreds of specific diagnostic categories. Partly because this classification system has been adopted by major health insurance companies, its terms and definitions have become standard for all mental health professionals. According to the APA, the DSM-5 chapter on anxiety disorder no longer includes obsessive-compulsive disorder or PTSD (posttraumatic stress disorder). Instead, these disorders have been relocated to their own respective chapters.[18]

psychotherapeutic drugs: drugs that are prescribed for their effects in relieving symptoms of anxiety, depression, or other mental disorders.

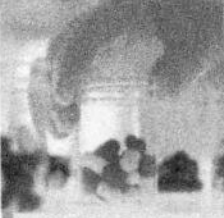

DRUGS IN THE MEDIA

Mental Illness at the Movies

Most of us know at least one person who is being treated with medication for depression or for ADHD (Chapter 6). In fact, one in every five Canadians (20% of Canadians) will have a mental health problem at some point in his or her life.[19] As a group, mood disorders are one of the most common mental illnesses in the general population. Canadian studies looking at lifetime incidence of major depression found that 7.9–8.6% of adults over the age of 18 and living in the community met the criteria for diagnosis of major depression at some time in their lives.[20] Because these and most other mental disorders can be controlled to some degree with medication, we do not experience firsthand many of the most troubling behaviour problems that lead to a diagnosis of a serious mental disorder. Films and television programs have attempted to portray characters struggling with mental disorders, and some of these portrayals can be informative. The book *Movies and Mental Illness* uses the viewing of popular films as an instructional aid to learning about abnormal psychology.[21]

These films can also teach us about how medications are used in treating those disorders. Two of the best film depictions of mental institutions are *The Snake Pit* (1948), starring Olivia de Havilland, and *One Flew Over the Cuckoo's Nest* (1975), starring Jack Nicholson. Both films are available on video and provide an interesting contrast. Although neither portrays the mental institution in a positive light, one is set in the period before antipsychotic and antidepressant medications were available, and the later film is set at a time when some of the early drugs of those types were widely used.

A more recent portrayal of mental illness by actor Jack Nicholson can be found in the 1998 film *As Good as It Gets*. Nicholson's character has obsessive-compulsive disorder, and for most of the film he refuses to treat the problem with medication. Although the medication itself plays a minor role, it is shown to be an important part of his later improvement. In the 2001 film *A Beautiful Mind*, a Princeton math professor and Nobel laureate's lifelong struggle with schizophrenia is portrayed in convincing fashion, along with the usefulness, limitations, and side effects of the antipsychotic medications he used to control the symptoms.

Next time you are discussing movies with your friends, see if you can come up with other examples of films or television programs that depict the use of psychoactive drugs in the treatment of mental disorders. Are the medications generally treated inappropriately as either cures or as a way to force conformity and compliance? Or are they treated more realistically as beneficial in some ways, yet with both limited effectiveness and unwanted side effects?

Anxiety Disorders and Phobias Anxiety is a normal and common human experience; anticipation of potential threats and dangers often helps us avoid them. However, when these worries become unrealistic, resulting in chronic uneasiness, fear of impending doom, or bouts of terror or panic, they can interfere with the individual's daily life. Physical symptoms may also be present, often associated with activation of the autonomic nervous system (e.g., flushed skin, dilated pupils, gastrointestinal problems, increased heart rate, or shortness of breath).[22] The DSM-5 refers to these and other problems as **anxiety disorders** (see the DSM-5 box).

anxiety disorders: mental disorders characterized by excessive worry, fears, or avoidance.

Perhaps because these disorders all seem to have some form of anxiety associated with them, and perhaps because for many years psychiatrists classified benzodiazepines and other depressants as *antianxiety drugs* (see Chapter 7), we tend to think of anxiety not as a behavioural symptom but rather as an internal state that *causes* the disorders. That view fits well with the medical model, but we should guard against easy acceptance of the view that these disorders are caused by anxiety and that therefore we can treat them by using antianxiety drugs. In recent years, psychiatrists have increasingly used selective reuptake inhibitors, classified as antidepressants, to treat obsessive-compulsive disorder

DSM-5

Anxiety Disorders and Phobias

Agoraphobia, Specific Phobia, and Social Anxiety Disorder (Social Phobia)
Panic Attack
Panic Disorder and Agoraphobia
Specific Phobia (also known as Simple Phobia)
Social Anxiety Disorder (also known as Social Phobia)

Generalized Anxiety Disorder
Generalized anxiety disorder is characterized by excessive anxiety and worry about a number of events or activities, such as school, work performance, or finances, and lasting for a period of six months or longer.

Panic Disorder (with or without Agoraphobia)
Panic disorder is defined by recurring, unexpected panic attacks and by subsequent concern about future attacks or about the meaning of the attacks.

The agoraphobia (*fear of the marketplace*) that often accompanies panic disorders is a fear of being in places or situations from which escape might be difficult or where help might not be available in the event of either a panic attack or some other incapacitating or embarrassing situation (e.g., fainting or losing bladder control). The person with agoraphobia might avoid going outside the home alone or be afraid of being in a public place or standing in a line.

Specific Phobia
Specific phobia is excessive or unreasonable fear of a specific situation or object (e.g., elevators, flying, enclosed spaces, or some type of animal).

Social Phobia
Social phobia is an overwhelming, persistent fear of social or performance situations (e.g., speaking in public, entering a room full of strangers, or using a public restroom).

Source: Reprinted with permission from the Diagnostic and Statistical Manual of Mental Disorders, Fourth Edition (Copyright © 2000) and the Diagnostic and Statistical Manual of Mental Disorders, Fifth Edition (Copyright © 2013). American Psychiatric Association. All Rights Reserved.

and other anxiety disorders. Since 1987, hospitalization rates for anxiety disorders in general hospitals have decreased by 49%.[20] The prevalence rates for anxiety disorders in Canada are listed in Table 8.1.

Table 8.1 One-Year Prevalence of Anxiety Disorders in Canada

Specific phobias (6.2%–8%) and social phobia (6.7%) are the most prevalent anxiety disorders in Canada.

Type of Anxiety Disorder	Population Ages 15–64 Years, % with an Anxiety Disorder
Generalized anxiety disorder	1.1
Specific phobia	6.2–8.0
Social phobia	6.7
Panic disorder	0.7

Source: Health Canada. *A Report on Mental Illnesses in Canada.* Ottawa, Ontario, Canada, 2002. © Health Canada Editorial Board Mental Illnesses in Canada. Canadian Cataloguing in Publication data: ISBN H39-643/2002E; 0-662-32817-5.

Obsessive-Compulsive Disorder (OCD) Obsessions are unwanted and repeated thoughts, feelings, or images that are intrusive and inappropriate and that cause marked distress. Compulsions are urgent, repetitive behaviours, such as hand washing, counting, or repeatedly "checking" to make sure that some dreaded event will not occur (e.g., checking that all doors and windows are locked, then checking again and again).

Posttraumatic Stress Disorder (PTSD) The person has been exposed to an event that involved actual or threatened death or serious injury, and the person reacted with intense fear or helplessness. The person persistently re-experiences the event through recollections, dreams, or a sudden feeling as if the event were occurring.

Psychosis **Psychosis** refers to a major disturbance of normal intellectual and social functioning in

psychosis: a serious mental disorder involving loss of contact with reality.

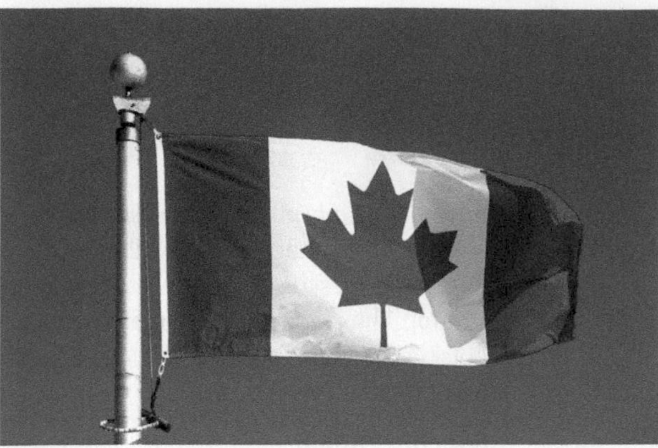

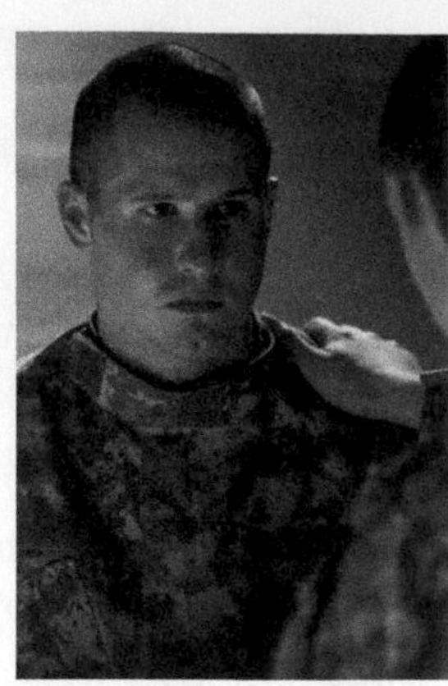

Troubling events on the front line can sometimes trigger PTSD for soldiers. PTSD is a common psychiatric disorder in Canada, with a prevalence rate of experiencing PTSD in one's lifetime estimated at almost 10% (i.e., one in ten Canadians). With PTSD are also increased rates of drug use and addiction.

which there is loss of contact with reality. Not knowing the current date, hearing voices that aren't there, and believing that you are Napoleon or Christ are some examples of this withdrawal from reality. Many people refer to psychosis as reflecting a primary disorder of *thinking*, as opposed to mood or emotion. However, individuals with schizophrenia do exhibit perturbations in mood and emotion secondary to alterations in limbic system function (see Figure 8.4).

Psychotic behaviour may be viewed as a group of symptoms that can have many possible causes. One important distinction is between the *organic* psychoses and the *functional* psychoses. An organic disorder is one that has a known physical cause. Psychosis can result from many things, including brain tumours or infections, metabolic or endocrine disorders, degenerative neurological diseases, chronic alcohol use, and high doses of stimulant drugs, such as amphetamine or cocaine. Functional disorders are simply those for which there is no known or obvious physical cause. A person who has a chronic (long-lasting) psychotic condition for which there is no known cause will probably receive the diagnosis of **schizophrenia**. There is a popular misconception that schizophrenia means "split personality" or refers to individuals exhibiting multiple personalities. Instead, schizophrenia should probably be translated as *shattered mind*. See the DSM-5 box for the diagnostic criteria for schizophrenia.

schizophrenia: a type of chronic psychosis.

DSM-5

Diagnosis of Schizophrenia

A. Characteristic symptoms: Two or more of the following:
   1. Delusions (irrational beliefs)
   2. Hallucinations (e.g., hearing voices)
   3. Disorganized speech (incoherent, frequent changes of topic)
   4. Grossly disorganized behaviour (inappropriate, unpredictable) or catatonic (withdrawn, immobile)
   5. Negative symptoms (lack of emotional response, little or no speech, doesn't initiate activities)

B. Interference with social or occupational function

C. Duration of at least six months

Source: Reprinted with permission from the Diagnostic and Statistical Manual of Mental Disorders, Fourth Edition (Copyright © 2000) and the Diagnostic and Statistical Manual of Mental Disorders, Fifth Edition (Copyright © 2013). American Psychiatric Association.

Figure 8.4 Brain Areas Affected by Schizophrenia

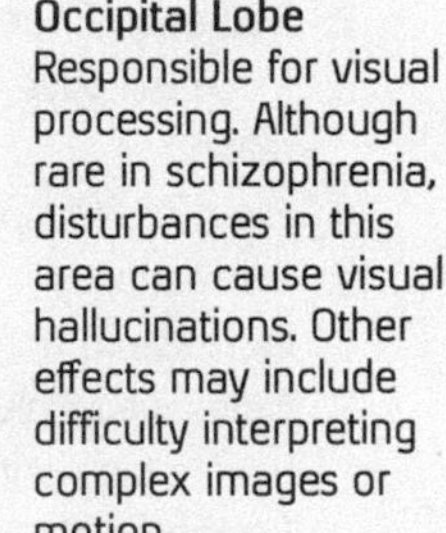

Basal Ganglia
Related to movement, emotions, and the integration of sensory information. Abnormal function of the basal ganglia is thought to contribute to hallucinations and paranoia. Traditional antipsychotic medications can excessively blockade dopamine receptors in the basal ganglia, which can cause motor-related side effects.
Auditory System
Allows humans to hear and understand speech. Overactivity of Wernicke's area, the area responsible for speech, can cause auditory hallucinations in people with schizophrenia.
Occipital Lobe
Responsible for visual processing. Although rare in schizophrenia, disturbances in this area can cause visual hallucinations. Other effects may include difficulty interpreting complex images or motion.
Frontal Lobe
Performs problem solving, insight, and other high-level reasoning. Disruptions caused by schizophrenia create difficulties in organizing thoughts and planning.
Limbic System
Critical to emotion. Disturbances to the limbic system are thought to relate to the agitation often exhibited in cases of schizophrenia.
Hippocampus
Coordinates memory function and learning, which are related functions that can be disrupted in cases of schizophrenia.

Mood Disorders *Mood disorder* refers to the appearance of depressed or manic symptoms. Mood disorders have no single cause, but several factors, such as a biochemical imbalance in the brain, psychological factors, and socioeconomic factors, tend to make some individuals prone to such disorders.[20] Refer to Figure 6.5 in Chapter 6 for one schematic representation of mood in which depression is shown as an abnormally low mood and mania as an abnormally high mood. The important distinction in the DSM-5, and in the drug treatment of mood disorders, is between **bipolar disorder**, in which both manic and depressive episodes have been observed at some time, and major **depression**, in which only depressive episodes are reported. See the DSM-5 box for diagnostic criteria for manic episode and major depressive episode.

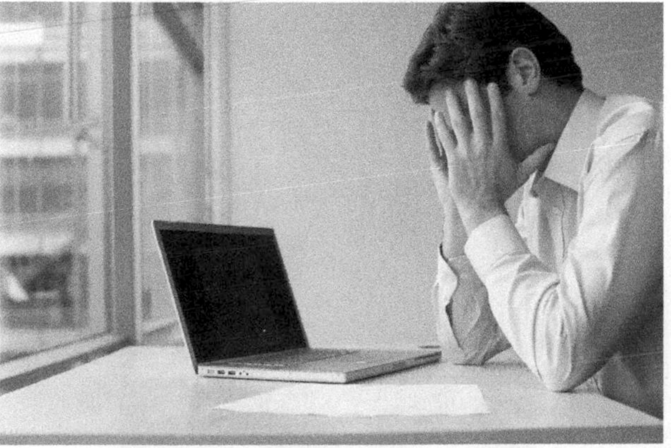

bipolar disorder: a type of mood disorder also known as manic-depressive disorder.

depression: a major type of mood disorder.

Depressive Disorders The DSM-5 diagnostic criteria for major depressive disorder are the same as the

DSM-5

Bipolar and Related Disorders

I. Manic Episode
   A. Abnormally and persistently elevated, expansive, or irritable mood
   B. At least three of the following:
      1. Inflated self-esteem or grandiosity
      2. Decreased need for sleep
      3. More talkative than usual or pressure to keep talking
      4. Flight of ideas or feeling that thoughts are racing
      5. Distractibility
      6. Increase in activity
      7. Excessive involvement in pleasurable activities that have a high potential for painful consequences (shopping, sex, foolish investments)
   C. Mood disturbance is sufficiently severe to cause marked impairment in functioning

II. Major Depressive Episode
   A. Five or more of the following, including either No. 1 or No. 2:
      1. Depressed mood most of the day, nearly every day
      2. Markedly diminished interest or pleasure in most activities
      3. Significant changes in body weight or appetite (increased or decreased)
      4. Insomnia or hypersomnia nearly every day
      5. Psychomotor agitation (increased activity) or retardation (decreased activity)
      6. Fatigue or loss of energy
      7. Feelings of worthlessness or excessive guilt
      8. Diminished ability to think or concentrate
      9. Recurrent thoughts of death or suicide, or a suicide attempt or plan for committing suicide
   B. The symptoms cause clinically significant distress or impairment
   C. Not due to a drug or medical condition

Source: Reprinted with permission from the Diagnostic and Statistical Manual of Mental Disorders, Fourth Edition (Copyright © 2000) and the Diagnostic and Statistical Manual of Mental Disorders, Fifth Edition (Copyright © 2013). American Psychiatric Association. All Rights Reserved.

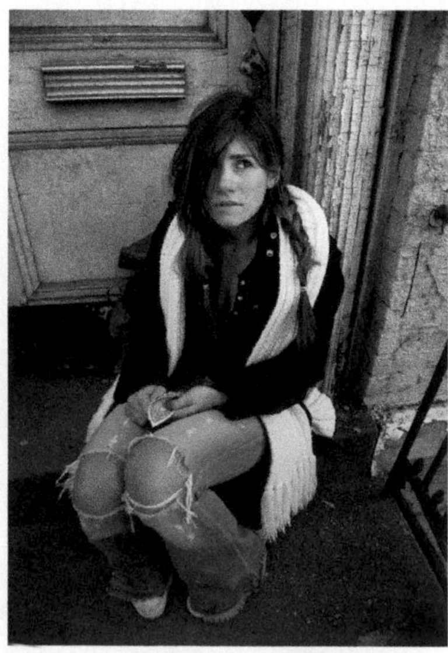

Mental disorders are typically categorized by behavioural symptoms; for example, schizophrenia is characterized by delusions, hallucinations, and disorganized speech and behaviour. Many successful people are now speaking out, to show the diverse faces and lives of those suffering from mental illness.

criteria listed in the DSM-5 box for major depressive episode in bipolar and related disorders, with two additional criteria:

D. The occurrence of the major depressive episode is not better explained by other psychotic disorders.
E. There has never been a manic episode or hypomanic episode.[23]

Individual human beings often don't fit neatly into one of these diagnostic categories, and in many cases assigning a diagnosis and selecting a treatment are as much a matter of experience and art as they are of applying scientific descriptions. For example, suppose a person displays both abnormal mood states and bizarre thinking. If it is assumed that the disturbance of thinking is the primary problem and that the person is elated or depressed because of a bizarre belief, then the individual may be diagnosed as having schizophrenia. Another professional might see the mood disorder as primary, with the "crazy" talk supporting a negative view of the world, and give the individual a primary diagnosis of depression.

BOX 8.1

PANIC DISORDER

The symptoms of panic attacks may include shortness of breath, dizziness or faintness, palpitations or accelerated heart rate, trembling, sweating, choking, numbness, fear of dying, or fear of going crazy or doing something uncontrolled.[24] There are no inclusive models of panic disorder in animals. Consideration of parallels between behavioural profiles drawn from animal models of anxiety and clinical panic symptoms should focus on behaviours that reflect comparable aspects of anxiety. Conditioned fear and exploratory tendencies of animals in new environments provide a parallel for the agoraphobic symptoms in people with panic disorder. A neuropeptide found in the gut and in the brain, cholecystokinin (CCK), appears to play a fundamental role in panic that can be modelled in animals. Injection of CCK in control subjects and people with panic disorder can cause a panic attack. Some people with an anxiety disorder need a lower dose than do control subjects, suggesting they are more sensitive to the anxiogenic (anxiety-producing) effects of CCK. It is interesting that people with panic disorders are also more sensitive to life events (e.g., going out in public), which may suggest they have higher levels of CCK in their brains. These studies are important because drugs that work in these animal models may also have an important role in treating or controlling the symptoms associated with panic disorder in people. For example, diazepam is relatively ineffective in the long-term management of panic disorder and is ineffective in animal models of panic symptoms. We don't know what causes some people to develop panic disorder, but we do know that some people with panic disorder report increased anxiety in their lives that led to depression before their first panic attack. We also know that some people just have panic attacks (uncomplicated panic), while others have other symptoms at the same time (comorbid). Anxiety and depression are important to the development of panic disorder (see part I in Figure 8.5, which summarizes Hebb's model of the progression of panic disorder). Reciprocal influences on individual states of anxiety and depression may be further influenced by subjective factors, including age of onset, chronic illness in the family, subject history, or other stressors.

Panic disorder is diagnosed according to DSM-5 criteria, and comorbid disturbances associated with panic (part II in Figure 8.5) are affected by panic duration, frequency, and severity. Panic evolves at some point following repeated depressive and anxiety episodes. The temporal parameters associated with the appearance of panic symptoms among various clinical populations or specific individuals have not been clearly determined.

Panic symptoms (part II in Figure 8.5), once present, may consist primarily of autonomic symptoms, including cardiovascular disturbances (such as palpitation) or cognitive symptoms, including depersonalization (a loss of the sense of personal identity and external reality) and fear of losing control, accompanied by phobic or depressive symptoms (uncomplicated panic). More commonly panic disorder is complicated with depression of varying severity (mild to severe depression), mild phobia, hypochondriasis, or severe avoidance behaviour. The varying types of panic classifications may represent different developmental stages of panic. Moreover, age of onset, illness in the family, and panic duration, frequency, and severity may influence the progression of panic from uncomplicated panic episodes to panic with comorbid symptoms of depression and phobia. Such factors may influence pharmacological management of panic. Depending on the person's clinical history and the brain regions involved, different psychotherapeutics can be prescribed for treatment (see Figure 8.5).

Research suggests that the amygdala, a structure deep within the brain, serves as a communication hub that signals the presence of a threat and triggers a fear response or anxiety. It also stores emotional memories and may play a role in the development of anxiety disorders. The developmental stages of panic (part III in Figure 8.5) appear to be characterized by prominent symptoms that may involve brain-stem structures, mesolimbic areas, or cortical areas. Uncomplicated panic, for example, may be primarily associated with cardiovascular and respiratory disturbances (brainstem), although anxiety (amygdala) and rumination (nucleus accumbens, ventral tegmental area [VTA], prefrontal cortex) are also present. Comorbidity with depression or phobia would typically involve mesencephalic (e.g., VTA), mesolimbic (e.g., nucleus accumbens, amygdala), and cortical areas (e.g., prefrontal cortex and cingulate gyrus) (see Figure 8.5).

The children of adults with anxiety disorders are at much greater risk of an anxiety disorder than is the general population, which may imply a genetic factor, an effect of parenting practices, or both.[20,25] In panic disorder, different brain regions may support specific symptomatology. Clinical history, such as the age of onset and familial illness, also plays a role, although the delineation between genetics and environment is not clear.

continued

BOX 8.1

PANIC DISORDER
continued

Figure 8.5 A General Schematic of Panic Disorder

This schematic illustration of the involvement of repeated anxiety episodes in panic (I) shows the developmental stage or course of panic, the precipitating variables that affect its course (II), and some of the central sites hypothesized to be involved in panic disorder (III). Repeated anxiety (part I) may bring on major affective disorder, while depression may lead to further increases in anxiety.

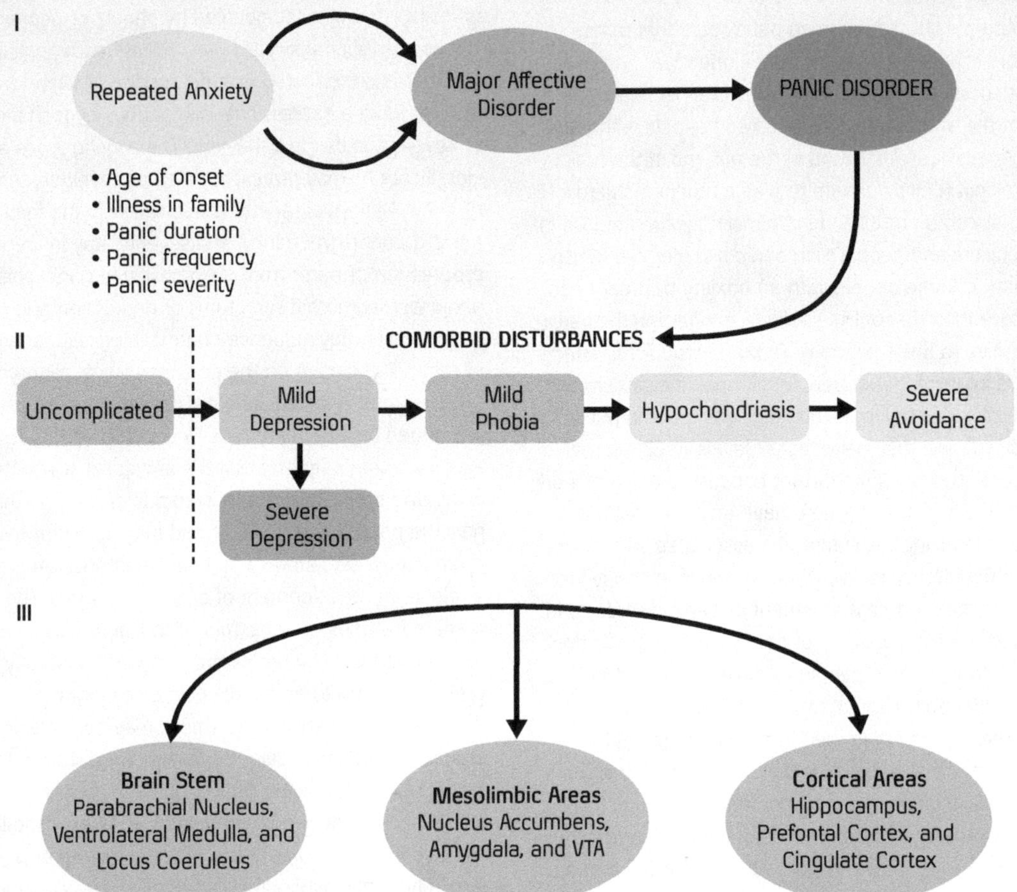

Source: Fig. (2), Schematic Illustration of the Involvement of Repeated Anxiety Episodes in Panic, on p. 8 in Hebb, A.L.O., G.J. Anger, P.D. Mendella, F.M. Sirois, R.W. Gilbert, and R.M. Zacharko. "The Myth of Panic Spontaneity: Consideration of Behavioural and Neurochemical Sensitization." *The Open Psychiatry Journal* 1 (2007), pp. 1–25.

LO5, LO6, LO7, LO8, LO9, LO10

Treatment of Mental Disorders

Over the centuries, people with mental illnesses have been subjected to various kinds of treatment, depending on the views held at the time regarding the causes of mental illness.

Before 1950

Because we are concerned with drug therapy a good place to begin our history is in 1917, when a physical treatment was first demonstrated to be effective in serious mental disorders. In those days a great proportion of the patients with psychosis had *general paresis*, a syphilitic infection of the nervous system.

It was noticed that the fever associated with malaria often produced marked improvement, and so in 1917 "malaria therapy" was introduced in the treatment of general paresis. The later discovery of antibiotics that could cure syphilis virtually eliminated this particular type of treatment.

In the 1920s, wealthier patients could afford a course of "narcosis therapy," in which barbiturates and other depressants were used to induce sleep for as long as a week or more. Another use for sedative drugs was in conjunction with psychotherapy. An intravenous dose of thiopental sodium, a rapid-acting barbiturate, would relax a person and produce more talking during psychotherapy. The theory was that such a reduction in inhibitions would enable the patient to express repressed thoughts; thus, the term *truth serum* came to be used for thiopental sodium and for scopolamine, an anticholinergic drug used similarly. Anyone who has ever listened to a person who has drunk a good bit of alcohol will tell you that although the talk might be less inhibited, it isn't always more truthful. So-called truth serum apparently worked about as well.

In 1933, Manfred Sakel of Vienna induced comas in some people with schizophrenia by administering insulin. The resulting drop in blood glucose level caused the brain's neurons to first increase their activity and produce convulsions and then decrease their activity and leave the patient in a coma. A course of 30 to 50 of these treatments over two to three months was believed to be highly effective, and discharge rates of 90% were reported in the early years of insulin-shock therapy. Later studies demonstrated that the relapse rate was quite high, and this treatment was abandoned.

Ladislas von Meduna believed, incorrectly, that no person with epilepsy also had schizophrenia and no person with schizophrenia also had epilepsy. Reasoning that epileptic convulsions prevented the development of schizophrenia, he felt that inducing convulsions might have therapeutic value for people with schizophrenia. His first convulsant drug was camphor, but it had the disadvantage of a lag time of several hours between injection and the convulsions. In 1934, he started using pentylenetetrazol, which induced convulsions in less than 30 seconds, and he reported improvement in 50–60% of patients.

The use of a drug was not ideal for inducing convulsions, because even a 30-second interval between injection and loss of consciousness (with the convulsion) produced much anguish in the patient. Ugo Cerletti, after experimenting on pigs in a slaughterhouse, developed the technique of using electric shock to induce convulsions. This method has the advantage of inducing loss of consciousness and convulsion at the moment the electric shock is applied. **Electroconvulsive therapy (ECT)** involves passing electrical currents though the brain to trigger seizures, and although early work in the 1930s and 1940s suggested high improvement rates, later studies found a reduction of schizophrenic symptoms in only about half of the patients, and the relapse rates were quite high.

At the University of Toronto in the 1980s, Shugar and colleagues analyzed ECT use for schizophrenia in 57 hospitals across Ontario. ECT was used when drugs failed to achieve a satisfactory response, although there was very little uniformity or standardization in the use of ECT for schizophrenia. ECT use was higher among individuals who had comorbid symptoms of depression (schizoaffective).[26] ECT may remain the only treatment alternative for some psychiatric patients, as concluded by a study commissioned by the Quebec government, but many uncertainties still surround its efficacy and use. In-hospital data indicate that about 3000 patients receive ECT per year, including 700 in Quebec. In 2007, the procedure was used more than 15 000 times in Canada.[27]

Antipsychotic drugs are still the first choice for schizophrenia treatment, although recent data show that ECT clearly works in some patients, and combining both treatments can accelerate benefits to these patients. The side effects of shock therapy may be more tolerable to patients than those of antipsychotic drugs.[28,29] ECT is still widely used with severely depressed patients who do not respond to medication. Scientists are unsure how the treatment works, but it appears to produce many changes in the chemistry and functioning of the brain, including stabilization of monoamines (dopamine, serotonin, and norepinephrine), which are thought to underlie symptoms of depression and schizophrenia.[30] ECT is still a controversial form of treatment, but the controversy surrounding ECT may stem from the impression people had when it was administered in earlier days without anaesthesia, as was portrayed in the movie *One Flew Over the Cuckoo's Nest*. ECT has evolved to include the administration of anaesthesia, muscle relaxants, and oxygen, so it is considered to be quite a safe form of treatment.[31] The new Irene and Leslie Dubé Centre

electroconvulsive therapy (ECT): a medical procedure in which a cerebral seizure is induced by a brief electrical stimulus under controlled conditions; purpose is to treat major mental disorders.

for Mental Health at the Royal University Hospital in Saskatoon, Saskatchewan, has a new ECT facility with seven beds. ECT is also done typically on the nondominant hemisphere of the brain, as opposed to bilaterally, in an effort to minimize loss of recent memories.[32]

In its first updated position statement on ECT since 1992, the Canadian Psychiatric Association says that while the mechanism of action of ECT still can't be fully explained, extensive research and more than 70 years of experience support the view that ECT "should remain readily available as a treatment option" for major depression, bipolar disorder, and schizophrenia.[28]

Antipsychotics

A number of people were involved in the discovery that a group of drugs called the **phenothiazines** had special properties when used by people with mental illnesses. Credit is usually given to a French surgeon, Henri Laborit, who first tested these compounds in conjunction with surgical anaesthesia. He noted that the most effective of the phenothiazines, chlorpromazine, did not by itself induce drowsiness or a loss of consciousness, but it seemed to make the patients unconcerned about their upcoming surgery. He reasoned that this effect might reduce emotionality in psychiatric patients and encouraged his psychiatric colleagues to test the drug. The first report of these French trials of chlorpromazine in people with mental illnesses mentioned that not only were the patients calmed, but the drug also seemed to act on the psychotic process itself. This new type of drug action attracted a variety of names: in Canada the drugs were generally called tranquillizers, which some now think is an unfortunate term that focuses on the calming action and seems to imply sedation. Another term used was **neuroleptic**, meaning "taking hold of the nervous system," a term implying an increased amount of control. Although both of these terms are still in use, most medical texts now refer to this group of drugs as **antipsychotics**, reflecting their ability to reduce psychotic symptoms without necessarily producing drowsiness and sedation. The tremendous impact of phenothiazine treatment on the management of hospitalized patients is clear from a 1955 statement by the director of the Delaware State Hospital:

> We have now achieved . . . the reorganization of the management of disturbed patients. With rare exceptions, all restraints have been discontinued. The hydrotherapy department, formerly active on all admission services and routinely used on wards with disturbed patients, has ceased to be in operation. Maintenance EST (electroshock treatment) for disturbed patients has been discontinued. . . . There has been a record increase in participation by these patients in social and occupational activities.
>
> These developments have vast sociological implications. I believe it is fair to state that pharmacology promises to accomplish what other measures have failed to bring about—the social emancipation of the mental hospital.[33]

Treatment Effects and Considerations Along with an increase in the use of phenothiazines in the treatment of people with mental illnesses came an increase in the sophistication of experimental programs that evaluate the effectiveness of various drugs. Results of these studies show clearly that phenothiazine-treated patients improve more than patients receiving placebo or no treatments. In a National Institute of Mental Health (NIMH) study, after six weeks 75% of people with acute schizophrenia receiving phenothiazines showed either moderate or marked improvement, whereas of those receiving placebos only 23% improved. Over the years many more studies have demonstrated consistently that although phenothiazines are far from a complete cure for every patient, they are significantly better than placebo treatments in reducing psychotic behaviours.

Another aspect of evaluating the effectiveness of drug treatment is determining the incidence of relapse, or symptom recurrence, when treatment is discontinued. It is most likely that discontinuation of drug therapy will lead to relapse in 75–95% of patients within a year and in more than 50% of patients in six months. Almost all studies report that when medication is resumed, there is again a reduction in symptoms.

In the years since 1950, many new phenothiazines have been introduced and several completely new types of antipsychotic drugs have been discovered. The therapeutic effects of antipsychotic medications target the positive symptoms, particularly agitation, aggression, delusions, and hallucinations, effectively. The negative symptoms of chronic psychotic illness, including social withdrawal, lack of motivation, and impaired cognition, including deficient working memory, are typically less responsive to treatment and contribute to the long-term disability associated with

phenothiazines: a group of drugs used to treat psychosis.

neuroleptics: a general term for antipsychotic drugs.

antipsychotics: a group of drugs used to treat psychosis; same as neuroleptics.

Table 8.2 Atypical and Conventional Antipsychotic Drugs: Routes of Administration, Dosage, and Cost in Canada

Antipsychotic Agent (year marketed in Canada)	Forms Available	Usual Target Doses (in mg/d)	Monthly Cost ($*)
Modern Atypical Antipsychotics			
aripiprazole (2013)	T	10–30	370–740
clozapine (1991)	T	300–450	310–740
olanzapine (1996)	T, W, IM_S	10–20	265–515
quetiapine (1998)	T	300–600	145–275
risperidone (1993)	T, L	2–6	100–250
risperidone depot (2004)	IM_D	25–50‡	640–1250
ziprasidone (2008)	T, IM_S	80–160	–
Representative Conventional Antipsychotics			
chlorpromazine (1953)	T, L, IM_S	75–400	25–50
flupenthixol (1983)	T, L	9–24	65–160
flupenthixol decanoate (1983)	IM_D	20–60†	40–80
fluphenazine (1960)	T, L, IM_S, IM_D	4–20	25–35
haloperidol (1966)	T, L, IM_S, IM_D	4–12	15–35
loxapine (1978)	T, L, IM_S	20–100	30–45
perphenazine (1957)	T, L	16–48	10–15
thiothixine (1968)	C	15–30	20–60
trifluoperazine (1958)	T	5–20	15–35

T = tablet; W = rapid-dissolving water; IM_S = short-acting intramuscular injection; L = oral liquid; IM_D = long-acting intramuscular depot; C = capsule; *Prescription retail price in Canadian dollars rounded to closest $5; includes $10 pharmacy professional fee (Source: Shopper's Drug Mart, Halifax, NS, May 2005); † Available only through special access in Canada; ‡ Risperidone and flupenthixol depot formulations are usually administered every two weeks.

Source: Garner, D.M., R.J. Baldessarini, and P. Waraich. Table 1, "Modern Antipsychotic Drugs: A Critical Overview." *Canadian Medical Association Journal* 172, no. 13 (2005), pp. 1703–1711.

psychosis. Table 8.2 lists routes of administration, dosages, and costs of antipsychotic medications in Canada.

First-generation antipsychotics (FGAs), also known as *typical* or *conventional* antipsychotics, can be classified according to their chemical structure (e.g., phenothiazines, such as fluphenazine, or butyrophenones, such as haloperidol and most of the other drug types introduced before the mid-1990s) or potency (low, intermediate, high) as determined by dopamine D2 receptor binding affinity (D2 is one of many subtypes of dopamine receptors).[34] All antipsychotics introduced in the past ten years are second-generation antipsychotics (SGAs) or *atypical* antipsychotics (aripiprazole, clozapine, olanzapine, paliperidone, quetiapine, risperidone, and ziprasidone) that have greater serotonin (5-HT) affinity relative to dopamine D2 receptor affinity.

Ziprasidone (Zeldox) was discovered and developed by Pfizer. It is a serotonin and dopamine antagonist that is reported to treat symptoms characterized as both positive (e.g., visual and auditory hallucinations) and negative (lack of motivation and social withdrawal), as well as the overall psychopathology of the disorder.[35,36] In patients with chronic schizophrenia treated over five years, ziprasidone treatment was associated with lower health care costs, the lowest predicted number of type 2 diabetes cases and cardiovascular disease events, and the highest quality of life relative to risperidone, olanzapine, and quetiapine treatments.[37] The length of time a drug binds to dopamine D2 receptors may explain clinical differences in dosing requirements and side effects among SGAs.

Second-generation or atypical antipsychotic agents (ATAs) became available on the Canadian market in the 1990s for the treatment of schizophrenia and related psychotic disorders. They include risperidone, olanzapine, quetiapine, and clozapine, which are less likely to cause extrapyramidal side effects and carry a significantly lower risk of tardive dyskinesia (discussed below) than do typical agents.[38]

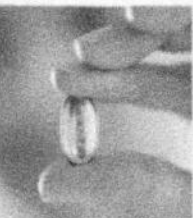

DRUGS IN DEPTH

Thioridazine Use in Canada

Thioridazine is a phenothiazine that has been used in Canada for the treatment of schizophrenia since 1959. The original brand name of thioridazine was Mellaril. In July 2000, Novartis Pharma Canada Inc., the manufacturer of Mellaril, distributed a letter to Canadian health care professionals that discussed potentially life-threatening changes in heart rhythm caused by Mellaril. In response to these safety issues and as requested by Health Canada, Novartis withdrew the drug from the Canadian market in July 2001.

Health Canada issued an advisory that sales of thioridazine were to be stopped by September 30, 2005. The safety concerns (benefits versus risks) arose from rare occurrences of heart rhythm changes that could be life threatening. Novartis subsequently advised Health Canada that the company would voluntarily discontinue Mellaril worldwide by June 30, 2005. The move by Health Canada to stop the sale of thioridazine followed the Novartis decision. Some of the benefits and risks of modern and conventional antipsychotic agents are listed in Table 8.3.

Sources: Health Canada: Media Advisory. *Sales of Antipsychotic Drug Thioridazine to Be Stopped.* 2005. Retrieved September 26, 2011, from http://www.hc-sc.gc.ca/ahc-asc/media/advisories-avis/_2005/2005_95-eng.php; and Health Canada. "Thioridazine (Mellaril) and Mesoridazine (Serentil): Prolongation of the QTC Interval." *Adverse Drug Reaction Newsletter* 11 (2001), p. 1. Retrieved September 26, 2011, from http://dsp-psd.pwgsc.gc.ca/Collection/H12-38-11-1E.pdf.

Table 8.3 Benefits and Risks of Modern and Conventional Antipsychotic Agents*

	Modern Antipsychotic Agents						Conventional Antipsychotic Agents by Potency†		
Property	**aripiprazole**	**clozapine**	**olanzapine**	**quetiapine**	**risperidone**	**ziprasidone**	**High**	**Moderate**	**Low**
Efficacy in terms of									
positive symptoms	++	++++	+++	++	+++	+++	+++	+++	+++
negative symptoms	+	++	+	+	+	+	+	+	+
relapse	++	++++	+++	?	+++	?‡	++	++	++
Adverse effects									
Anticholinergic	0	+++	+	0	0	0	0	++	+++
Cardiac repolarization	0	0	0	0	0	+	0	0	++
Hypotension	+	+++	++	++	+++	+	+	++	+++
Hyperprolactinemia	0	0	+	0	++	+	++	++	++
Type 2 diabetes mellitus	+	++	++	+	+	+	+	+	+
Sexual dysfunction	+	++	++	+	++	+	++	++	+++
Weight gain	0	+++	+++	++	+	0	0	+	++
EPS§	+	0	+	0	++	+	++++	+++	++
NMS	?	+	+	+	+	+	+++	++	+

Note: EPS = extrapyramidal signs or symptoms (dystonia, bradykinesia tremor, akathisia, dyskinesia); NMS = neuroleptic malignant syndrome (fever, delirium, unstable vital signs, variable rigidity); *Benefit or risk: ++++ = very high, +++ = high, ++ = moderate, + = low, 0 = negligible, ? = poorly defined; †Examples of high-potency conventional agents are flupenthixol, fluphenazine, haloperidol, trifluoperazine; moderate-potency agents include loxapine and zuclopenthixol; and low-potency agents include chlorpromazine, methotrimeprazine and thioridazine; ‡The risk of relapse was reduced when compared with placebo over 1 year. No long-term data are available for comparison with other antipsychotic agents; §Akathisia (anxious restlessness) can occur with modern antipsychotic agents.

Source: Garner, D.M., R.J. Baldessarini, and P. Waraich. Table 1, "Modern Antipsychotic Drugs: A Critical Overview." *Canadian Medical Association Journal* 172, no. 13 (2005), pp. 1703–1711.

Second-generation antipsychotics are not without side effects, however (see Table 8.4). The number of antipsychotic medications dispensed over ten years in Manitoba and the costs associated with them are presented in Figure 8.6 and Figure 8.7.

The use of ATAs in treating children has been increasing exponentially, raising concerns as to the appropriateness of this practice. In a Canadian survey, 89% of developmental pediatricians ($N = 198$) and 94% of child psychiatrists prescribed ATAs. Most commonly prescribed to children were risperidone (69%) for diagnoses that include psychotic, mood, anxiety, externalizing, and pervasive developmental disorders. Also common among practitioners was prescribing ATAs for such symptoms as aggression, low frustration tolerance, and affect (emotion) dysregulation. Children under the age of nine received 12% of all prescriptions. Without clear guidelines for indications, dosing, and monitoring, these medications are currently being used off-label in children. There were wide variations in the type and frequency of patient monitoring among clinicians.[39]

Until recently there have been no approved indications for ATA use in children and adolescents in Canada. Based on U.S. Food and Drug Administration approvals and a review of randomized controlled trials, seven indications for ATA use were identified that target specific symptoms in youth diagnosed with schizophrenia, bipolar I disorder, autism, pervasive developmental disorder, disruptive behaviour disorders (including conduct disorder and ADHD), developmental disabilities, and Tourette syndrome. Canada has outlined national clinical practice guidelines for ATA treatment based on a hierarchy of evidence (see Figure 8.8) for this vulnerable population.[40] Abilify is the first and only medication in Canada approved to treat schizophrenia in adolescents 15 to 17 years of age.[41]

Table 8.4 Side Effects of Second-Generation Antipsychotics

Side Effects	Drugs Most Likely to Have These Effects
Weight gain, diabetes	Clozapine, olanzapine, quetiapine, risperidone, ziprasidone, aripiprazole
Movement effects (e.g., tremors, stiffness, agitation)	Risperidone, olanzapine, quetiapine, ziprasidone, aripiprazole, clozapine
Sedation (e.g., sleepiness, low energy)	Clozapine, olanzapine and quetiapine, risperidone, ziprasidone, aripiprazole
Decreased sex drive and function, missed periods, discharge from breasts	Risperidone, olanzapine, quetiapine, clozapine, ziprasidone

Source: Adapted from *Physician's Desk Reference*. Oradell, NJ: Medical Economics, 2004.

Figure 8.6 Annual Number of Antipsychotic Prescriptions Dispensed in Manitoba between 1996 and 2006

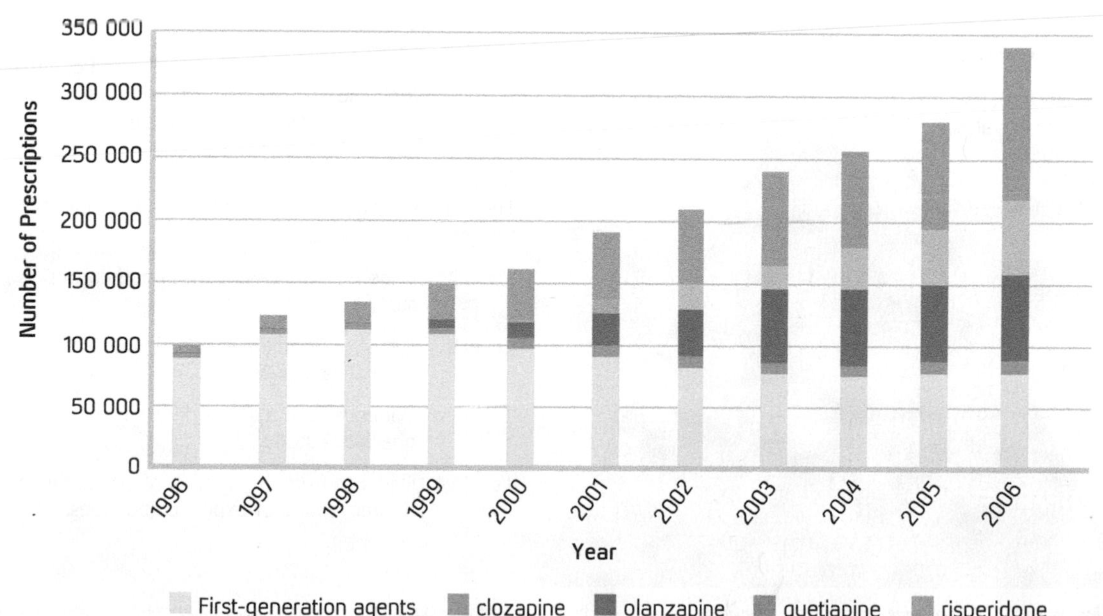

Source: Alessi-Severini, S., R.G. Biscontri, D.M. Collins, A. Kozyrskyj, J. Sareen, and M.W. Enns. Figure 1, "Utilization and Costs of Antipsychotic Agents: A Canadian Population-Based Study, 1996–2006." *Psychiatric Services* 59, no. 5 (2008), pp. 547–553. www.ps.psychiatryonline.org. © American Psychiatric Association.

Figure 8.7 Annual Total Costs of First-Generation versus Second-Generation Antipsychotics between 1996 and 2006

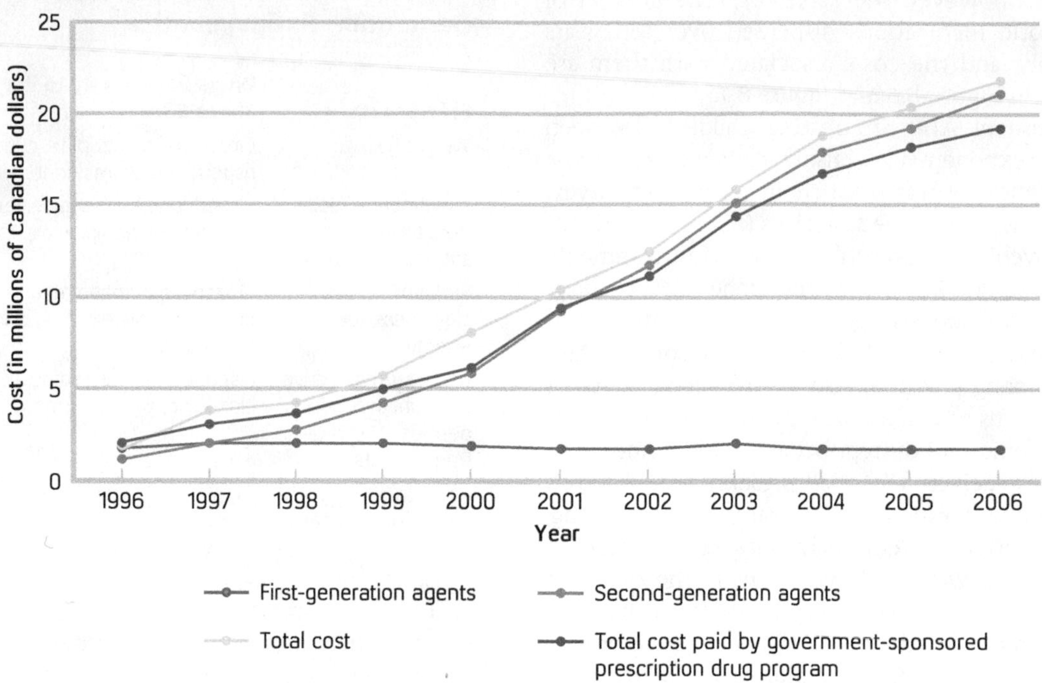

Source: Alessi-Severini, S., R.G. Biscontri, D.M. Collins, A. Kozyrskyj, J. Sareen, and M.W. Enns. Figure 1, "Utilization and Costs of Antipsychotic Agents: A Canadian Population-Based Study, 1996–2006." *Psychiatric Services* 59, no. 5 (2008), pp. 547–553. www.ps.psychiatryonline.org. © American Psychiatric Association.

Figure 8.8 Hierarchy of Evidence Summary

Recommendations for the treatment of schizophrenia are based on existing scientific evidence as developed by the Schizophrenia Patient Outcomes Research Team in the United States. Based on exhaustive reviews of the treatment outcomes literature, the treatment recommendations focus on treatments for which there is substantial evidence of efficacy. This procedure constitutes evidence-based practice.

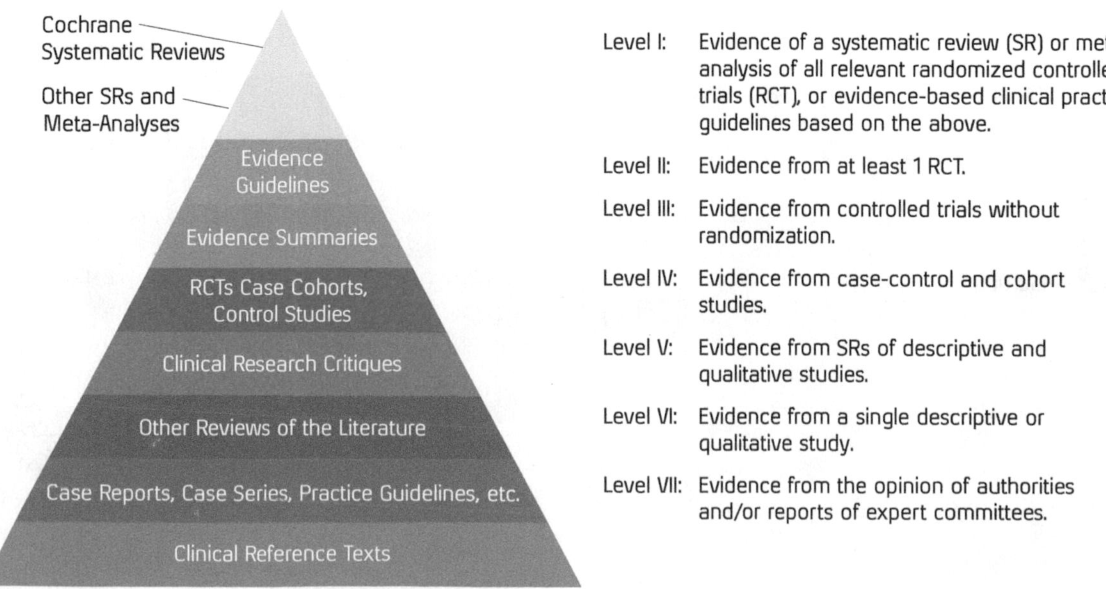

Source: *Navigating the Maze*, University of Virginia, Health Sciences Library, modified by University of Washington Health Sciences Library. *Evidence-Based Practice Tools Summary.* http://healthlinks.washington.edu/ebp/ebptools.html

Mechanism of Antipsychotic Action The first clue to the mechanism of action for antipsychotics was that virtually all of the phenothiazines and other typical antipsychotics produce *pseudoparkinsonism*. Patients treated with these medications exhibit symptoms similar to Parkinson's disease (tremors and muscular rigidity). Because Parkinson's disease is known to be caused by a loss of dopamine neurons in the nigrostriatal dopamine pathway (see Chapter 4), scientists focused on the ability of antipsychotic drugs to block dopamine receptors. Although the typical antipsychotics are generally fairly "dirty" drugs pharmacologically (they block other types of receptors as well), the doses required for the different drugs to produce antipsychotic effects do not correlate well with the ability of the different drugs to bind to any receptor except dopamine receptors (specifically, the D2 type of dopamine receptor). It is now well accepted that the initial effect of antipsychotic drugs is to block D2 dopamine receptors. This effect occurs with the first dose, but the antipsychotic effect of these drugs is not seen for at least 10 to 14 days (the lag period). Thus, the ultimate mechanism of antipsychotic action is some (as yet unknown) response of the nervous system to repeated administration of dopamine antagonists.

When clozapine was introduced, it differed from the other antipsychotics in two interesting ways. First, it produced much less pseudoparkinsonism than the other drugs. Second, some patients who had failed to improve with the other antipsychotics showed improvement when treated with clozapine. Clozapine was very promising, but it unfortunately has a risk of producing a deadly suppression of white blood cell production. The drug was withdrawn from the market but then made available again, as long as patients have periodic blood samples taken to monitor their white blood cells. Clozapine produces effects on a wide range of receptor types, but eventually it was determined that its unique properties were probably related to its ability to block both dopamine D2 and serotonin 5-HT2A receptors. Risperidone, olanzepine, and the other atypical antipsychotics were developed with these two actions in mind, and none of the newer drugs carries the risk of suppressing white blood cell production. The atypical antipsychotics are sometimes referred to as serotonin-dopamine antagonists. Pseudoparkinsonism is reduced because of serotonin-dopamine interactions in the nigrostriatal pathway. These drugs are also said to be capable not only of reducing the *positive* symptoms of schizophrenia (hallucinations, delusions, disorganized speech and behaviour) but also of improving the *negative* symptoms (lack of emotion, social isolation, lack of initiative). In contrast, the typical antipsychotics were known primarily for reducing positive symptoms.[42]

Side Effects of Antipsychotics Two positive aspects of the antipsychotics are that they do not produce drug dependence and it is extremely difficult to use them to commit suicide. Some allergic reactions might be noted, such as jaundice or skin rashes. Some patients exhibit photosensitivity, a tendency for the skin to darken and burn easily in sunlight. These reactions have a low incidence and usually decrease or disappear with a reduction in dosage. *Agranulocytosis*, low white blood cell count of unknown origin, can develop in the early stages of treatment. Because white blood cells are needed to fight infection, this disorder has a high mortality rate if it is not detected before a serious infection sets in. It is extremely rare with most of the antipsychotics other than clozapine.

The most common side effect of antipsychotic medication involves the nigrostriatal dopamine pathway (see Chapter 4). The major effects include a wide range of movement disorders from facial tics to symptoms that resemble those of Parkinson's disease (tremors of the hands when they are at rest; muscular rigidity, including a masklike face; and a shuffling walk). As noted above, this pseudoparkinsonism is less of a problem with the newer atypical antipsychotics.

Tardive dyskinesia is the most serious complication of antipsychotic drug treatment. Although first observed in the late 1950s, it was not viewed as a major problem until the mid-1970s, 20 years after these drugs were introduced. The term *tardive dyskinesia* means "late-appearing abnormal movements" and refers primarily to rhythmic, repetitive sucking and smacking movements of the lips; thrusting of the tongue in and out ("fly-catching"); and movements of the arms, toes, or fingers. The fact that this syndrome usually occurs only after years of antipsychotic drug treatment, and that the symptoms persist and sometimes increase when medication is stopped, raised the possibility of irreversible changes. The current belief is that tardive dyskinesia is the result of supersensitivity of the dopaminergic receptors. Although reversal of the symptoms is possible in most cases, the best treatment is prevention, which can be accomplished through early detection and an immediate lowering of the medication level.

A meta-analysis of several large trials of long-term typical antipsychotic drug treatment using more than 1600 patients found that pseudoparkinsonism was reported as an adverse reaction in about 20% of the patients, whereas tardive dyskinesia was reported for only about 2%.[43]

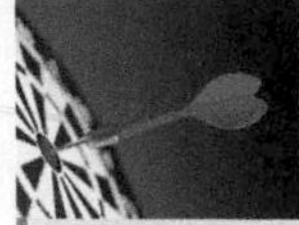

TARGETING PREVENTION

Black-Box Warnings: Treating Older Adults with Antipsychotics

Antipsychotics are used as drug therapies for people with dementia to manage difficult behaviours, such as agitation or aggression.[44] Both conventional and atypical antipsychotics may be associated with an increased risk for death in older adults with dementia. Second-generation antipsychotic (SGA) medications are also associated with an increased risk of death in older adults with dementia. Health Canada and the U.S. Food and Drug Administration (FDA) instituted a black-box warning for all SGA medication use in seniors, which was followed by similar warnings for first-generation antipsychotics (FGAs), such as haloperidol and perphenazine. Health Canada's warning also extended to risperidone (Risperdal), quetiapine (Seroquel), olanzapine (Zyprexa), and clozapine (Clozaril).

The black-box warnings followed a study by Sebastian Schneeweiss and colleagues, who reported the mortality rate in FGA-treated older adult patients was 1.47 times that of SGA-treated patients within three months of starting the antipsychotic prescription. The study, published in the February 2007 *Canadian Medical Association Journal*, included more than 37 000 people in British Columbia aged 65 and older who were started on antipsychotic medications. About one-third of these patients received FGA prescriptions, and the rest were given the newer SGAs.[45]

Another study conducted by Gill and colleagues and published in the June 5, 2007 *Annals of Internal Medicine* was conducted in patients with dementia aged 66 years and older in Ontario. From public health databases, the authors constructed and compared three cohorts of FGA users, SGA users, and nonusers of antipsychotics based on dementia patients' status as community-dwelling or long-term-care (LTC) residents. Included in the study were 27 259 pairs of antipsychotic-using and nonusing patients matched in demographics and clinical status. The researchers found that starting atypical antipsychotics was associated with a statistically significant increase in the risk for death at 30 days, and this increased risk was still present three months after the start of use. Typical antipsychotic use was associated with a higher risk for death 30, 60, 120, and 180 days after start of a new prescription. Following the publication of these studies, the prescribing labels of all antipsychotics are now required to carry a standard warning: "Elderly patients with dementia-related psychosis and treated with antipsychotics have an increased risk of death." However, the black-box warning is not a contraindication, and clinicians can still use these drugs for people with dementia.[46]

Although recent Canadian population-based reports suggest that antipsychotics are associated with increased risk for death in older adults with dementia, their impact on prescription rates is unclear. Between October 2002 and June 2005, Health Canada issued three warnings of increased risk of death or stroke in senior patients with dementia who take atypical antipsychotic drugs, such as risperidone. Dr. Paula Rochon, vice-president of research at Women's College Hospital in Toronto, concluded that the warnings failed to reduce the prescription rates of those drugs.[47] Other drugs that should be avoided by seniors are included in the Beers List, a list originally compiled by Dr. Mark Beers in 1991 and most recently updated in 2003.[48] The Beers List includes drugs that are either ineffective in seniors or put them at an unnecessarily high risk when safer alternatives are available.[47]

Significant weight gain has been seen with many of the new atypical agents, along with increased blood lipids and other indications of a "metabolic syndrome" that is associated with increased risk for diabetes. This is a significant public health concern because so many patients are now receiving these medications. Another concern is the use of antipsychotic medications in older adults (see the Targeting Prevention box).

Although antipsychotic drugs were first developed in the early 1950s to treat schizophrenia, they have become widely used in long-term-care (LTC) facilities to manage behavioural disturbances and agitation associated with dementia. Several studies conducted in the United States during the 1970s and 1980s found that close to 40% of nursing home residents were receiving antipsychotics.[49] The widespread use and growing perceptions that antipsychotics were being used as chemical restraints prompted the U.S. Congress to introduce the Omnibus Budget Reconciliation Act of 1987 (OBRA), which legislated standards for care in LTCs, including the use of psychotropic drugs. The OBRA regulations, implemented in the 1990s, appear to have been effective, and use of antipsychotics in LTC residents declined by approximately one-third.

Canada, unlike the United States, has no mandatory regulations limiting the use of antipsychotics in LTC facilities. Three LTC facilities in Western Canada participated in a study where it was recognized that atypical antipsychotics represented 73.4% of all prescriptions.[50] Hagen's study of LTC facilities in Alberta indicated that the overall rate of antipsychotic prescriptions for LTC residents in Canada (30.8%) is higher than the rates in comparable studies in Europe and the United States, and it is much higher than the 7.5% rate in Japan.[51] Albertan rates are also approximately double that of most U.S. rates (approximately 15%) since the introduction of OBRA federal regulations and approximately double the rate of 17% found in one other Canadian study.[52]

Long-Term Effectiveness It was mentioned earlier that drug dependence is not a problem with antipsychotic agents. In fact, it has long been known that even patients who clearly benefit from their use tend to dislike the drugs and often stop taking them. This noncompliance in drug therapy may result in hospitalization (see Figure 8.9). The drug trials that demonstrate the benefits of antipsychotic medications typically last six or eight weeks. This is long enough to allow for some dosage adjustment and for the lag period for the antipsychotic effect, and so these studies are optimal for the drug companies' purpose—to show that their drug works better than a placebo. But patients are typically treated with these drugs for long periods—in many cases, for the remainder of their lives. The NIMH funded a long-term study, "Clinical Antipsychotic Trials of Intervention Effectiveness," that followed 1400 patients with chronic schizophrenia taking four different atypical antipsychotics and one typical antipsychotic for up to 18 months.[53] The most surprising finding was that three-fourths of the patients quit taking the assigned medication before reaching 18 months of treatment. Some stopped because the drug did not appear to be helping and some stopped because the side effects became intolerable, but the biggest single reason for stopping was "patient's decision." In other words, in spite of short-term evidence of the efficacy of these drugs, their real-world effectiveness in chronic schizophrenia is considerably less than we had previously thought. The other surprising finding was that there was no clear evidence that the newer atypical agents worked any better than

Figure 8.9 Hospitalizations for Schizophrenia* in General Hospitals per 100 000 People by Age Group, Canada, 1999/2000

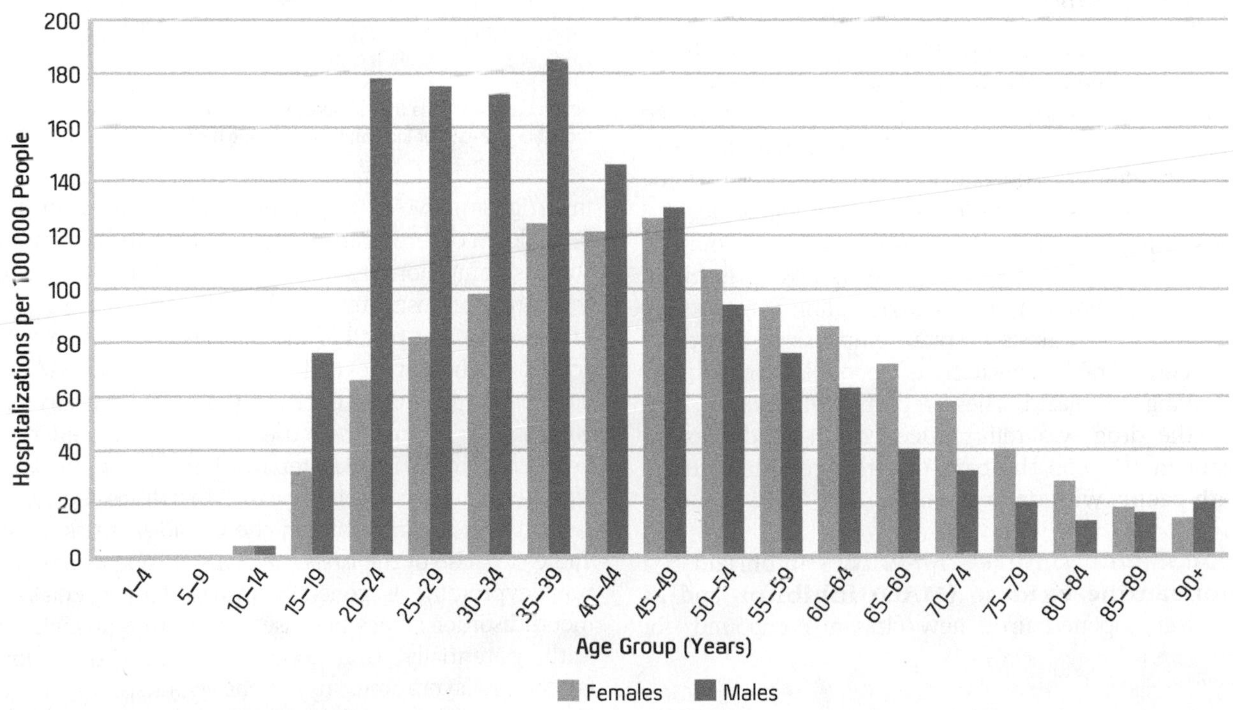

* Using most responsible diagnosis only.

Source: Health Canada. *A Report on Mental Illnesses in Canada*. Ottawa, Ontario, Canada, 2002. © Health Canada Editorial Board Mental Illnesses in Canada. Canadian Cataloguing in Publication Data: ISBN H39-643/2002E; 0-662-32817-5.

the typical drug, nor were there significant differences in extrapyramidal symptoms. Given the greater cost of the newer drugs, it is now being questioned whether there is any real benefit to prescribing them.[54]

Drug approval is under the jurisdiction of the Therapeutics Products Program, a division of Health Canada that reviews the safety and efficacy data for each new drug submission. If a new drug submission is found to be acceptable on the basis of clinical trial efficacy and toxicity data, the Therapeutics Products Program issues a notice of compliance and the associated product labelling. The drug is then approved and may be prescribed by physicians and dispensed by pharmacies in Canada. However, such approval does not mean that provincial drug plans or other third-party payers will pay for the approved drug. The decision regarding who pays is made by each province. It will be interesting to see how clinical practice responds to this new information about antipsychotics and whether subsequent research can demonstrate any long-term benefit for the newer and more expensive atypical antipsychotics. It needs to be emphasized that a new drug may or may not be better than the older generic medication because often it is not on the market long enough before use to collect information about side effects.

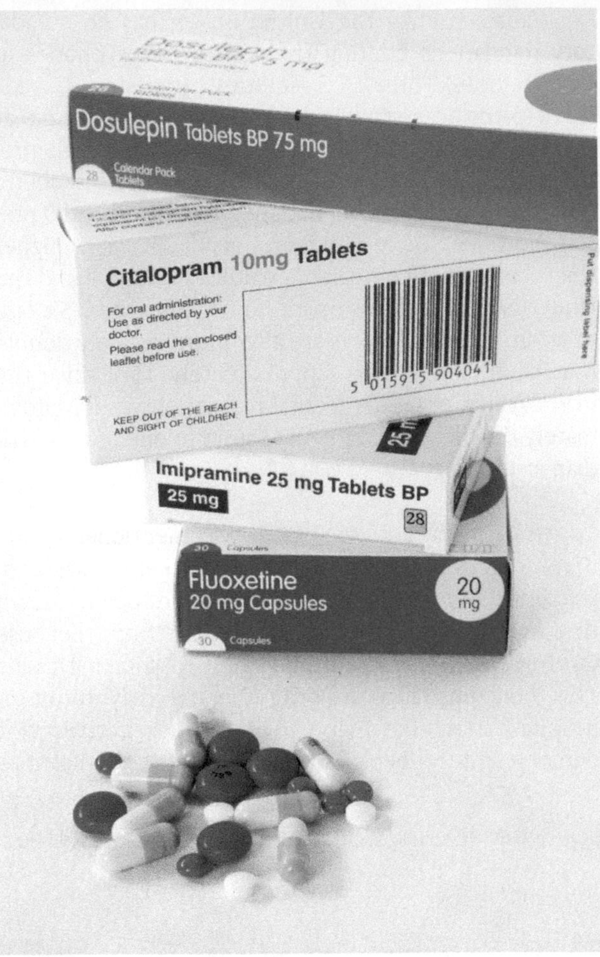

Health Canada warns that antidepressants may trigger suicidal thoughts in 2–3% of kids and teens taking them.

Antidepressants

The story of the antidepressant drugs starts with the fact that tuberculosis was a major chronic illness until about 1955. In 1952, preliminary reports suggested that a new drug, isoniazid, was effective in treating tuberculosis; isoniazid and similar drugs that followed were responsible for the emptying of hospital beds. One of the antituberculosis drugs was iproniazid, which was introduced simultaneously with isoniazid but was withdrawn as too toxic. Clinical reports on its use in tuberculosis hospitals emphasized that there was considerable elevation of mood in the patients receiving iproniazid. These reports were followed up, and the drug was reintroduced as an antidepressant agent in 1955 on the basis of early promising studies with people with depression.

Monoamine Oxidase Inhibitors Iproniazid is a **monoamine oxidase (MAO) inhibitor**, and its discovery opened up a new class of compounds for investigation. MAO is an enzyme involved in the breakdown of serotonin, norepinephrine, and dopamine, and its inhibition results in increased availability of these neurotransmitters at the synapse. This was the first clue to the possible mechanism of antidepressant action. Although several MAO inhibitors (MAOIs) have been introduced over the years, toxicity and side effects have limited their use and have reduced their number. Iproniazid was removed from sale in 1961 after being implicated in at least 54 fatalities. Currently two MAOIs are available on the Canadian market (see Table 8.5). Use of the *irreversible* MAOIs phenelzine and tranylcypromine is generally managed by specialized mood disorder clinics because of the drugs' association with potentially fatal food and drug interactions (serotonin syndrome, hypertensive crisis). A major limitation of the use of the MAOIs is that they alter the normal metabolism of a dietary amino acid, tyramine, such that if an individual consumes foods with a high

monoamine oxidase (MAO) inhibitor: a type of antidepressant drug.

Table 8.5 Antidepressant Drugs Available in Canada

Generic Name	Examples of Brand Names	Usual Dose Range (mg/day)
MAO Inhibitors		
phenelzine	Nardil	45–75
tranylcypromine	Parnate	20–30
moclobemide (not available in U.S.)	Apo-Moclobemide	300–600
Tricyclics		
amitriptyline	Elavil	100–200
desipramine	Apo-Desipramine	75–200
doxepin	Sinequan	100–200
imipramine	Apo-Imipramine	100–200
nortriptyline	Apo-Nortriptyline	25–200
Selective Reuptake Inhibitors		
citalopram	Celexa	20–40
escitalopram	Cipralex	10–20
fluoxetine	Prozac	20–40
paroxetine	Paxil	20–50
sertraline	Zoloft	50–200
venlafaxine	Effexor	75–375
duloxetine	Cymbalta	40–60
Others		
bupropion	Wellbutrin	200–300
mirtazapine	Remeron	15–45
trazodone	Desyrel	150–200

tyramine content while taking MAOIs, a hypertensive (high blood pressure) crisis can result. Because aged cheeses are one source of tyramine, this is often referred to as the "cheese reaction." A severe headache, palpitations, flushing of the skin, nausea, and vomiting are some symptoms of this reaction, which has in some cases ended in death from a stroke (cerebrovascular accident). Besides avoiding foods and beverages that contain tyramine (aged cheeses, chianti wine, smoked or pickled fish, and many others), patients taking MAO inhibitors must also avoid sympathomimetic drugs, such as amphetamines, methylphenidate, and ephedrine.

However, all prescribers and pharmacists should be aware of these risks (and how to avoid them) and explain them to patients taking an irreversible MAOI. Despite the potential risks, under careful conditions phenelzine 30-90 milligrams daily or tranylcypromine 20-60 milligrams daily may prove effective where other antidepressants have not. Moclobemide is a *reversible* and selective MAOI that does not require the same dietary restrictions as irreversible MAOIs. Moclobemide is a well-tolerated alternative to selective serotonin reuptake inhibitors or serotonin norepinephrine reuptake inhibitor agents, particularly in people with a significant anxiety component to their depressive episode. Though moclobemide is often perceived as being less effective than irreversible MAOIs, this perception is not substantiated by clinical trials.[55]

Tricyclic Antidepressants Sometimes when you are looking for one thing, you find something entirely different. The MAOIs were found among antituberculosis agents, and the phenothiazine antipsychotics were found while looking for a better antihistamine. The **tricyclic** antidepressants were found in a search for better phenothiazine antipsychotics. The basic phenothiazine structure consists of three rings, with various side chains for the different antipsychotic drugs. Imipramine resulted from a slight change in the middle of the three rings and was tested in 1958 on a group of patients. The drug had little effect on psychotic symptoms but improved the mood of people with depression. This was the first

tricyclic: a type of antidepressant drug.

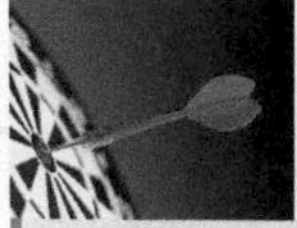

TARGETING PREVENTION

Black-Box Warnings: Treating Adolescents and Children with Antidepressants

On June 10, 2003, the United Kingdom (UK) Committee on Safety of Medicines published a report advising physicians and patients not to use paroxetine for depression in patients younger than 18 years. On October 27, 2003, the U.S. FDA issued a public health advisory that emphasized all newer antidepressants should be used with caution in pediatric patients. On October 15, 2004, the FDA issued another public health advisory that included a black-box warning and an expanded statement about a possible increased risk of suicidal ideation and behaviour in children and adolescents who were being treated with all antidepressants. These warnings were issued in response to reports of increased suicidal ideation in children who had been prescribed paroxetine. On March 22, 2004, the FDA issued a public health advisory about the need to closely monitor patients of all ages for worsening depression or suicidality after the initiation of antidepressant therapy or changes in dose. On June 3, 2004, Health Canada issued a similar advisory.

New monthly antidepressant prescriptions in Ontario were analyzed from January 2001 to January 2005, before and after the issue of these five warnings. Four of the five antidepressant warnings had no effect on new prescriptions for SSRIs as a group in any age category (under 20, 20–65, over 65 years of age); see Figure 8.10. The June 10, 2003, warning in the UK about the use of paroxetine resulted in a statistically significant 54% decrease ($p = .03$) in new prescriptions of paroxetine issued to patients younger than 20 years in Ontario.[56]

The warning issued by Health Canada mandated wording in antidepressant labels differ substantially from that issued by the FDA. The FDA revised the black-box warning in prescription labels in 2007 to state that patients up to 24 years old are at risk of suicidal thoughts and behaviours, but there is no evidence of increased risk in adults older

Figure 8.10 New SSRI Prescription Rates among Individuals Younger Than 20 Years, 20–65 Years, and Older Than 65 Years, Ontario, 2001–2005

Arrows indicate the dates of the five antidepressant warnings: June 10, 2003 (UK), October 27, 2003 (U.S. FDA); March 22, 2004 (FDA); June 3, 2004 (Health Canada); and October 15, 2004 (FDA).

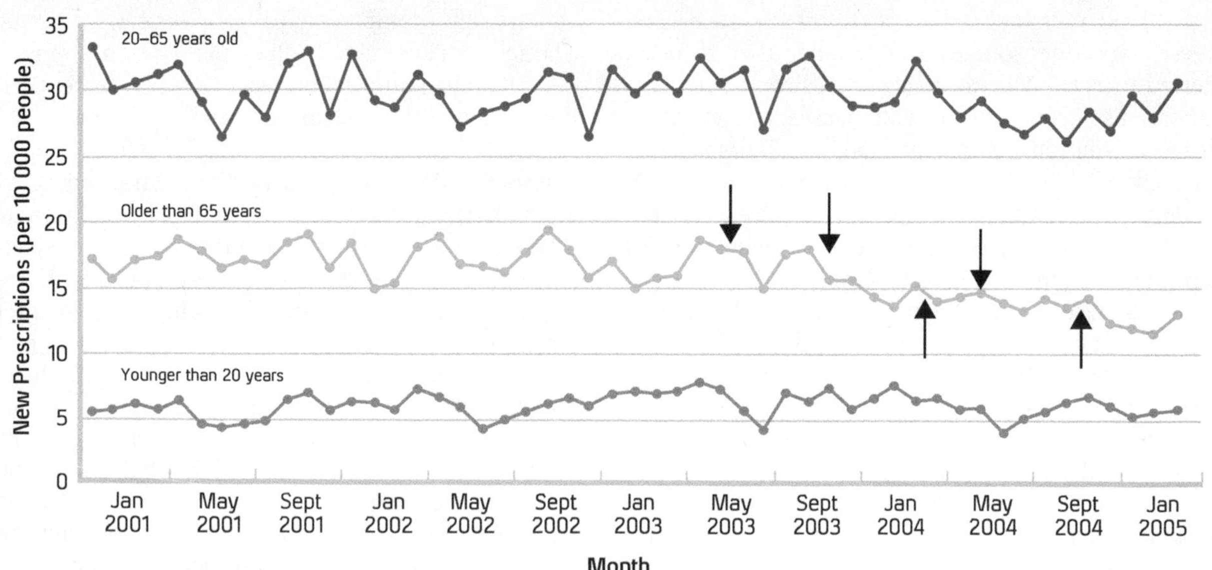

Source: Kurdyak, P.A., D.N. Juurlink, and M.M. Mamdani. "The Effect of Antidepressant Warnings on Prescribing Trends in Ontario, Canada." *American Journal of Public Health* 97, no. 4 (2007), pp. 750–54.

continued

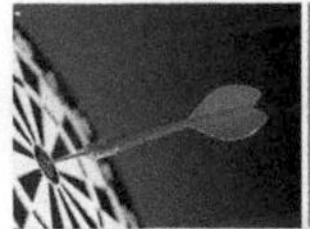

TARGETING PREVENTION

Black-Box Warnings: Treating Adolescents and Children with Antidepressants *continued*

than 24. The agency requires all antidepressants, including the older tricyclic drugs, to carry this warning. Health Canada, in contrast, applies the warning to patients of all ages but specifically to SSRIs and SSNRIs. It also requires drug labels and patient-information sheets to describe the increased risks of "agitation and hostility or anxiety, or impulsive or disturbing thoughts that could involve self-harm or harm to others" after a patient initiates antidepressant therapy. During the same period of declining prescriptions for depression (Figure 8.11a), the rate of completed suicides saw a statistically significant increase in children and adolescents aged 17 and younger, from 0.04 a year per 1000 individuals before the Health Canada warning to 0.15 a year per 1000 after the warning. A total of 99 children and adolescents and 136 young adults completed suicide between 1995 and 2005 in Manitoba, for example (Figure 8.11b).[57]

Figure 8.11 After the Black-Box Warnings

(a) In the two years after the Canadian regulatory agency issued a warning about the use of antidepressants in children and adolescents, researchers found a decrease in medical treatment for depression in children, adolescents, and young adults and a parallel increase in the rate of completed suicides among children and adolescents, according to a study in the *Canadian Medical Association Journal.* (b) Crude annual rates of completed suicide per 1000 children and adolescents (8–17 years) and young adults (19–24 years), by year, are shown here, before and after Health Canada issued a warning about antidepressant use in children and adolescents (date indicated by red line). People age 18 years were excluded because of the unclear impact of the warning on prescribing in this age group. Data for years with fewer than six suicides, although included in the outcome analysis, are not portrayed in the figure for confidentiality purposes. The dates are indicated for similar warnings issued in the United Kingdom (dashed line) and the United States (dotted line).

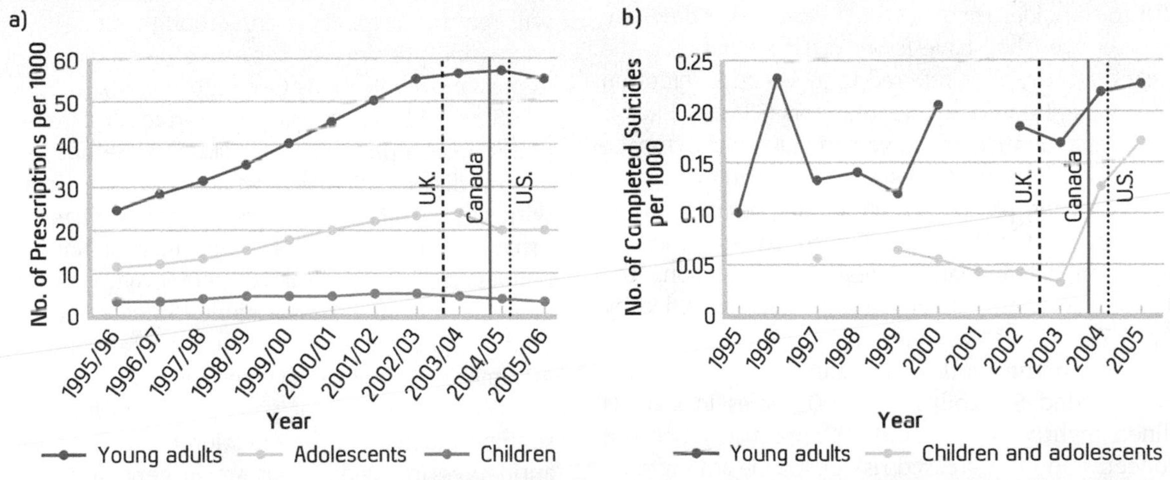

Source: Laurence Katz, M.D., Kozyrskyj, Prior, Enns, Cox, and Sareen. "Effect of Regulatory Warnings on Antidepressant Prescription Rates, Use of Health Services and Outcomes among Children, Adolescents and Young Adults." *Canadian Medical Association Journal* 178, no. 8 (April 8, 2008), pp. 1005–1011.

tricyclic antidepressant, and many more have followed (refer to Table 8.2). Although these drugs are not effective for all people, most controlled clinical trials do find that depressive episodes are less severe and resolve more quickly if the people are treated with one of the tricyclic antidepressants than if they are given a placebo.

The first tricyclics were discovered to interfere with the reuptake into the terminal of the neurotransmitters norepinephrine, dopamine, and serotonin. This results in an increased availability of these neurotransmitters at the synapse. Because MAO inhibition also results in increased availability of the same neurotransmitters, there has been considerable speculation that the antidepressant actions of both classes of drugs result from increased synaptic availability of one or more of these neurotransmitters. One of the effective antidepressants, desipramine, was found to have a much greater effect on the reuptake of norepinephrine than on the reuptake of either dopamine or serotonin, so for a time most theories of antidepressant action focused on norepinephrine.

Selective Reuptake Inhibitors The introduction in 1987 of fluoxetine (Prozac) ushered in the era of the **selective serotonin reuptake inhibitors (SSRIs)**. Trazodone had already been available and was known to have a greater effect on serotonin than on norepinephrine reuptake, calling the norepinephrine theory into question. Prozac soon became the most widely prescribed antidepressant drug ever marketed. Prozac is safer than the tricyclic antidepressants in that it is less likely to lead to overdose deaths, so physicians felt more confident about prescribing it. Despite some reports in the early 1990s of unusual violent or suicidal reactions, sales of Prozac continued at a high rate, and several other SSRIs were introduced by other companies. Drugs have also been developed that are reuptake inhibitors for both serotonin and norepinephrine. In that sense they are similar to the older tricyclics, but these newer drugs are more selective (they have fewer other actions than the tricyclics) and are thus referred to as selective serotonin and norepinephrine reuptake inhibitors (SSNRIs). Effexor was the first of these, followed in 2004 by Cymbalta (Table 8.5). Sales of antidepressants continued to increase, and the growing practice of prescribing antidepressants to children and adolescents helped to fuel sales. In 2006, seven different antidepressants were among the 100 most prescribed drugs in the United States, led by Lexapro, Zoloft, and Effexor.

Although the worldwide value of antidepressant sales exceeded $15 billion in 2003, sales in Canada declined slightly in 2004 and 2005, primarily because of concerns about increased risk of suicide among children and adolescents. Analysis of data submitted to the FDA for approval of nine drugs found higher rates of suicidal thoughts among the drug groups than among the placebo controls, and so Health Canada and the FDA began requiring a printed black-box warning about the increased risk of suicidal tendencies in children and adolescents.[58] Sales of SSRIs in Canada seemed back on track for further increases by 2006, led partly by their increasing use to treat generalized anxiety disorder. In 2007, Health Canada and the FDA proposed to extend the black-box warning on suicidal thoughts to include young adults ages 18–24, but industry analysts felt this would not significantly change overall sales.[59]

selective serotonin reuptake inhibitor (SSRI): a type of antidepressant drug.

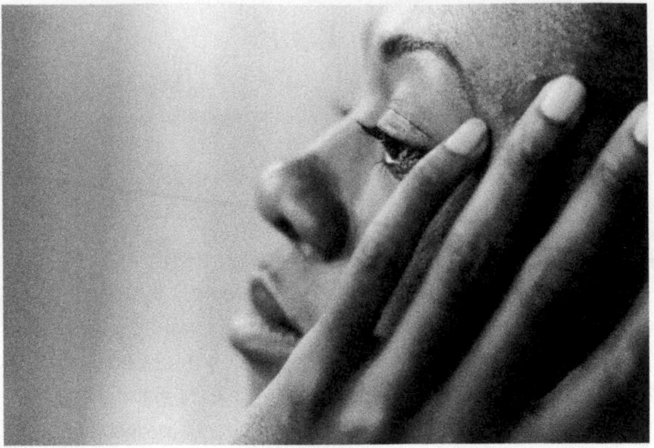

Depression is a serious, debilitating disorder that often responds to antidepressant medication.

Approximately 8% of Canadian adults will experience major depression at some time in their lives and will require hospitalization, although rates have been decreasing presumably because of the efficacy of antidepressant medications (see Figure 8.12).

Suicidal behaviour is an important and preventable public health problem in Canada. While not in itself a mental illness, suicidal behaviour is highly correlated with mental illness and raises many similar issues. It usually marks the end of a long road of hopelessness, helplessness, and despair. All people who consider suicide feel life to be unbearable. Suicide rates among young Inuit men in Nunavut are astronomical, at 40 times the Canadian average for young men.[60]

Another factor that perhaps should influence prescribing practices is the question of just how effective antidepressant medications are in general. It had been noticed in an earlier, not widely read Internet journal article that the data submitted to the FDA for approval of the SSRIs often showed very small, or sometimes no, differences between the tested drug and placebo. Because the FDA requires the company to submit records of all studies, even the unsuccessful ones, analysis of the overall set of results seemed to indicate that the majority of the effectiveness produced by these drugs can be attributed to a placebo effect. Professor Irving Kirsch at the University of Hull in the United Kingdom and colleagues in Canada and the United States

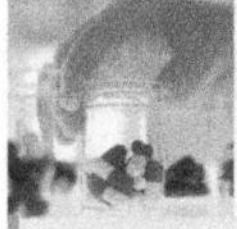

DRUGS IN THE MEDIA

The Use of Antidepressants in Pregnancy

The use of SSRIs by pregnant women may be contraindicated, not because of increased suicidal thoughts but because of harm to the fetus. Ongoing research shows evidence that SSRIs can be harmful to pregnant women or their babies. Chambers and colleagues found a 15.5% incidence of more than three minor genetically related anomalies among infants of women who were exposed to Prozac during pregnancy.[61] Health Canada issued an advisory on August 9, 2004, warning pregnant women taking SSRIs during the third trimester of pregnancy that their newborns may experience withdrawal problems. The advisory states that newborns whose mothers took SSRIs during pregnancy have developed complications at birth requiring prolonged hospitalization, breathing support, and tube feeding. Reported symptoms include feeding and breathing difficulties, seizures, muscular rigidity, jitteriness, and constant crying. The symptoms may be due to "discontinuation effects" (withdrawal from the drug) or other effects of SSRIs.[62]

Bérard and colleagues at Pfizer Canada in Montreal measured the association between the class of antidepressant used according to trimester of exposure during pregnancy and infants born small for their gestational age. They found that the use of venlafaxine (Effexor, an antidepressant of the SSNRI class) during the second trimester of pregnancy may increase the risk of infants being born small for their gestational age. Regardless of the trimester of use, no association was found between SSRIs or tricyclics and the risk of babies being small for their gestational age.[63]

analyzed data from 47 clinical trials that had been submitted to the FDA and reported that new generation SSRI antidepressants, such as Prozac and Paxil, mostly fall "below the recommended criteria for clinical significance."[64] In other words, the most modern drugs prescribed for depression generally don't work.[64,65]

A similar study published in a widely respected medical journal confirms this finding and will perhaps get more attention.[65] This 2008 report compared the results of the FDA-reported studies that were never published in medical journals to those that were published, and found that among the published studies,

Figure 8.12 Rates of Hospitalization for Major Depressive Disorder* in General Hospitals by Sex, Canada, 1987/88–1999/2000

Overall, between 1987 and 1999 hospitalization rates for major depressive disorder decreased by 33% among both men and women.

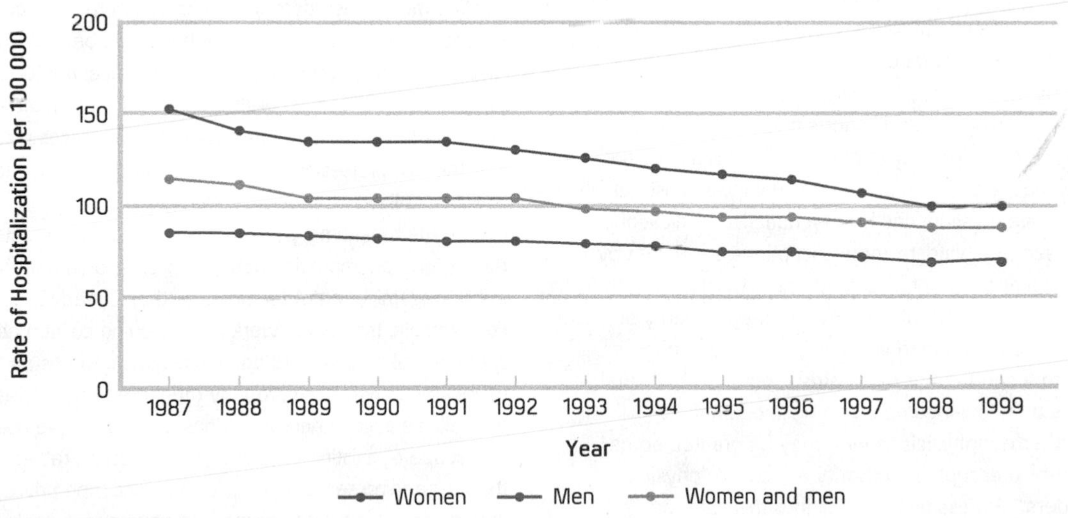

* Using most responsible diagnosis only.

Note: Age standardized to 1991 Canadian population.

Source: Health Canada. *A Report on Mental Illnesses in Canada.* Ottawa, Canada © 2002 ISBN H39-643/2002E 0-662-32817-5. Figure 2-5. Retrieved from http://www.cmha.ca/bins/content_page.asp?cid=4-42-215.

94% found a favourable effect of the tested drug compared with placebo. Most of the studies that found no effect were never published. Overall, only about half of the 74 studies submitted to the FDA since 1987 in support of the new drug applications for 12 antidepressants found positive results in favour of the tested drug. The selective publication of only the positive findings means that practising physicians who read the medical literature get an inflated picture of the overall effectiveness of this type of medication. At this point, the best evidence we have indicates that these antidepressant drugs are probably slightly better than placebos but are certainly not as effective overall as most people, including most physicians, have believed. However, if you are currently taking one of these medications, please do not simply stop taking it abruptly. There are major withdrawal effects associated with abrupt cessation of most of these medications, so if you are trying to decide what to do about continued use, be sure to consult your physician.

Mechanism of Antidepressant Action Most antidepressants seem to work by increasing the availability of either norepinephrine or serotonin at their respective synapses.[66] However, the antidepressant effect of MAOIs, tricyclics, and SSRIs exhibits a lag period. People must be treated for about two weeks before improvement is seen, even though the

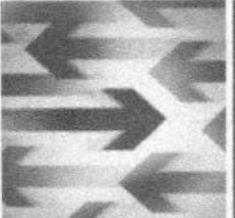

TAKING SIDES

Should Psychologists Be Allowed to Prescribe?

Health Canada decides how drugs are sold, and provincial and territorial legislatures determine which professions may prescribe. The debate over whether clinical psychologists should be granted the right to prescribe psychoactive medication has received considerable attention over the last two decades in the United States, but relatively little discussion of this controversial topic has occurred among Canadian mental health professionals, namely, psychologists and psychiatrists.[67]

Currently, the professionals who are best prepared to understand the complexities of prescribing psychoactive medications for mental disorders are psychiatrists. Following their medical training, these specialists have intensive training in the diagnosis and treatment of mental disorders, and especially in the use of medications, such as antipsychotics and antidepressants. However, most patients who receive prescriptions for psychoactive medications do not see psychiatrists; the prescriptions are written by family practitioners, internal medicine specialists, or other nonpsychiatrist medical doctors. This may be partly because patients are unwilling to visit a psychiatrist, but often it is due to a shortage of psychiatrists, particularly in rural settings or in low-income urban neighbourhoods.

Other nonphysicians who may be granted some degree of prescriptive authority are called "physician extenders." Professions that fall into this category include nurse practitioners, pharmacists, and physician assistants, whose prescriptive authority depends on physician supervision and is limited to specific drugs or drug formularies. Advocates assert that because doctoral-level psychologists have more education than do other professionals who have secured various degrees of prescriptive authority (for example, nurse practitioners and pharmacists), psychologists should qualify for privileges.[67]

Basic medical training includes very little formal coursework or experience in understanding, diagnosing, and treating mental disorders. Sometimes patients are seeing the medical doctor for prescriptions and also seeing a psychologist. Professional clinical psychologists have extensive training in understanding, diagnosing, and treating mental disorders with behavioural therapy or psychotherapy, but they typically have little background in medicine. If the psychologist and the medical doctor have developed an effective collaboration, this arrangement can often work well for the patient. But in many cases it seems that the two professions have so little common ground that effective collaboration is difficult.

In the meantime, psychologists could concentrate their efforts on improving both the professional and the public dissemination of the services they already provide. For example, they could work on improving collaboration with general practitioners and psychiatrists to ensure that medicated patients are properly monitored and advised of available psychotherapy options. Expanding the quality and scope of existing psychological therapies, rather than expanding services to include prescription privileges, may represent more promising and appropriate goals for psychology at the present time.[67] What are the critical questions that should be answered by proponents of prescription privileges for psychologists?

biochemical effects on MAO or on reuptake occur in a matter of minutes. Although it has been suggested that some patients might benefit more from one type than from another, experiments have so far failed to reveal any rational basis for choosing among the drugs in any individual case, and overall the effectiveness of the drug does not seem to depend on which of the neurotransmitters is more affected.

Current theories of the antidepressant action of these agents focus less on the initial biochemical effects of the drugs than on the reaction of the neurons to repeated drug exposure. As is the case with antipsychotics, we do not yet know the complete story of how long-term exposure to antidepressant drugs eventually results in improvement of the symptoms of depression. In addition to the MAOIs, tricyclics, and selective reuptake inhibitors, such drugs as Wellbutrin and Remeron act through somewhat different mechanisms. The fact that drugs with a wide variety of initial biochemical effects are all about equally effective (they reduce depressive symptoms for some people, but not for all) means it is possible that no single biochemical mechanism explains the effects of all these drugs.

Electroconvulsive Therapy

Probably the single most effective treatment for the depressed patient is electroconvulsive shock therapy (ECT). One report summarized the available good studies and showed that in seven of eight studies ECT was more effective in relieving the symptoms of depression than was placebo. Further, in four studies ECT was more effective than the most effective class of antidepressant drugs, and in three other studies the two treatments were equal. One factor that makes ECT sometimes the clear treatment of choice is its more rapid effect than that found with current antidepressant drugs. Reversal of depression might not occur for two or three weeks with drug treatment, but with ECT results sometimes are noticed almost immediately. When there is a possibility of suicide, ECT is thus the obvious choice, and it is possible to use both drug and ECT treatment simultaneously.[68]

Mood Stabilizers

In the late 1940s, two medical uses were proposed for salts of the element **lithium**. In the United States, lithium chloride, which tastes much like sodium chloride (table salt), was introduced as a salt substitute for heart patients. However, above a certain level lithium is quite toxic, and because there was no control over the dose, many users became ill and several died. This scandal was so great in the minds of American physicians that a proposed beneficial use published in 1949 by an Australian, John Cade, produced little interest in the United States.[69]

Cade had been experimenting with guinea pigs, examining the effects of lithium on urinary excretion of salts. Lithium appeared to have sedative properties in some of the animals, and so he administered the compound to several of his patients. The patients with mania all improved, whereas there seemed to be no effect on those with depression or people with schizophrenia. This was followed up by several Danish studies in the 1950s and early 1960s, and it became increasingly apparent that the large majority of manic individuals showed dramatic remission of their symptoms after a lag period of a few days when treated with lithium carbonate or other salts.[69] The first published study on lithium use in Canada was conducted by Edward Kingstone at the Department of Psychiatry, McGill University, Montreal.[70] In 1970, Canada and the United States admitted lithium to the marketplace.[69,71]

Three factors slowed the acceptance of lithium in North America and FDA approval in 1970. First was the salt-substitute poisonings, which gave lithium a bad reputation as a potentially lethal drug. Second, mania was not seen as a major problem in Canada and the United States.[69] Manic patients feel energetic and have an unrealistically positive view of their own abilities, and such people are unlikely to seek treatment on their own. Also, patients who became quite manic and lost touch with reality would probably have been diagnosed with schizophrenia in those days, perhaps at least partly because a treatment existed for schizophrenia. The antipsychotic drugs can control mania in most cases. The third and possibly most important factor is economic and relates to the way new drugs are introduced: by companies that hope to make a profit on them. Lithium is one of the basic chemical elements (number 3 on the periodic chart) and its simple salts had been available for various purposes for many years, so it would be impossible for a drug company to receive an exclusive patent to sell lithium. A company generally must go to considerable expense to conduct the research necessary to demonstrate safety and effectiveness to Health Canada and the FDA. If one company

lithium: a drug used in treating mania and bipolar disorder.

had done this, as soon as the drug was approved any other company could also have sold lithium, and it would have been impossible for the first company to recoup its research investment. After several years of frustration, the weight of the academically conducted research and the clinical experience in Europe was such that several companies received approval to sell lithium in 1970.

Treatment with lithium requires 10 to 15 days before symptoms begin to change, and once again the ultimate mechanism for its action is not yet known. Lithium is both safe and toxic. It is safe because the blood level can be monitored routinely and the dose adjusted to ensure therapeutic, but not excessive, blood levels. Patients develop tolerances to the minor side effects of gastrointestinal disturbances and tremors. Excessively high levels in the blood cause confusion and loss of coordination, which can progress to coma, convulsions, and death if lithium is not stopped and appropriate treatment instituted.

Of primary importance in the therapeutic use of lithium is the realization that lithium acts as a mood-normalizing agent in individuals with bipolar (manic-depressive) illness. Lithium will prevent both manic and depressed mood swings. It has only moderate effects on univocal depressions (see Table 8.6).

The biggest limitation to the usefulness of lithium is that patients simply do not like to take it and most will discontinue its use at some point. This high rate of noncompliance is the major reason that, although lithium is perhaps the single most effective psychotherapeutic agent available, alternative medications have been developed.

An International Consensus Group comprising Canadian, American, and international researchers formulated treatment guidelines for the management of depression associated with bipolar disorder (bipolar depression). Most importantly, they identified common misconceptions about bipolar depression and established that lithium is effective for both depression and mania phases of bipolar disorder.[72] Among these misconceptions was the belief that bipolar disorder is not a chronic condition, that treatment of only acute episodes is warranted, and that the frequency of bipolar episodes does not dictate therapy selection. Moreover, first-line treatments should include antidepressant medications and a **mood stabilizer** only if manic

mood stabilizer: an agent that has efficacy in treating acute manic and depressive symptoms.

Table 8.6 Drug Treatment Two-Year Outcome in Univocal and Bipolar Patients

Percentage of Patients with Relapses during Treatment		
	First 4 Months	**Next 20 Months**
Univocal Patients		
Lithium	30	41
Imipramine	32	29
Placebo	73	85
Bipolar Patients		
Lithium	22	18
Imipramine	46	67
Placebo	54	67

Sources: Prien, R.F., E.M. Caffey Jr., and C.J. Klett. "Prophylactic Efficacy of Lithium Carbonate in Manic-Depressive Illness: Report of the Veteran's Administration and National Institute of Mental Health Collaborative Study Group." *Archives of General Psychiatry* 28 (1973), pp. 337–41; Calabrese, J.R., and others. "International Consensus Group on Bipolar I Depression Treatment Guidelines." *Journal of Clinical Psychiatry* 65, no. 4 (2004), pp. 571–79; and Prien, R.F., and others. "Drug Therapy in the Prevention of Recurrences in Unipolar and Bipolar Disorders: Report of the NIMH Collaborative Study Group Comparing Lithium Carbonate, Imipramine, and a Lithium Carbonate-Imipramine Combination." *Archives of General Psychiatry* 41 (1984), pp. 1095–1104.

symptoms appear. A combination of an antidepressant and a mood stabilizer was believed to have a quicker onset than a mood stabilizer, such as lithium, alone.[72]

In Canada, in 2003–2004, 37% of patients with a mental illness discharged from acute care hospitals were readmitted within a year (see Figure 8.13), compared with 27.3% of patients discharged with a non-mental illness.[73] Probabilities were highest among those diagnosed with schizophrenia and personality disorders. The risk of readmission among individuals diagnosed with schizophrenia and a co-occurring substance disorder was 53.3%. This was 14.2% higher than the risk among those diagnosed with schizophrenia but no substance disorder. Alcohol and illicit drug use have been demonstrated to compromise the efficacy of schizophrenia treatment by degrading the effect of antipsychotic medications and have been associated with less compliance with regimens of medication use and rehabilitation.[74] It should be noted that the transition from acute care to community-based services can be positive for some individuals. There is evidence that suggests patients in a 24/7 treatment program versus those in a 24/5 have similar treatment outcomes. Therefore, by reducing resources for residential services and providing additional community-based services we are able to reach more clients, address

Figure 8.13 One-Year Acute Care Hospital Readmission Rates for Patients with Mental Illness by Condition and Co-occurring Disorder, Canada, 2003–2004

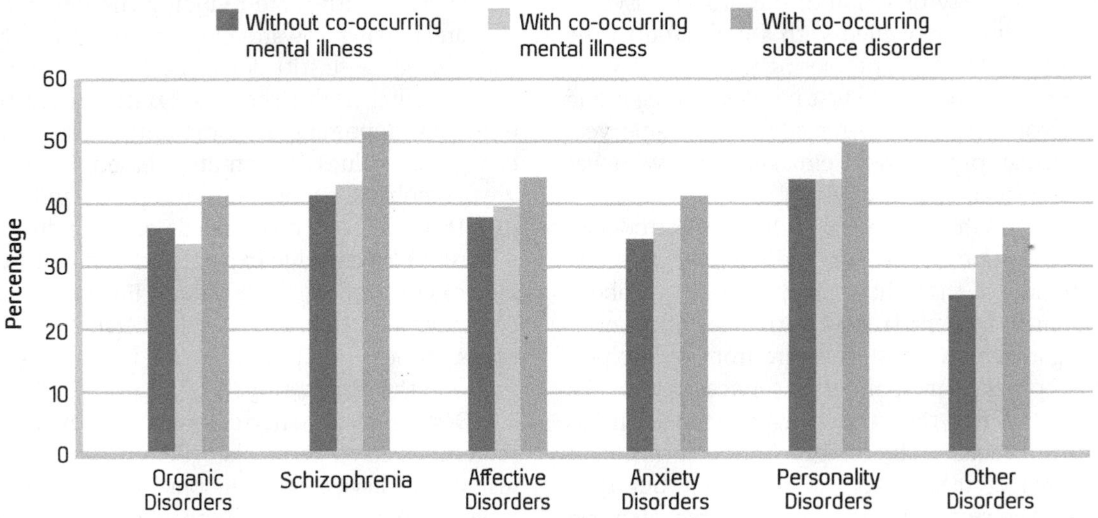

Source: Madi, N., H. Zhao, and J.F. Li. "Canadian Institute for Health Information (CIHI) Survey: Hospital Readmissions for Patients with Mental Illness in Canada." *Healthcare Quarterly* 10, no. 2 (2007), pp. 30–32.

issues earlier, focus more upstream, explore challenges within communities, and provide more direct support for families.

In addition to lithium, alternatives include anticonvulsants and antipsychotics. Three drugs that were initially developed as anticonvulsants (to treat epileptic seizures) are being used as mood stabilizers (to treat bipolar disorder). Valrico acid (Epicene), carbamazepine (Tegretol), and lamotrigine (Lamictal) have received Health Canada approval for use in bipolar disorder, based on published evidence of their effectiveness. These drugs are particularly useful in people who might be susceptible to epileptic seizures. They are probably not quite as effective as lithium, but they have the advantage that monitoring of blood levels is not required.[75] Treatment of bipolar disorder leads to improvement in a significant proportion of patients, but most drugs rarely produce full remissions. Clinically controlled randomized trials produce significant results that are often not found in the real world. In contrast to controlled clinical trials, in a naturalistic study that did not exclude subjects with comorbid conditions or substance abuse, Alda and colleagues at Capital Health Nova Scotia reviewed the health records of 120 patients to analyze the ability of drug regimes to prevent symptoms. Alda reported that rates of full response to individual mood stabilizers were low: lithium, 30%; carbamazepine, 0%; valproate, 13%; lamotrigine, 11%; and olanzapine, 25%.[76] These mood-stabilizing anticonvulsants are also thought to be better accepted by patients than is lithium, but noncompliance is an issue with these drugs as well (but perhaps not as much as with lithium). Patients with bipolar disorder who clearly improve while on medication but who relapse because they stop taking it may go through this cycle repeatedly, often with tragic consequences (suicide, arrest, homelessness; see the next section).

LO11 Consequences of Drug Treatments for Mental Illness

The use of modern psychopharmaceuticals, which began in the mid-1950s in Canada, has affected the lives of millions of people who have been treated with them. But the availability of these effective medications has also brought about revolutionary changes in our society's treatment of and relationship with people with mental illnesses. In May 1954, chlorpromazine (Thorazine) hit the market and within eight short months it was administered to over two million patients worldwide. Chlorpromazine was discovered in France in 1950 by Henri Laborit and was initially developed and synthesized in the search for a better antihistamine.[77] Chlorpromazine was the first antipsychotic drug (known under the trade name Largactil in Europe and Thorazine in Canada and in the United

States). Pierre Deniker, a psychiatrist of the Saint-Anne Psychiatric Centre in Paris, is credited with first recognizing the specificity of action of the drug in psychosis in 1952. Deniker travelled with a colleague to the United States and Canada, promoting the drug at medical conferences in 1954. The first publication regarding its use in North America was made in the same year by the Canadian psychiatrist Heinz Lehmann, who was based in Montreal.

The year in which chlorpromazine was introduced in the United States, 1955, was the last year in which the population of these hospitals increased. At about the same time in Canada, psychiatric deinstitutionalization began with a transfer of care from public psychiatric hospitals to mental health services within the community.[13] Since then the average population has continued to decline. The antipsychotics do not cure schizophrenia or other forms of psychosis, but they can control the symptoms to a great degree, allowing the patients to leave the hospital, live at home, and often earn a living. These drugs began the liberation of people with mental illnesses from hospitals, where many of them had previously stayed year after year, committed for an indefinite time. Drugs do help individuals move forward and live enhanced and positive successful lives.

The trend toward deinstitutionalization in Canada was as marked with massive reductions in the hospital populations. The movement out of psychiatric hospitals was accelerated in the 1960s with the establishment of federally supported community mental health centres. In Canada, between 1961 and 1976, 34 000 patients were discharged from psychiatric facilities, with similar trends occurring across Europe, although perhaps at a more gradual pace.[78] The idea was to treat people with mental illnesses closer to home in a more natural environment, at lesser expense, and on an outpatient basis.

The stigma attached to mental illnesses presents a serious barrier not only to diagnosis and treatment but also to acceptance in the community. The Canadian Alliance on Mental Illness and Mental Health (CAMIMH) has identified combatting the stigma of mental illnesses and preventing discrimination against people with mental illnesses as one of the most pressing priorities for improving the mental health of Canadians. Educating the public and the media about mental illness is a first step toward reducing the stigma and encouraging greater acceptance and understanding of mental illness. The opportunity for such a program to work was greatly enhanced by the availability of potent, effective psychopharmaceuticals, especially the antipsychotics. Their success, however, is being questioned.

Many countries are reducing the number of beds and are moving toward closing psychiatric hospitals and replacing institutional care with community-based mental health services. Strategies are therefore especially important to communicate the underlying change in values. Community-based services place great emphasis on people's autonomy and providing care that is based on the needs of the individuals and is sensitive to their life experiences and culture. Strategies have to reflect these values. Further, introducing community-based services considerably changes the rights, duties, and protection of individuals, families, staff, and the community.[79]

Despite these shortcomings, the mental health professions have been changed by these drugs. The majority of psychiatrists in practice today spend less time doing psychotherapy than did their colleagues in the 1950s. In fact, for many psychiatrists the first issue is to establish an appropriate drug regimen, and only after the initial symptoms are controlled will they engage in much talk therapy. For some psychiatrists the prescription pad has replaced the couch as their primary tool. This may be sensible in terms of overall cost effectiveness, but it has altered the doctor–patient relationship.

Concomitant with the liberation of patients from hospitals and their return to the communities came a concern for their civil rights. Indefinite commitment to a hospital had been declared unconstitutional, and all provinces and territories have since developed procedures to protect the rights of individual patients. Hearings are required before a person can be committed for treatment against his or her will, and it is usually necessary to demonstrate a clear and present danger to the patient's own person or to others. Periodic reviews of the patient's status are called for, and if at any time the immediate danger is not present, the patient must be released. No one would want to argue that people with mental illnesses should not have these rights, but the availability of psychoactive medications helps create difficult situations. A patient who is dangerously psychotic might be admitted for treatment, and after a few weeks on an antipsychotic drug might be sufficiently in control to be allowed to leave the hospital. However, if the patient remains suspicious or simply doesn't like to take the medication, he or she will eventually stop taking it and again become psychotic. Or patients might be released into the community, perhaps functioning with medication or perhaps not, too sick to really take care of themselves but not sick

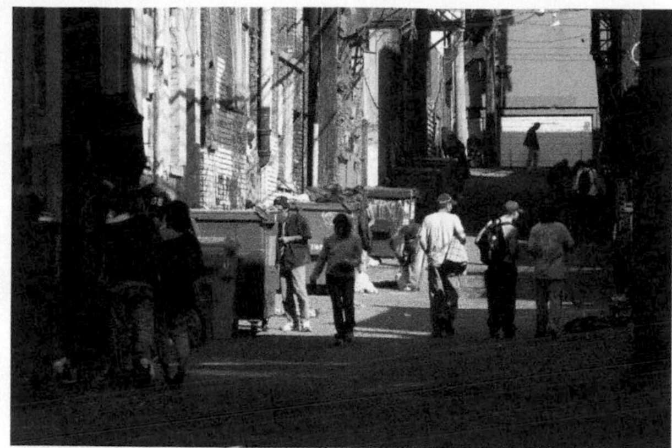

Poverty in Downtown East Vancouver contributes to homelessness and addiction.

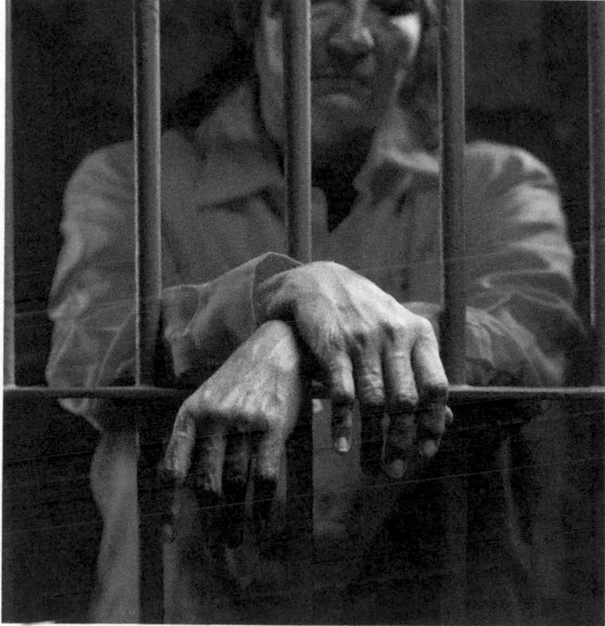

The number of people with mental illnesses is increasing in Canadian prisons.

enough to present an immediate danger. Often, the eventual result is violation of a law, leading to imprisonment. In fact, more people with mental illnesses are jailed each year than are admitted to psychiatric hospitals. The high prevalence of mental illness among incarcerated populations in Canada has been explained in a number of specific ways.[80] Offenders with mental disorders may be arrested at a disproportionately high rate compared with offenders without mental disorders. People with mental illness may also be less skilful at crime or more easily caught. Or, once arrested, they may be more likely to plead guilty because of an inability to pay for or inability to understand legal representation.[81]

About one-third of all homeless people in Canada have some form of mental illness. In Canada the percentage of homeless people who have had either a mental illness or a substance abuse diagnosis is approximately 86%.[82] Seventy-five percent of homeless women have a mental illness.[83] Individuals with schizophrenia are greatly overrepresented in Canadian prison and homeless populations.[18,83]

> In no other field, except perhaps leprosy, has there been as much confusion, misdirection and discrimination against the patient as in mental illness.. . . Down through the ages they have been estranged by society and cast out to wander in the wilderness. Mental illness, even today, is all too often considered a crime to be punished, a sin to be expiated, a possessing demon to be exorcized, a disgrace to be hushed-up, a personality weakness to be deplored or a welfare problem to be handled as cheaply as possible.[84]

The plight of our homeless, rootless people with mental illnesses has been the subject of magazine and television reports, and efforts are being made to change the way these people are treated. In British Columbia there is an increased visibility of homelessness, addictions, and poverty in downtown Vancouver. Among the political responses to the visibility of mental illness in B.C. has been the opening of a new 100-bed facility for people with mental health and addiction problems and the establishing of Vancouver's Downtown Community Court.[13] The Mental Health Commission of Canada has allocated $110 million to support homelessness projects focused on people with mental illness in Vancouver, Toronto, Montreal, and Moncton. Eighty-five percent of the funding will go to housing and 15% to research on its effectiveness.

In 1998, data from Correctional Services Canada found 1000 inmates out of 14 000 in the prison population were diagnosed with mental health disorders. In 2004, that number soared to 1500 in a prison population of 12 500. Women have an even higher prevalence rate, with 25% identified on admission as having a mental illness in 2007—an increase of 100% over ten years ago.[84]

The Regional Psychiatric Centre in Saskatoon is Canada's only psychiatric prison taking female offenders. The prison houses both men and women with severe mental illnesses. The poor treatment of women offenders with mental issues has been featured in the media, most notably the death and inquest of Ashley Smith.

Summary

- Diagnosis of mental disorders is difficult and controversial, but the DSM-5 provides a standard diagnostic approach for most purposes.
- Panic disorder evolves at some point following repeated episodes of depression and anxiety. Treatment of panic attacks with specific pharmacological treatment depends on the person's clinical history and the brain regions suspected to be involved.
- The medical model of mental illness has been widely opposed as mental illness cannot always be equated with other illness of the body, yet psychotherapeutic drugs are often discussed in the context of this model.
- The introduction of antipsychotics in the mid-1950s started a revolution in mental health care and increased interest in psychopharmacology.
- The antipsychotics are helpful for the majority of people with schizophrenia, but they often produce movement disorders, some of which resemble Parkinson's disease.
- Chlorpromazine, a phenothiazine, was the first antipsychotic drug used to treat schizophrenia in the 1950s.
- Phenothiazine treatment had a tremendous impact on the management of hospitalized patients.
- Chlorpromazine is a typical antipsychotic drug while clozapine is an atypical antipsychotic drug used in the treatment of schizophrenia.
- Antipsychotic drugs are thought to reverse neurotransmitter system changes underlying schizophrenia.
- There are limited data on the efficacy of antipsychotic drug action in children, adolescents, and older adults. Typical and atypical antipsychotics are associated with increased risk of death in older adults.
- The major groups of antidepressant drugs are the MAOIs, the tricyclics, and the SSRIs.
- Many antidepressant medications work to increase serotonin or norepinephrine levels within the brain. Other antidepressant medications work through different biochemical pathways. Most antidepressant medications are equally effective, suggesting that no single biochemical mechanism, including serotonin activity, can explain their effects.
- Fluoxetine (Prozac) quickly became the largest-selling antidepressant drug in history.
- Although black-box warnings by Health Canada on treating adolescents and children with antidepressants did result in fewer prescriptions, suicide rates increased.
- Lithium acts as a mood-normalizing agent in people with bipolar disorder, preventing both manic and depressed mood swings. Lithium's mechanism of action is unknown.
- The number of people occupying beds in psychiatric hospitals has declined since 1955, largely because psychotherapeutic drugs allow people to be released after shorter stays.
- The number of people in Canadian prisons and on the streets with a mental illness is increasing.

Review Questions

1. Give two examples of an anxiety disorder.
2. Is schizophrenia a functional or an organic psychosis?
3. Besides sadness, what are some other indicators of a major depressive episode?
4. What type of drug is chlorpromazine, and where was it first tested on patients?
5. What is tardive dyskinesia, and how does it respond to a reduction in the dose of an antipsychotic drug?
6. Which type of drug was discovered while testing an antituberculosis agent?
7. How do the SSRIs differ from the older tricyclics in terms of their actions in the brain?
8. What were two of the three reasons it took so long for lithium to be available for use?
9. If clozapine is so dangerous, why is it prescribed at all?
10. Why was Prozac the most widely prescribed antidepressant drug ever marketed?
11. How has deinstitutionalization contributed to the increasing numbers of people with mental illnesses in our prisons and on Canadian streets?

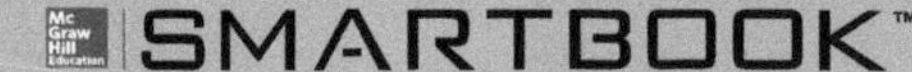

SECTION

4

DRUGS, BEHAVIOUR, AND SOCIETY

CHAPTER 9

Alcohol

In this section we will look at the fascinating drug called alcohol. We say fascinating because it is a very small molecule that can have broad effects on the individual and the individual's role in society. What is alcohol and how does it affect the body and brain? How does alcohol influence an individual's relationship with others, and what is its impact on society?

ALCOHOL

Alcohol: social lubricant, adjunct to a fine meal, or demon rum? People today are no different from people throughout the centuries; many use alcohol, and many others condemn its use. This love-hate relationship with alcohol has been ongoing for a long time. The last two decades have brought a slight swing of the pendulum: Health-conscious Canadians are opting for low-alcohol or no-alcohol drinks, consumption of hard liquor is down, and we receive frequent reminders to use alcohol responsibly, not to drink and drive, and not to let our friends drive if they've been drinking. Let's take a closer look at the world's number-one psychoactive substance.

CHAPTER 9

ALCOHOL

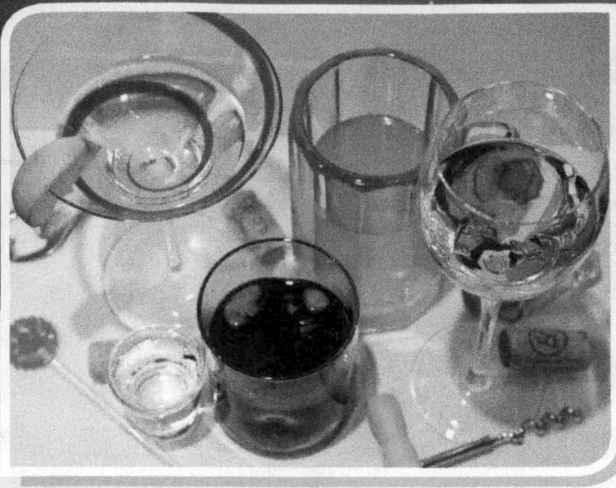

OBJECTIVES

When you have finished this chapter, you should be able to

- **LO1** Describe the production and approximate alcohol content of the major alcoholic beverage types.
- **LO2** Summarize the history and effectiveness of the temperance and prohibition movements in North America.
- **LO3** Describe recent alcohol consumption trends in Canadian youth and adults.
- **LO4** Discuss the absorption, distribution, metabolism, and mechanism of action of alcohol.
- **LO5** Describe the range of behavioural effects of alcohol.
- **LO6** Describe the toxic effects of alcohol on the brain, liver, heart, and other organ systems of the body.
- **LO7** Describe the effects of alcohol on the unborn child.
- **LO8** Describe the symptoms seen during alcohol withdrawal in dependent individuals.

LO1 Alcoholic Beverages

Fermentation and Fermentation Products

Many thousands of years ago Neolithic humans discovered "booze." Beer and berry wine were known and used about 6400 BC and grape wine dates from 300 to 400 BC. Mead, which is made from honey, might be the oldest alcoholic beverage; some authorities suggest it appeared in the Paleolithic age, about 8000 BC. Early use of alcohol seems to have been worldwide: Beer was drunk by the Native people whom Columbus met.

fermentation: the production of alcohol from sugars through the action of yeasts.

distillation: the evaporation and condensing of alcohol vapours to produce beverages with higher alcohol content.

Fermentation forms the basis for all alcoholic beverages. Certain yeasts act on sugar in the presence of water, and this chemical action is fermentation. Yeast recombines the carbon, hydrogen, and oxygen of sugar into ethyl alcohol and carbon dioxide. Chemically, $C_6H_{12}O_6$ (glucose) is transformed into C_2H_5OH (ethyl alcohol) + CO_2 (carbon dioxide).

Most fruits, including grapes, contain sugar, and the addition of the appropriate yeast (which is pervasive in the air wherever plants grow) to a mixture of crushed grapes and water will begin the fermentation process. The yeast has only a limited tolerance for alcohol; when the concentration reaches 15%, the yeast dies and fermentation ceases. While up to 15% is theoretically possible, in practice the standard alcohol content for wine is about 12%.

Cereal grains can also be used to produce alcoholic beverages. However, cereal grains contain starch rather than sugar, and before fermentation can begin the starch must be converted to sugar. This is accomplished by making *malt,* which contains enzymes that convert starch into sugar. In Canadian beer the primary grain is barley, which is malted by steeping it in water and allowing it to sprout. The sprouted grain is then slowly dried to kill the sprout but preserve the enzymes formed during the growth. This dried, sprouted barley is called malt, and when crushed and mixed with water, the enzymes convert the starch to sugar. Only yeast is needed then to start fermentation. The lower sugar content of these grain-based beverages results in somewhat lower alcohol content: the typical Canadian commercial beer contains about 5% alcohol.

Distilled Products

To obtain alcohol concentrations above 15%, distillation is necessary. **Distillation** is a process in which the solution containing alcohol is heated, and the vapours are collected and condensed into liquid form again. Alcohol has a lower boiling point than water, so there is a higher percentage of alcohol in the distillate (the condensed liquid) than there was in the original solution.

There is still debate over who discovered the distillation process and when the discovery was made, but many authorities place it in Arabia around AD 800. The term *alcohol* comes from an Arabic word meaning "finely divided spirit" and originally referred to that part of the wine collected through distillation–the essence, or "spirit," of the wine. In Europe, only fermented beverages were used until the 10th century, when the Italians first distilled wine, thereby introducing "spirits" to the Western world. These new products were studied and used in the treatment of many illnesses, including senility. The initial feeling about their medicinal value is best seen in the Latin name given these condensed vapours by a thirteenth-century French professor of medicine: *aqua vitae*, "the water of life."

On the continent, Europeans distilled wine into "brandywine" (derived from the Dutch term "burnt wine"), while the Irish and Scots distilled their malted-grain beverages (beer) into whisky (the Gaelic term *uisgebaugh* also means "water of life").

In North America the alcoholic content of distilled beverages may be indicated by the term **proof**. The percentage of alcohol by volume is one-half of the proof number: for instance, 90-proof whisky is 45% alcohol. The word *proof* developed from a British Army procedure to gauge the alcohol content of distilled spirits before there were modern techniques.

proof: a measure of a beverage's alcohol content; twice the alcohol percentage.

DRUGS IN THE MEDIA

Advertising Alcohol on Television

When it comes to the world portrayed on television, both in programs and in advertising, it seems that beer is okay (there are lots of beer ads and a few more or less positive references to beer drinking on some programs), wine is a little less okay, but distilled spirits are apparently not okay. Advertising of beer on television has not been particularly restricted. But, depending on where you live, and especially if you live in the United States, you might never see television ads for distilled spirits.

After Prohibition, purveyors of distilled spirits did not advertise on radio, and later they did not advertise on television. This was a voluntary ban by the radio, television, and liquor industries, not something mandated by any federal agency. In 1996, Seagram became the first liquor manufacturer to break the voluntary ban, and a few other companies followed suit. The ads are shown on local TV stations in several large cities, usually later at night. According to a December 7, 2000, article in *The New York Times*, in 1999 $18 million was spent to advertise liquor on television and radio combined—not much in comparison to beer advertising or to the amount spent to advertise distilled spirits in magazines and newspapers.

In December 2001 the American broadcaster NBC announced it would begin "limited" advertising for liquor, only after 9 p.m., and only on shows with primarily adult viewers. The plan was to start the ads in April 2002. This announcement generated quite a response from a wide variety of watchdog groups. Several of NBC's local affiliates promised to block those ads when they appeared, public opinion polls showed most people opposed the idea of televised liquor ads, 13 members of Congress wrote NBC a letter promising to hold hearings on the matter. In March, only a couple of weeks before the first ads were to appear, NBC reversed its earlier decision and agreed not to advertise hard liquor. Apart from the embarrassment of explaining how these ads target mature adults rather than those under 21, the networks and their current advertisers worry that federal legislation might restrict the advertising of wine and beer along with hard liquor.

Today, liquor advertising on Canadian television is regulated by the Code for Broadcast Advertising of Alcoholic Beverages. Its guidelines are fairly loose; spirits advertisements appear during prime time and are not confined to late-night television. However, before 1996 it too limited advertising for any liquor containing more than 7% alcohol by volume.

The liquid was poured over gunpowder and ignited. If the alcohol content was high enough, the alcohol would burn and ignite the gunpowder, which would go "poof" and explode. That was proof that the beverage had an acceptable alcohol content, about 57%. Typical distilled beverages sold commercially (whisky, vodka, gin, etc.) range between 40% and 50% alcohol content (80 to 100 proof).

Beer

Beer is made by adding barley malt to other cereal grains, such as ground corn or rice. The enzymes in the malt change the starches in these grains into sugar; then the solids are filtered out before the yeast is added to the mash to start fermentation. Hops (dried blossoms from only the female hop plant) are added with the yeast to give beer its distinctive, pungent flavour. Although there are many varieties of beer, they fall into two broad types: ale and *lager*. Most of the beer sold today in America is lager, from the German word *lagern*, meaning "to store." The fermentation process originally took place in alpine caves, where the cooler temperatures made for slower fermentation, and the yeasts tended to drop to the bottom of the mash. Over the years, this resulted in a selection process for types of yeast that work well as "bottom fermenters." So, modern lagers are made using bottom-fermenting yeasts, cool temperatures, and slower fermentation. Ale is made using a top-fermenting yeast and slightly warmer temperatures, and the shorter fermentation time results in more of the flavour of the malt being retained in the final product. In general, ales have a stronger taste and lagers the lighter taste favoured by most Canadian beer drinkers.

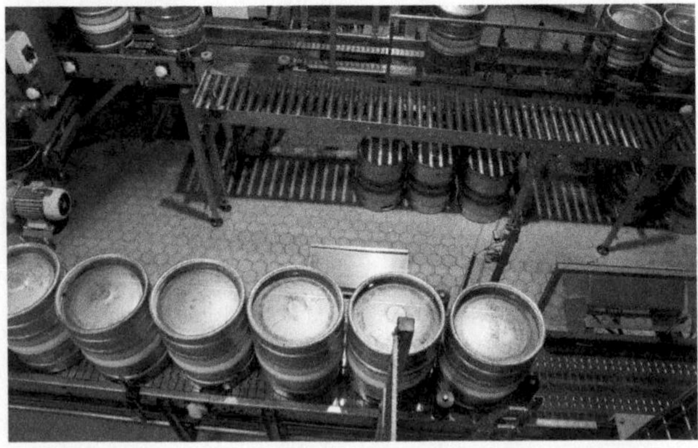

Although breweries are becoming increasingly popular in Canada, most beer consumed is produced domestically by foreign-owned brewers.

Because most Canadian beer is sold in bottles or cans, the yeast must be removed to prevent it from spoiling after packaging. This is usually accomplished by heating it (pasteurization), but some brewers use microfilters to remove the yeasts while keeping the beer cold. The carbonation is added at the time of packaging. Standard brands of commercial Canadian beer contain about 5% alcohol.

If you were asked to produce a "light" beer, with fewer calories, a lighter taste, and less alcohol, what would you do–add water? That's only part of the answer, because light beers have about 10% less alcohol and 25 to 30% fewer calories. The mash is fermented at a cooler temperature for a longer time, so that more of the sugars are converted to alcohol. *Then* the alcohol content is adjusted by adding water, resulting in a beverage with considerably less remaining sugar and only a bit less alcohol.

Canadian-produced beer accounts for 88% of domestic beer sales and can be divided into three categories: draught, bottled, and canned. Labatt (Anheuser-Busch InBev), Sleeman (Sapporo Brewery), and Molson (Molson Coors Brewing Company) dominate the Canadian market. Once purely Canadian institutions, Labatt and Sleeman are now owned by foreign interests while Molson is jointly owned in Canada and the United States. The largest fully Canadian-owned brewer, Moosehead Breweries, controls about 5.5% of the Canadian market.

Competition among national brands for Canadian market share is high. In recent years, many national brewers have seen declines in sales, while local or regional favourites have experienced growth. This change may reflect a growing demand for specialty and premium brews, some of which are imported while others are domestic.[1]

Beer is the top choice of alcoholic beverage for Canadians, although in terms of volume and sales its dominance has seen decline as consumers increase their wine consumption.[2]

Wine

Wine is one of humankind's oldest beverages, a drink that for generations has been praised as a gift from heaven and condemned as a work of the devil. Although a large volume of wine is now produced in mechanized, sterilized wine "factories," many small wineries operate alongside the industry giants, and the tradition continues that careful selection and cultivation of grapevines, good weather, precise timing of the harvest, and careful monitoring of fermentation and aging can result in wines of noticeably higher quality.

There are two basic types of North American wines. *Generics* usually have names taken from European land areas where the original wines were produced: Chablis, Burgundy, and Rhine are examples. These are all blended wines, made from whatever grapes are available, and during processing they are made to taste something like the traditional European wines from those regions. *Varietals* are named after one variety of grape, which by law must make up at least 51% of the grapes used in producing the wine. Chardonnay, merlot, and zinfandel are some examples. There are many varietal wines, and traditionally they have been sold in individual bottles and are more expensive than the generics. Most white wines are made from white grapes, although it is possible to use red grapes if the skins are removed before fermentation. Red wines are made from red grapes by leaving the skins in the crushed grapes while they ferment. "Blush" wines such as white zinfandel have become quite popular. With the zinfandel grape, which is red, the skins are left in the crushed grapes for a short while, resulting in a wine that is just slightly pink.

Besides red versus white and generic versus varietal, another general distinction is dry versus sweet. The sweeter wines are likely to have a "heavier" taste overall, with the sweetness balancing out flavours that might be considered harsh in a dry wine.

Because carbon dioxide is produced during fermentation, it is possible to produce naturally carbonated sparkling wines by adding a small amount of sugar as the wine is bottled and then keeping the bottle tightly corked. French champagnes are made in this way, as are the more expensive champagnes, which might be labelled "naturally fermented in the bottle," or "*methode Champagnoise*." A cheaper method is used on inexpensive sparkling wines: Carbon dioxide gas is injected into a generic wine during bottling. Champagnes vary in their sweetness, also, with brut being the driest. Sweet champagnes are labelled "extra dry." The *extra* means "not," as in *extraordinary*.

Most wines contain about 12% alcohol. It was discovered many years ago in Spain that if enough brandy is added to a newly fermented wine the fermentation will stop and the wine will not spoil (turn to vinegar). Sealing the wine in charred oak casks for aging further refined its taste, and soon *sherry* was in great demand throughout Europe. Other fortified wines, all of which have an alcohol content near 20%, include port, Madeira, and Muscatel.

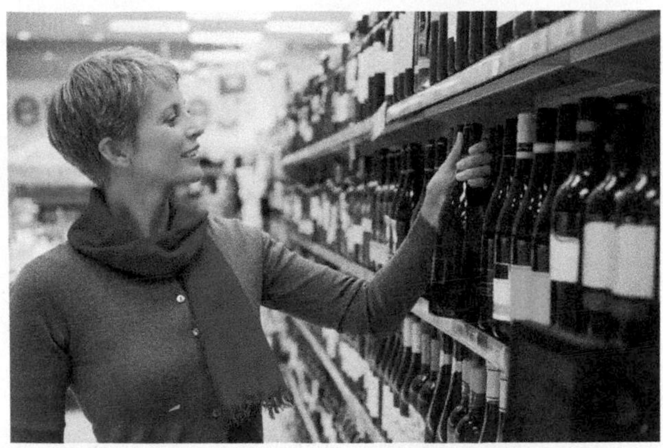

Wine consumption has increased considerably during the past 35 years.

Distilled Spirits

Although brandy, distilled from wine, was probably the first type of spirits known to Europeans, the Celts of Ireland and the Scottish highlands were distilling a crude beverage known as *uisgebaugh* before 1500. If you try to pronounce that, you'll see that it was the origin of the word *whisky*. Today's Scotch whisky is distilled from fermented barley malt (a strong beer).

One of the early distillers who established a good reputation was Elijah Craig, a Baptist minister living in what was then Bourbon County, Kentucky. He began storing his whisky in charred new oak barrels, originating a manufacturing step still used with American bourbon whiskies.

By the seventeenth century, improved distillation techniques had made possible the production of relatively pure alcohol. Today's standard product from many large commercial distilleries is 95% pure ethyl alcohol (ethanol) (190 proof). Into the process goes whatever grain is available at a cheap price and tank loads of corn syrup or other sources of sugars or starches. Out the other end come *grain neutral spirits*, a clear liquid that is essentially tasteless (except for the strong alcohol taste), which might be sold in small quantities as Everclear or for use in medicine or research. More often, it is processed in bulk in various ways. For example, large quantities of ethanol are added to gasoline to produce a less polluting fuel, which also helps out the farmer. Besides other industrial uses for ethanol, such as in cleaners and solvents, bulk grain neutral spirits are also used in making various beverages, including blended Scotch whiskies. One of the first beverages to be made from straight grain neutral spirits was gin. By filtering the distillate through juniper berries and then diluting it with water, a medicinal-tasting drink was produced. First called "jenever" by the Dutch and "genievre" by

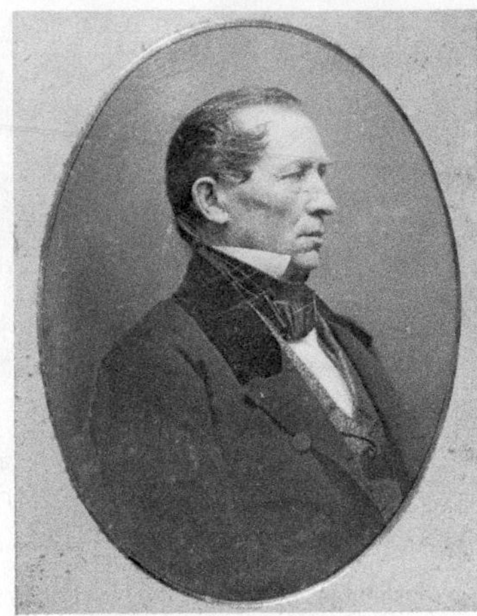

Canadian Club Whisky is a distilled spirit produced since 1858 by Hiram Walker.

the French, the British shortened the name to "gin." Gin became a popular beverage in England and now forms the basis for many a martini.

Another major use for bulk grain neutral spirits is in the production of *vodka.* Vodkas are simply a mixture of grain neutral spirits and water, adjusted to the desired proof.

The proof at which distillation is carried out influences the taste and other characteristics of the liquor. When alcohol is formed, other related substances, known as **congeners**, are also formed. These may include alcohols other than ethanol, oils, and other organic matter. Luckily they are present only in small amounts, because some of them are quite toxic. Grain neutral spirits contain relatively few congeners and none of the flavour of the grains used in the mash. Whisky is usually distilled at a lower proof, not more than 160, and thus the distillate contains more congeners and some of the flavour of the grain used. Whisky accumulates congeners during aging, at least for the first five years, and the congeners and the grain used provide the variation in taste among whiskies.

Until Prohibition, almost all whisky consumed in North America was straight rye or bourbon. Prohibition introduced smuggled Canadian and Scotch whisky to American drinkers, and they liked them. World War II sent men around the world, further exposing them to this different type of liquor. Scotch and Canadian whiskies are lighter than American whiskey, which means lighter in colour and less heavy in taste. They are lighter because Canadian and Scotch whiskies are typically *blended* whiskies, made from about two-thirds straight whisky and one-third grain neutral spirits. After World War II, U.S. manufacturers began selling more blended whisky. Seagram's 7-Crown has been one of the most popular blended whiskies.

congeners: other alcohols and oils contained in alcoholic beverages.

Liqueurs, or cordials, are similar in some ways to the fortified wines. Originally the cordials were made from brandy mixed with flavourings derived from herbs, berries, or nuts. After dilution with sugar and water, the beverages are highly flavoured, sweet, and usually about 20–25% alcohol. Some of the old recipes are still closely guarded secrets of a particular group of European monks. The late twentieth century saw an increase in popularity for these drinks, which are usually consumed in small amounts and have only about half the alcohol content of vodka or whisky. Many new types were introduced, from Bailey's Irish Cream to varieties of schnapps. Peppermint, peach, and other types of schnapps are made from grain neutral spirits, which are diluted, sweetened, and flavoured with artificial or natural flavourings.

LO2 Alcohol Use and "The Alcohol Problem"

Historians seem to agree that most North Americans drank alcoholic beverages and most people favoured these beverages compared with drinking water, which was often contaminated. The per capita consumption of alcohol was apparently much greater than current levels, and little public concern was expressed. Even the early Puritan ministers, who were moralistic about all kinds of behaviour, referred to alcoholic drink as "the Good Creature of God." They denounced drunkenness as a sinful misuse of the "Good Creature" but clearly placed the blame on the sinner, not on alcohol itself.[3]

A new view of alcohol as the *cause* of serious problems began to emerge in America soon after the Revolution. That view took root and still exists as a major influence in American culture today. It is so pervasive that some people have a hard time understanding what is meant by the "demonization" of alcohol (viewing alcohol as a demon, or devil). The concept is important, partly because alcohol was the first psychoactive substance to become demonized in American culture, leading the way for similar views of cocaine, heroin, and marijuana in this century. We are referring to a tendency to view a substance as an *active* (sometimes almost purposeful) source of *evil,* damaging everything it touches. Whenever harmful consequences result from the use of something (firearms and nuclear energy are other possible examples), some people find it easiest to simply view that thing as "bad" and seek to eliminate it.

The Temperance Movement

The first writings indicating a negative view of alcohol itself are attributed to a prominent Philadelphia physician named Benjamin Rush, one of the signers of the Declaration of Independence. Rush's 1784 pamphlet, "An Inquiry into the Effects of Ardent Spirits on the Mind and Body," was aimed particularly at distilled spirits (*ardent* means "burning," "fiery"), not at the weaker beverages, such as beer and wine. As a physician, Rush had noticed a relationship between heavy drinking and jaundice (an indicator of liver disease), "madness" (perhaps the delirium tremens of withdrawal, or perhaps what we now call Korsakoff's psychosis), and "epilepsy" (probably the seizures seen during withdrawal). All of those are currently accepted and well-documented consequences of heavy alcohol use. However, Rush also concluded that hard liquor damaged the drinker's morality, leading to a variety of antisocial, immoral, and criminal behaviours. Although the correlation between these types of behaviour and alcohol use had been documented many times, Rush believed that this was a direct toxic action of distilled spirits on the part of the brain responsible for morality. Rush then introduced for the first time the concept of "addiction" to a psychoactive substance, describing the uncontrollable and overwhelming desires for alcohol experienced by some of his patients. For the first time this condition was referred to as a *disease* (caused by alcohol), and he recommended total abstinence from alcohol for those who were problem drinkers.[4]

Other physicians readily recognized these symptoms in their own patients, and physicians became the first leaders of the **temperance** movement. What Rush proposed, and most early followers supported, was that everyone should avoid distilled spirits entirely, because they were considered to be toxic, and should consume beer and wine in a *temperate*, or moderate, manner. Temperance societies were formed in many parts of the country, at first among the upper classes of physicians, ministers, and businesspeople. In the early 1800s, it became fashionable for the middle classes to join the elite in this movement, and hundreds of thousands of American businesspeople, farmers, lawyers, teachers, and their families "took the pledge" to avoid spirits and to be temperate in their use of beer or wine.

In the second half of the nineteenth century, things changed. Up to this time there had been little consumption of commercial beer in the Americas. It was only with the advent of artificial refrigeration and the addition of hops, which helped preserve the beer, that the number of breweries increased. The waves of immigrants who entered Canada and the United States in this period provided the necessary beer-drinking consumers. At first, encouraged by temperance groups that preferred beer consumption to the use of liquor, breweries were constructed everywhere. However, alcohol-related problems did not disappear. Instead, disruptive, drunken behaviour became increasingly associated in the public's mind with the new wave of immigrants–Irish, Italians, and eastern Europeans, more often Catholic than Protestant–and they drank beer and wine. Temperance workers now advocated total abstinence from all alcoholic beverages, and pressure grew to prohibit the sale of alcohol altogether.

Prohibition

The first North American prohibition period began in 1851 when Maine passed its prohibition law. Legislative steps toward prohibition were first initiated in Canada with the passage of the Dunkin Act in 1864, which permitted Upper Canadian jurisdictions to forbid the sale of liquor by majority vote. The Canada Temperance Act, enacted by Parliament in 1878, after Confederation, provided an option for Canadian jurisdictions to opt in by plebiscite to prohibition. In 1898, a federal referendum on prohibition won by a slim majority. Sir Wilfrid Laurier, the prime minister at the time, failed to introduce it into federal bill due to strong antipathy for prohibition in Quebec.[5]

In 1899, a group of educators, lawyers, and clergymen described the saloon as the "workingman's club, in which many of his leisure hours are spent, and in which he finds more of the things that approximate luxury than in his home. . . ." They went on to say: "It is a centre of learning, books, papers, and lecture hall to them. It is the clearinghouse for common intelligence, the place where their philosophy of life is worked out, and their political and social beliefs take their beginnings."[6] Truth lay

temperance: the idea that people should drink beer or wine in moderation but drink no hard liquor.

somewhere between those statements and the sentiments expressed in a sermon:

> The liquor traffic is the most fiendish, corrupt and hell-soaked institution that ever crawled out of the slime of the eternal pit. It is the open sore of this land. . . . It takes the kind, loving husband and father, smothers every spark of love in his bosom, and transforms him into a heartless wretch, and makes him steal the shoes from his starving babe's feet to find the price for a glass of liquor. It takes your sweet innocent daughter, robs her of her virtue and transforms her into a brazen, wanton harlot. . . .
>
> The open saloon as an institution has its origin in hell, and it is manufacturing subjects to be sent back to hell.[7]

Prohibition was not just a matter of "wets" versus "drys" or a matter of political conviction or health concerns. Intricately interwoven with these factors was a middle-class, rural, Protestant, evangelical concern that the good and true life was being undermined by ethnic groups with a different religion and a lower standard of living and morality. One way to strike back at these groups was through prohibition. The temperance movement can be credited for strengthening the political power of women's groups, such as the WCTU. Acting as protectors of the family, women marched, organized letter-writing campaigns, raised money, and had a major influence on decisions to outlaw the sale of alcohol.

Between 1907 and 1919, 34 U.S. states enacted legislation enforcing statewide prohibition, whereas only 2 states repealed their prohibition laws. By 1917, 64% of the U.S. population lived in dry territory, and between 1908 and 1917 over 100 000 licensed bars were closed. In Canada, Prince Edward Island became the first province to establish prohibition in 1901. By the end of World War I, all remaining provinces and Yukon had joined prohibition.[5]

But provincial and state prohibition laws did not mean that the residents did not drink. They did, both legally and illegally. They drank illegally in speakeasies and other private clubs. They drank legally from a variety of the many patent medicines that were freely available. A few of the more interesting ones were Whisko, a "nonintoxicating stimulant," at 55 proof; Colden's Liquid Beef Tonic, "recommended for treatment of alcohol habit," with 53 proof; and Kaufman's Sulfur Bitters, which "contains no alcohol" but was in fact 20% alcohol (40 proof) and contained no sulphur. Although prohibition laws were in effect until 1927, numerous exceptions were permitted by the Ontario government, including exemption of wineries, distilleries, and numerous breweries from closure allowing continued contribution to Canada's export market.[5]

In August 1917, the U.S. Senate adopted a resolution, authored by Andrew Volstead, that submitted the national prohibition amendment to the states. The U.S. House of Representatives concurred in December, and 21 days later, on January 8, 1918, Mississippi became the first state to ratify the 18th Amendment. A year later, January 16, 1919, Nebraska was the thirty-sixth state to ratify the amendment, and the deed was done.

As stated in the amendment, a year after the thirty-sixth state ratified it, national **Prohibition** came into effect on January 16, 1920. The amendment was simple, with only two operational parts:

> Section 1. After one year from the ratification of this article the manufacture, sale or transportation of intoxicating liquors within, the importation thereof into, or the exportation thereof from the United States and all territory subject to the jurisdiction thereof for beverage purposes is hereby prohibited.
>
> Section 2. The Congress and the several States shall have concurrent power to enforce this article by appropriate legislation.

The beginning of Prohibition was hailed in a radio sermon by popular preacher Billy Sunday:

> The reign of tears is over. The slums will soon be a memory. We will turn our prisons into factories and our jails into storehouses and corncribs. Men will walk upright now, women will smile, and the children will laugh. Hell will be forever for rent.[3]

The law did not result in an alcohol-free society, and this came as quite a surprise to many people. Apparently the assumption was that Prohibition would be so widely accepted that little enforcement would be necessary. Along with saloons, breweries, and distilleries, hospitals that had specialized in the treatment of alcohol dependence closed their doors, presumably because there would no longer be a need for them.

It soon became clear that people were buying and selling alcohol illegally and that enforcement was not going to be easy. The majority of the population might have supported the idea of Prohibition, but such a large minority insisted on continuing to drink that *speakeasies*, *hip flasks*, and *bathtub gin* became household words. Organized crime became both more organized and vastly more profitable as a result of Prohibition.

Prohibition: laws prohibiting all sales of alcoholic beverages from 1920 to 1933.

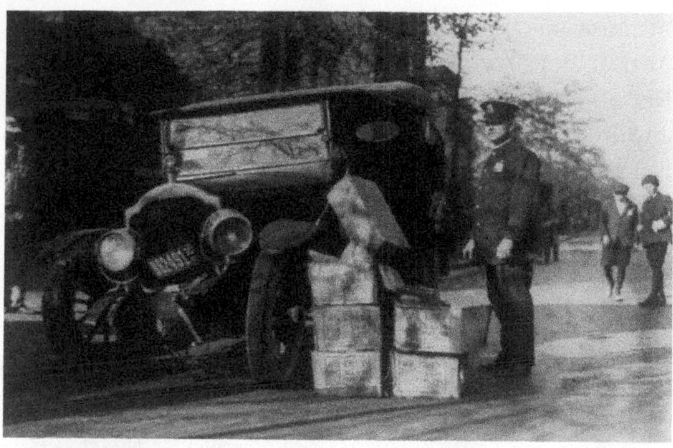

Prohibition laws were frequently violated, and enforcement was an ongoing problem.

Prohibition Worked!

The popular conception is that Prohibition was a total failure, leading to its repeal. That is not the case. Prohibition did reduce overall alcohol intake. Hospital admissions for alcohol dependence and deaths from alcohol declined sharply at the beginning of Prohibition. But during the 1920s, it appears that the prohibition laws were increasingly violated, and the rates of alcohol dependence and alcohol-related deaths began to increase. However, even toward the end of the "noble experiment," as Prohibition was called by its detractors, alcohol dependence and alcohol-related deaths were still lower than before Prohibition.

Prohibition Is Repealed

If Prohibition did reduce alcohol-related problems, why was it repealed? In Canada it was the realization that the prohibition laws were unenforceable. Throughout the course of Prohibition the sale of alcohol continued to flourish nationwide, under several different guises. Illicit stills and "moonshine" proliferated, bootlegging rose dramatically, and speakeasies became commonplace. Consequentially, most provinces repealed their prohibition laws by 1930. Prince Edward Island was the last province to repeal prohibition, doing so in 1948.[5]

There was also fear that the widespread and highly publicized disrespect for the Prohibition law encouraged a sense of "lawlessness," not just among the bootleggers and gangsters but also in the public at large. The Great Depression, which began in 1929, not only made more people consider the value of tax revenues but also increased fears of a generalized revolt. If Prohibition weakened respect for law and order, it had to go. Although women's groups had played a big role in getting Prohibition passed and lobbied against repeal, other women's groups (again acting as protectors of the family) argued that Prohibition's dangers were too great and supported repeal. Realizing that they could not stop people from drinking entirely, temperance groups turned their efforts to curtailing the sale of liquor through the establishment of Liquor Control Boards.

The prohibition of alcohol, much like the current prohibitions of marijuana and heroin, did work in that it reduced alcohol availability, alcohol use, and related problems. On the other hand, even at its best it did not allow us to close all the jails and mental hospitals, and it encouraged organized crime and created expensive enforcement efforts.

Regulation after 1933

After national Prohibition, control over alcohol was returned to the provinces and states. Each jurisdiction has since had its own means of regulating alcohol. Although a few jurisdictions remained dry after prohibition, most allowed at least beer sales. Thus, the temperance sentiment that beer was a safer beverage continued to influence policy. In many cases, beer containing no more than 3.2% alcohol by weight was allowed as a "nonintoxicating" beverage.

Over the years the general trend was for a relaxation of laws: provinces and states that did not allow sales of liquor became fewer, until in 1966 the last dry state, Mississippi, became wet. The minimum age to purchase alcoholic beverages was set at 21 in all provinces and states, except Ontario, Prince Edward Island, Quebec, Saskatchewan, New York, and Louisiana.

During the 1970s, many provinces and states lowered the drinking age to 18 or 19. Per capita consumption rates, which were relatively stable during the 1950s, increased steadily from 1965 through 1980. However, pushed by concerns over young people dying in alcohol-related traffic accidents, in the 1980s the U.S. Congress authorized the Transportation Department to withhold a portion of the federal highway funds for any state that did not raise its minimum drinking age to 21. In 1988, the final state raised its drinking age, making 21 the uniform drinking age all across the United States. Today in Canada, the drinking age is 19 in all provinces and territories except Manitoba, Quebec, and Alberta, where it is 18.[3,8]

LO3 Who Drinks? And Why?

Cultural Influences on Drinking

Comparing alcohol use in various cultures around the world allows us to look at ethnic and social factors that lead to differences in patterns of alcohol use. For example, both the Irish and the Russian cultures are associated with heavy drinking, especially of distilled spirits, and with high rates of intoxication and alcohol-related problems. By contrast, Mediterranean countries like Italy and Spain have been characterized by wine consumption, often in a family environment and associated with meals. In these cultures, children are introduced to wine drinking within the family at an early age, but drunkenness is discouraged. A report from the International Center for Alcohol Policies examined young people's attitudes toward drunkenness and their experience with drinking and becoming drunk in several countries around the world. They reported that 17-year-olds in Sweden and other northern European countries were five times as likely to report having been drunk, compared to 17-year-olds in Italy, France, and Greece.[9]

It is important to note that the culture of "extreme drinking" does not necessarily correlate well with overall alcohol consumption. The French and Italians may drink wine in moderation with their meals and in family settings, but they manage to drink a lot of wine. Luxembourg, France, Ireland, and Italy are all among the top countries for total per capita alcohol consumption, but the drinking patterns and alcohol-related problems vary considerably among these countries. It should be pointed out that these comparative statistics are based on reported sales, and Russia is not included because so much alcohol is sold on the black market in that country. As for beer consumption, the Czech Republic leads this list, followed by Germany, Austria, and Ireland.[10] Canada ranks 24th and the United States is 13th in per capita beer consumption.[11]

Figure 9.1 Sales of Alcoholic Beverages per Capita 15 Years and Older by Volume in Canada, 2003 and 2013

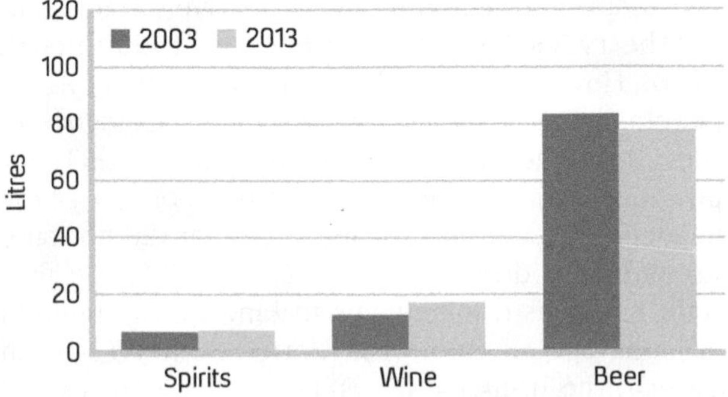

Source: Statistics Canada (2014). Control and Sale of Alcoholic Beverages, for the Year Ending March 31, 2013. Retrieved June 12, 2014 from http://www.statcan.gc.ca/daily-quotidien/140410/dq140410a-eng.htm.

Prevalence and Patterns of Alcohol Use in Canada

In 2013, $21.4 billion worth of alcoholic beverages, equating to approximately 265.4 million litres of absolute alcohol, were sold in Canadian beer stores, liquor stores, and establishments. An estimate of Canadian alcohol consumption may be made based on the volume sales of beer, wine, and spirits. Sales in Canada between 2003 and 2013 are depicted in Figure 9.1. Beer is the number-one choice, both in terms of amount sold (volume) and sales. In 2013 Canadians aged 15 years and older, recognizing the illegal sale to minors, bought just more than 78 litres of beer per person per year (2.3 billion litres).[12]

Canadian Alcohol and Drug Use Monitoring Survey (CADUMS)

The *Canadian Alcohol and Drug Use Monitoring Survey* (CADUMS) is a yearly survey of alcohol and illicit drug use among Canadians aged 15 years and older for which data from 2008 through 2012 are readily available. The most recent results gathered in 2012 from telephone interviews of respondents across all ten provinces represent over 27 million Canadian residents. Although similar to the *Canadian Addiction Survey* (CAS) of 2004, CADUMS has a twofold purpose: first, to determine how many Canadians use alcohol, drugs, and other substances, and second, to determine the influence of substance use both on the user as well as its effects on the nonuser.

Alcohol consumption in the past year (2012) was reported by 78.4% of Canadians surveyed, a trend similar to the previous year (2011) (see Table 9.1). Similar trends were observed in that 82.7% of males (relative to 74.4% of females) and 80% of adults aged 25 years and older (relative to 70% of youth) reported past-year consumption of alcohol (see Table 9.2).

Alcohol Use among Postsecondary Students

Traditionally, the postsecondary years have been associated with increased alcohol use, misuse, and abuse. There is an increased number of individuals consuming

Table 9.1 Prevalence of Alcohol Use and Exceeding Low-Risk Alcohol Drinking Guidelines (LRDG), Total Population, CAS 2004, CADUMS 2008–2012

	CAS			CADUMS		
	2004	**2008**	**2009**	**2010**	**2011**	**2012**
	Overall	Overall	Overall	Overall	Overall	Overall
N	13 909	16 640	13 082	13 615	10 076	11 090
Lifetime Use	92.8 [91.6–93.9]	90.2* [89.2–91.1]	88.6(^) [87.5–89.6]	88.9(*) [87.9–89.9]	89.7^ [88.4–91.0]	91.0 [89.9–92.2]
Past-Year Use	79.3 [78.1–80.5]	77.3 [76.0–78.6]	76.5(^) [75.1–77.8]	77.0(*) [75.6–78.3]	78.0 [76.4–79.5]	78.4 [77.0–79.9]
Average Age of Initiation for Youth 15–24 Years	17.9 [17.8–18.1]	18.0 [17.9–18.2]	18.0 [17.9–18.2]	18.2 [18.0–18.3]	18.1 [18.0–18.3]	18.3 [18.1–18.5]
Exceeding low-risk drinking guidelines[1]						
Exceeds LRDG Chronic	14.3 [13.2–15.3]	15.0 [13.9–16.2]	14.5 [13.3–15.7]	14.5 [13.4–15.6]	14.4 [13.1–15.8]	14.4 [13.1–15.7]
Exceeds LRDG Acute	10.2 [9.2–11.1]	10.9 [9.8–11.9]	11.7 [10.5–12.9]	10.5 [9.5–11.5]	10.1 [8.9–11.2]	9.9 [8.8–11.0]
Exceeds LRDG Chronic—among Drinkers	18.0 [16.7–19.4]	19.8 [18.3–21.2]	19.1 [17.6–20.7]	19.1 [17.6–20.5]	18.7 [17.0–20.4]	18.6 [16.9–20.2]
Exceeds LRDG Acute—among Drinkers	12.9 [11.7–14.0]	14.3 [12.9–15.6]	15.5 [14.0–17.0]	13.8 [12.6–15.1]	13.1 [11.6–14.5]	12.8 [11.4–14.2]

N = Sample size

[95% Confidence Interval]

*Indicates the difference between 2008 and 2004 is statistically significant.

(^)Indicates the difference between 2009 and 2004 is statistically significant.

(*)Indicates the difference between 2010 and 2004 is statistically significant.

^Indicates the difference between 2011 and 2004 is statistically significant.

[1]Based on alcohol consumption in the previous seven days

Source: Canadian Alcohol and Drug Use Monitoring Survey, 2012. Health Canada, 2013. Reproduced with permission from the Minister of Health, 2014.

alcohol during university undergraduate years compared to Canadian youth in general. For example, among undergraduate students, average age 22 years, 85.7% reported drinking within the past year, compared to 82.9% of Canadian youth 15–24 years of age.[13]

Patterns of use for university students differ from those of youth in general: 14.5% and 16.1% of youth and 16.1% and 22.1% of university students report binge drinking (more than four to five drinks in a row for an extended period of time) and light frequent drinking, respectively.

Despite societal pleas for sobriety and the laws and rules supporting such pleas, drinking behaviour itself has not changed much in the past few years. Indeed, increased incidence of alcohol-mediated aggression, vandalism, poor grades, trouble with the police, and absenteeism due to alcohol withdrawal toxicity (i.e., hangover) have been reported.[14] It has been surmised that these unfavourable results of alcohol use are in part influenced by the environment, with more students drinking off campus in drinking establishments that are less controlled and less friendly. Keg parties and alcohol use during recruitment or rush activities have been banned by many fraternities, partly due to legal liability in the event a guest was injured under the influence of alcohol. One ray of hope is that today's postsecondary students are less likely than those of the early 1980s to drive after drinking, although sadly it still occurs.

Two influential national surveys were released in 2004 to assess patterns of alcohol and drug use among undergraduate university and college students (Canadian Campus Survey) and among the general population (Canadian Addiction Survey).[15,16] The *Canadian*

Table 9.2 Canadian Alcohol Consumption (CADUMS 2012), by Sex and Age

	Overall	Male	Female	15–24	25+
N	11 090	4386	6704	687	10 403
Lifetime Use	91.0 [89.9–92.2]	92.9 [91.2–94.5]	89.3* [87.6–90.9]	79.5 [74.7–84.3]	93.1** [92.1–94.1]
Past 12-Month Use	78.4 [77.0–79.9]	82.7 [80.6–84.8]	74.4* [72.4–76.4]	70.0 [64.5–75.5]	80.0** [78.6–81.4]
Past 30 Days Use	63.3 [61.6–65.1]	69.8 [67.1–72.4]	57.2* [55.0–59.5]	49.9 [44.1–55.7]	65.8** [64.1–67.6]
Age of Initiation (years)	18.3 [18.1–18.5]	17.3 [17.1–17.6]	19.2* [19.0–19.5]	16.2 [16.0–16.5]	18.6** [18.4–18.8]

N = Sample size

[95% Confidence Interval]

*Significant difference between males and females

**Significant differences between youth age 15–24 and adults age 25+

Source: Canadian Alcohol and Drug Use Monitoring Survey, 2012. Health Canada, 2013. Reproduced with permission from the Minister of Health, 2014.

Campus Survey included a random sample of over 6200 full-time undergraduate students (fewer than 50% of students eligible to partake) from 40 universities (64 eligible universities) across the country. Students completed questionnaires by mail (56%) or online (44%) during the period between March and April of 2004. Table 9.3 compares the results from identical questions asked in the *Canadian Campus Survey* and the *Canadian Addiction Survey* reporting the same measures for comparison of different populations (therefore, not adding to 100% within rows or columns).

Young adults, especially males, irrespective of university enrollment, are more likely to engage in risky alcohol consumption, hazardous consumption, and harmful consumption (as defined in Table 9.3) than are Canadians 25 years of age or older. The data suggest that weekly, or more often, university students irrespective of gender participate in harmful alcohol consumption

Table 9.3 Patterns of Risky Alcohol Use, Undergraduate Students, General Population Age 18/19–24 and General Population Age 25+, Canada, 2004–05

Measure	Undergraduate Students (Canadian Campus Survey)		General Population Age 18/19–24 (Canadian Addiction Survey)		General Population Age 25+ (Canadian Addiction Survey)	
	Male	Female	Male	Female	Male	Female
5+ drinks on a single occasion at least weekly (4+ for females)	20.6%	12.5%	15.7%	10.3%	6.0%	1.5%
Hazardous consumption (AUDIT 8+)	37.6%	27.5%	36.8%	24.5%	16.5%	4.0%
Harmful consumption (reporting at least one harmful consequence from the AUDIT)	45.9%	42.4%	44.0%	35.7%	19.3%	9.2%

Source: Adapted from Adlaf, E., P. Begin, and E. Sawka (Eds.). (2005). *Canadian Addiction Survey (CAS): A National Survey of Canadians' Use of Alcohol and other Drugs: Prevalence of Use and Related Harms: Detailed Report.* Ottawa: Canadian Centre on Substance Abuse. Retrieved December 2, 2013, from http://www.ccsa.ca/2005%20CCSA%20Documents/ccsa-004028-2005.pdf; and Adlaf, E., A. Demers, and L. Gliksman (Eds.). (2005). *Canadian Campus Survey, 2004.* Toronto: Centre for Addiction and Mental Health. Retrieved December 2, 2013 from http://www.camh.ca/en/research/research_areas/community_and_population_health/Documents/CCS_2004_report.pdf

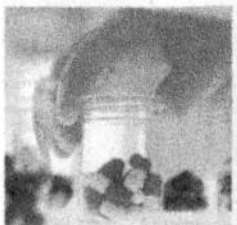

DRUGS IN THE MEDIA

Heavy Drinking a Problem at Most Canadian Campuses—Report: But Many Universities Are Taking Measures to Counter Binge Drinking

It's come to be seen as a rite of passage among students. Each year, along with the start of classes, are the inevitable pub crawls, keg parties and excessive drinking that often accompany frosh week events. But this fall, more universities are cracking down on these behaviours and putting policies in place to discourage binge drinking. Excessive drinking is a common problem at most colleges and universities, sometimes precipitating incidents that make national headlines. St. Patrick's Day festivities sparked a riot last March near Fanshawe College in London, Ontario. Two alcohol-related deaths at Queen's University in 2010 led to a coroner's investigation. And last fall, a student at Acadia University died of alcohol poisoning during orientation week.

Now, a report conducted in response to the death at Acadia says, "Harmful drinking by university students is a problem for most, if not every university." The report by the Nova Scotia Department of Health and Wellness says, "The university environment has a significant role in shaping student behaviours, and as such, the campus context needs to be altered so that it does not support a heavy drinking culture." The report, "Reducing Alcohol Harms among University Students," was published in the spring and recently made available online.

According to one estimate, almost 90 percent of Canadian university students drink alcohol, while 32 percent reported drinking heavily at least once a month. Men drink more than women but the gap is narrowing, the report said. A recent trend among young people is to mix alcohol with caffeinated beverages, which can exacerbate health risks associated with heavy drinking. The study recommends that universities take a comprehensive approach to combat binge drinking. No single intervention, such as a public awareness campaign, is effective in changing student drinking habits, said Lisa Jacobs, the report's author. Focusing on the individual drinker in a university context has a limited impact, she said, "because the actual drinking environment on campus supports, and in some cases promotes, heavy drinking."

Many schools have taken measures to restrict drinking in student dorms, with a growing trend to make residences alcohol-free during orientation week. Western, Guelph, Queen's and others have done so in recent years, and anecdotal evidence suggests the measures are working. Last year, Queen's banned alcohol in its residences during orientation week, reduced the volume of alcohol that of-age students are allowed to have in residence and banned alcohol in residences' common areas. Queen's is also reviewing its campus alcohol policy and developing a new disciplinary system for violations.

University of Alberta recently announced a ban on drinking in common areas of its undergraduate student residences starting in September on a year-round basis. Last year, pathways below dorm rooms were routinely littered with broken glass from students tossing bottles out of windows and several drunk students, found lying in vomit, had to be taken to hospital. "It's incomprehensible to defend a culture and a system that fosters and celebrates this type of behaviour," said Frank Robinson, U of A's vice-provost and dean of students. The university is moving ahead with the measures despite vigorous opposition from students.

At the University of Saskatchewan, students launched the Student Binge Drinking Prevention Initiative last year. The research project, which evolved from a senior-year sociology class on addiction, recruits student volunteers to conduct surveys and focus groups. They plan to use the data to create an advertising and social media campaign to discourage students from binge drinking and to produce a how-to guide for other universities.

Carleton University controls who is admitted to its undergraduate pub and what can be served there. "Thursday nights were like fight night," said Ryan Flannagan, Carleton's director of student affairs, as large numbers of non-Carleton patrons would flock to the pub. Carleton's campus safety officers were routinely assaulted and Ottawa Police were often on site. When someone was stabbed six years ago, said Mr. Flannagan, "that was basically the last straw." Since then, Carleton students must sign in any off-campus guests to the pub, and only one at a time. In the pub, there is a ban on shots, a limit of one pitcher of beer per person and no sales of pitchers after midnight. Regular meetings with student union representatives and campus bar managers review incidents to identify what went wrong. The changes, though initially opposed by students, have turned things around. "It's dramatically different,"

continued

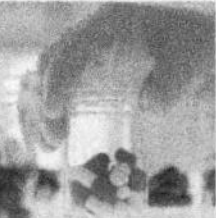

DRUGS IN THE MEDIA

Heavy Drinking a Problem at Most Canadian Campuses—Report: But Many Universities Are Taking Measures to Counter Binge Drinking

continued

Mr. Flannagan said. "It's a safe place for students to go so they can have fun with their peers." Carleton is now developing a broader alcohol strategy to address responsible drinking on campus, with built-in accountability measures, said Mr. Flannagan. He would like to see a marketing campaign to educate students on what constitutes responsible drinking. Behavioural change takes time, but past efforts have helped reduce rates of both smoking and drinking and driving, he noted. "We need the same type of effort to combat binge drinking by students."

Source: Adapted from University Affairs (2012). Heavy Drinking a Problem at Most Canadian Campuses: Report. But many universities are taking measures to counter binge drinking. By Rosanna Tamburri, Previously published in the October 2012 issue of *University Affairs*. Reprinted with permission of *University Affairs*.

as indicated by the World Health Organization's Alcohol Use Disorder Identification Test (AUDIT). AUDIT is a simple, reliable screening tool sensitive to early detection of risky and problematic (hazardous and harmful) alcohol use. The ten AUDIT questions survey alcohol consumption (three questions), drinking behaviour and dependence (three questions), and consequences or problems related to drinking (four questions). A score of 8 or higher is indicative of hazardous drinking.

Regional Differences in Alcohol Use in Canada

Regional differences exist across Canada with regard to alcohol consumption, at least as estimated by alcohol sales. The value of sales of alcoholic beverages per capita (combining beer, wine, and spirits) for the provinces and territories in 2013 is shown in Table 9.4.

The highest per capita sales occur in Yukon, followed by Newfoundland and Labrador; New Brunswick has the lowest. The differences in per capita sales may loosely reflect differences in the proportion of drinkers in various parts of the country. It does not account for homemade brews and wines, however.

More than 75% of Canadians reported alcohol consumption in 2012, similar to the rates the previous year as per the CADUMS. The lowest reported rates were in Nova Scotia at 72.3% and the highest in Quebec at 82.1%. When compared with the average for the nine remaining provinces, Nova Scotia, New Brunswick (73.8%), and Prince Edward Island (74.0%) fell below average, while alcohol use in Quebec was higher than the national average. These patterns were unchanged from 2011.[17]

Table 9.4 Sales of Alcoholic Beverages per Capita, Age 15 Years and Over, 2013

	Beer	Wine	Spirits	Total
		dollars		
Canada	**314.1**	**233.9**	**185.7**	**733.7**
Newfoundland and Labrador	518.0	147.1	316.3	981.4
Prince Edward Island	356.6	141.3	229.8	727.7
Nova Scotia	365.8	160.7	244.5	771.0
New Brunswick	329.5	132.8	169.0	631.3
Quebec	337.4	339.2	104.2	780.7
Ontario	282.9	201.9	184.6	669.4
Manitoba	308.1	144.3	247.1	699.6
Saskatchewan	332.3	103.3	271.1	706.7
Alberta	332.6	193.3	235.9	761.7
British Columbia	302.9	273.1	225.6	801.5
Yukon	646.8	282.1	403.1	1,332.1
Northwest Territories and Nunavut	408.6	146.0	399.8	954.4

Source: Statistics Canada (2014). Control and Sale of Alcoholic Beverages, for the Year Ending March 31, 2013. Retrieved June 5, 2014 from http://www.statcan.gc.ca/daily-quotidien/140410/dq140410a-eng.htm

LO4 Alcohol Pharmacology

Absorption

Some alcohol is absorbed from the stomach, but the small intestine is responsible for most absorption. In an empty stomach, the overall rate of absorption depends primarily on the concentration of alcohol. Alcohol taken with or after a meal is absorbed more slowly because the food remains in the stomach for digestive action, and the protein in the food retains the alcohol with it in the stomach. Plain water, by decreasing the concentration, slows the absorption of alcohol, but carbonated liquids speed it up. The carbon dioxide acts to move everything quite rapidly through the stomach to the small intestine. It is because of this emptying of the stomach and the more rapid absorption of alcohol in the intestine that champagne has a faster onset of action than noncarbonated wine.

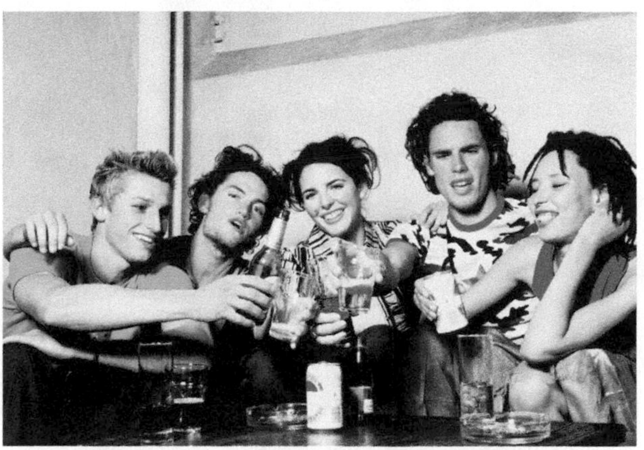

Alcohol abuse by postsecondary students usually occurs through binge drinking, which is defined as having five or more drinks in a row.

Distribution

The relationship between **blood alcohol concentration** (BAC) and alcohol intake is relatively simple and reasonably well understood. When taken into the body, alcohol is distributed throughout the body fluids, including the blood. However, alcohol does not distribute much into fatty tissues, so a 180-pound lean person will have a lower BAC than a 180-pound fat person who drinks the same amount of alcohol.

Table 9.5 demonstrates the relationships among alcohol intake, BAC, and body weight for hypothetical,

blood alcohol concentration (blood alcohol level): a measure of the concentration of alcohol in blood, expressed in grams per 100 mL (percentage).

Table 9.5 Relationships among Gender, Weight, Alcohol Consumption, and Blood-Alcohol Concentration

		Blood-Alcohol Concentrations (g/100 mL)					
Absolute Alcohol (grams/ounces)	**Beverage Intake***	**Female (45 kg/ 100 lb)**	**Male (45 kg/ 100 lb)**	**Female (70 kg/ 150 lb)**	**Male (70 kg/ 150 lb)**	**Female (90 kg/ 200 lb)**	**Male (90 kg/ 200 lb)**
14/0.5	28 g (1 oz) spirits† 1 glass wine 1 can beer	0.045	0.037	0.03	0.025	0.022	0.019
28/1	56 g (2 oz) spirits† 2 glasses wine 2 cans beer	0.090	0.075	0.06	0.050	0.045	0.037
56/2	112 g (4 oz) spirits† 4 glasses wine 4 cans beer	0.180	0.150	0.12	0.100	0.090	0.070
84/3	168 g (6 oz) spirits† 6 glasses wine 6 cans beer	0.270	0.220	0.18	0.150	0.130	0.110
112/4	224 g (8 oz) spirits† 8 glasses wine 8 cans beer	0.360	0.300	0.24	0.200	0.180	0.150
140/5	280 g (10 oz) spirits† 10 glasses wine 10 cans beer	0.450	0.370	0.30	0.250	0.220	0.180

*In one hour

†100-proof

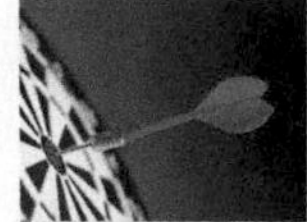

TARGETING PREVENTION

Estimating Blood-Alcohol Concentration

Table 9.5 is one way to estimate blood alcohol level based on gender, weight, and number of drinks. However, more dynamic blood-alcohol calculators are now available on the Internet. An Internet search for "blood alcohol calculator" turns up several. Whether or not you consume alcohol, it is instructive to understand how your own body (and brain) will respond to various numbers of alcoholic drinks. Try a few of the Internet calculators to see how their results compare with each other and with Table 9.5. An important thing for you to learn is how many drinks it is likely to take to bring your BAC to 0.08%, which is the legal limit for driving in Canada and the United States.

Compared with men, women absorb a greater proportion of the alcohol they drink. Some metabolism of alcohol actually occurs in the stomach, where the enzyme alcohol dehydrogenase is present. Because this stomach enzyme is more active, on the average, in men than in women, women might be more susceptible to the effects of alcohol.[18]

Notice that several beverages are equated to 0.5 ounce of absolute alcohol. A 12-ounce can or bottle of beer at about 4% alcohol contains $12 \times 0.04 = 0.48$ ounce of alcohol. The same amount is found in a glass containing about 4 ounces of wine at 12% alcohol, 1 ounce of 100-proof spirits, or 1.25 ounces of 80-proof spirits. Each of these can be equated as a standard "drink."

We have not yet considered metabolism, but we can do so with one more simple calculation. Alcohol is removed by the liver at a constant rate of 0.25 to 0.30 ounce of ethanol per hour. Most people fall within this range no matter what their body size or drinking experience, unless they have consumed so much alcohol that the liver is damaged. To be on the safe side, estimate that you can metabolize about 0.25 ounce per hour, and note that this is one-half of one of our standard drinks (1 beer, 1 shot, or 1 glass of wine). Over the course of an evening, if your rate of intake equals your rate of metabolism, you will maintain a stable BAC. If you drink faster than one drink every two hours, your BAC will climb.

Figure 9.2 The Relationship between Blood Alcohol Concentration and Alcohol Intake

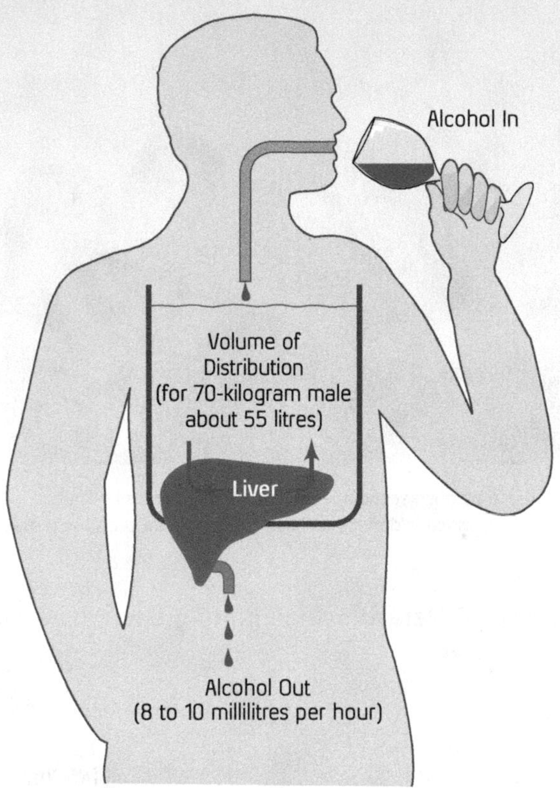

Compared with men, women absorb a greater proportion of the alcohol they drink. Some metabolism of alcohol actually occurs in the stomach, where the enzyme alcohol dehydrogenase is present. Because this stomach enzyme is more active, on the average, in men than in women, women might be more susceptible to the effects of alcohol.[18] Most alcohol is administered orally. However, other models of administration are being experimented with.

average females and males. The chart distinguishes between the sexes because the average female has a higher proportion of body fat and therefore, for a given weight, has less volume in which to distribute the alcohol. Understanding this table and trying one of the blood alcohol calculators on the Internet (see Targeting Prevention) could reveal how much you can probably drink to avoid going above a specified BAC.

Table 9.5 makes the simplifying assumption that all of the alcohol is absorbed quickly so there is little opportunity for metabolism. If the 150-pound female had a tank of water weighing about 100 pounds (12.5 gallons, or 45 litres) and just dumped 1 ounce (28.3 g) into it and stirred it, the concentration would be about 0.6 g/L, or 0.06 g/100 mL (0.06%). Figure 9.2 shows a schematic of such a tank. The 150-pound average male has a tank with more water in it, so his alcohol concentration after 1 ounce is about 0.05%. The major factor determining individual differences in BAC is the volume of distribution, so find your own weight on Table 9.5 and estimate how many drinks could be poured into your tank to obtain a BAC of 0.05%.

Metabolism

Once absorbed alcohol remains in the bloodstream and other body fluids until it is metabolized, and more than 90% of this metabolism occurs in the liver. A small amount of alcohol, less than 2%, is normally excreted unchanged–some in the breath, some through the skin, and some in the urine.

The primary metabolic system is a simple one: the enzyme *alcohol dehydrogenase* converts alcohol to *acetaldehyde*. Acetaldehyde is then converted fairly rapidly by aldehyde dehydrogenase to acetic acid. With most drugs a constant *proportion* of the drug is removed in a given amount of time, so that with a high blood level the amount metabolized is high. With alcohol, the *amount* that can be metabolized is constant at about 0.25 to 0.30 ounces per hour regardless of the BAC. The major factor determining the rate of alcohol metabolism is the activity of the enzyme alcohol dehydrogenase. Exercise, coffee consumption, and so on have no effect on this enzyme, so the sobering-up process is essentially a matter of waiting for this enzyme to do its job at its own speed.

Acetaldehyde might be more than just an intermediate step in the oxidation of alcohol. Acetaldehyde is quite toxic; though its blood levels are only one-thousandth of those of alcohol, this substance might cause some of the physiological effects now attributed to alcohol. One danger in heavy alcohol use might be in the higher blood levels of acetaldehyde.

The liver responds to chronic intake of alcohol by increasing the activity of metabolic enzymes (see Chapter 5). This gives rise to some interesting situations. In a person who drinks alcohol heavily over a long period, the activity of the metabolic enzymes increases. As long as there is alcohol in the system, alcohol gets preferential treatment and the metabolism of other drugs is *slower* than normal. When heavy alcohol use stops and the alcohol has disappeared from the body, the high activity level of the enzymes continues for four to eight weeks. During this time other drugs are metabolized more *rapidly*. To obtain therapeutic levels of other drugs metabolized by this enzyme system (e.g., the benzodiazepines), it is necessary to administer less drug to a chronic heavy drinker and more drug to one who has recently stopped drinking. Thus, alcohol increases the activity of one of the two enzyme systems responsible for its own oxidation. The increased activity of this enzyme is a partial basis for the tolerance to alcohol that is shown by heavy users of alcohol.

Mechanism(s) of Action

Alcohol is like any other general anaesthetic: It depresses the CNS. It was used as an anaesthetic until the late nineteenth century, when nitrous oxide, ether, and chloroform became more widely used. However, it was not just new compounds that decreased alcohol's use as an anaesthetic; alcohol itself has some major disadvantages. In contrast to the gaseous anaesthetics, alcohol metabolizes slowly. This gives alcohol a long duration of action that cannot be controlled. A second disadvantage is that the dose effective in surgical anaesthesia is not much lower than the dose that causes respiratory arrest and death. Finally, alcohol makes blood slower to clot.

The exact mechanism for the CNS effect of alcohol is not clear. Until the mid-1980s, the most widely accepted theory was that alcohol acted on all neural membranes, perhaps altering their electrical excitability. However, with increased understanding of the role of the GABA receptor complex in the actions of other depressant drugs (see Chapter 7), researchers began to study the effects of alcohol on GABA receptors. As with the barbiturates and benzodiazepines, alcohol enhances the inhibitory effects of GABA at the GABA-A receptor. This would explain the similarity of behavioural effects among these three different

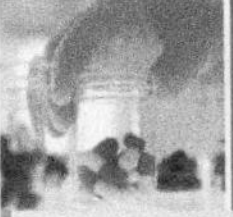

DRUGS IN THE MEDIA

Bottoms Up: Risky Alcohol Abuse Practices of Canadian Youth

Alcohol abuse in adolescent and university-aged student populations is a significant problem in North America.[19,20] For example, the minimum legal drinking age (MLDA) in Ontario is 19 years old; from April 2002 to March 2007, in the months after reaching the MLDA, there were significant associated increases in alcohol-use disorders and assaults related to alcohol use among young adults that warranted treatment in an emergency department or inpatient setting.[21]

Urban myths and trends related to substance abuse are not uncommon. The accessibility and popularity of social media allows videos or stories of substance abuse practices to go viral and be viewed around the world. Unusual examples of alcohol abuse include vodka being poured over an open eyeball[22]; vodka-soaked tampons being inserted into the vagina or rectum[23]; and alcohol being funnelled into the rectum.[23] These atypical routes of administration can be harmful: the application of alcohol could cause pain, damage mucosal tissue, and possibly compromise innate antimicrobial environments.[24,25] Why are young adults attempting these risky practices? Accurately studying the true incidence and prevalence of university students' drinking habits is difficult, because alcohol abuse is likely underrecognized or underreported by the students.[20]

One trend, the consumption of alcohol mixed with energy drinks (AmED), is associated with increased risk-taking behaviours compared to university students consuming alcohol alone.[20] AmED use was associated with increased heavy episodic drinking, drinking more alcohol than on a typical drinking occasion, and more negative consequences related to drinking.[20] One study[26] found that university students who had consumed AmED at a bar had a fourfold increased risk of intending to drive while intoxicated compared to their peers who consumed only alcohol.

The potential harms associated with non-oral routes of administering alcohol aren't the only risk. After an alcoholic beverage is swallowed, the ethanol diffuses from the gut into the bloodstream, elevating the blood alcohol concentration (BAC), and is subsequently circulated and distributed throughout organs and tissues.

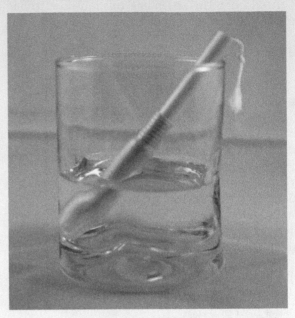

Alcohol absorbs through mucous membranes including vaginal and rectal membranes with significant risk of damage to tissue.

Several enzymes throughout the body, mostly in the liver, metabolize the majority of ethanol; the remainder is eliminated in the breath, urine, feces, sweat, and breast milk. Intra-rectal alcohol diffuses directly into the bloodstream, theoretically resulting in a higher BAC and more immediate effect than if the alcohol were ingested. Light physical exercise can also increase BAC, because systemic blood flow is diverted away from the liver, gastrointestinal tract, spleen and pancreas, and redirected to skeletal muscle.[27] A sustained high BAC can significantly impair brain function, which can manifest as a decreased level of consciousness and impaired airway reflexes, such as coughing to clear the airway after vomiting.[28] Alcohol can also interact with medications or substances in the blood, potentially affecting bioavailability, intended therapeutic effects, and causing harm secondary to substance toxicity.[29,30] Plenty of inherent risk is associated with ingesting alcohol, but oral consumption can be enjoyed responsibly in moderation.

The authors thank Ryan J. Mitchell, BScN, RN for article contribution.

kinds of chemicals. But alcohol has many other effects in the brain, so it has been very difficult to pin down a single mechanism. No matter what neurotransmitter or receptor or transporter is examined, alcohol appears to alter its function in some way. Because alcohol's ability to enhance GABA inhibition at the GABA-A receptor occurs at very low doses, this mechanism probably has special importance. Remember that GABA is a widespread inhibitory neurotransmitter, so alcohol tends to have widespread inhibitory effects on neurons in the brain. Chronic alcohol use incites adaptations in $GABA_A$ receptor function, expression, and trafficking. These changes may underlie alcohol-related tolerance, dependence, and withdrawal hyperexcitability.[31,32]

At higher doses alcohol also blocks the effects of the excitatory transmitter glutamate at some of its receptors, so this may enhance its overall inhibitory actions. Glutamate is the major excitatory neurotransmitter in the brain. How does alcohol affect glutamate? Alcohol has been shown to inhibit glutamate's excitatory action by inhibiting the N-methyl-D-aspartate (NMDA) receptor. It is not known precisely the mechanism by which alcohol inhibits NMDA receptor function, yet a direct interaction of alcohol with the NMDA receptor regulating channel gating is suspected.[33] NMDA receptors are found in the cortex, hippocampus, and nucleus accumbens, areas implicated in cognition and reward.

Alcohol also produces a variety of effects on dopamine, serotonin, and acetylcholine neurons, and researchers continue to explore these various actions with an eye to understanding not only the acute intoxicating effects of alcohol, but also the long-term changes that occur when the brain is exposed to alcohol on a chronic basis. One of the oldest and chemically simplest psychoactive drugs also seems to have the most complicated set of effects on the nervous system.

LO5 Behavioural Effects

At the lowest effective blood levels, complex, abstract, and poorly learned behaviours are disrupted. As the alcohol dose increases, better learned and simpler behaviours are also affected. Inhibitions can be reduced, with the result that the overall amount of behaviour

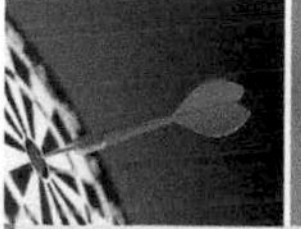

TARGETING PREVENTION

Signs of Alcohol Poisoning

Although most alcohol-related deaths among postsecondary students are due to accidents, every year we hear of tragedies involving students who simply drink themselves to death. You might be in a position to save someone's life if you know the signs of alcohol poisoning and what to do.

Signs

1. The person is unconscious or semiconscious (unable to answer simple questions).
2. Breathing rate is slow (less than 8 breaths per minute) or irregular (10 seconds between any two breaths).
3. The person's skin is cold and clammy, pale, or has a bluish tinge.
4. Vomiting and then losing consciousness.

What to Do

1. NEVER leave someone who is this drunk alone to "sleep it off."
2. Call 911 if the person is unconscious or incoherent.
3. If you have been drinking, try to get someone who is sober to help. BUT, don't be afraid to call for help yourself. Many postsecondary institutions have formal "medical amnesty" policies, meaning you can't get in trouble for helping someone who is in a medical emergency. Even without such a policy, campus officials will be happy that you took action.
4. Monitor breathing while waiting for help, and roll the person on his or her side to keep vomit from drowning them. If the person does vomit, be sure to clear the airway.

Adapted from the University of Arizona's StepUp program.

increases under certain conditions. Even though alcohol can result in an increase in activity, most scientists would not call alcohol a stimulant. Rather, the increased behavioural output is usually attributed to decreased inhibition of behaviour.

If the alcohol intake is "just right," most people experience euphoria, a happy feeling. Below a certain BAC there are no mood changes, but at some point we become uninhibited enough to enjoy our own "charming selves" and uncritical enough to accept the "clods" around us. We become witty, clever, and quite sophisticated, or at least it seems we are.

Another factor contributing to the feeling of well-being is the reduction in anxieties as a result of the disruption of normal critical thinking. The reduction in concern and judgment can range from not worrying about who'll pay the bar bill to being sure that you can take that next curve at 60 mph.

These effects depend on the BAC–also called blood alcohol level (BAL). As noted previously, BAC is reported as the number of grams of alcohol in 100 mL of blood and is expressed as a percentage. For example, 100 g in 100 mL is 100%, and 100 mg of alcohol in 100 mL of blood is reported as 0.10%.

Before suggesting relationships between BAC and behavioural change, two factors must be mentioned. One is that the rate at which the BAC rises is a factor in determining behavioural effects. The more rapid the increase, the greater the behavioural effects. Second, a higher BAC is necessary to impair the performance of a chronic, heavy drinker than to impair a moderate drinker's performance.

Performance differences might reflect only the extent to which experienced drinkers have learned to overcome the disruption of nervous system functioning. Another explanation might be that the CNS in the regular drinker develops a tolerance to alcohol. It is established that neural tissue becomes tolerant to alcohol, and tolerance can apparently develop even when the alcohol intake is well spaced over time.

Table 9.6 describes some general behavioural effects of increasing doses of alcohol. These relationships are approximately correct for moderate drinkers. There are some reports that changes in nervous system function have been obtained at concentrations as low as 0.03 to 0.04%.

The surgical anaesthesia level and the minimum lethal level are perhaps the two least precise points in the table. In any case, they are quite close, and the safety margin is less than 0.1% blood alcohol. Death resulting from acute alcohol intoxication usually is the result of respiratory failure when the medulla is depressed.

Scientific study of the behavioural effects of alcohol is made difficult by the importance of placebo effects. With a substance as pervasive as alcohol, we have a long history of learning about what to expect from this substance, even before taking a drink (and even for those who never drink). Culture passes along a rich set of ideas about how alcohol is supposed to affect people, and we need to be sure which of the many behavioural changes we see after people drink are actually due to the pharmacological effects of having alcohol in the system. A number of laboratory studies have focused on alcohol effects using the *balanced placebo* design. Half the study participants are given mixed drinks that contain alcohol, while the other half get similar-tasting drinks without alcohol. Each of those groups is divided in half, with some being told they are getting alcohol (whether they are or not) and

Table 9.6 Blood Alcohol Concentration and Behavioural Effects

Percent BAC	Behavioural Effects
0.05	Lowered alertness, usually good feeling, release of inhibitions, impaired judgment
0.10	Slower reaction times and impaired motor function, less caution
0.15	Large, consistent increases in reaction time
0.20	Marked depression in sensory and motor capability, intoxication
0.25	Severe motor disturbance, staggering, sensory perceptions, great impairment
0.30	Stuporous but conscious—no comprehension of what's going on
0.35	Surgical anaesthesia; about LD_1, minimal level causing death
0.40	About LD_{50} BAC known to cause death in 50% of people

others being told they are testing a nonalcohol drink. By analyzing the behavioural effects seen in the four conditions, it is possible to determine which effects are actually produced by alcohol and which by the belief that one has consumed alcohol (alcohol expectancy effects). Many of the effects on social behaviour (increased laughter, talkativeness, flirtation) are strongly influenced by expectancy even when no alcohol has been consumed, whereas such things as impairment in reaction times and driving simulators result from actual alcohol consumption even when the participant is not aware of the alcohol in the drink. Clearly such studies are limited to the effects of fairly low doses, because if enough alcohol is consumed the participants can detect its effects.

Time-Out and Alcohol Myopia

Many of the effects experienced by drinkers are based on what they expect to happen, which interacts somewhat with the pharmacological effects of alcohol. One important component of alcohol use is that drinking serves as a social signal, to the drinker and others, indicating a "time-out" from responsibilities, work, and seriousness. Sitting down with a drink indicates "I'm off duty now" and "Don't take anything I say too seriously." Steele and Josephs proposed that alcohol induces a kind of social and behavioural myopia, or nearsightedness.[34] After drinking, people tend to focus more on the here and now and to pay less attention to peripheral people and activities, and to long-term consequences. That might be why some people are more violent after drinking, whereas others become more helpful even if there is personal risk or cost involved. The idea is that alcohol releases people from their inhibitions, largely because the inhibitions represent concerns about what might happen, whereas the intoxicated individual focuses on the immediate irritant or the person who needs help right now.

Driving under the Influence

Attention was focused in the early 1980s on the large number of traffic fatalities involving alcohol. As an example, 60% of traffic fatalities in Canada in 1982 were alcohol related. Although the percentage dropped in 2007 to approximately 40%, societal costs of alcohol-related traffic deaths and injuries remained significant; this is exemplified by the estimated 1054 fatalities and 60 000 injuries related to driving while intoxicated reported in Canada in 2007.

Several studies have demonstrated that the danger of combining alcohol with automobiles is dose-related. At a BAC of 0.08% the relative risk of being involved in a fatal crash is about three times as great as for a sober driver. A British study on younger, less experienced drivers (and drinkers) found that the relative risk at 0.08% was about five times as great. The risk rises sharply for all drivers with a BAC above 0.10. Similarly, the risk of involvement in a personal injury crash increases with BAC, as does the risk of involvement in a fatal pedestrian accident.

With respect to age, drinking drivers come from all age groups but younger drivers have more than their share of alcohol-related accidents. Table 9.7 shows a

Table 9.7 Percentage of Drinking Drivers in Fatal Crashes Compared with Licensed Drivers by Age Group for Canada, 2003–2005

Age Group	% of Drinking Drivers in Fatal Crashes	% of Licensed Drivers
16–19 years	10.7%	4.8%
20–24 years	21.6%	8.1%
25–34 years	25.1%	17.7%
35–44 years	19.6%	21.7%
45–54 years	13.2%	20.6%
55–64 years	6.2%	14.2%
65+ years	3.7%	12.9%

Source: Transport Canada. *Road Safety and Motor Vehicle Regulation Directorate Fact Sheet TP 2436E: A Quick Look at Alcohol-Related Crashes in Canada.* 2008. Retrieved October 2, 2011, from http://www.tc.gc.ca/eng/roadsafety/tp-tp2436-rs200809-menu-397.htm.

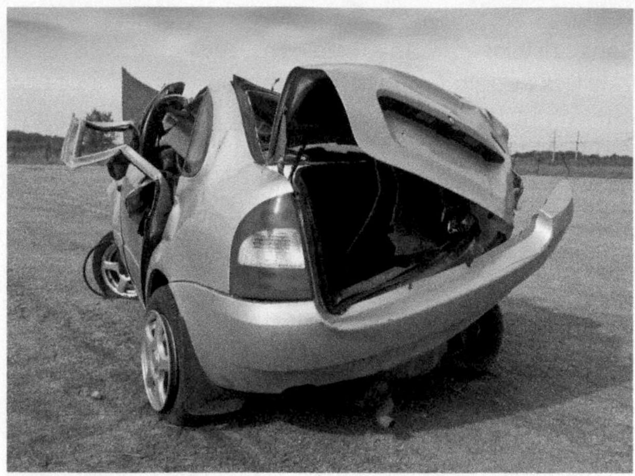

The risk of crashes rises with increasing BAC, with a sharp increase at BACs above 0.10.

breakdown of the number of drinking drivers involved in fatal crashes by age group.

More than 75% of drinking drivers involved in fatal crashes between the years 2003 and 2005 were under the age of 45, with the highest rate of alcohol involvement in traffic fatalities being among 21–24-year-olds. Figure 9.3 depicts a change consistent with the general aging of the population in Canada. Between 1996 to 2001 and 2003 to 2005, more middle-aged drivers who consumed alcohol were involved in fatal crashes.

Figure 9.3 Drinking Drivers in Fatal Crashes by Age Group, Percentage Increase or Decrease in Number from 1996–2001 to 2003–2005

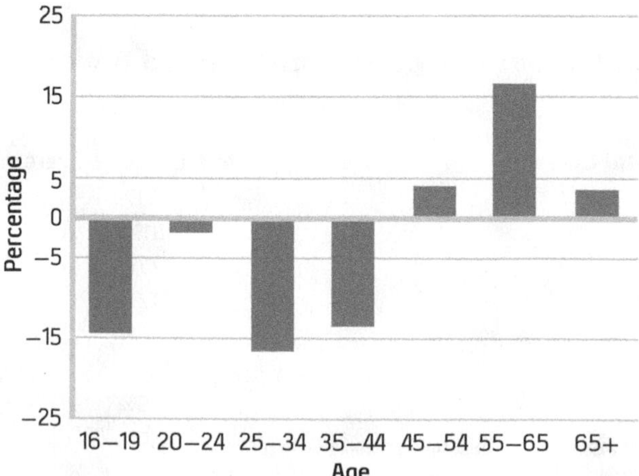

Source: Transport Canada. *Road Safety and Motor Vehicle Regulation Directorate Fact Sheet TP 2436E: A Quick Look at Alcohol-Related Crashes in Canada.* 2008. Retrieved October 2, 2011, from http://www.tc.gc.ca/eng/roadsafety/tp-tp2436-rs200809-menu-397.htm.

What can be done about this problem? Current efforts focus mainly on three fronts: identifying repeat offenders and keeping them off the roads, publicizing in the mass media the dangers of drinking and driving, and targeting younger drinkers for special prevention efforts. The "breathalyzer law" in 1969 criminalized drivers with a BAC greater than 0.08%; it has effectively reduced alcohol fatality rates by 18%. Mothers Against Drunk Driving (MADD) and its predecessor, People to Reduce Impaired Driving Everywhere, resulted in a 19–23% reduction in drinking-driver fatality rates.[35,36]

Other interesting facts have emerged from studies of alcohol and accidents. Alcohol-related traffic fatalities are not a random sample of all fatalities. Single-vehicle fatalities are more likely to involve alcohol than are multiple-vehicle fatalities. Alcohol-related fatalities are a greater proportion of the fatalities occurring during dark hours than of those occurring in daylight and are a greater proportion of fatalities occurring on the weekend than of those occurring during the week. Fatally injured drivers in accidents occurring between midnight and 3 AM are 8 times as likely to have a BAC above 0.08% as drivers in accidents occurring between 9 AM and noon.

When you hear that about 85% of all the fatally injured drivers who had been drinking were male, that sounds like a big difference, and it is. But it is important to remember that 70% of all fatally injured drivers are male, whether or not drinking is involved. That men are more likely to be involved in alcohol-related traffic fatalities reflects three important facts: Any given car is more likely to have a male than a female driver, men might take more chances when driving even when they're sober, and male drivers are more likely than female drivers to have been drinking.

What's a safe BAC? If you are going to drink and want to remain in reasonable control of your faculties, you should probably stay below 0.05%. Individuals differ considerably in their sensitivities to alcohol, however, so the best rule is to learn about your own sensitivity and not to feel compelled to keep up with anyone else's drinking. Alcohol-induced impairment is dose-related and depends on what you're trying to do. Carrying on bar conversation places fewer demands on your nervous system than driving on a crowded freeway during rush hour, where any alcohol at all might interfere.

BAC gives a good estimate of the alcohol concentration in the brain, and the concentration of alcohol in the breath gives a good estimate of the alcohol concentration in the blood. The concentration in the blood is almost 2100 times the concentration in air expired from the lungs, making breath samples accurate indicators of BAC. Such breath samples are easily collected by police and can be the basis for conviction as a drunk driver in most jurisdictions. It is a criminal offence in both Canada and the United States to drive a vehicle with a BAC of 0.08% or higher, and the penalties are severe.[35,37] Licence suspension and administrative fines are issued to drivers with BAC levels of 0.05% or lower in many Canadian provinces, with many having established zero tolerance (BAC level of zero) for novice drivers.[35]

Sexual Behaviour

No psychoactive substance has been as closely linked to sexuality as alcohol. Movies tell us that a romantic occasion is enhanced with wine or champagne, and the use of sexual attraction in beer ads on television is so common we are barely aware of it. The association has been noted for generations–400 years ago Shakespeare wrote about alcohol in *Macbeth:* "Lechery, sir, it provokes and unprovokes; it provokes the desire, but it takes away the performance."

Was Shakespeare right? It certainly seems that alcohol does make people less inhibited, and more likely to desire sex, but can we demonstrate that this is a real effect? If so, how much of the enhancement of sexual interest after drinking is really due to the pharmacological effects of the alcohol, and how much is a placebo response based on our expectancies about alcohol's effects? The importance of understanding alcohol's ability to provoke desire is enormous. On one hand, many people of both sexes for many generations and across many cultures have viewed alcohol's ability to enhance sexual interest and pleasure as a great benefit, and many will continue to do so. On the other hand, the use of alcohol is linked with risky sexual behaviour (early sexual experience; unprotected sex) as well as with increased likelihood of sexual assault. The analogy to "playing with fire" is an apt one–under the right circumstances both fire and alcohol are beneficial, but both are risky and can lead to destructive outcomes.

And what about the other half of Shakespeare's statement, that alcohol takes away the performance? Anecdotal evidence shows that men with high BACs are unable to attain or maintain an erection, and there is clinical evidence that chronic alcohol abuse can lead to more permanent impotence in men. But are these effects consistent, and are they limited to high doses or long-term exposure?

Human sexual response is complex, but we can somewhat artificially divide our questions about sexuality into psychological effects (ratings of sexual arousal or interest) versus physiological effects (measurements of penile tumescence or vaginal blood volume; measurements of time to orgasm). Also, we should assume that men and women may differ considerably with respect to both dimensions of sexuality and alcohol's effects on them.

A review of the available literature on alcohol and sex points out some still unresolved questions, but also some reliable findings reported by different sets of researchers.[38] First, both men and women tend to agree with the expectancy statements that alcohol enhances or disinhibits sexuality. In balanced-placebo laboratory experiments, men who had stronger expectancies that alcohol would enhance sexuality also reported experiencing more arousal after being given a placebo drink. Therefore, at least some of the subjective arousal that men experience after drinking is a psychological reaction to the belief that alcohol enhances sexuality. There have been fewer such experiments with women, and the results have been inconsistent.

When men and women have been given alcohol in a laboratory setting and then exposed to erotic films, both sexes report more sexual arousal after alcohol, and there is a correlation between their ratings of feeling intoxicated and their self-reported arousal. These studies have not usually explored BACs above 0.15%, and most have used lower BACs. In men, physiological measures of penile tumescence are correlated with self-reports of arousal, whereas in women there is no consistent relation between self-reported arousal and vaginal blood volume.

Many studies have reported that alcohol reduces penile tumescence in men, sometimes even at fairly low doses. The long-standing assumption has been that this is a direct pharmacological effect on the physiological mechanisms responsible for penile erection. However, several studies have found no effect on this measure, even at fairly high doses. Studies on animals and on nocturnal penile tumescence in men who are asleep have generally not found that alcohol suppresses erection. Therefore, attention is now shifting to the idea that when men become less aroused at higher BACs it might be due to impaired attention to or processing of erotic information. Alcohol can also impair the ability to suppress an erection when men are instructed to avoid becoming aroused.

Several studies have reported that when men believe that a woman has been drinking, they rate her as being more interested in sex and more sexually available. A similar finding has been reported for women's perceptions of men who have been drinking.

Surveys typically find that people are more likely to have sex on a date (including first dates) when they drink on that date. With respect to risky sex, both men and women given alcohol in laboratory situations report more willingness to engage in unprotected sex, and more agreement with justifications for not using condoms.

We know that alcohol is a frequent presence in sexual assaults, and laboratory studies on college students have reported some related findings. When a date rape scene is described to either men or women, less blame is assigned to the perpetrator if he has been described as drinking before the rape, and more blame is assigned to the victim if she has been described as drinking. Men are generally more aroused by nonviolent erotic films than by erotic films that contain violence, but after consuming alcohol in the laboratory, they were less discriminating and more likely to be aroused by the violent films.

Many of these effects of alcohol on sexual behaviour are consistent with the alcohol myopia theory mentioned previously—alcohol impairs information processing in such a way that people are more likely to attend to what's right in front of them at the time. In a conflicting sexual situation, the person affected by alcohol will be more likely to tend toward immediate gratification and less likely to be inhibited by concerns about outcomes that are uncertain or delayed.

Blackouts

Alcohol-induced blackouts are periods during alcohol use in which the drinking individual appears to function normally but later, when the individual is sober, he or she cannot recall any events that occurred during that period. The drinker might drive home or dance all night, interacting in the usual way with others. When the individual cannot remember the activities, the people, or anything else, that's a blackout. Most authorities include it as one of the danger signs suggesting excessive use of alcohol. The limited amount of recent research on this topic is probably related to ethical concerns about giving such high doses of alcohol to experimental subjects. An article from 1884 titled "Alcoholic Trance" referred to the syndrome: "This trance state is a common condition in inebriety, where . . . a profound suspension of memory and consciousness and literal paralysis of certain brain-functions follow."[39] This trance state may last from a few moments to several days, during which the person may appear and act rationally, and yet be actually a mere automaton, without consciousness or memory of his actual condition.

Crime and Violence

Homicide The correlation between alcohol use and homicides is well known to police and judicial systems around the world. Based on several studies of police and court records, the proportion of murderers who had been drinking before the crime ranged from 36% in Baltimore to 70% in Sweden.[40] In Canada statistics describing the correlation between homicide and alcohol use have been derived through federal prison surveys. Among homicide offenders, 34% reported being under the influence of alcohol at the time of the crime.[41] Across all these studies, about 50% of the murder victims had been drinking. These data certainly imply that homicide is more likely to occur in situations in which drinking also occurs, but they leave open the question as to whether alcohol plays a causal role in homicides.

A recent study has suggested that membership in Alcoholics Anonymous may reduce alcohol-related homicide mortality rates, particularly among males who consume spirits and wine.[42]

Assault and Other Crimes of Violence As with homicide, studies of assault, spousal abuse, and child abuse reveal correlations with drinking: Heavier drinkers are more likely to engage in such behaviours, and self-reports by offenders indicate a high likelihood that they had been consuming alcohol before the violent act. However, scientists are still cautious in trying to determine how much of a causal role alcohol plays in such activity. For example, if fights are likely to occur when men get together in groups at night, and drinking is likely to occur when men get together in groups at night, how much of a role does alcohol itself play in increasing the chances of violence? Similarly, if both heavy drinking and violent arguments are characteristics of dysfunctional family situations, how much of the ensuing family violence can be blamed on the use of alcohol? Unfortunately, it has proven difficult to perform controlled experimental studies on these complex problems, so the answers remain unclear.

Date Rape In spite of widespread concern about drugs being slipped into someone's drink, by far the most significant date-rape drug is and always has been alcohol. For most postsecondary women who report having been sexually assaulted by a date, the assault happened after the woman had consumed alcohol[43]; this is why many campuses now combine sexual assault prevention education with alcohol education. (For more on this topic, see the date rape discussion in Chapter 7.)

Suicide Most studies show that alcohol is involved in about one-third of all suicides. Suicide *attempts* seem to have a different background than successful suicides, but alcohol abuse is second only to depression as the diagnosis in suicide attempters. The relationship between alcohol abuse and depression is a strong one and has been the subject of many studies. A recent study of almost 2000 suicide attempts in Germany again found that acute alcohol consumption was present in about one-third of the cases, and in about one-sixth of the total cases the person could be diagnosed with an alcohol use disorder (alcohol abuse or dependence).[44]

Physiological Effects

Peripheral Circulation One effect of alcohol on the CNS is the dilation of the peripheral blood vessels. This increases heat loss from the body but makes the drinker feel warm. The heat loss and cooling of the interior of the body are enough to cause a slowdown in some biochemical processes. This dilation of the peripheral vessels argues against giving alcohol to individuals in shock or extreme cold. Under these conditions blood is needed in the central parts of the body, and heat loss must be diminished if the person is to survive.

Fluid Balance One action of alcohol on the brain is to decrease the output of the antidiuretic hormone (ADH, also called vasopressin) responsible for retaining fluid in the body. It is this effect, rather than the actual fluid consumption, that increases the urine flow in response to alcohol. This diuretic effect can lower blood pressure in some individuals.

Hormonal Effects Even single doses of alcohol can produce measurable effects on a variety of hormonal systems: Adrenal corticosteroids are released, as are catecholamines from the adrenal medulla, and the production of the male sex hormone testosterone is suppressed. It is not known what significance, if any, these effects have for occasional, moderate drinkers. However, chronic abusers of alcohol can develop a variety of hormone-related disorders, including testicular atrophy and impotence in men and impaired reproductive functioning in women.

LO6 Alcohol Toxicity

Alcohol consumption can result in toxicity, both acute and chronic. We have already discussed the problem of alcohol-related traffic accidents, which we would consider to be examples of acute behavioural toxicity. In a similar vein are other alcohol-related accidents and adverse effects, such as falls, drowning, cycling and boating accidents, and accidents associated with operating machinery. The Centers for Disease Control estimate that acute alcohol-related problems cause more than 20 000 deaths annually in the United States (about 13 000 from automobile accidents).[45]

Acute physiological toxicity in the form of alcohol overdose occurs quite often if you include people who drink enough to become physically ill and/or to experience hangovers. In addition, more than 1000 people die in the United States each year from accidental alcohol poisoning (high blood alcohol level). As the DAWN data in Chapter 2 revealed, many drug-related deaths include alcohol in combination with some other substance, so it is difficult to know exactly how many overdose deaths are primarily due to alcohol versus another drug, or to the specific combination. Several well-publicized drinking deaths of young postsecondary students have occurred in recent years. These students had been drinking for many hours before their deaths, and as a result colleges and universities began re-examining their alcohol-use policies. Two pieces of advice are worth mentioning: (1) If one of your friends drinks enough to pass out, DO NOT simply leave her or him alone to sleep it off. The person should be placed on his or her side so that any vomit is less likely to be aspirated, and someone who is sober needs to monitor the person's breathing until he or she can be aroused and begins to move. If this is not possible, take the victim to the emergency room. Don't worry about getting in trouble for helping out a friend–the alternative can be much worse. (2) It is particularly dangerous to drink to the point of vomiting and then begin drinking again after vomiting. The vomiting reflex is triggered by rapidly rising BAC, usually above 0.12%. But the vomiting reflex is inhibited when the BAC rises above 0.20 or so, and it is then possible to continue drinking and reach lethal concentrations.

Hangover

The Germans call it "wailing of cats" (*Katzenjammer*), the Italians "out of tune" (*stonato*), the French "woody mouth" (*gueule de boise*), the Norwegians "workmen in my head"

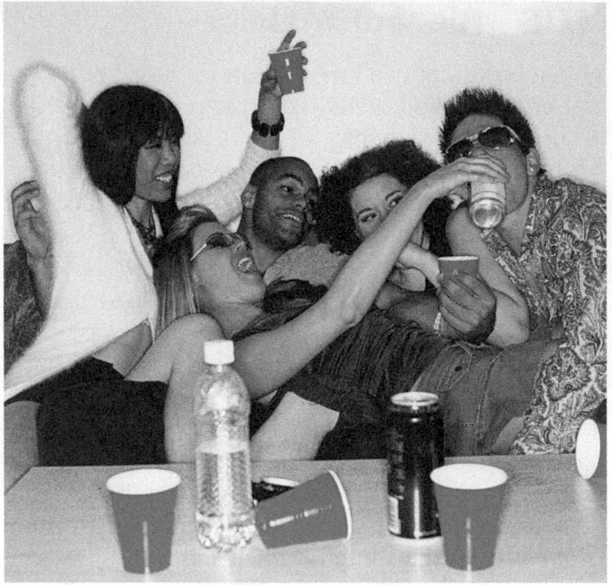

Rapid consumption of alcohol can lead to acute toxicity.

(*jeg har tommeermenn*), and the Swedes "pain in the roots of the hair" (*hont i haret*). Hangovers aren't much fun. And they aren't very well understood, either. Even moderate drinkers who only occasionally overindulge are well acquainted with the symptoms: upset stomach, fatigue, headache, thirst, depression, anxiety, and general malaise.

Some authorities believe that the symptoms of a hangover are the symptoms of withdrawal from a short- or long-term dependence on alcohol. The pattern certainly fits. Some people report continuing to drink just to escape the pain of the hangover. This behaviour is not unknown to moderate drinkers, either: Many believe that the only cure for a hangover is some of "the hair of the dog that bit you"–alcohol. And it might work to minimize symptoms, because it spreads them out over a longer time. There is no evidence that any of the "surefire-this'll-fix-you-up" remedies are effective. The only known cures are an analgesic for the headache, rest, and time.

Some hangover symptoms are probably reactions to congeners. Congeners are natural products of the fermentation and preparation process, some of which are quite toxic. Congeners make the various alcoholic beverages different in smell, taste, colour, and, possibly, hangover potential.

Still other factors contribute to the trials and tribulations of the "morning after the night before." Thirst means that the body has excreted more fluid than was taken in with the alcoholic beverages. However, this does not seem to be the only basis for the thirst experienced the next day. Another cause might be that alcohol causes fluid inside cells to move outside the cells. This cellular dehydration, without a decrease in total body fluid, is known to be related to, and might be the basis of, an increase in thirst.

The nausea and upset stomach typically experienced can most likely be attributed to the fact that alcohol is a gastric irritant. Consuming even moderate amounts causes local irritation of the mucosa lining the stomach. It has been suggested that the accumulation of acetaldehyde, which is quite toxic even in small quantities, contributes to the nausea and headache. The headache can also be a reaction to fatigue. Fatigue sometimes results from a higher than normal level of activity while drinking. Increased activity frequently accompanies a decrease in inhibitions, a readily available source of energy, and a high blood sugar level. One effect of alcohol intake is to increase the blood sugar level for about an hour after ingestion. This can be followed several hours later by a low blood sugar level and an increased feeling of fatigue.

Recently several products that are supposed to prevent hangovers have been advertised on TV and through the Internet, and sold in bars, liquor stores, and convenience stores. Although one of these products claims to have been tested in a placebo-controlled study, the study has not been published in a scientific journal and the product's ingredients, including a small amount of activated charcoal meant to absorb congeners, seems unlikely to have much real effect. The best way to avoid a hangover is still to drink in moderation, regardless of the beverage.

Chronic Disease States

The relationship of alcohol use to many diseases has been studied extensively. As a general rule, heavy alcohol use, either directly or indirectly, affects every organ system in the body. The alcohol or its primary metabolite, acetaldehyde, can irritate and damage tissue directly. Because alcohol provides empty calories, many heavy drinkers do not eat well, and chronic malnutrition leads to tissue damage. Separating the effects of alcohol exposure from those of malnutrition relies to a great extent on experiments with animals. Some animals can be fed adequate diets and exposed to high concentrations of alcohol, whereas other animals are fed diets deficient in certain vitamins or other nutrients.

Brain Damage

Perhaps the biggest concern is the damage to brain tissue that is seen in chronic alcohol abusers. It has been reported for years that the brains of deceased heavy drinkers demonstrate an obvious overall loss of brain tissue: the ventricles (internal spaces) in the brain are enlarged, and the fissures (sulci) in the cortex are widened. Modern imaging techniques have revealed this tissue loss in living alcohol abusers as well. This generalized loss of brain tissue is probably a result of direct alcohol toxicity rather than malnutrition and is associated with *alcoholic dementia*, a global decline of intellect. Patients with this type of organic brain syndrome might have difficulty swallowing in addition to impaired problem solving, difficulty in manipulating objects, and abnormal electroencephalograms. Another classical alcohol-related organic brain syndrome has two parts, which so often go together that the disorder is referred to as **Wernicke-Korsakoff syndrome**. *Wernicke's disease* is associated with a deficiency of thiamine (vitamin B_1) and can sometimes be corrected nutritionally. The symptoms include confusion, ataxia (impaired coordination while walking), and abnormal eye movements. Most patients with Wernicke's disease also exhibit *Korsakoff's psychosis*, characterized by an inability to remember recent events or to learn new information. Korsakoff's psychosis can appear by itself in patients who maintain adequate nutrition, and it appears to be mostly irreversible. There has been great controversy about the specific brain areas that are damaged in Wernicke-Korsakoff syndrome, as well as about the relationship between the two parts of the disorder.

Important practical questions include the following. Exactly how much alcohol exposure is required before behavioural and/or anatomical evidence can be found indicating brain damage? And how much of the cognitive deficit seen in alcoholic dementia can be reversed when drinking is stopped and adequate nutrition is given? Both have been the subject of several experiments. There is no definitive answer for the first question. Some of the studies on moderate drinkers have included individuals who consume up to 10 drinks per day! Most studies with lower cutoffs for moderate drinking have not found consistent evidence for anatomical changes in the brain. As for recovery, several studies have reported both behavioural improvement and apparent regrowth of brain size in chronic alcohol abusers after some months of abstinence. However, not all such studies find improvement, and some have found improvement in some types of mental tasks but not in others.

Liver Disease

Fatty acids are the usual fuel for the liver. When present, alcohol has higher priority and is used as fuel instead. As a result, fatty acids (lipids) accumulate in the liver and are stored as small droplets in liver cells. This condition is known as alcohol-related *fatty liver*, which for most drinkers is not a serious problem. If alcohol input ceases, the liver uses the stored fatty acids for energy. Sometimes the droplets increase in size until they rupture the cell membrane, causing death of the liver cells. Before the liver cells die, a fatty liver is completely reversible and usually of minor medical concern.

Sometimes, with prolonged or high-level alcohol intake, another phase of liver damage is observed. Alcoholic hepatitis is a serious disease and includes both inflammation and impairment of liver function. Usually this occurs in areas of the liver where cells are dead and dying, but it is not known if an increasingly fatty liver leads to alcoholic hepatitis. Alcoholic hepatitis does exist in the absence of a fatty liver, so this form of tissue damage might be due to direct toxic effects of alcohol.

Cirrhosis is the liver disease everyone knows is related to high and prolonged levels of alcohol consumption. It's not easy to get cirrhosis from drinking alcohol—you have to work at it. Usually it takes about 10 years of steady drinking of the equivalent of a pint or more of whisky a day. Not all cirrhosis is alcohol-related, but a high percentage is, and cirrhosis is the eleventh leading cause of death in Canada. In large urban areas it is the fourth or fifth leading cause of death in men aged 25 to 65. In cirrhosis, liver cells are replaced by fibrous tissue (collagen), which changes the structure of the liver (see Figure 9.4). These changes decrease blood flow and, along with the loss of cells, result in a decreased ability of the liver to function. When the liver does not function properly, fluid accumulates in the body, jaundice develops, and other infections or cancers have a better opportunity to establish themselves in the liver. Cirrhosis is not reversible, but stopping the intake of alcohol will retard its development and decrease the serious medical effects. In drinkers with severely damaged livers, liver transplants have been quite successful—a 64% survival rate after two years. Most of these recipients do not resume drinking after the transplant.

Heart Disease

Another area of concern is the effect of alcohol on the heart and circulation. Heavy alcohol use is associated

Wernicke-Korsakoff syndrome: chronic mental impairments produced by heavy alcohol use over a long period of time.

cirrhosis: an irreversible, frequently deadly liver disorder associated with heavy alcohol use.

Figure 9.4 (a) Normal liver; (b) Cirrhotic liver

(a)

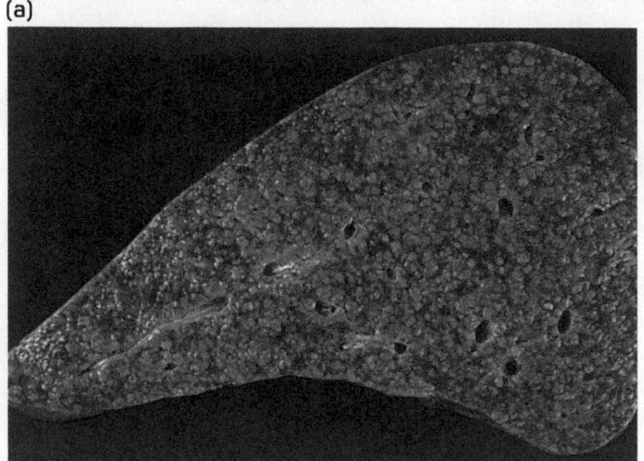

(b)

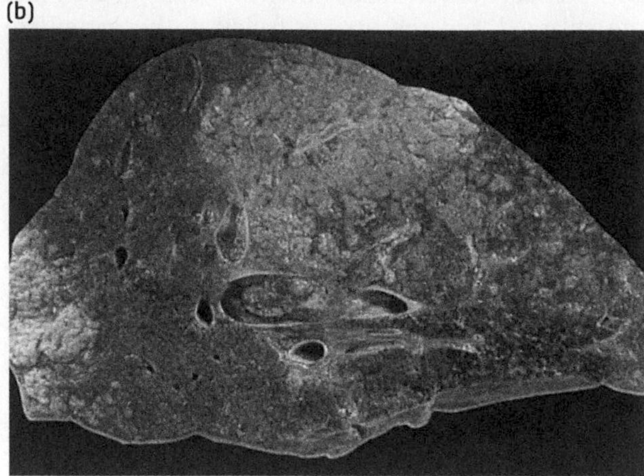

with increased mortality resulting from heart disease. Much of this is due to damage to the heart muscle (cardiomyopathy), but the risk of the more typical heart attack resulting from coronary artery disease also increases. Heavy drinkers are also more likely to suffer from high blood pressure and strokes. An interesting twist to this story is that several studies have found a *lower* incidence of heart attacks in moderate drinkers than in abstainers, and for several years this protective effect of moderate alcohol consumption and the possible mechanism for it have been discussed. It has been pointed out that the abstainers in such studies might include both abstaining alcohol abusers who once drank heavily and others who quit on their doctor's advice because of poor health. However, one study separated those who never drank from the "quitters" and still reported fewer heart attacks and lower overall mortality in moderate drinkers, with increased mortality for both abstainers and heavy drinkers.[46] It has been proposed that alcohol increases high-density lipoproteins (HDL, sometimes called "good cholesterol"), some of which seem to protect against high blood pressure. The reduced blood clotting produced by alcohol could also play a role. There has been speculation that red wine might have better effects than other forms of alcohol due to the presence of antioxidants in the grapes from which the wine is made. But the scientific evidence supports only a beneficial effect of regular alcohol use, with an increased risk for those who "binge" drink (heavy use once a week or so).[47]

Cancer

Alcohol use is associated with cancers of the mouth, tongue, pharynx, larynx, esophagus, stomach, liver, lung, pancreas, colon, and rectum. There are many possible mechanisms for this, from direct tissue irritation to nutritional deficiencies to the induction of enzymes that activate other carcinogens. A particularly nasty interaction with cigarette smoking increases the incidence of cancers of the oral cavity, pharynx, and larynx. Also, suppression of the immune system by alcohol, which occurs to some extent every time intoxicating doses are used, probably increases the rate of tumour growth.

The Immune System

The immune deficits seen in chronic alcohol abusers are associated with at least some increase in the frequency of various infectious diseases, including tuberculosis, pneumonia, yellow fever, cholera, and hepatitis B. Alcohol use might be a factor in AIDS, for several reasons: loss of behavioural inhibitions probably increases the likelihood of engaging in unprotected sex; alcohol could increase the risk of HIV infection in exposed individuals; and alcohol could suppress the immune system and therefore increase the chances of developing full-blown AIDS once an HIV infection is established. Although one epidemiological study did not find an acceleration of HIV-related disease in infected individuals who drank, heavy alcohol use is probably not a good idea for anyone who is HIV-positive.

Canadian Recommended Guidelines for Low-Risk Drinking

In November 2011 the Canadian federal and provincial/territorial health ministers received Canada's Low-Risk Alcohol Drinking Guidelines (LRDG), which comprise five guidelines and a series of tips (see Table 9.8). Low-risk alcohol use involves consumption of no more than

Table 9.8 Recommended Guidelines for Low-Risk Drinking

These Guidelines are not intended to encourage people who choose to abstain for cultural, spiritual or other reasons to drink, nor are they intended to encourage people to commence drinking to achieve health benefits. People of low bodyweight or who are not accustomed to alcohol are advised to consume below these maximum limits.

Guideline 1 Do not drink in these situations:	When operating any kind of vehicle, tools or machinery; using medications or other drugs that interact with alcohol; engaging in sports or other potentially dangerous physical activities; working; making important decisions; if pregnant or planning to be pregnant; before breastfeeding; while responsible for the care or supervision of others; if suffering from serious physical illness, mental illness or alcohol dependence.
Guideline 2 If you drink, reduce *long-term* health risks by staying within these **average** levels:	**Women** • 0–2 standard drinks* per day • No more than 10 standard drinks per week **Men** • 0–3 standard drinks* per day • No more than 15 standard drinks per week Always have some non-drinking days per week to minimize tolerance and habit formation. Do not increase drinking to the upper limits as health benefits are greatest at up to one drink per day. Do not exceed the daily limits specified in Guideline 3.
Guideline 3 If you drink, reduce ***short-term*** risks by choosing safe situations and restricting your alcohol intake:	Risk of injury increases with each additional drink in many situations. For both health and safety reasons, it is important not to drink more than: • Three standard drinks* in one day for a woman • Four standard drinks* in one day for a man Drinking at these upper levels should only happen ***occasionally*** and always be consistent with the ***weekly*** limits specified in Guideline 2. It is especially important on these occasions to drink with meals and not on an empty stomach; to have no more than two standard drinks in any three-hour period; to alternate with caffeine-free, non-alcoholic drinks; and to avoid risky situations and activities. Individuals with reduced tolerance, whether due to low bodyweight, being under the age of 25 or over 65 years old, are advised to never exceed Guideline 2 upper levels.
Guideline 4 When pregnant or planning to be pregnant:	***The safest option during pregnancy or when planning to become pregnant is to not drink alcohol at all.*** Alcohol in the mother's bloodstream can harm the developing fetus. While the risk from light consumption during pregnancy appears very low, there is no threshold of alcohol use in pregnancy that has been definitively proven to be safe.
Guideline 5 Alcohol and young people:	Alcohol can harm healthy physical and mental development of children and adolescents. ***Uptake of drinking by youth should be delayed at least until the late teens and be consistent with local legal drinking age laws.*** Once a decision to start drinking is made, drinking should occur in a safe environment, under parental guidance and at low levels (i.e., one or two standard drinks* once or twice per week). From legal drinking age to 24 years, it is recommended women never exceed two drinks per day and men never exceed three drinks in one day.

*A "standard drink" is equal to a 341 ml (12 oz.) bottle of 5% strength beer, cider or cooler; a 142 ml (5 oz.) glass of 12% strength wine; or a 43 ml (1.5 oz.) shot of 40% strength spirits (NB: 1 Canadian standard drink = 17.05 ml or 13.45 g of ethanol)

Source: Reproduced with permission from the Canadian Centre on Substance Abuse.

the recommended quantity of alcohol within the number of days specified. In comparison, high-risk alcohol use involves consuming more alcohol than recommended within the stated time frame. Low-risk alcohol use is predicted to reduce alcohol-related deaths by approximately 4600 per year in Canada. Unfortunately, at least half of consumers fall in the high-risk group.[48] It is naïve to presume that the mere presentation of guidelines will be sufficient to change drinking behaviour, but it is hoped that in collaboration with other evidence-based regulatory and preventive interventions the initiative will incite change.[49,50]

Of those Canadians who consumed alcohol in the past 12 months (see Table 9.8), 18.6% exceeded guideline 1 for chronic effects of alcohol and 12.8% (9.9% of the total population) exceeded guideline 2 for acute effects of alcohol. Males were more likely than females to violate both guidelines. The chronic-risk guideline was exceeded by 21.2% of male drinkers and 15.9% of female drinkers, while 15.8% of male drinkers and 9.7% of female drinkers drank in excess of the acute-risk guideline.

In youth aged 15 to 24 years, drinking patterns exceeded their adult (25 years and older) counterparts. Approximately 25% of youth drinkers versus 17.6% of adult drinkers exceeded the guideline for chronic risk, while 17.9% of youth drinkers and 11.9% of adult drinkers drank to excess of that recommended by the acute-risk guideline. Year-to-year comparisons failed to reveal differences that could be attributed to age or sex.

LO7 Fetal Alcohol Syndrome

There is no evidence that the occasional consumption of one or two drinks has overall negative effects on the physical health of most individuals. An important exception to this statement might be drinking during pregnancy. Fetal alcohol spectrum disorder (FASD) is a term used to describe a range of cognitive, behavioural, and physical disabilities that can occur in persons exposed to alcohol during gestation. Included under the FASD umbrella are three diagnostic terms: **fetal alcohol syndrome** (FAS), partial fetal alcohol syndrome (PFAS), and alcohol-related neurodevelopmental disorder (ARND). FASD is considered to be the leading cause of developmental and cognitive disabilities in Canadian children. It is preventable.

The unfortunate condition of infants born to alcohol-abusing mothers was noted in an 1834 report to the British Parliament: They have a "starved, shriveled, and imperfect look." Until fairly recently most scientists and physicians believed that any effects on the offspring of heavy alcohol users were the result of poor nutrition or poor prenatal care. Those beliefs changed, however, when a 1973 report described eight children who displayed a particular pattern of craniofacial and other defects. All of these children had been born to alcohol-dependent mothers. This article was the first to describe the symptoms of FAS. There are three primary criteria for diagnosing FAS, at least one of which *must* be present:

1. Growth retardation occurring before and/or after birth.
2. A pattern of abnormal features of the face and head, including small head circumference, small eyes, or evidence of retarded formation of the midfacial area, including a flattened bridge and short length of the nose and flattening of the vertical groove between the nose and mouth (the philtrum).
3. Evidence of CNS abnormality, including abnormal neonatal behaviour, mental retardation, or other evidence of abnormal neurobehavioural development.

fetal alcohol syndrome: facial and developmental abnormalities associated with the mother's alcohol use during pregnancy.

Each of these features can be seen in the absence of alcohol exposure, and other features might also be present in FAS, such as eye and ear defects, heart murmurs, undescended testicles, birthmarks, and abnormal fingerprints or palmar creases. Research also found a high frequency of various abnormalities of the eyes, often associated with poor vision. Thus, the diagnosis of FAS is a matter of judgment, based on several symptoms and often on the physician's knowledge of the mother's drinking history.

Many animal studies have been done in a variety of species, and they indicate that FAS is related to peak BAC and to duration of alcohol exposure, even when malnutrition is not an issue. In mice and other animal models, increasing amounts of alcohol yield an increase in mortality, a decrease in infant weight, and increased frequency of soft-tissue malformation. The various components of the complete FAS reflect damage occurring

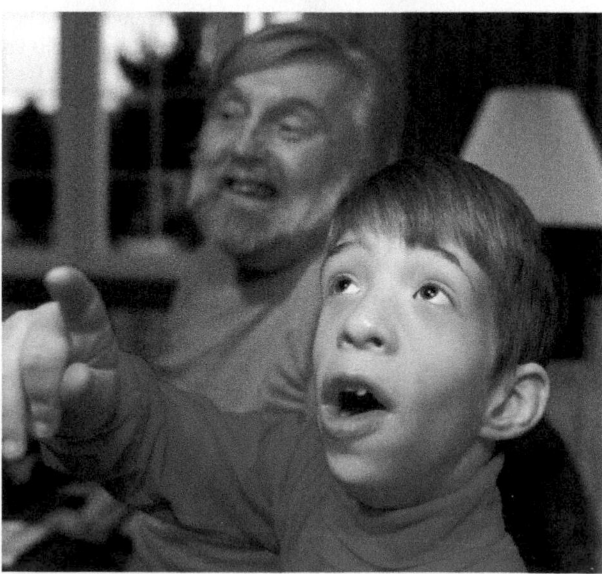

This boy shows typical features of fetal alcohol syndrome, including small eyes, flattened bridge of the nose, and flattening of the vertical groove between the nose and mouth.

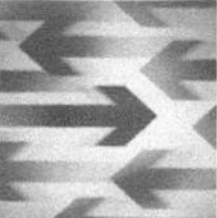

TAKING SIDES

Protecting the Unborn from Alcohol

Increased concern about fetal alcohol syndrome has led to some significant changes in the status of pregnant women, at least in certain instances and locations. Waiters have refused to serve wine to pregnant women, women have been arrested and charged with child abuse for being heavily intoxicated while pregnant, and others have been charged with endangerment for breastfeeding while drunk. These social interventions represent concerns for the welfare of the child. However, to women already concerned about their own rights because of the issue of government regulation of abortion, such actions seem to be yet another infringement, yet another signal that the woman's rights are secondary to the child's.

We know that heavy alcohol consumption during pregnancy does increase the risk to the child of permanent disfigurement and mental retardation. We also know that, even among the heaviest drinkers, the odds still favour a normal-appearing baby (less than 10% of the babies born to the heaviest-drinking 5% of mothers exhibit full-blown FAS).

Do you think that men are more likely than women to support limiting the rights of pregnant women to drink while they are pregnant? You might ask a group of both men and women to give you answers to the following questions.

How strongly do you agree (5 = strong agreement, 1 = strong disagreement) with the following statements?

1. Women who repeatedly get drunk while they are pregnant should be kept in jail if necessary until the baby is born.
2. All bartenders should be trained not to serve any drinks at all to a woman who is obviously pregnant.
3. If a man and a pregnant woman are drinking together and both become intoxicated, both the man and the woman should be arrested for child abuse.

at different developmental stages, so heavy alcohol exposure throughout pregnancy is the most damaging situation, followed by intermittent high-level exposure designed to imitate binge drinking.

Not all infants born to drinking mothers show abnormal development. If they did, it would not have taken so long to recognize FAS as a problem. Estimates of the prevalence of FAS in the overall population range from 0.2 per 1000 births to 1.5 per 1000.[51] Estimating the prevalence among problem drinkers or alcohol abusers is more of a problem. There is the difficulty not only of diagnosing FAS but also of diagnosing alcohol abuse. If the physician knows that the mother is a heavy drinker, this can increase the probability of noticing or diagnosing FAS, thus inflating the prevalence statistics among drinking mothers. FAS seems to occur in 23 to 29 per 1000 births among women who are problem drinkers. If all alcohol-related birth defects (referred to as **fetal alcohol effect**, or FAE) are counted, the rate among heavy-drinking women is higher, from 80 to a few hundred per 1000. Maternal alcohol abuse might be the most frequent known environmental cause of mental retardation in the Western world.

In addition to the risk of FAS, the fetus of a mother who drinks heavily has a risk of not being born at all. Spontaneous abortion early in pregnancy is perhaps twice as likely among the 5% of women who are the heaviest drinkers. The data on later pregnancy loss (stillbirths) are not as clearly related to alcohol for either animals or humans.

An important question, and one that can never be answered in absolute terms, is whether there is an acceptable level of alcohol consumption for pregnant women. The data on drinking during pregnancy rely on self-reports by the mothers, who are assumed to be at least as likely as everyone else to underreport their drinking. In addition, almost every study has used different definitions of heavy drinking, alcohol abuse, and problem drinking. The heaviest drinkers in each study are the most at risk for alcohol-related problems with their children, but

fetal alcohol effect: individual developmental abnormalities associated with the mother's alcohol use during pregnancy.

we don't really know if the large number of light or moderate drinkers are causing significant risks. Based on the dose-related nature of birth problems in animal studies, one might argue that any alcohol use at all produces some risk, but at low levels the increased risk is too small to be revealed except in a large-scale study. In 1981, the U.S. surgeon general recommended that "pregnant women should drink absolutely no alcohol because they may be endangering the health of their unborn children." Maybe that went a bit too far. The bottom line is this: Scientific data do not demonstrate that occasional consumption of one or two drinks definitely causes FAS or other alcohol-related birth defects. On the other hand, neither do the data prove that low-level alcohol use is safe nor do they indicate a safe level of use. Remember from Chapter 5 that it is not within the realm of science to declare something totally safe, so it will be impossible to ever set a safe limit on alcohol use. Most women decrease their alcohol use once they have become pregnant, and many decrease it further as pregnancy progresses.

LO8 Alcohol Dependence

Withdrawal Syndrome

The physical dependence associated with prolonged heavy use of alcohol is revealed when alcohol intake is stopped. *The abstinence syndrome that develops is medically more severe and more likely to cause death than withdrawal from opioid drugs.* In untreated advanced cases, mortality can be as high as one in seven. For that reason it has long been recommended that the initial period of **detoxification** (allowing the body to rid itself of the alcohol) be carried out in an inpatient medical setting, especially for people who have been drinking very heavily or have other medical complications. The progression of withdrawal, the abstinence syndrome, has been described in the following way:

- Stage 1: tremors, excessively rapid heartbeat, hypertension, heavy sweating, loss of appetite, and insomnia.
- Stage 2: hallucinations–auditory, visual, tactile, or a combination of these; and, rarely, olfactory signs.
- Stage 3: delusions, disorientation, delirium, sometimes intermittent and usually followed by amnesia.
- Stage 4: seizure activity.

Medical treatment is usually sought in stage 1 or 2, and rapid intervention with a sedative drug, such as diazepam, will prevent stage 3 or 4 from occurring. The old term **delirium tremens** is used to refer to severe cases including at least stage 3.

Tremors are one of the most common physical changes associated with alcohol withdrawal and can persist for a long period after alcohol intake has stopped. Anxiety, insomnia, feelings of unreality, nausea, vomiting, and many other symptoms can also occur.

The withdrawal symptoms do not develop all at the same time or immediately after abstinence begins. The initial signs (tremors, anxiety) might develop within a few hours, but the individual is relatively rational. Over the next day or two, hallucinations appear and gradually become more terrifying and real to the individual. One common feature of alcohol-withdrawal hallucinations includes the sensation of ants or snakes crawling on the skin. You might remember that this also occurs after high doses of stimulant drugs. In the context of alcohol withdrawal, it is an indication that the nervous system is rebounding from constant inhibition and is hyperexcitable.

Optimal treatment of patients during the early stages involves the administration of a benzodiazepine, such as chlordiazepoxide or diazepam (see Chapter 7). Because of the high degree of cross-dependence between alcohol and chlordiazepoxide, one drug can be substituted for the other and withdrawal continued at a safer rate.[52]

Some withdrawal symptoms can last for up to several weeks. Unstable blood pressure, irregular breathing, anxiety, panic attacks, insomnia, and depression are all reported during this period. These phenomena have been referred to as a protracted withdrawal syndrome, and they can trigger intense cravings for alcohol. Thus, some chronic drinkers might benefit from residential or inpatient treatment for up to six weeks, simply to prevent relapse during this critical period. Preventing relapse for longer periods is a difficult task that is discussed in Chapter 17.

Dependent Behaviours

Probably the most significant influence on Canadian attitudes about alcohol dependence was a 60-year-old

detoxification: an early treatment stage, in which the body eliminates the alcohol or other substance.

delirium tremens: an alcohol withdrawal syndrome that includes hallucinations and tremors.

book called *Alcoholics Anonymous.* This book described the experiences of a small group of people who formed a society whose "only requirement for membership is a desire to stop drinking." That society has now grown to include more than 1.5 million members in over a hundred countries. A central part of their belief system is that alcohol dependence is a progressive disease characterized by a loss of control over drinking and that the disease can never be cured. People who do not have the disease might drink and even become intoxicated, but they do not "lose control over alcohol." There is a suspicion that the dependent drinker is different even before the first drink is taken. The only treatment is to arrest the disease by abstaining from drinking. This *disease model* of alcohol dependence has received support from many medical practitioners and has been endorsed by the Canadian Medical Association and other professional groups. In one sense, this description of alcohol dependence as a disease is a reaction against long-held notions that excessive drinking is only a symptom of some other underlying pathology, such as depression, or some type of personality defect. Traditional psychoanalysts practising many years ago might have treated alcohol abusers by trying to discover the unconscious conflicts or personality deficiencies that caused the person to drink. One important consequence of defining alcohol dependence as a *primary* disease is to recognize that the drinking itself might be the problem and that treatment and prevention should be aimed directly at alcohol abuse/dependence.

However, there are many scientific critics of the disease concept. If alcohol dependence is a disease, what is its cause? How are alcohol abusers different from others, except that they tend to drink a lot and have many alcohol-related problems? Although sequential stages have been described for this "progressive disease," most individual drinkers don't seem to fit any single set of descriptors. Some don't drink alone, some don't drink in the morning, some don't go on binges, some don't drink every day, and some don't report strong cravings for alcohol. Experiments have shown that alcohol-dependent individuals do retain considerable control over their drinking, even while drinking—it's not that they completely lose control when they start drinking, but they might

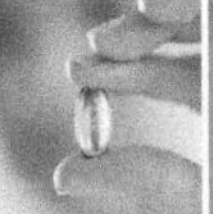

DRUGS IN DEPTH

Is Alcoholics Anonymous a Religion?

For many young adults, occasional bouts of alcohol abuse appear to be symbolic of their freedom from the constraints and values imposed by their parents. For some, part of the separation from parental authority includes less involvement in the religious practices traditional to the family. And for some whose abuse of alcohol eventually begins to interfere significantly in their lives, getting sober may also involve "getting religion" back into their lives. One good example of this type of change is former President George W. Bush, who in 1986 decided to quit drinking and who also became much more involved in religion, both without any direct involvement with Alcoholics Anonymous.

The original founders of Alcoholics Anonymous (AA) were strongly influenced by the Oxford Group, a Christian religious movement that involved reflecting on your own shortcomings (sins), admitting them to another, and helping others as a way of improving yourself. These became the central ideas behind AA, and certainly its first members were expected to "accept Jesus Christ as your Lord and Savior." But how does that history relate to AA as practised today and all over the world? Is it essentially a religion?

Most AA members would say no. AA is not intended to replace anyone's church or other religious practices, and the 12 steps (see Chapter 18) include the phrases "God as we understood Him," and "a Power greater than ourselves." For many AA members, this means the traditional Christian view of God, but adherents of Judaism and Islam also find their religions to be compatible with AA's beliefs. Many who are quite firm adherents of AA are even agnostics or atheists, and they are able to interpret this "Power greater than ourselves" in terms of the power of the 12-step program, or the power of the group. For them, taking a "moral inventory" (step 4), confessing their shortcomings to another individual (step 5), and then helping others to maintain sobriety represent their "spiritual awakening," implying perhaps a change of focus from being self-centred to being more responsible to others and for others.

have either less ability or less desire to limit their drinking because they do drink excessively. Although an "alcoholic personality" has been defined that characterizes many drinkers who enter treatment, the current belief is that these personality factors (impulsive, anxious, depressed, passive, dependent) reflect the years of intoxication and the critical events that led to the decision to enter treatment rather than preexisting abnormalities that caused the problem drinking.

The American Psychiatric Association's *Diagnostic and Statistical Manual of Mental Disorders*[53] is the closest thing there is to a single official, widely accepted set of labels for behavioural disorders, including substance use disorders. The DSM-5 lists 11 possible criteria for alcohol use disorder, including drinking more than intended, desire to cut down or stop, craving, drinking causing disruption of major life roles, social problems, giving up other activities, repeated hazardous use, tolerance, and withdrawal. The severity of the disorder is then ranked based on the number of these criteria, with six or more of the symptoms indicating a severe alcohol use disorder.

Why are some people able to drink in moderation all their lives, whereas others repeatedly become intoxicated, suffer from alcohol-related problems, and continue to drink excessively? So far, no single factor and no combination of multiple factors has been presented that allows us to predict which individuals will become alcohol abusers. Multiple theories exist, including biochemical, psychoanalytic, and cultural approaches. At this period of scientific history, probably the most attention is being focused on understanding two types of factors: cognitive and genetic. Two important tools have been used in the cognitive research: the Alcohol Expectancy Questionnaire (asking people what effects they think alcohol has on people), and the balanced placebo design.[54] Both alcohol-dependent drinkers and social drinkers report more intoxication and consume more drinks when they are told the drinks have alcohol, regardless of the actual alcohol content. It is important that alcohol-dependent people actually given small amounts of alcohol (equivalent to one or two drinks) do not report becoming intoxicated and do not increase their drinking if they are led to expect that the drink contains no alcohol. Therefore, it would seem that, if alcohol abusers do lose control when they begin drinking, it might be because they have come to *believe* that they will lose control if they drink (this is sometimes referred to as the *abstinence violation effect*). These balanced placebo experiments have been replicated several times by others. The most obvious interpretation of such results is that alcohol use provides a social excuse for behaving in ways that would otherwise be considered inappropriate, and it is enough for one to believe that one has drunk alcohol for such behaviours to be released.

Considerable evidence supports the idea that some degree of vulnerability to alcohol dependence might be inherited. Alcohol dependence does tend to run in families, but some of that could be due to similar expectancies developed through similar cultural influences and children learning from their parents. Studies on twins provide one way around this problem. Monozygotic (one-egg, or identical) twins share the same genetic material, whereas dizygotic (two-egg, or fraternal) twins are no more genetically related than any two nontwin siblings. Both types of twins are likely to share very similar cultural and family learning experiences. If one adult twin is diagnosed as alcohol dependent, what is the likelihood that the other twin will also receive that diagnosis (are the twins concordant for the trait of alcohol dependence)? Almost all such studies report the concordance rate for monozygotic twins is higher than that for dizygotic twins, and in some studies it is as high as 50%. These results imply that inheritance plays a strong role but is far from a complete determinant of alcohol dependence. Another important type of study looks at adopted sons whose biological fathers were alcohol dependent. These reports consistently find that such adoptees have a much greater than average chance of becoming alcohol dependent, even though they are raised by "normal" parents. Although these studies again provide clear evidence for a genetic influence, most children of alcohol abusers do not become alcohol dependent—they simply have a statistically greater risk of doing so. For example, in one study, 18% of the adopted-away sons of alcohol-dependent drinkers became dependent on alcohol, compared with 5% of the adopted-away sons whose parents had not received the diagnosis.

Alcohol dependence is a complicated feature of human behaviour, and even if genetic influences are critical, more than one genetic factor could be involved. Probably it is too much to hope that a single genetic marker will ever be found to be a reliable indicator of alcohol dependence in all individuals.

Summary

- Alcohol is made by yeasts in a process called fermentation. Distillation is used to increase the alcohol content of a beverage.
- National Prohibition of alcohol was successful in reducing alcohol consumption and alcohol-related problems, but also led to increased law-breaking and a loss of alcohol taxes.
- Alcohol use has decreased since 1980, and consumption varies widely among different cultural groups and in different regions of Canada.
- In 2013, Canada sold $21.4 billion worth of alcoholic beverages equating to approximately 265.4 million litres of absolute alcohol.
- The Canadian Alcohol and Drug Use Monitoring Survey (CADUMS) is an annual general population survey (from 2008 through 2012) of alcohol and illicit drug use among Canadians aged 15 years and older.
- Men are more likely than women to be heavy drinkers, and college students are more likely to drink than others of the same age.
- Alcohol is metabolized by the liver at a constant rate, which is not much influenced by body size.
- The exact mechanism(s) by which alcohol exerts its effects in the central nervous system is not known, but probably its interactions with the GABA receptor are important.
- Knowing a person's weight, gender, and the amount of alcohol consumed it is possible to estimate the blood alcohol content (BAC), and from that to estimate the typical effects on behaviour.
- The balanced placebo design has helped to separate the pharmacological effects of alcohol from the effects of alcohol expectancies.
- Alcohol tends to increase the user's focus on the "here and now," a kind of alcohol myopia.
- Alcohol-related traffic fatalities have decreased considerably since 1980, but there are still thousands every year in North America.
- Alcohol appears to enhance interest in sex, but to impair physiological arousal in both sexes.
- Alcohol use is statistically associated with homicide, assault, family violence, and suicide.
- Chronic heavy drinking can lead to neurological damage, as well as damage to the heart and liver. However, moderate drinking has been associated with a decrease in heart attacks.
- Canada's Low-Risk Alcohol Drinking Guidelines (LRDG) consist of five guidelines and a series of tips.
- Fetal alcohol syndrome is seen in about 3% of babies whose mothers drink heavily.
- Withdrawal from heavy alcohol use can be life-threatening when seizures develop.
- The notion that alcohol dependence is a disease in its own right goes back at least to the 1700s, but did not become popular until Alcoholics Anonymous began to have a major influence in the 1940s and 1950s.
- Although many studies have indicated a likely genetic influence on susceptibility to alcohol dependence, the exact nature and extent of this genetic link is not known.

Review Questions

1. What is the maximum percentage of alcohol obtainable through fermentation alone? What would that be in "proof"?
2. Did Prohibition reduce alcohol abuse?
3. In about what year did apparent consumption of alcohol reach its peak?
4. About how much more likely are men than women to engage in frequent heavy drinking?
5. About how many standard drinks can the typical human metabolize each hour?
6. For your own gender and weight, about how many standard drinks are required for you to reach the legal BAC limit for driving under the influence?
7. Alcohol enhances the action of which neurotransmitter at its receptors?
8. What is the typical behaviour of a person with a BAC of 0.20%?
9. What term is used to describe the fact that drinkers tend to focus on the "here and now"?
10. About what proportion of traffic fatalities are considered to be alcohol related?
11. What is the role of expectancy in males' increased interest in sex after drinking?
12. If alcohol did not actually increase violent tendencies, how might we explain the statistical correlation between alcohol and such things as assault and homicide?
13. Why is it dangerous to drink alcohol to "stay warm" in the winter?

14. If someone you know has drunk enough alcohol to pass out, what are two things you can do to prevent a lethal outcome?
15. Can brain damage be reversed if someone has been drinking heavily for many years?
16. About what percentage of the heaviest-drinking women will have children diagnosed with FAS?
17. What is the most dangerous withdrawal symptom from alcohol?
18. Did the early founders of AA view alcohol dependence as a disease?
19. If one identical twin is diagnosed with alcohol dependence, what is the likelihood that the other twin will also receive this diagnosis?

SECTION

5

DRUGS, BEHAVIOUR, AND SOCIETY

CHAPTER 10

Tobacco

Why do people smoke, and why do they have such a hard time quitting?

CHAPTER 11

Caffeine

How much of an effect does caffeine really produce? What are the relative strengths of coffee, tea, and soft drinks?

CHAPTER 12

Natural Health Products and Over-the-Counter Drugs

Which of the common drugstore drugs are psychoactive?

FAMILIAR DRUGS

Some drugs are seen so often that they don't seem to be drugs at all, at least not in the same sense as cocaine or marijuana. However, tobacco and its ingredient nicotine, as well as caffeine in its various forms, are psychoactive drugs that meet any reasonable definition of the term *drug*. Both caffeine and nicotine also fall under the category of stimulant drugs. Certainly the drugs sold over the counter (OTC) in pharmacies are drugs, and many of them have their primary effects on the brain and behaviour. In Section 5, we learn about the psychological effects of all these familiar drugs, partly because they are so commonly used.

CHAPTER 10

TOBACCO

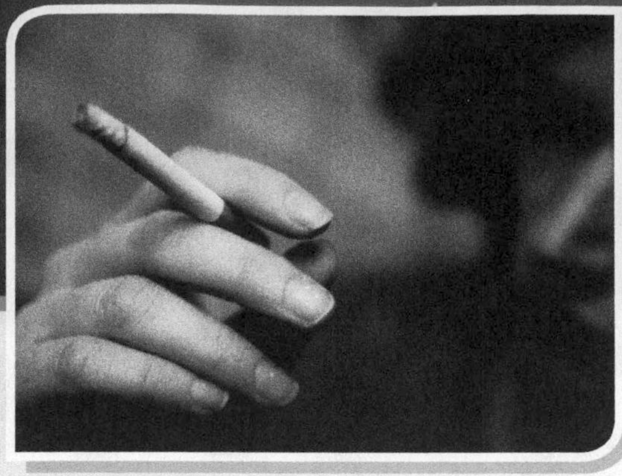

OBJECTIVES

When you have finished this chapter, you should be able to

- **LO1** Describe how Europeans spread tobacco use around the world.
- **LO2** Explain the historical importance of tobacco to Canada.
- **LO3** Summarize the history of anti-tobacco efforts and the response from the tobacco companies.
- **LO4** Explain the difficulties in marketing "safer" cigarettes as related to government regulation.
- **LO5** List the most important adverse health consequences of smoking and the total annual smoking-attributable mortality in Canada.
- **LO6** Examine the controversy over second-hand smoke as both a social issue and a public health issue.
- **LO7** Describe the effects of cigarette smoking on a developing fetus and a newborn.
- **LO8** Describe how nicotine affects cholinergic receptors in the brain and throughout the body, and describe the most common physiological and behavioural effects of nicotine.
- **LO9** Describe the roles of counselling, nicotine replacement therapy, and bupropion in smoking cessation.

The sale and use of tobacco products has always generated controversy, but never at greater levels than it does today. Tobacco represents an interesting social dilemma—a product that is legal for adults to use, and that a significant proportion of adults enjoy using and expect to continue using (although these numbers are decreasing), yet a substance that is responsible for more adverse health consequences and death than any other. This chapter examines how we arrived at tobacco's current status, and what changes lie on the horizon for this agricultural commodity, dependence-producing substance, and topic for policy discussions from local city councils to federal government.

LO1, LO2 Tobacco History

Long before Christopher Columbus voyaged across the Atlantic, the Aboriginal peoples here were using tobacco. It was one of many contributions the New World made to Europe: tobacco, corn, sweet potatoes, white potatoes, chocolate, and—so you could lie back and enjoy it all—the hammock. Columbus recorded that the people of San Salvador presented him with tobacco leaves on October 12, 1492, a fitting birthday present.

In 1497, a monk who had accompanied Columbus on his second trip wrote a book on First Nations customs that contained the first printed report of tobacco smoking. It wasn't called tobacco, and it wasn't called smoking. Inhaling smoke was called drinking. In that period you either "took" (used snuff) or "drank" (smoked) tobacco.

The word *tobacco* came from one of two sources. *Tobacco* referred to a two-pronged tube used by Aboriginal people to take snuff. But some early reports confused the issue by incorrectly applying the name to the plant being used. Another idea is that the word developed its current usage from the province of Tobacos in Mexico, where everyone used the herb. In 1598, an Italian-English dictionary published in London translated the Italian *Nicosiana* as the herb tobacco, and that spelling and usage gradually became dominant.

One member of Columbus's party, Rodrigo de Jerez, was the poor fellow who introduced tobacco drinking to Europe. When he returned with his habit to Portugal, his friends were convinced the devil had possessed him when they saw smoke coming out his mouth and nose. The priest agreed, and Rodrigo spent the next several years in jail, only to find on his release that many people were doing the same thing for which he had been jailed.

Early Medical Uses

Tobacco was formally introduced to Europe as a herb useful for treating almost everything. A 1529 report indicated tobacco was used for "persistent headaches," "cold or catarrh," and "abscesses and sores on the head."[1] Between 1537 and 1559, 14 books mentioned the medicinal value of tobacco.

French physician Jean Nicot became enamoured of the medical uses of tobacco. He tried it on enough people to convince himself of its value and sent glowing reports of the herb's effectiveness to the French court. He was successful in "curing" the migraine headaches of Catherine de Medici, queen of Henry II of France, which made tobacco use very much "in." It was called the *herbe sainte,* "holy plant," and the *herbe à tous les maux,* "the plant against all evils." By 1565, the plant had been called *nicotiane,* after Nicot. In 1753, Linnaeus, the Swedish "father of taxonomy," named the

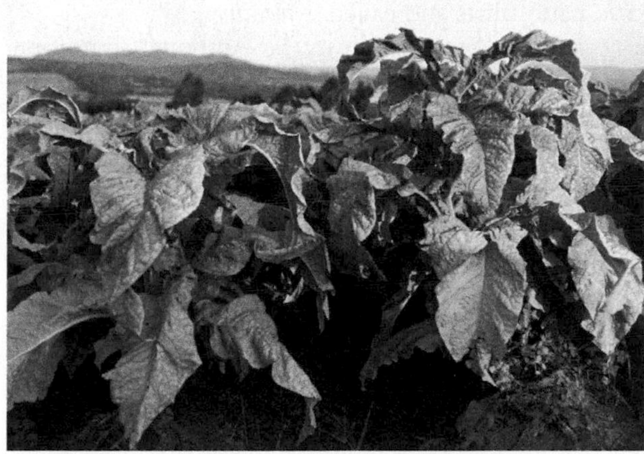

Tobacco was in use by indigenous peoples in North America long before it was introduced into Europe. In 1535, Jacques Cartier encountered natives on the island of Montreal using tobacco.

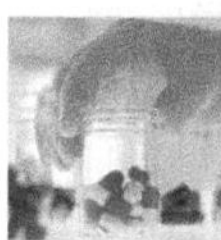

DRUGS IN THE MEDIA

Tobacco Use in the Movies

In 1989, U.S. tobacco companies voluntarily agreed to halt the long-standing practice of directly paying film producers for what is known as "product placement" in popular films. All sorts of companies do this, and at times, the practice is fairly obvious once you know about it. For example, you might notice that in one movie a particular brand of new automobile appears with unusual frequency. In another, one type of soft drink can or billboard (and never a competing brand) might be seen in the background of several shots. Despite all the efforts to control more explicit advertising of cigarettes to young people, this practice is especially insidious because research indicates that tobacco use by an adolescent's favourite actor does influence the adolescent's smoking behaviour. Thus, this type of product placement is likely to be a very potent form of advertising for cigarette manufacturers. Did the 1989 voluntary ban work?

Apparently not, according to a study reported in the medical journal *The Lancet* in 2001.[2] Researchers from Dartmouth College studied the top 25 U.S. films each year for 10 years (1988–1997, a total of 250 films). The first three of those years should have reflected pre-ban film production, compared with the later seven years. They found that 85% of the films portrayed tobacco use. Specific brands were identified in 28% of the films. Neither of these statistics varied from before to after the voluntary ban on direct payments for product placement. Films considered suitable for adolescent audiences (those with PG or PG-13 ratings) contained as many brand appearances as films for adult audiences.

One important difference noted was an increase, rather than a decrease, in the frequency of use of an identified brand by an actor, as opposed to the appearance of a package or billboard in the background. This suggests that this effective form of hidden advertising in movies is actually increasing rather than decreasing. Ironically, the 2005 film *Thank You for Smoking,* about a tobacco company spokesperson, contains no scenes of actual smoking behaviour.

Canadian youth, because of Canada's film rating system, are exposed to 60% more images of tobacco than are American youth.[3] A study released in August 2010 by the World Health Organization and Physicians for a Smoke-Free Canada estimated that about 130 000 of 300 000 youth smokers began smoking as a result of exposure to on-screen tobacco use: "Non-smoking teens whose favourite stars frequently smoke on screen are sixteen times more likely to have positive attitudes about smoking in the future." Smoke Free Movies BC is calling for restricted ratings on movies in which smoking is featured.[4]

plant genus *Nicotiana*. When a pair of French chemists isolated the active ingredient in 1828, they acted like true nationalists and called it *nicotine*.

In the sixteenth century, Sir Anthony Chute summarized much of the available information and said, "Anything that harms a man inwardly from his girdle upward might be removed by a moderate use of the herb." Others, however, felt differently: "If taken after meals the herb would infect the brain and liver," and "Tobacco should be avoided by (among others) women with child and husbands who desired to have children."[1]

In 1617, Dr. William Vaughn phrased the last thought a little more poetically:

> Tobacco that outlandish weede
> It spends the braine and spoiles the seede
> It dulls the spirite, it dims the sight
> It robs a woman of her right.[5]

Dr. Vaughn may have been ahead of his time. Current research verifies tobacco's adverse effects on reproductive functioning in both men and women, as we discuss later in the chapter. The slow advance of medical science through the eighteenth and nineteenth centuries gradually removed tobacco from the doctor's black bag, and nicotine was dropped from the United States *Pharmacopoeia* in the 1890s.

Canada has three major tobacco companies: Imperial Tobacco Canada Limited; Rothmans, Benson & Hedges Incorporated; and JTI-Macdonald Corporation. Imperial Tobacco was founded in the nineteenth century in Montreal. About 90% of the tobacco grown in Canada is produced in a highly concentrated area in southwestern Ontario, close to the north shore of Lake Erie near the towns of Delhi and Tillsonburg. Tillsonburg, a town located about 50 kilometres southeast of London, Ontario, was once home to Canadian singer Stompin' Tom Connors, who wrote a song about working in the tobacco fields and named it after the town. The remainder of the tobacco grown in Canada is grown in Quebec (98 farms), Prince Edward Island (35 farms), Nova Scotia (9 farms), and New Brunswick (5 farms).[6]

Chewing Tobacco

The popularity of chewing tobacco gradually increased and annual production peaked at 578 metric tons in Canada in 1980.[7] Chewing was a suitable activity for a country on the go; it freed the hands, and the wide-open spaces made an adequate spittoon.

The start of the twentieth century was the approximate high point for chewing tobacco, the sales of which slowly declined through the early part of that century, as other tobacco products became more popular. Chewing tobacco has remained a big part of Major League Baseball over the years. Today there is a push to ban chewing tobacco on and off the field, both for the health of the players and to promote them as positive role models for young fans.[8]

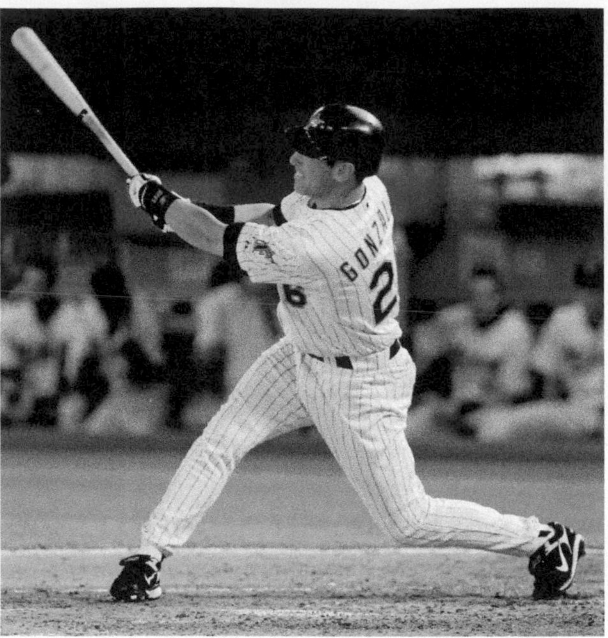

Major League Baseball player Luis Gonzalez is an active advocate against the use of tobacco products both on the field and off.

Cigars

The transition from chewing to cigarettes had a middle point, a combination of both smoking and chewing: cigars. Cigarette smoking was becoming popular, and cigar manufacturers did their best to keep cigarettes under control. They suggested that cigarettes were drugged with opium and people could not stop using them, and that the paper was bleached with arsenic and, thus, was harmful. They had some help from Thomas Edison in 1914:

> The injurious agent in Cigarettes comes principally from the burning paper wrapper. . . . It has a violent action in the nerve centers, producing degeneration of the cells of the brain, which is quite rapid among boys. Unlike most narcotics, this degeneration is permanent and uncontrollable. I employ no person who smokes cigarettes.[9]

The efforts of the cigar manufacturers worked for a while, and cigar sales reached their highest level in 1920, when 8 billion were sold. As sales increased, though, so did the cost of the product. Lower cost and changing styles led to the emergence of cigarettes as the leading form of tobacco use.

Cigarettes

Thin reeds filled with tobacco had been seen by the Spanish in Yucatan in 1518. In 1844, the French were using them, and the Crimean War circulated the cigarette habit throughout Europe. The first British cigarette factory was started in 1856 by a returning veteran of the Crimean War, and in the late 1850s an English tobacco merchant, Philip Morris, began producing handmade cigarettes.

In Canada and the United States, cigarettes were being produced during the same period (14 million in 1870), but their popularity increased rapidly in the 1880s. The date of the first patent on a cigarette-making machine was 1881, and by 1885 more than 1 billion cigarettes a year were being sold. Not even that great he-man, boxer John L. Sullivan, could stem the tide, though in 1905 his opinion of cigarette smokers was pretty clear:

> Smoke cigarettes? Not on your tut-tut. . . . You can't suck coffin-nails and be a ring-champion. . . . You never heard of . . . a bank burglar using a cigarette, did you? They couldn't do it and attend to biz. Why, even drunkards don't use the things. . . . Who smokes 'em? Dudes and college stiffs–fellows who'd be wiped out by a single jab or a quick undercut. It isn't natural to smoke cigarettes. An American ought to smoke cigars. . . . It's the Dutchmen, Italians, Russians, Turks and Egyptians who smoke cigarettes and they're no good anyhow.[6]

The years from 1920 to 1950 were three golden decades for cigarette consumption in Canada. Cigarettes were custom packaged and shipped to Canadian soldiers overseas. Macdonald's Tobacco created a series of cards that were distributed to Canadian soldiers and organizations to support the consumption of Macdonald's Tobacco. The card shown here told families and organizations how they could order cigarette packages to be shipped to Canadian soldiers overseas.

LO3, LO4, LO5, LO6, LO7

Tobacco under Attack

As with every other psychoactive substance, use by some raises concerns on the part of others, and many efforts have been made over the years to regulate tobacco use.

The long and slowly developing attack on tobacco as a major health problem had its seeds in reports in the 1930s and 1940s indicating a possible link between smoking and cancer. A 1952 article in *Readers' Digest* called "Cancer by the Carton" drew public attention to the issue and led to a temporary decline in cigarette sales. The major tobacco companies recognized the threat and responded vigorously in two important ways. One was the formation of the supposedly independent Council for Tobacco Research to look into the health claims (later investigations revealed this council was not independent of tobacco company influence and served largely to try to undermine any scientific evidence demonstrating the negative health consequences of tobacco use). The other response was the mass marketing of filter cigarettes and cigarettes with lowered tar and nicotine content. The public apparently had faith in these "less hazardous" cigarettes, because cigarette sales again began to climb.

In the early 1960s, the U.S. surgeon general's office formed an Advisory Committee on Smoking and Health. Its first official report, released in 1964, stated clearly that cigarette smoking was a cause for increased lung cancer in men (at the time, the evidence for women was less extensive). Per capita sales of cigarettes in Canada began a decline that continued over the next 20 years (see Figure 10.1). In 1965, cigarette packages were required to include the surgeon general's warning. All television and radio advertising of cigarettes was banned in 1971, and smoking was banned on intercity buses and domestic airline flights in 1989. The list of provincial, territorial, and local laws prohibiting smoking in public buildings, offices, restaurants, and even bars grows every year. Clearly, momentum is behind efforts to restrict smoking–and exposure to second-hand smoke. Almost 6300 nonsmokers die each year in Canada from exposure to second-hand smoke.[10] In Canada, a key target of harm reduction measures in smoking is the protection of nonsmokers from second-hand smoke in workplaces, restaurants, cars, and even homes.[11]

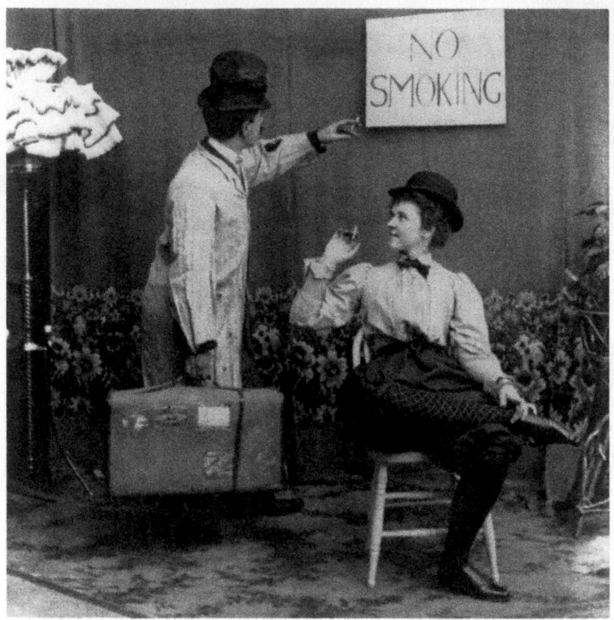

Some early tobacco control efforts focused on women, associating tobacco use with immoral behaviour.

The National Clearinghouse on Tobacco and Health (NCTH) and Health Canada are the Canadian hosts for Guildford Depository materials relating to the Canadian tobacco industry. The book *Smoke and Mirrors* by Rob Cunningham provides a historical account of the evolution of tobacco in Canada, the major tobacco control issues, the failures and successes of tobacco control efforts, and a plan to reduce tobacco use in the future. The Canadian Council for Tobacco Control is the national organization that specializes in tobacco and health. Table 10.1 provides a chronology of key tobacco-related events in Canada.

Figure 10.1 Trends in Cigarette Sales in Canada since 1980

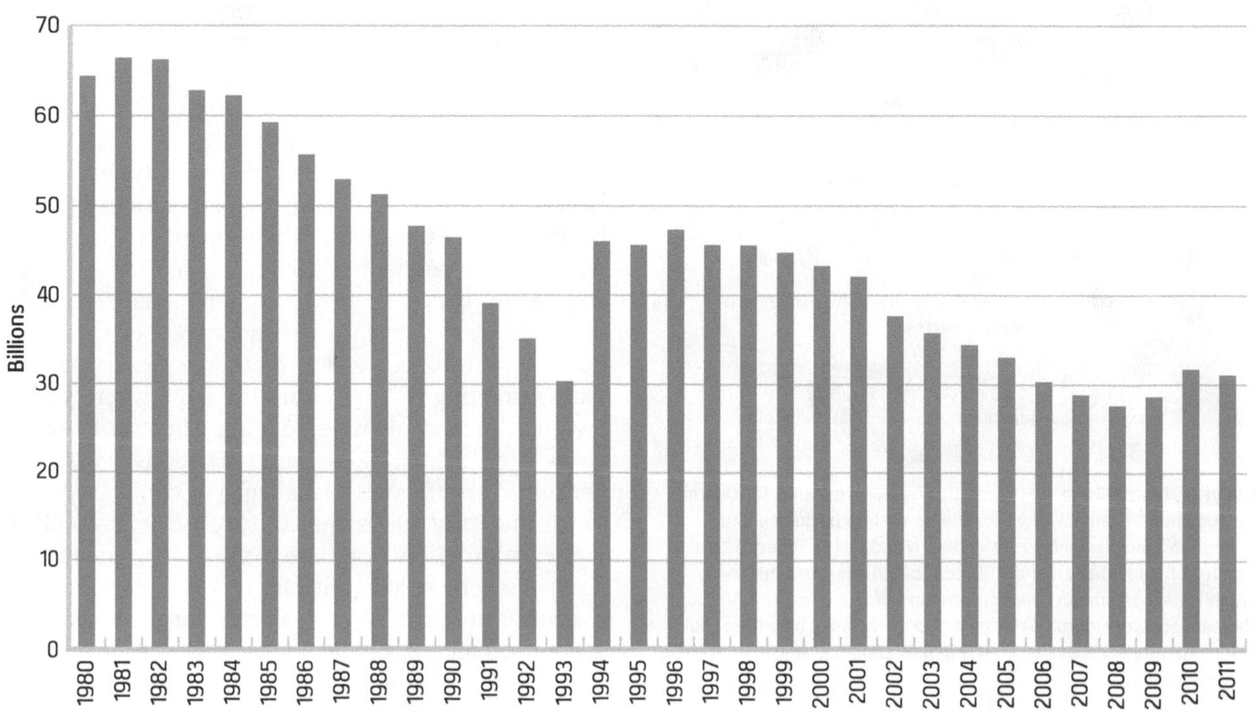

Table 10.1 Timeline of Key Canadian Facts Related to Tobacco

1670: New France's Sovereign Council imposes duties on tobacco.

1676: New France's residents are prohibited from smoking or carrying tobacco on the streets.

1739: Canada exports tobacco to France.

1858: Macdonald Tobacco is established in Montreal.

1878: House of Commons defeats resolution to abolish tobacco taxes.

1891: British Columbia prohibits the sale of tobacco to minors, followed by Ontario and Nova Scotia, New Brunswick (1893), and Northwest Territories (1896).

1906: Federal Department of Agriculture establishes the Tobacco Branch.

1908: Tobacco Restraint Act makes it illegal to sell tobacco products to anyone under 16 years of age; this Act was never enforced.

1912: Imperial Tobacco of Canada is incorporated to produce and market tobacco products across Canada.

1914: House of Commons Select Committee on Cigarette Evils conducts public hearings.

1927: First Canadian advertisement showing a woman smoking a cigarette appears in *Montreal Gazette*.

1950: Large-scale epidemiological studies showing a statistical association between lung cancer and smoking are published.

1952: Federal government reduces tobacco taxes in response to a rise in cigarette smuggling.

1954: Canadian Medical Association issues first public warning on the hazards of smoking. The link between smoking and lung cancer was established in the medical literature in the 1950s, yet the tobacco industry cast doubt and made great strides to publicly hide the negative health effects of tobacco.[12]

1957: Ontario Flue-cured Tobacco Growers' Marketing Board is established.

1961: Results published of major Health and Welfare study, initiated in 1954, on the effects of smoking on Canadian war veterans; 60% more deaths among cigarette smokers than nonsmokers are reported, and an association is made between cigarette smoking and an increase in lung cancer and heart disease.

1962: Report of the Royal College of Physicians in London, England, provides research evidence of the harmful consequences of smoking.

1963: Federal Minister of Health and Welfare Judy LaMarsh draws attention to the link between cigarette smoking and lung cancer, coronary heart disease, and chronic bronchitis. Canadian Tobacco Manufacturers Council is established.

1964: Report of the Advisory Committee to the United States Surgeon General concludes that lung cancer and chronic bronchitis are medical consequences of smoking. Canadian tobacco industry adopts first voluntary code on marketing practices.

1965: Federal Department of National Health and Welfare commissions national survey on smoking.

1967: Federal Cabinet approves preparation of legislation to require statements of tar and nicotine levels on cigarette packages and in advertising; however, no bill is introduced.

1969: A report by the House of Commons Committee on Health, Welfare and Social Affairs (Isabelle Report) contains recommendations on restricting the advertising and promotion of tobacco products.

1970: In its first anti-smoking resolution, the World Health Assembly calls upon governments to act against smoking as an avoidable cause of death.

1971: The government introduces Bill C-248 to ban advertising of tobacco products; however, the bill is not debated. Instead, the tobacco industry and the government agree to voluntary guidelines.

1974: The Canadian Council on Smoking and Health is formed. Charter members include the Canadian Cancer Society, the Canadian Heart Foundation, the Heart and Stroke Foundation of Canada, and the Canadian Lung Association. Non-Smokers' Rights Association also is formed.

1976: City of Ottawa passes first municipal bylaw restricting smoking in public places.

1979: Nicotine gum is made available in Canada on a prescription basis.

Continued

Table 10.1 *Continued*

1985: National Strategy to Reduce Tobacco Use is established with representation from federal and provincial/territorial governments and eight health organizations. Physicians for a Smoke-Free Canada is established. Treasury Board announces voluntary guidelines for federal public servants on workplace smoking.

1988–89: Federal laws are enacted to prohibit tobacco advertising and ensure smoke-free workplaces. The government also begins requiring cigarette manufacturers to list the additives and their amounts in each brand. The Tobacco Products Control Act (TPCA), which prohibits all tobacco advertising, requires health warnings on tobacco packaging and restricts promotional activities, comes into effect[13]; covers smoking and smokeless tobacco.[14]

1993: Federal law enacted to raise the legal age for buying tobacco to 18.

1994: Bigger and stronger warning messages required on cigarette packs. Canadian scientists report finding evidence of cigarette smoke in fetal hair, the first biochemical proof that the offspring of nonsmoking mothers can be affected by passive cigarette smoke.[14]

1995: Supreme Court of Canada squashes the federal ban on tobacco advertising; tobacco companies launch an aggressive advertising campaign using billboards, newspaper ads, and event sponsorships. Ottawa releases *A Blueprint to Protect the Health of Canadians,* an outline of proposed legislation to reinstate the advertising ban, but no bill is introduced in Parliament.

1997: The Tobacco Act is passed; its associated regulations impose general restrictions on manufacturers and distributors; restrict promotion, packaging, and products; and impose point-of-sale restrictions.[14]

1999: Toronto starts its anti-smoking campaign by eliminating smoking in public spaces and workplaces.

2001: Restaurants are included in the Toronto ban, followed by bars in 2004, whereupon clubgoers are forced to become extra-vigilant about their body odours.

2000: New regulations require cigarette packages to be emblazoned with large explicitly visceral warning labels.

2009: Ontario drivers who smoke with children in the car become subject to a fine.

2010: Sale of flavoured tobacco products is banned. Teens are forced to experiment with far less delicious, but equally addictive, tobacco-flavoured tobacco.

2013: Emerging use of herbal tobacco-free hookah.

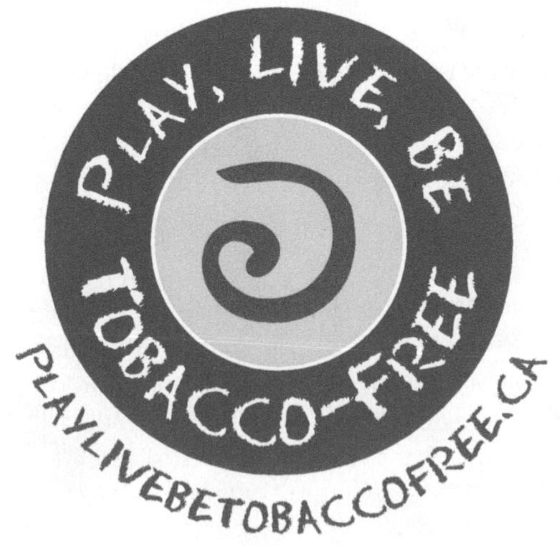

Just as smoking ads have targeted specific groups, so too do current anti-smoking campaigns.

The Quest for "Safer" Cigarettes

Nicotine appears to be the constituent in tobacco that keeps smokers coming back for more–if the nicotine content of cigarettes is varied, people tend to adjust their smoking behaviour, taking more puffs and inhaling more deeply when given low-nicotine cigarettes, and reporting no satisfaction if all the nicotine is removed.[15] Another complex product of burning tobacco is something called tar, the sticky brown stuff that can be seen on the filter after a cigarette is smoked. Beginning in the mid-1950s with the mass marketing of filter cigarettes, the tobacco companies began to promote the idea of a "safer" cigarette, without actually admitting that there was anything unsafe about their older products. Because the companies were advertising their cigarettes as being lower in tar and nicotine, for many years the Federal Trade Commission (with

MIND/BODY CONNECTION

A Foggy Future: The Adverse Effects of Shisha Consumption or Hookah Use

Is Canada winning the war on smoking? Data suggest that young Canadians are smoking fewer cigarettes. New data suggest young Canadians are turning to water pipes with the belief that smoke from water pipes is safe—while in reality the fumes they're inhaling may be even more toxic than those from cigarettes. Water pipes, the new tobacco trend of the twenty-first century, are also called shisha or hookah. Originating from the Middle East and India in the sixteenth century, they are gaining popularity in Canada. According to the 2013 Ontario Drug Use and Health Survey performed by the Centre for Addiction and Mental Health (CAMH), almost 10% of Ontario students between Grades 7 and 12 smoked a hookah in the last year, while only 8.5% of this age group reported cigarette use; similar trends are being reported across the country. Perceived as a lesser version of cigarette smoking, young adults are taking on some of the following beliefs that are proving to be quite controversial.

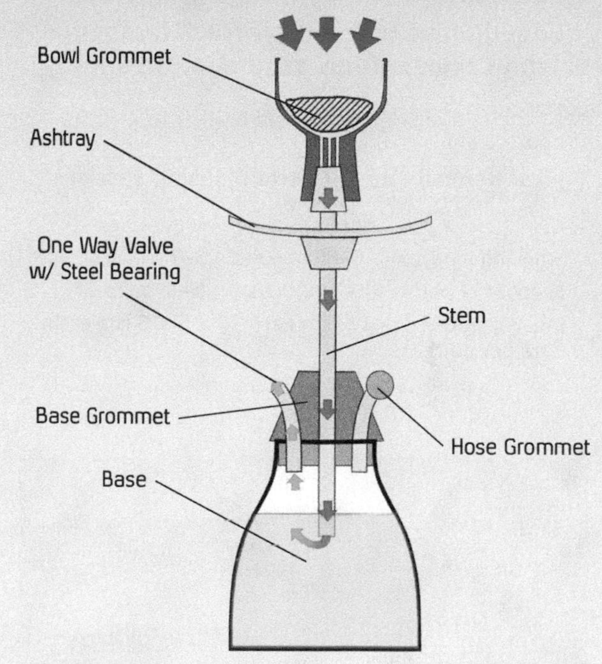

Some Common Misconceptions Surrounding Hookah Use

- Smoking water pipes is safer because the water will filter toxic chemicals
- Shisha is all natural; there are no added chemicals as in cigarettes
- Tobacco-free shisha is composed only of plant matter
- Second-hand smoke from water pipes has no effect on those around us or our environment[16]

Product and Method of Consumption

Herbal and tobacco shisha, commonly known as hookah or narghile, has become an increasingly popular alternative to cigarettes. Shisha is often made by a base of tobacco or marijuana leaves with added flavouring for improved taste. These substances are consumed through a pipe connected to a tall structure containing a water container, a bowl, and a charcoal chamber. Shisha is placed in the bowl, where it becomes heated by charcoal just above. The smoke is pushed downward toward the water jug, where the smoke's temperature is reduced significantly. The smoke then exits the main system and is spread throughout the individual pipes for consumption.[16]

Chemical Compounds

Due to the lack of regulation, shisha is packaged with no informative labels warning users of the harmful effects. Traditional tobacco cigarettes contain cancer-causing chemicals such as formaldehyde, benzene, tar, hydrogen cyanide, and high levels of carbon monoxide. Both herbal and tobacco shisha are found to contain chromium, nickel, arsenic, tar, chrysene, and naphthalene, a known carcinogen.[17] Second-hand smoke also poses a problem, as herbal shisha contains formaldehyde and PAH compounds equal to or in excess of what's found in second-hand tobacco smoke.[17]

Hookah Sessions

Shisha users often inhale more deeply and attend longer sessions of smoking than a regular cigarette smoker. When smoked, one gram of tobacco shisha contains 11 times more carbon monoxide than a single gram of cigarette tobacco.[18] Longer exposure time results in increased effects on participants. Smoke produced from herbal and tobacco shisha is known to contain cancerous agents such as carcinogens. The levels of agents released from first- and second-hand smoke are equal to or greater than the amount of toxins released from cigarettes.[19] University students also attend hookah bars regularly. The downtown scene attracts many university students, and hookah bars are building on the increased demand. This increases exposure time to all participants, also increasing the risk of cancer and other diseases.[20]

Continued

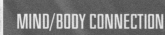

MIND/BODY CONNECTION

A Foggy Future: The Adverse Effects of Shisha Consumption or Hookah Use

continued

Typical Hookah and Cigarette Smoking Sessions[21]

	Hookah	Cigarettes
Smoking time	28–80 minutes	5–7 minutes
Number of puffs	50–200 puffs	8–12 puffs
Inhaled smoke (litre per puff)	0.15 litre each	0.5–0.6 litre each

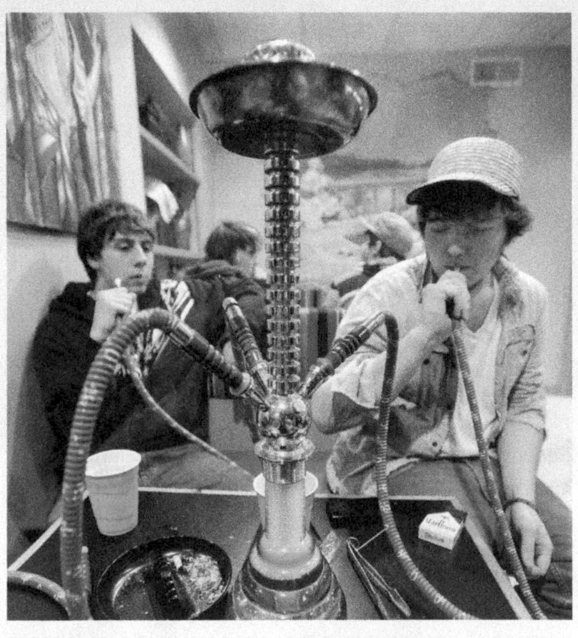

Adverse Effects of Shisha[22]

- Increased blood pressure and heart rate[23]
- Lung disease including chronic obstructive pulmonary disease (COPD)[23]
- Increased risk of oral disease, oral cancer, and lung cancer[23]
- Harm to the fetus including low birthweight and other effects similar to smoking cigarettes[23]
- Communicable disease due to pipe sharing, such as influenza, herpes, hepatitis, tuberculosis, and meningitis[23]

Raising Awareness

Smoking tobacco indoors is not allowed in most places in Canada—bars serve "herbal" tobacco-free hookah using a mixture of flavours and herbs. There are more than 80 hookah bars in Toronto alone. Because they serve tobacco-free herbal hookah, hookah bars in Canada aren't required to have age restrictions, and do not fall under anti-tobacco smoking laws. The charcoal used to heat tobacco or herbal hookah in water pipes emits high levels of carbon monoxide, metals, and cancer-causing chemicals, prompting educators and lawmakers across Canada to take action. Alberta and Ontario have since banned hookah smoking in public places altogether. The University of Saskatchewan and Alberta have joined forces in increasing awareness, education, and dispelling myths around this "healthier" alternative through student health services. It is hoped that the hazardous health effects of herbal hookah will become as well known as the saying "cancer by the carton."

The authors thank Taylor Conrad of Saint Mary's University for article contribution.

Source: Based on "A Foggy Future: The Adverse Effects of Shisha Consumption or Hookah Use." University of Saskatchewan Health Services. (May 13, 2014). University of Saskatchewan. Hookah: What You Need to Know. Retrieved from: http://students.usask.ca/current/life/health/stayhealthy/brochures/hookah.php.

industry support and cooperation) monitored the tar and nicotine yields of the various cigarette brands and made those results public. The U.S. Congress and the National Cancer Institute promoted research to develop safer cigarettes. The public listened to all this talk about safer cigarettes and bought in–sales of filter cigarettes took off, and by the 1980s low tar and nicotine cigarettes dominated the market.

The problem with all this is that *safer* doesn't mean "safe," and it wasn't at all clear how much safer these low tar and nicotine cigarettes actually are for people over a lifetime of smoking. Some early studies had indicated that those who had smoked lower-yield cigarettes for years were at less risk for cancer and heart disease than those who smoked high-yield brands. But other studies seemed to show that if a smoker switched from a high-yield to a low-yield cigarette, changes in puff rate and depth of inhalation would compensate for the lower yield per puff, and there might be no advantage to switching.

Current Cigarette Use

Cigarette use by Canadians ages 12 and older is presented in Table 10.2. Compared with the national

Table 10.2 Cigarette Use in the Provinces and Territories, 1999–2011

YEAR	1999	2000	2001	2002	2003	2004	2005	2006	2007	2008	2009	2010	2011
CANADA	25.2	24.4	21.7	21.4	20.9	19.6	18.7	18.6	19.2	17.9	17.5	16.7	17.3
BRITISH COLUMBIA	20.0	19.6	16.7	16.5	16.4	15.2	14.7	16.4	14.4	14.7	14.9	14.3	14.2
ALBERTA	26.0	22.6	25.1	22.8	20.0	20.1	20.6	21.3	21.0	20.4	18.0	18.8	17.7
SASKATCHEWAN	25.9	28.1	25.4	21.2	24.1	21.7	22.0	23.7	24.0	20.4	22.3	21.1	19.2
MANITOBA	23.3	25.7	25.9	21.1	20.9	20.6	22.3	20.1	19.9	20.8	18.9	20.5	18.7
ONTARIO	23.2	23.1	19.7	19.7	19.6	18.7	16.4	16.6	18.3	16.8	15.4	15.2	16.3
QUEBEC	30.3	28.2	24.1	25.8	24.6	22.2	22.2	20.1	21.7	19.1	20.7	17.8	19.8
NEW BRUNSWICK	26.5	26.6	25.0	21.1	24.3	24.2	21.8	22.6	21.2	19.9	21.3	19.3	18.8
NOVA SCOTIA	28.9	29.8	24.9	25.3	22.1	20.2	21.0	21.8	20.4	19.7	19.8	20.8	18.1
PRINCE EDWARD ISLAND	25.6	25.7	25.6	23.1	21.4	21.2	19.9	19.2	18.4	19.2	17.7	16.2	19.1
NFLD. & LABRADOR	28.5	27.7	25.7	24.1	23.0	21.8	20.6	21.7	21.2	20.2	20.7	20.0	19.0

*INCLUDES DAILY AND NON-DAILY SMOKERS

DATA SOURCE: CTUMS, 1999–2011

Source: © All rights reserved. Canadian Tobacco Use Monitoring Survey (CTUMS), 2012. Health Canada, 2013. Reproduced with permission from the Minister of Health, 2014.

estimate of 12.7%, the prevalence of smoking is above average among those attending university in Quebec (18.3%) and the Atlantic provinces (16.9%) and lowest among those from British Columbia (9.6%) and the Prairies (8.9%). Current smoking is not significantly related to gender or extracurricular orientation.[24] There is an almost perfectly inverse linear relationship between number of years of education and the percentage of that group that smokes cigarettes.[25]

Current smoking prevalence by age is presented in Figure 10.2. Since 1985, smoking prevalence has significantly decreased in all age groups, with an overall average decrease of 14%. Despite anti-smoking education, 8% of young people ages 15-19 still become regular smokers.[26] In 2008-2009, 3% of students in Grades 6-9 smoked, and 13% of students in Grades 10-12 were regular smokers.[27] Aboriginal peoples have a long history of using tobacco in ritual ceremonies and prayer. However, traditional use of tobacco does not include smoking cigarettes. A 2005 study of a First Nations community in Manitoba revealed that 82% of adolescents ages 15-19 years and 70% of Inuit ages 18-45 years are current smokers.[28]

Smokeless Tobacco

In the early 1970s, many cigarette smokers apparently began to look for alternatives that would reduce the risk of lung cancer. Pipe and cigar smoking enjoyed a brief, small increase, followed by a long period of decline. Sales of **smokeless tobacco** products—specifically, different kinds of chewing tobacco—began to increase. Once limited to western movies and the baseball field in terms of public awareness, smokeless tobacco use grew to become a matter of public concern.

The most common types of oral smokeless tobacco are loose-leaf (Red Man, Levi Garrett, Beech Nut), which is sold in a pouch, and **moist snuff** (Copenhagen, Skoal), which is sold in a can. When you see a baseball player on TV with a big wad in his cheek, it is probably composed of loose-leaf tobacco. With all

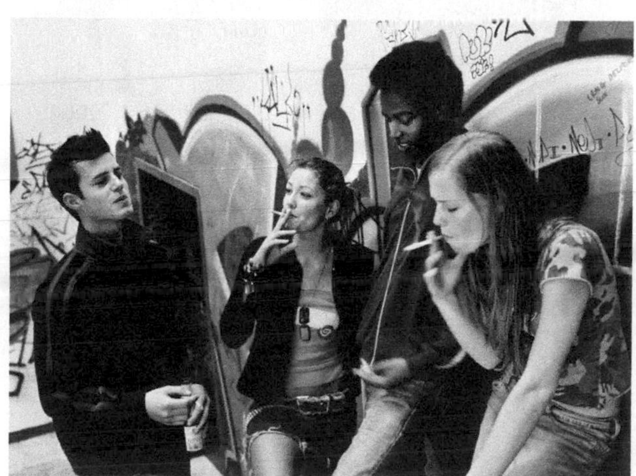

Canada is considered to be at the forefront of anti-smoking legislation.

smokeless tobacco: a term used for chewing tobacco.

moist snuff: finely chopped tobacco, held in the mouth rather than snuffed into the nose.

Figure 10.2 Current Smoking Prevalence from 1985 to 2012 for Canadians Aged 15 Years and Older, Youth Aged 15–19, and Young Adults Aged 20–24

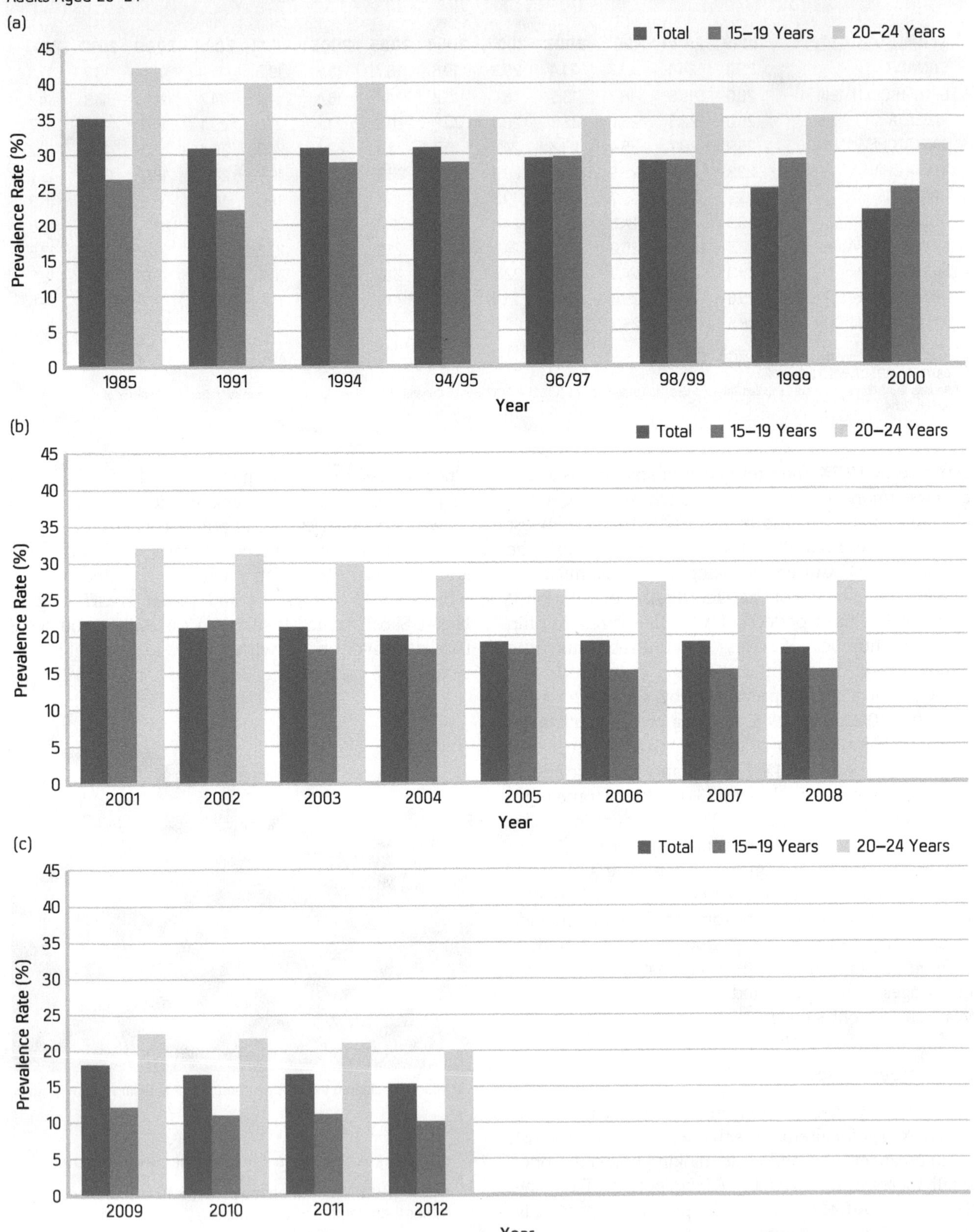

Source: Canadian Tobacco Use Monitoring Survey (CTUMS), 2012. Health Canada, 2013. Reproduced with permission from the Minister of Health, 2014

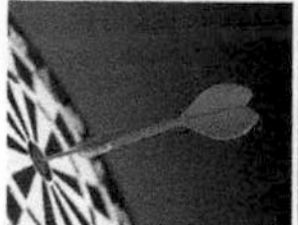

TARGETING PREVENTION

Smoking among First Nations Adolescents

Tobacco use is the leading preventable cause of death and disease in Canada, killing 47 000 Canadians each year.[29] Smoking in adolescents is especially troubling. The *2007 Nova Scotia Student Drug Use Survey* reported that the average age for first smoking a whole cigarette was 12.9 years and that 28% of students in Grades 7–12 reported they had smoked at least one whole cigarette in their lifetime.[30] Cigarette smoking prevalence has decreased significantly, from 36% in 1998 to 24% in 2007. Sixteen percent of students reported smoking during the year, with 13% smoking 1 to 10 cigarettes per day, and 3% of all students smoking 11 or more. Males and females were equally likely to have smoked cigarettes during the year, although cigarette smoking was more common among older (25% in Grade 12) than younger students (4% in Grade 7).

In the six months before the survey, 54% of students who smoked cigarettes during the year tried to quit. To obtain tobacco products, 6% of students in Grade 7, 9, and 10 and 13% of Grade 12 students lied about their age or used fake identification.[30] In Alberta and Nova Scotia, people under age 18 who are caught smoking or in possession of tobacco products can have their cigarettes seized by police, but only in Alberta can minors also be fined up to $100.[31,32] In Canada, selling tobacco products to minors may result in fines of up to $4000 for a store owner and $10 000 for a corporation for a first offence; subsequent offences can result in fines of up to $150 000, and retailers with two or more convictions risk being banned from selling cigarettes for a period.[33,34,35]

According to Statistics Canada, in 2009 the smoking rate was 13% among teens 15–19 years of age, down from 15% in 2008, although in 2009 smoking rates were 15% for Canadian teens and 17% for Quebec teens.[36] Rates of smoking are highest among First Nations and Inuit youth.[37] For thousands of years tobacco was a sacred part of First Nations traditional ceremonies, rituals, and prayers, providing a conduit to communicate with the spiritual world of their ancestors.[37] In its original form, tobacco has honour, purpose, and medicinal attributes, cleansing and healing the body and soul. The Haudenosaunee First Nations speak of tobacco in their Creation story, while the Cree profess tobacco to be a natural product and not just one plant; plants had to be combined in offerings to the spiritual world.[38] The smoking of cigarettes and chewing of tobacco have no place in Aboriginal ceremonies. The chemical additives found in commercial tobacco and the addictive incentive detract from its spiritual purpose.[37] Evidently, the differences between traditional and nontraditional uses of tobacco are not clear because of the high prevalence of smoking in youths and elders.[38] Compounding the problem is the fact that First Nations people have been allowed to purchase up to three cartons of cigarettes a week from on-reserve stores without having to pay the provincial or territorial tobacco tax.[39] Canadian First Nations are almost three times as likely to smoke (see Figure 10.3) and less likely—although they self-report being more willing (see Table 10.3)—to use a smoking cessation aid, such as the nicotine patch, relative to other Canadians.[40] The Canadian government is concerned about high smoking rates among First Nations people, so it is cutting back on the number of tax-free cigarettes they can buy.

Figure 10.3 Smoking among First Nations Youth

This figure shows the prevalence of current smoking among 236 youths ages 10–19 in the Oji-Cree community of Sandy Lake, in northwestern Ontario, and the age-specific national averages from Health Canada's *1994 Youth Smoking Survey*.

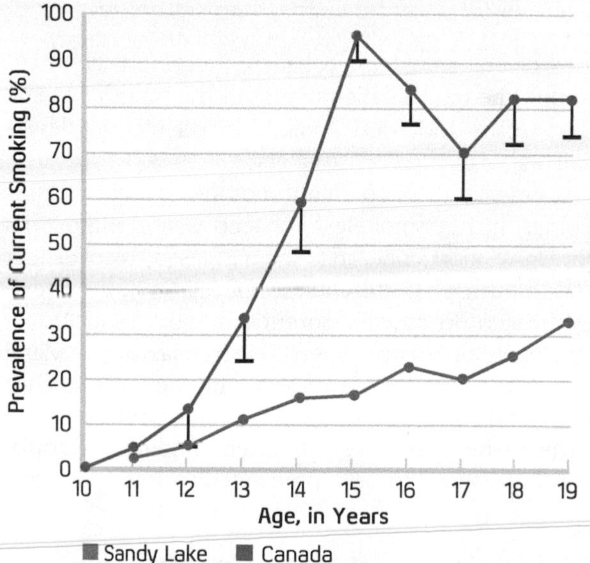

Source: Retnakaran, R., and others. "Cigarette Smoking and Cardiovascular Risk Factors among Aboriginal Canadian Youths." *Canadian Medical Association Journal* 173 (2005), pp. 885–89.

Continued

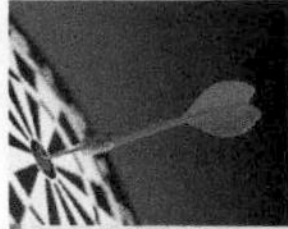

TARGETING PREVENTION

Smoking among First Nations Adolescents

continued

Table 10.3 Smoking Cessation Behaviours and Attitudes toward Cessation Drug Therapy

Characteristic	Aboriginal Number of Subjects (%)	Non-Aboriginal Number of Subjects (%)
Female	260 (63.8)	53 (52.0)
Daily smoker	211 (51.8)	58 (56.9)
Occasional smoker	122 (30.0)	9 (8.8)
Ex-smoker	70 (17.1)	35 (34.3)
Saw a physician in the past year	135 (35.1)	48 (54.5)
Received cessation advice from a physician	94 (69.6)	28 (58.3)
If discussed cessation, received drug therapy advice from physician	56 (57.7)	17 (60.7)
Attempted to stop or reduce	189 (47.9)	33 (36.7)
Willing to use at least one agent	162 (39.8)	51 (50.0)
Willing to use nicotine patch	114 (30.9)	40 (42.9)
Willing to use nicotine gum	98 (27.5)	28 (29.8)
Willing to use bupropion	60 (16.9)	27 (29.0)

Source: Nicotine and tobacco research: official journal of the Society for Research on Nicotine and Tobacco by SOC FOR RES ON NICOTINE & TOBACCO. Reproduced with permission of TAYLOR & FRANCIS LTD in the format reuse in a book/e-book via Copyright Clearance Center.

forms of oral smokeless tobacco, nicotine is absorbed through the mucous membranes of the mouth into the bloodstream, and users achieve blood nicotine levels comparable to those of smokers.

Chewing tobacco might not be as unhealthy as smoking it, but smokeless tobacco is not without its hazards. Of most concern is the increased risk of cancer of the mouth, pharynx, and esophagus. Snuff and chewing tobacco do contain potent carcinogens, including high levels of tobacco-specific **nitrosamines**. Many users experience tissue changes in the mouth, with **leukoplakia** (a whitening, thickening, and hardening of the tissue) a relatively frequent finding. Leukoplakia is considered to be a precancerous lesion (a tissue change that can develop into cancer). The irritation of the gums can cause them to become inflamed or to recede, exposing the teeth to disease. The enamel of the teeth can also be worn down by the abrasive action of the tobacco. Dentists are also becoming more aware of the destructive effects of oral tobacco. The overall prevalence of smokeless tobacco use in Canada is low, at around 8% for those having *ever* used it and less than 1% for *recent* use in 2005.[41]

nitrosamine: a type of chemical that is carcinogenic; several are found in tobacco.

leukoplakia: a whitening and thickening of the mucous tissue in the mouth, considered to be a precancerous tissue change.

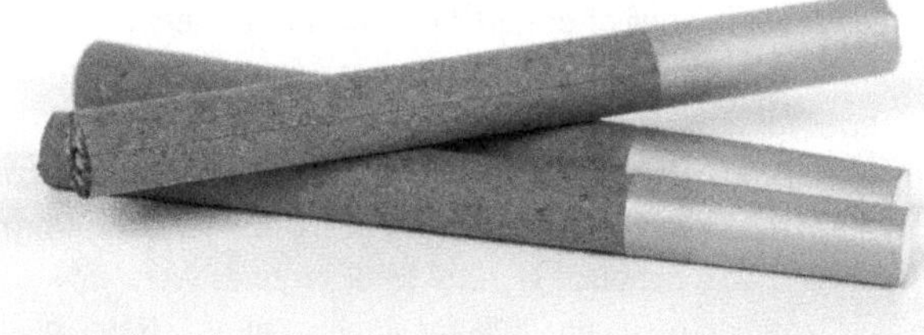

Cigarillos and flavoured cigarettes are illegal to sell individually in Canada.

Figure 10.4 Pipe Tobacco, Snuff, and Chewing Tobacco Consumption Is Low in Canada

Cigar use is steadily increasing. Cigarillos are popular among Canadian youth, and when cigarillo use was included in smoking prevalence statistics for youth ages 15–19, smoking rates increased from 15% to 20% in 2007.

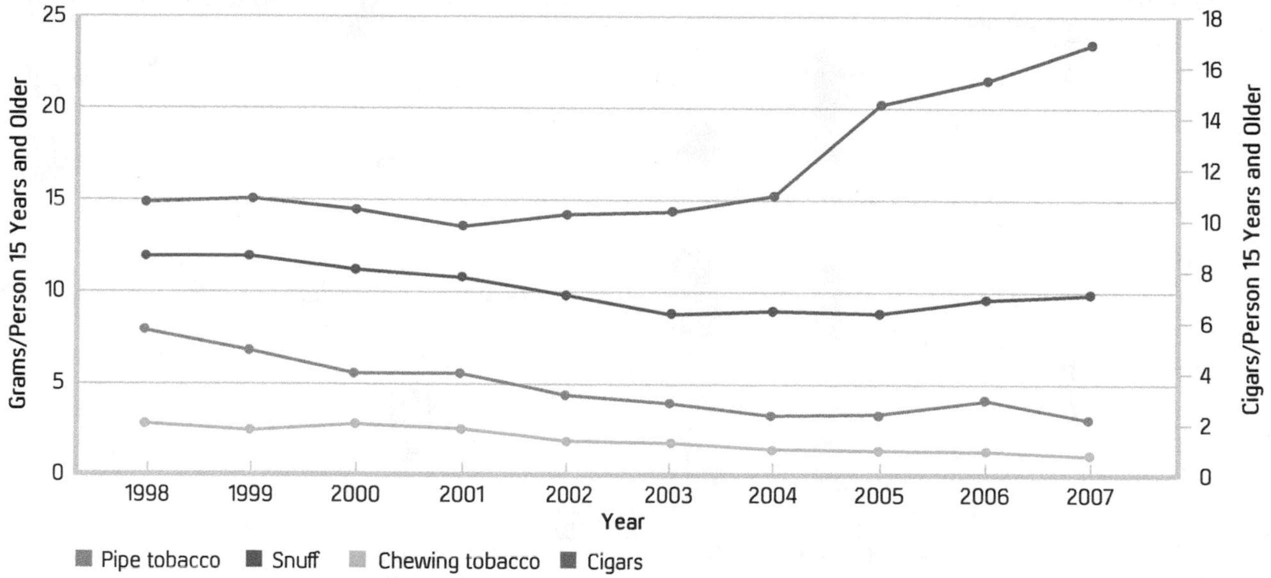

Source: Physicians for a Smoke-Free Canada. *Canadian Per-Capita Consumption of Pipe, Snuff, Chewing Tobacco and Cigars, 1998–2007.* 2008. Retrieved October 4, 2011, from http://www.smoke-free.ca/factsheets/pdf/cigars,%20snuff,%20chewing%20and%20pipe%20tobacco.pdf. Reprinted with permission of Physicians for a Smoke-Free Canada, www.smoke-free.ca.

Are Cigars Back?

After many years of declining popularity, cigar smoking reappeared on the cultural scene in the mid-1990s. Yuppies, businesspeople, and celebrities of both sexes began lighting up large, expensive cigars, many of which are made in Florida from tobacco supposedly grown from Cuban seeds. Magazines devoted to cigars, cigar bars, and radio talk-show discussions of the merits of specific brands all helped to spread the habit. Cigarillos and flavoured cigarettes have also become popular with Canadian youth (see Figure 10.4).

Adverse Health Effects

The smoke has now cleared after many government and other reports detailing the health hazards of tobacco use were revealed, and we can see the overall picture. Although lung cancer is not common, about 85% of all lung cancers occur in smokers. The cancer-causing agent in tobacco is likely not nicotine but rather the aromatics, such as benzo[a]pyrene, that arise from the burning of tobacco. They damage DNA, resulting in cancerous mutations. Every 11 minutes, a Canadian dies from tobacco use; that's 47 000 people every year. Almost 11 000 of these deaths are related to heart disease and stroke (Figure 10.5).[26]

Among deaths resulting from all types of cancer, smoking is estimated to be related to 17% and to an estimated 515 600 expected years of life lost in 2002.[42] It appears that mortality rate is predicated on the age at which smoking started and the number of cigarettes smoked. Clearly, smoking remains the chief single avoidable cause of cancer and death and the most important Canadian public health issue of our time.

Think of anything related to good physical health; the research says that cigarette smoking will impair it. The earlier the age at which you start smoking, the more smoking you do, and the longer you do it, the greater the impairment (see Figure 10.6). Smoking doesn't do any part of the body any good, at any time, under any conditions.

Passive Smoking: The Danger of Second-Hand Smoke

A great deal has been said and written about **passive smoking** or **second-hand smoke**—that is, the inhaling of cigarette smoke from the environment by nonsmokers. An epidemiological study published in

passive smoking, second-hand smoke: the inhalation of tobacco smoke by individuals other than the smoker.

Figure 10.5 Canadian Deaths Caused by Tobacco Use

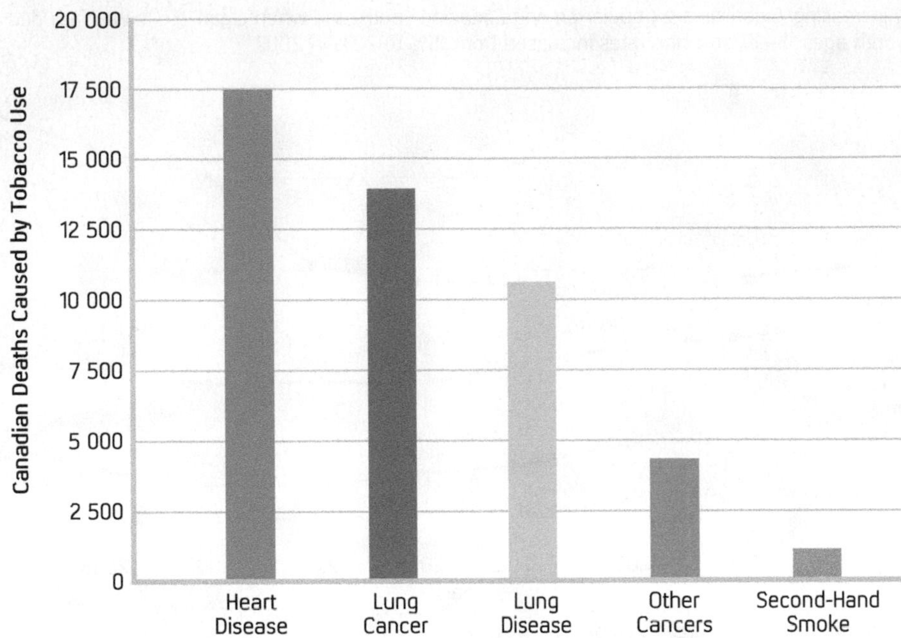

Source: Adapted from Physicians for a Smoke-Free Canada. Table entitled "Estimated Total Tobacco-Caused Deaths" from Fact Sheet "Estimated Tobacco-Caused Deaths in Canada, by Province and Gender." June 2004. Ottawa, ON.

Figure 10.6 Death Rates from Cancer of the Lung and Bronchus in Nonsmokers and Smokers of Various Numbers of Cigarettes per Day

Smoking contributes to more than 47 000 deaths a year in Canada, of which almost 11 000 (29%) are related to heart disease and stroke. Smoking is responsible for 14.54% of all heart disease and stroke deaths.[10] If current rates of tobacco use continue, approximately 1 million Canadians will die over the next 20 years as a direct result of smoking and second-hand smoke.[43]

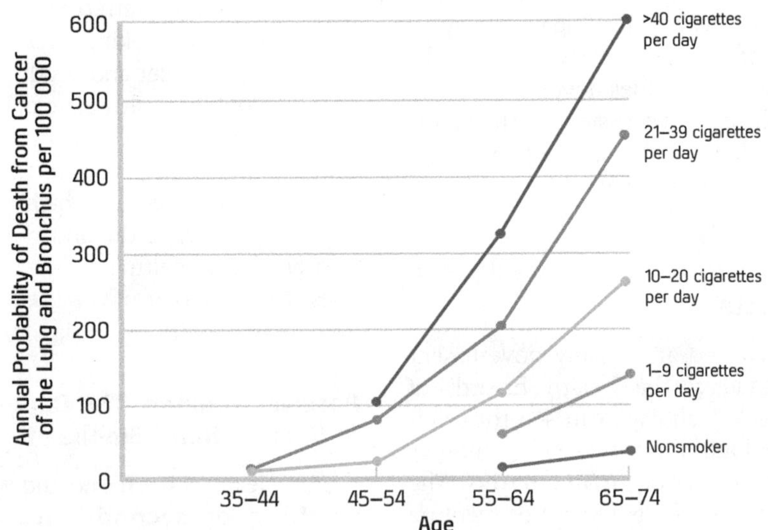

Source: Kahn, H.A. The Dorn Study of Smoking and Mortality among U.S. Veterans: Report on Eight and One-Half Years of Observation. In *Epidemiological Approaches to the Study of Cancer and Other Chronic Diseases*, W. Haenszel (Editor). National Cancer Institute Monograph No. 19. Bethesda, MD: U.S. Department of Health, Education, and Welfare, Public Health Service, National Institutes of Health, 1966, pp. 1–125.

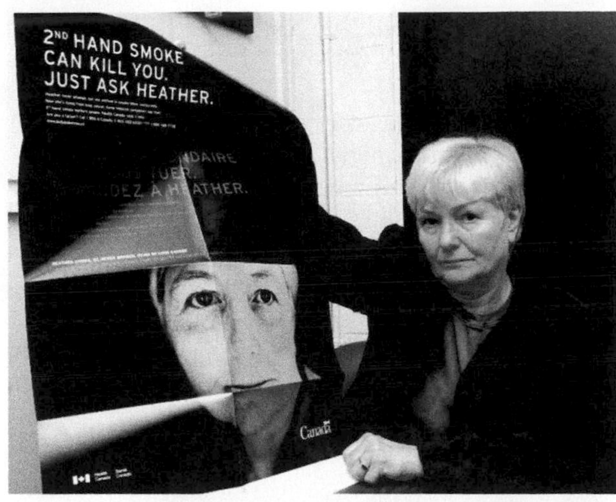

Heather Crowe fought to protect workers from second-hand smoke. A nonsmoker, her lung cancer was attributed to occupational exposure to cigarette smoke.

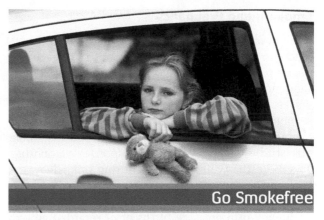

Breathing second-hand smoke subjects infants and children to dangerous carcinogens. Every day more than 1 million children are exposed to second-hand smoke, increasing their risk of pneumonia, asthma, and even cancer. In April 2008, Nova Scotia outlawed smoking in vehicles carrying children.

1981 by Takeshi Hirayama demonstrated that the risk of lung cancer was increased in nonsmoking Japanese women married to men who smoked compared with nonsmoking couples. He reported that this risk increased with the number of cigarettes smoked and the amount of second-hand smoke exposure.[44]

The importance of this issue can best be demonstrated by the death of Heather Crowe, a nonsmoking Ottawa server whose lung cancer was attributed to occupational exposure to cigarette smoke. Before her death she took her case to Workers' Compensation, and her claim was accepted. Health Canada asked her to appear in a campaign to relay the dangers of second-hand smoke to the public. Crowe demanded better laws to protect workers from second-hand smoke. At the time only about 5% of Canadians were protected from second-hand smoke; that number rose to 80% four years later with new laws in place to protect Canadians. Crowe convinced the Ontario government to pass the Smoke Free Ontario Act, but she died before it was in place.

Concerns about the effects of second-hand smoke have led to many more restrictions on smoking in the workplace and in public. Most provinces, territories, and municipalities now have laws prohibiting smoking in public conveyances and requiring the establishment of smoking and nonsmoking areas in public buildings and restaurants, and some communities have banned smoking in all restaurants. A few employers have gone so far as to either encourage or attempt to force their employees to quit smoking both on the job and elsewhere, citing health statistics that indicate that more sick days and greater health insurance costs are associated with smoking. The town of Truro, Nova Scotia, has even passed legislation banning smoking on Inglis Place, a street populated with numerous shops and restaurants.[45] This conflict between smoker and nonsmoker seems destined to get worse before it gets better. Although to some this battle might seem silly, it represents a very basic conflict between individual freedom and public health.

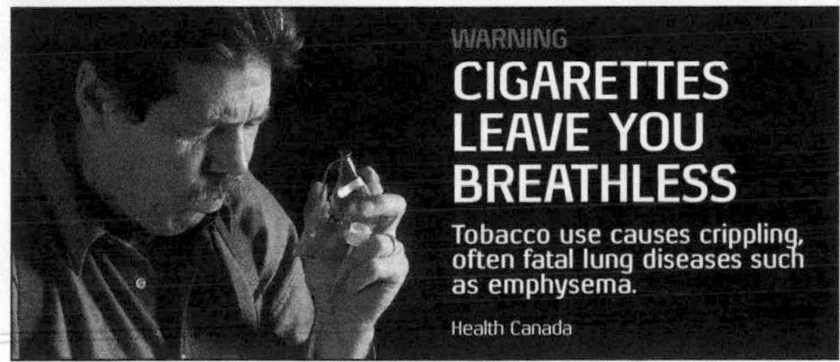
WARNING
CIGARETTES LEAVE YOU BREATHLESS
Tobacco use causes crippling, often fatal lung diseases such as emphysema.
Health Canada

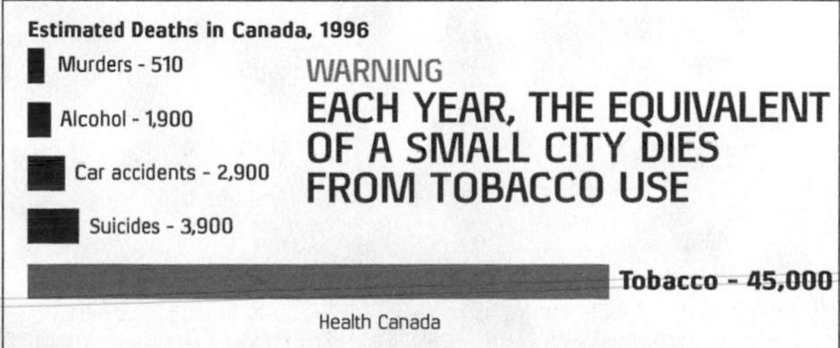

Photos licensed under Health Canada Copyright.

Under Canadian regulations, at least one of 16 different warnings must appear on cigarette packages. Health Canada is proposing larger warnings, with pictures, hoping to provoke greater emotional responses and better communicate health risks in hopes that tobacco users will be motivated to quit.

Smoking and Pregnancy

The nicotine, hydrogen cyanide, and carbon monoxide in a smoking mother's blood also reach the developing fetus and have significant negative consequences there. On average, infants born to smokers are about 250 grams lighter than infants born to nonsmokers. This basic fact has been known for almost 30 years and has been confirmed in numerous studies. There is a dose-response relationship. The more the woman smokes during pregnancy, the greater the reduction in her baby's birth weight. Is the reduced birth weight the result of an increased frequency of premature births or of retarded growth of the fetus? Smoking shortens the gestation period by an average of only two days, and when gestation length is accounted for, the smokers still have smaller infants. Ultrasonic measurements taken at various intervals during pregnancy show smaller fetuses in smoking women for at least the last two months of pregnancy. The infants of smokers are normally proportioned, but are shorter and smaller and have smaller head circumference than the infants of nonsmokers. The reduced birth weight of infants of women smokers is not related to how much weight the mother gains during pregnancy, and the consensus is that a reduced availability of oxygen is responsible for the diminished growth rate. Women who give up smoking early in pregnancy (by the fourth month) have infants with weights similar to infants of nonsmokers.[46]

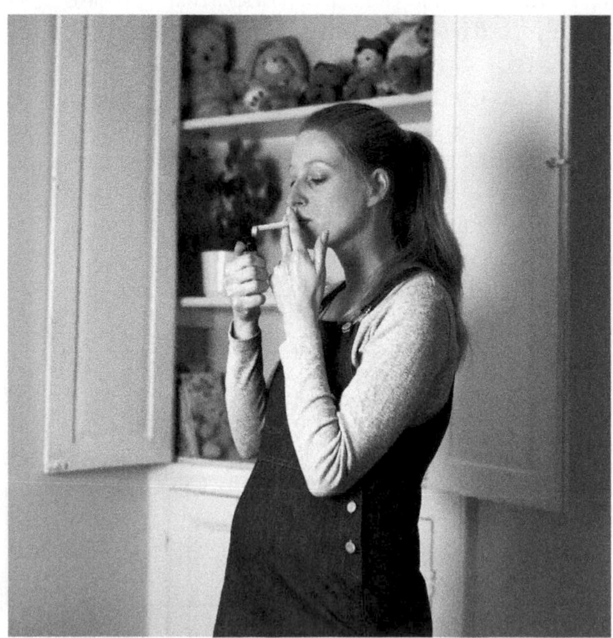

Smoking during pregnancy is associated with miscarriage, low birth weight, smaller head circumference, and later effects on the physical and intellectual development of the child.

Besides the developmental effects evident at birth, several studies indicate small but consistent differences in body size, neurological problems, reading and mathematical skills, and hyperactivity at various ages. It therefore appears that smoking during pregnancy can have long-lasting effects on both the intellectual and the physical development of the child. The increased perinatal (close to the time of birth) smoking-attributable mortality associated with sudden infant death syndrome (SIDS), low birthweight, and respiratory difficulties adds up to about 10 000 infant deaths per year.[47]

So far we have been talking about normal deliveries of babies. Spontaneous abortion (miscarriage) has also been studied many times in relation to smoking and with consistent results. Smokers have more spontaneous abortions than nonsmokers (perhaps 1.5 to 2 times as many). As for congenital malformations, the evidence for a relationship to maternal smoking is not as clear. If there is a small effect here, it could be either related to or obscured by the fact that many smokers also drink alcohol and coffee. One study indicated an increased risk of facial malformations associated with the father's smoking. Several studies have also found an increased risk of SIDS if the mother smokes, but it is not clear if this is related more to the mother's smoking during pregnancy or to passive smoking (the infant's breathing of smoke) after birth.

Several studies have reported an increased risk for nicotine dependence in adolescents whose mothers smoked during pregnancy. One obvious question is whether this relationship is due entirely to cultural and social similarities between the mothers and their offspring, but a number of animal studies have also demonstrated that prenatal nicotine exposure produces changes in brain chemistry in the offspring and differences in behavioural response to nicotine in adolescence.[48]

The overall message is very clear. Definite, serious risks are associated with smoking during pregnancy. In fact, the demonstrated effects of cigarette smoking on the developing child are of the same magnitude and type as those reported for babies born to mothers who used crack during their pregnancies, and many more pregnant women are smoking cigarettes than are using cocaine. If a female smoker discovers she is pregnant, she should quit smoking.

LO8 Pharmacology of Nicotine

Nicotine, a central nervous system (CNS) stimulant, is a naturally occurring liquid alkaloid that is colourless and volatile. On oxidation it turns brown and smells much like burning tobacco. Tolerance to its effects develops, along with the dependency that led Mark Twain to remark how easy it was to stop smoking–he'd done it several times!

Nicotine was isolated in 1828 and has been studied extensively since then. The structure of nicotine is shown in Figure 10.7. It is of some importance that nicotine in smoke has two forms, one with a positive charge and one that is electrically neutral. The neutral form is more easily absorbed through the mucous membranes of the mouth, nose, and lungs. In fact, the tobacco industry knows this and deliberately manipulates the pH of their products to shift more of the nicotine into the noncharged, easily absorbed state.[49]

Absorption and Metabolism

Inhalation is a very effective drug-delivery system; 90% of inhaled nicotine is absorbed. The physiological effects of smoking one cigarette have been mimicked by injecting about 1 milligram of nicotine intravenously.

Acting with almost as much speed as cyanide, nicotine is well established as one of the most toxic drugs known. In humans, 60 milligrams is a lethal dose, and death follows intake within a few minutes. A cigar contains enough nicotine for two lethal doses (who needs to take a second one?), but not all the nicotine is delivered to the smoker or absorbed in a short enough time to kill a person.

Nicotine is primarily deactivated in the liver, with 80-90% being modified before excretion through the kidneys. Part of the tolerance that develops to nicotine might result from the fact that either nicotine or the tars increase the activity of the liver microsomal enzymes that are responsible for the deactivation of drugs. These enzymes increase the rate of deactivation. The final step in eliminating deactivated nicotine from the body may be somewhat slowed by nicotine itself, since it acts on the hypothalamus to cause a release of the hormone that acts to reduce the loss of body fluids.

Figure 10.7 Nicotine (1-methyl-2-[3-pyridyl]pyrrolidone)

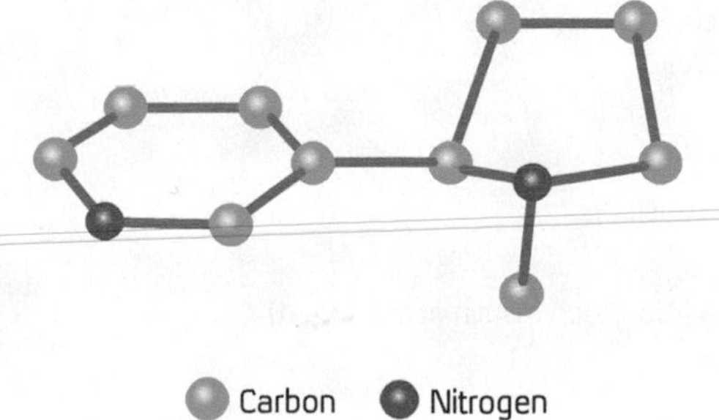

Physiological Effects

The effect of nicotine on areas outside the central nervous system has been studied extensively. Nicotine mimics acetylcholine by acting at several nicotinic subtypes of the cholinergic receptor site. Nicotine is not rapidly deactivated, and continued occupation of the receptor prevents incoming impulses from having an effect, thereby blocking the transmission of information at the synapse. Thus, the effects of nicotine are quite rapid because of the fast interaction with neuronal nicotinic receptors. But the reason that there appears to be a subsequent block is not because nicotine is preventing acetylcholine from further binding to the receptor but because occupancy of the receptor with an agonist converts it to a nonresponsive, desensitized state. These effects at cholinergic synapses are responsible for some of nicotine's effects, but others seem to be the result of an indirect action.

Nicotine also causes a release of adrenaline from the adrenal glands and other sympathetic sites and thus has, in part, a sympathomimetic action. Additionally, it stimulates and then blocks some sensory receptors, including the chemical receptors found in some large arteries and the thermal pain receptors found in the skin and tongue.

The symptoms of low-level nicotine poisoning are well known to beginning smokers and small children behind barns and in alleys: nausea, dizziness, and a general weakness. In acute poisoning, nicotine causes tremors, which develop into convulsions, terminated in many cases by death. The cause of death is suffocation resulting from paralysis of the muscles used in respiration. This paralysis stems from the blocking effect of nicotine on the cholinergic system that normally activates the muscles. With lower doses, respiration rate actually increases because the nicotine stimulates oxygen-need receptors in the carotid artery. At these lower doses of 6–8 milligrams, there is also a considerable effect on the cardiovascular system as a result of the release of adrenaline. Such release leads to an increase in coronary blood flow, along with vasoconstriction in the skin and increased heart rate and blood pressure. The increased heart rate and blood pressure raise the oxygen need of the heart but not the oxygen supply. Another action of nicotine with negative health effects is that it increases platelet adhesiveness, which increases the tendency to clot. Within the CNS, nicotine seems to act at the level of the cortex to increase somewhat the frequency of the electrical activity; that is, to shift the EEG toward an arousal pattern. Table 10.4 summarizes some of the physiological effects of nicotine.

Many effects of nicotine are easily discernible in the smoking individual. The heat releases the nicotine from the tobacco into the smoke. Inhaling while smoking one cigarette has been shown to inhibit hunger contractions of the stomach for up to an hour. That finding, along with a very slight increase in blood sugar level and a deadening of the taste buds, might be the basis for a decrease in hunger after smoking.

In line with the last possibility, it has long been said that a person who stops smoking begins to nibble food instead and thus gains weight. Carbohydrate-rich snack foods appear to be even more appealing when smokers are deprived of nicotine.[50] In addition, there is evidence that smoking increases metabolism rate, so that weight gain on quitting might be partially due to a decreasing metabolism rate or less energy utilization by the body.

In a regular smoker, smoking results in a constriction of the blood vessels in the skin, along with a decrease in skin temperature and an increase in blood pressure. The blood supply to the skeletal muscles does not change with smoking, but in regular smokers the amount of carboxyhemoglobin in the blood is usually abnormally high (up to 10% of all hemoglobin). All smoke contains carbon monoxide; cigarette smoke is about 1% carbon monoxide, pipe smoke, 2%, and cigar smoke, 6%. The carbon monoxide combines with the hemoglobin in the blood, so that it can no longer carry oxygen. This effect of smoking, a decrease in the oxygen-carrying ability of the blood, probably explains the shortness of breath smokers experience when they exert themselves.

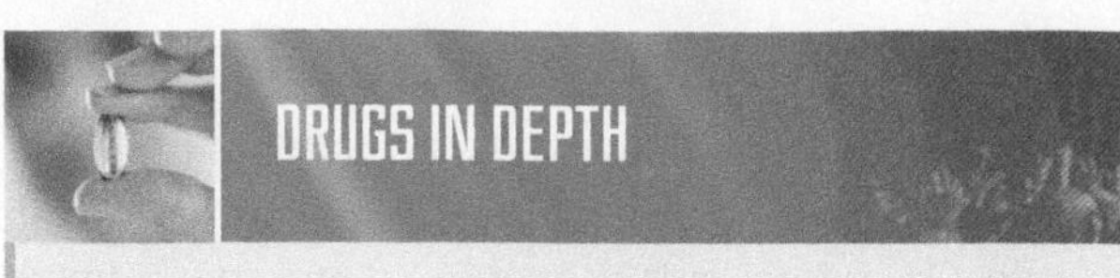

Possible New Painkiller?

One of the early uses of tobacco was as a painkiller. Nicotine itself does have some analgesic properties, but its toxicity limits its usefulness for this. The discovery of a pain-relieving substance in the skin of Ecuadorian "poison-arrow" frogs that binds strongly to nicotinic acetylcholine receptors (epibutadine) has led to the development and testing of several new nicotine analogues. Side effects, such as nausea and dizziness, have been a problem. It remains to be seen whether a related drug will someday be available for pain relief.

Table 10.4 Summary of the Physiological Effects of Nicotine on Various Organ Systems

Blood	**Central nervous system**
increased clotting tendency	light-headedness
Lungs	headache
bronchospasm	sleep disturbances
Muscular	abnormal dreams
tremors	irritability
pain	dizziness
Gastrointestinal	**Heart**
nausea	increased or decreased heart rate
dry mouth	increased blood pressure
dyspepsia	tachycardia
diarrhea	more (or less) arrhythmias
heartburn	coronary artery constriction
Joints	**Endocrine**
pain	hyperinsulinemia (too much insulin in the blood)
	insulin resistance

The decrease in the oxygen-carrying ability of the blood and the decrease in placental blood flow probably are related to the many results showing that pregnant women who smoke greatly endanger their unborn children.

Behavioural Effects

Despite all the protests and cautionary statements, the evidence is overwhelming that nicotine is the primary, if not the only, reinforcing substance in tobacco. Monkeys will work very hard when their only reward consists of regular intravenous injections of nicotine. The more nicotine in a cigarette, the lower the level of smoking. Intravenous injections and oral administration of nicotine will decrease smoking under some conditions–but not all.

An ongoing debate–among smokers as well as researchers–is whether nicotine acts to arouse and activate the smoker or whether it calms and tranquillizes the user. Smokers report seeking both effects, and experimental results are heavily influenced by the smoker's history and the situation.[51]

Most people smoke in a fairly consistent way, averaging one to two puffs per minute, with each puff lasting about two seconds and having a volume of 25 millilitres. This rate delivers to the individual about 1-2 micrograms of nicotine per kilogram of body weight with each puff. Smokers could increase the dose by increasing the volume of smoke with each puff or puffing more often, but this dose appears to be optimal for producing stimulation of the cerebral cortex.

Several studies have shown that smokers are able to sustain their attention to a task requiring rapid processing of information from a computer screen much better if they are allowed to smoke before beginning the task. This could be either because the nicotine produces a beneficial effect on this performance or because when the smokers are not allowed to smoke they suffer from some sort of withdrawal symptom.

Nicotine Dependence

Evidence that nicotine is a reinforcing substance in nonhumans, that most people who smoke want to stop and can't, that when people do stop smoking, they gain weight and exhibit other withdrawal signs, and that people who chew tobacco also have trouble stopping led to a need for a thorough look at the dependence-producing properties of nicotine. A 1988 U.S. surgeon general's report provided it, in the form of a 600-page tome.[52] This had been a traditionally difficult subject. Not many years ago, psychiatrists were arguing that smoking fulfilled unmet needs for oral gratification and therefore represented a personality defect. It has since come to light that the cigarette manufacturing company Philip Morris obtained evidence of the dependence-producing nature of nicotine with rats in the early 1980s, but, instead of publishing the results, the researchers were fired and the laboratory closed.[53] Industry executives in 1994 U.S. congressional hearings unanimously testified that nicotine was not addictive, still arguing that smoking was simply a matter of personal choice and that many people had been able to quit. A person can theoretically choose to stop using a drug, but that person may have a very difficult time doing so because of the potent reinforcing properties of the substance. That is the case with nicotine. The following conclusions of the surgeon general's report were pretty strong:

1. Cigarettes and other forms of tobacco are addictive.
2. Nicotine is the drug in tobacco that causes addiction.
3. The pharmacological and behavioural processes that determine tobacco addiction are similar to those that determine addiction to drugs such as heroin and cocaine.

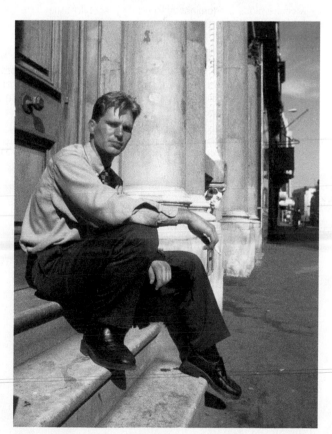

Nicotine is a dependence-producing substance, and users typically have a difficult time quitting.

Figure 10.8 Nicotinic Acetylcholine Receptors

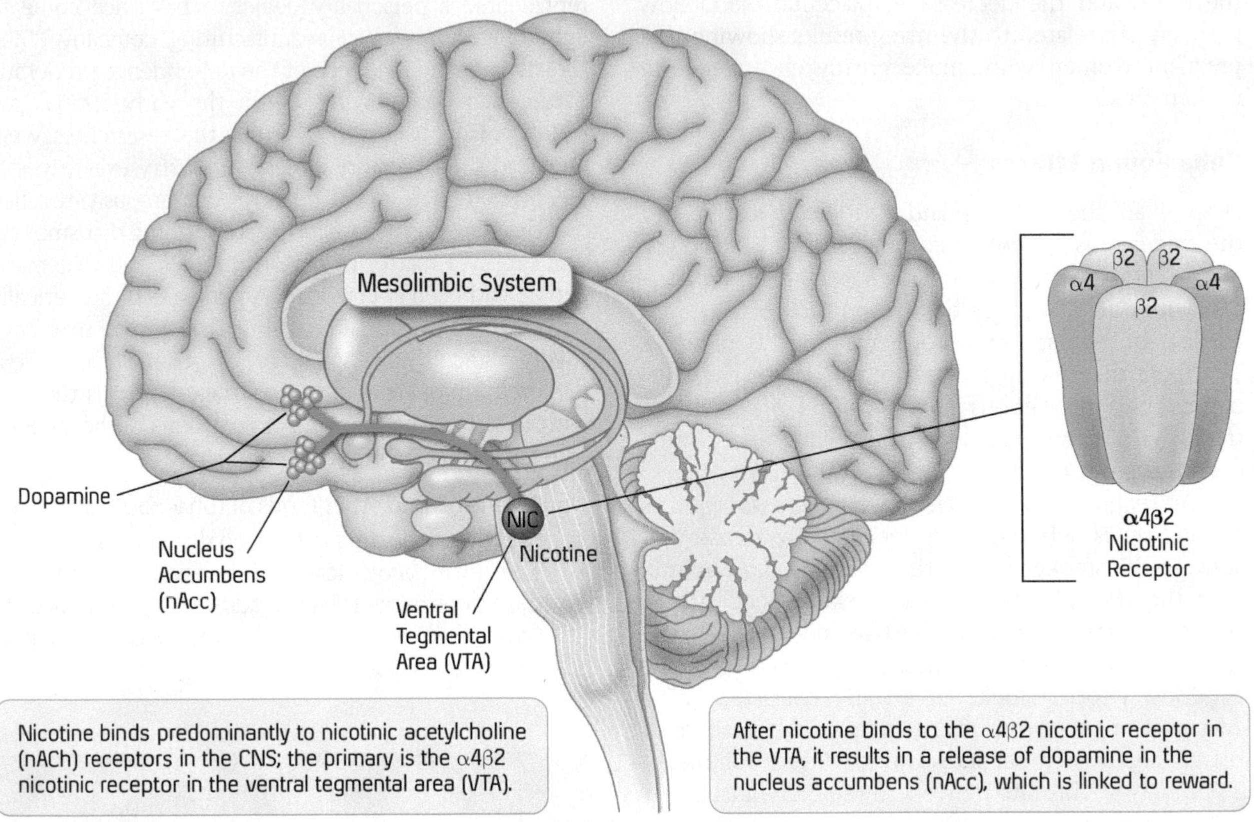
Mesolimbic System
Dopamine
Nucleus Accumbens (nAcc)
NIC
Nicotine
Ventral Tegmental Area (VTA)
β2
β2
α4
α4
β2
α4β2 Nicotinic Receptor
Nicotine binds predominantly to nicotinic acetylcholine (nACh) receptors in the CNS; the primary is the α4β2 nicotinic receptor in the ventral tegmental area (VTA).
After nicotine binds to the α4β2 nicotinic receptor in the VTA, it results in a release of dopamine in the nucleus accumbens (nAcc), which is linked to reward.

Nicotinic acetylcholine receptors are cholinergic receptors that form ligand-gated ion channels on neuronal membranes. Binding of nicotine (agonist) to the receptor results in opening of sodium channels (Na+) and depolarization of the neuronal membrane. A specific subtype of this receptor (α4β2 receptor) is thought to be one of the most important subtypes in facilitating the effects of nicotine on brain reward pathways.

Source: Adapted from ASH (Action on Smoking and Health). *ASH Guidance Notes: Varenicline—Guidance for Health Professionals on a New Prescription-Only Stop-Smoking Medication.* November 2006. London, UK: ASH. Retrieved December 2, 2011, from http://newash.org.uk/files/documents/ASH_447.pdf; Foulds, J. "The Neurobiological Basis for Partial Agonist Treatment of Nicotine Dependence: Varenicline." *International Journal of Clinical Practice* 60, no. 5 (2006), pp. 571–576; BBC News. Stop-*Smoking Drug Approved on NHS.* 2007. Retrieved December 2, 2011, from http://news.bbc.co.uk/2/hi/health/6705667.stm.

Nicotine, like heroin and cocaine, affects dopamine in the nucleus accumbens and mesolimbic system, which underlies the subjective reinforcing effects of nicotine (see Figure 10.8).

The U.S. surgeon general's message met with predictably negative reactions from the tobacco industry and from some tobacco-state politicians, and the debate continued until the late 1990s. Successful lawsuits by former smokers or their survivors finally convinced the tobacco companies that they were going to have to take seriously the issues of toxicity and dependence. In 1998, one company even faced criminal charges for growing a high-nicotine strain of tobacco with the presumed intent of manipulating nicotine levels to "hook" more smokers.

For the past several years, research into the mechanism of nicotine dependence has focused on the fact that nicotine affects dopamine in the nucleus accumbens,[54] a major target of the mesolimbic dopamine system, described in Chapter 4. The brains of chronic nicotine smokers also show a large reduction in one type of monoamine oxidase (MAO), the enzyme that breaks down dopamine and some other neurotransmitters.[55] This slowing of the breakdown of dopamine in chronic smokers might therefore enhance the effect of the dopamine released by each acute dose of nicotine, perhaps contributing to the strength of the dependence on nicotine experienced by most smokers.

The past decade has seen a great deal of research into the different subtypes of nicotinic cholinergic receptors, and several companies are developing new drugs targeted more specifically to certain subtypes. Although several such drugs are being tested in human trials, none is yet on the market.

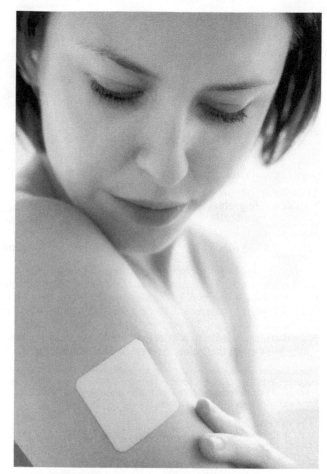

Nicotine replacement therapy—in the form of gum, a patch, lozenges, an inhaler, or a nasal spray—helps some smokers quit.

LO9 How to Stop Smoking

When you're young and healthy, it's hard to imagine dying, being chronically ill, or having **emphysema**, **bronchitis**, or **chronic obstructive pulmonary lung disease (COPD)** so that you can't get enough oxygen to walk across the room without having to stop to catch your breath. By the time you're old enough to worry about those things, it's difficult to change your health habits.

Many people want to stop smoking. Many people have already stopped. Are there ways to efficiently and effectively help those individuals who want to stop smoking to stop? With any form of pleasurable drug use, it is easier to keep people from starting to use the drug than it is to get them to stop once they have started. All the educational programs have had an effect on our society and on our behaviour. In an adult population, over a year, approximately 3–4% of people who smoke will quit without formal treatment, another 6–8% will quit with a brief counselling intervention (two to five minutes) and 12–16% will quit with an intensive intervention (15–30 minutes in four to eight sessions).[56] There is some indication that those who have quit on their own do better than those who have been in a treatment program, but then those who quit on their own also tend not to have been smoking as much or for as long.

One reason it is so hard for people to stop is that a pack-a-day smoker puffs at least 50 000 times a year. That's a lot of individual nicotine hits reinforcing the smoking behaviour. A variety of behavioural treatment approaches are available to help smokers who want to quit, and hundreds of research articles have been published on them. Although most of these programs are able to get almost everyone to quit for a few days, by six months 70–80% of participants are smoking again.

If nicotine is the critical thing, why not provide nicotine without the tars and carbon monoxide? Prescription nicotine chewing gum became available in 1984, after carefully controlled studies showed it to be a useful adjunct to smoking cessation programs. This gum is now available over the counter. In 1991, several companies marketed nicotine skin patches that allow slow release of nicotine to be absorbed through the wearer's skin. Nicotine lozenges are now available over the counter, and smokers can also get a prescription for a nicotine inhaler or nasal spray. Also, the prescription drug bupropion (Zyban) has been shown to help many people.

emphysema: a chronic lung disease characterized by difficulty breathing and shortness of breath.

bronchitis: inflammation of the main air passages to the lungs.

chronic obstructive pulmonary disease (COPD): a chronic lung disease in which airways swell and are partly blocked by mucus; includes chronic bronchitis and emphysema.

Figure 10.9 How Varenicline (Champix) Works

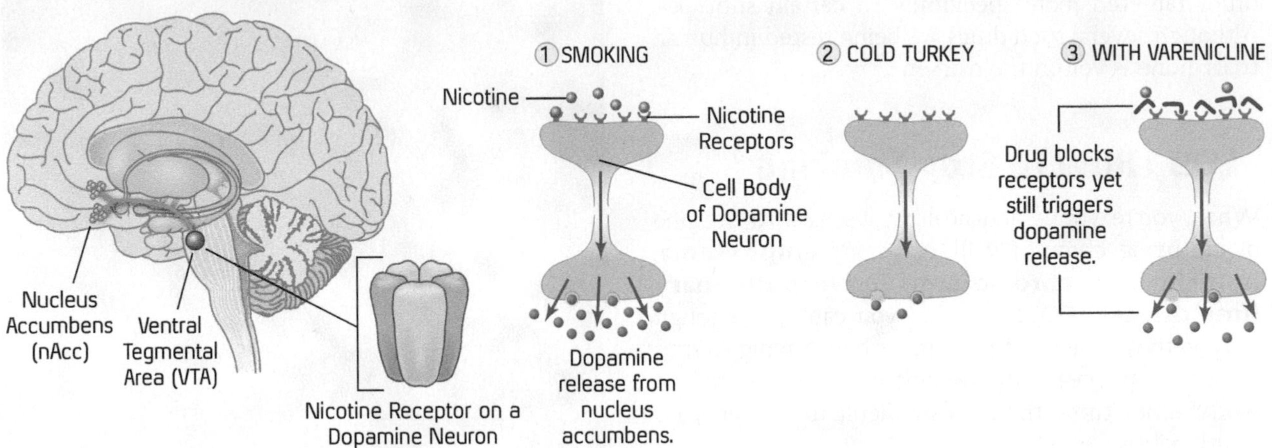

Varenicline stimulates the nicotine receptor on dopamine neurons, mimicking the effects of nicotine to reduce cravings. Varenicline also partially blocks the receptor, preventing nicotine from binding to it, resulting in a weaker response in people who give in to temptation and have a cigarette. **1.** Nicotine from a cigarette stimulates the release of dopamine, a substance produced by the body that triggers feelings of pleasure. **2.** When a smoker quits, the lack of nicotine leads to reduced levels of dopamine, causing feelings of craving and withdrawal. **3.** Varenicline both blocks the nicotine receptors (reducing the addictive power of the drug) and triggers moderate dopamine release to alleviate withdrawal symptoms. Varenicline has a warning about the possibility of psychiatric side effects reinforcing the fact that nicotinic receptors are involved in processes other than just facilitating nicotine addiction.

Source: Adapted from ASH (Action on Smoking and Health). *ASH Guidance Notes: Varenicline—Guidance for Health Professionals on a New Prescription-Only Stop-Smoking Medication.* November 2006. London, UK: ASH. Retrieved December 2, 2011, from http://newash.org.uk/files/documents/ASH_447.pdf; Foulds, J. "The Neurobiological Basis for Partial Agonist Treatment of Nicotine Dependence: Varenicline." *International Journal of Clinical Practice* 60, no. 5 (2006), pp. 571–576; BBC News. *Stop-Smoking Drug Approved on NHS.* 2007. Retrieved December 2, 2011, from http://news.bbc.co.uk/2/hi/health/6705667.stm.

In 2007, Health Canada approved varenicline (Champix), a nicotine partial-agonist drug (see Figure 10.9). In clinical trials it appears that this new drug may be slightly more effective than bupropion in helping people to remain abstinent for a year.[57] However, Health Canada has since issued a warning about heart-related side effects in people with cardiovascular disease who use Champix.[58]

There is money to be made from helping people quit smoking, especially if it can apparently be done painlessly with a substitute. In fact, given the harms associated with smoking, Ontario is about to add smoking cessation drugs to its list of drugs covered by health insurance.[59] The controlled studies done to demonstrate the usefulness of gum or skin patches have been carried out under fairly strict conditions, with a prescribed quitting period, several visits to the clinic to assess progress, and the usual trappings of a clinical research study, often including the collection of saliva or other samples to detect tobacco use. That's very different from buying nicotine gum and a patch off the shelf, with no plan for quitting, no follow-up interviews, and no monitoring. It's no wonder that some people have found themselves, despite warnings, wearing a nicotine patch and smoking at the same time. There is also belief and discussion surrounding the complete lack of effect of nicotine replacement therapy.[60]

Is there an effective nondrug program for quitting smoking? Yes and no. The effect of any program varies—some people do very well, some very poorly—and if one program won't work for an individual, maybe another one will. A new development is that nicotine vaccinations are in clinical trials, which, if they work, will revolutionize not only treatment of nicotine addiction but also its prevention.[61] Today, what we do know is that combining counselling and pharmacological treatments increases the odds of quitting.[62] We don't yet know which program will be best for any particular individual. If you want to stop smoking, keep trying programs; odds are you'll find one that works—eventually.

Summary

- Tobacco was introduced to Europe and the East after Columbus's voyage to the Americas.
- As with most other "new" drugs, Europeans either loved tobacco and prescribed it for all ailments or hated it and considered it responsible for many ills.
- In its original form, tobacco was used in ceremonies for its medicinal attributes by Aboriginal peoples. By 1800, tobacco was being commercially grown in Canada. In 1912, the Imperial Tobacco Company of Canada was incorporated to produce and market tobacco products across Canada.
- Anti-tobacco pamphlets have been around since 1604, with King James of England the first to state that tobacco was "harmefull to the braine, dangerous to the lungs."
- A 1952 article in *Readers' Digest* called "Cancer by the Carton" drew public attention to the issue and led to a temporary decline in cigarette sales.
- In 1988–1989 federal laws were enacted to prohibit tobacco advertising and ensure smoke-free workplaces, and the government began requiring cigarette manufacturers to list additives on packages.
- The Tobacco Products Control Act prohibited all tobacco advertising, required health warnings on tobacco packaging, and restricted promotional activities.
- In 1993, the legal age for buying tobacco was raised to 18; in 1994, bigger and stronger warning messages became required on cigarette packs; in 1997 the Tobacco Act imposed general restrictions on manufacturers and distributors; restricted promotion, packaging, and products; and imposed point-of-sale restrictions.
- Tobacco companies responded by forming a supposedly independent Council for Tobacco Research to look into the health claims, but later investigations revealed this council was not independent of tobacco company influence. They also mass marketed filter cigarettes and cigarettes with lowered tar and nicotine content.
- Around the mid-1950s, tobacco companies began to promote the idea of a "safer" cigarette, although *safer* doesn't mean "safe." Tobacco companies have tried to promote the idea of a "safer" cigarette with a filter, without actually admitting that there was anything unsafe about their older products.
- The typical modern cigarette is about half as strong in tar and nicotine content as a cigarette of 50 years ago.
- Cigarette smoking has declined considerably since the 1960s, but about 20% of young people still become regular smokers.
- The use of smokeless tobacco increased during the 1980s, causing concerns about increases in oral cancer.
- Although tobacco continues to be an important economic factor in North American society, it is also responsible for more annual deaths than all other drugs combined, including alcohol.
- Cigarette smoking is clearly linked to increased risk of heart disease, lung and other cancers, emphysema, heart disease, and stroke.
- Tobacco use kills 47 000 Canadians each year.
- Increased concern about the health consequences of passive smoking has led to many more restrictions on smoking in the workplace and in public.
- Almost 6300 nonsmokers die each year in Canada from exposure to second-hand smoke.
- On average, infants born to smokers are lighter, shorter, smaller, and have a smaller head circumference than the infants of nonsmokers. Differences in body size, neurological problems, reading and mathematical skills, and hyperactivity appear. Smokers have more miscarriages than nonsmokers.
- Nicotine, a central nervous system stimulant, mimics acetylcholine by acting at several nicotinic subtypes of cholinergic receptor site and blocks the transmission of information at the synapse.
- Nicotine causes a release of adrenaline, causes vasoconstriction in the skin, increases heart rate and blood pressure, increases platelet adhesiveness, inhibits hunger contractions of the stomach, and decreases the oxygen-carrying ability of the blood.
- Smoking cessation leads to immediate improvements in mortality statistics, and new products, including different types of nicotine replacement therapy, in combination with counselling, are being widely used by those who want to quit.

Review Questions

1. Why was nicotine named after Jean Nicot?
2. Which desired species of tobacco saved the English colonies in Virginia?
3. What techniques have been used to produce "safer" cigarettes?
4. About what proportion of 15- to 19-year-olds are smokers in Canada?
5. What is the significance of tobacco-specific nitrosamines?
6. What are the major causes of death associated with cigarette smoking?
7. What evidence is there that passive smoking can harm nonsmokers?
8. What are the effects of smoking during pregnancy?
9. Nicotine acts through which neurotransmitter in the brain? How does it interact with this neurotransmitter?
10. What is the evidence as to why cigarette smoking produces such strong dependence?

CHAPTER 11

CAFFEINE

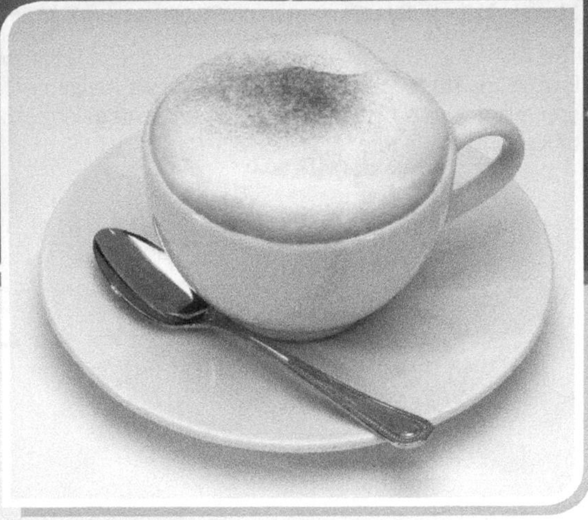

OBJECTIVES

When you have finished this chapter, you should be able to

- **LO1** Describe the early history of coffee, tea, and chocolate use.
- **LO2** Describe the methods for removing caffeine from coffee.
- **LO3** Explain the caffeine content of "energy drinks" in relation to colas and coffee.
- **LO4** Name the xanthines found in coffee, tea, and chocolate.
- **LO5** Describe caffeine's withdrawal symptoms.
- **LO6** Describe how caffeine exerts its actions on the brain.
- **LO7** Discuss the circumstances in which caffeine appears to enhance mental performance and those in which it does not.
- **LO8** Describe the concerns about high caffeine consumption during pregnancy.

LO1, LO2 Caffeine: The World's Most Common Psychostimulant

Caffeine, like nicotine, is a mild stimulant falling in the same classification as amphetamine and cocaine. Caffeine belongs to the methylxanthine (xanthine) biochemical family, which also includes theophylline, found in tea, and theobromine, found in chocolate.[1] On a daily basis, more people use caffeine than any other psychoactive drug.[2] Many people use it regularly, and there is evidence for dependence and some evidence that regular use can interfere with the very activities people believe that it helps them with. It is now so domesticated that most modern kitchens contain a specialized device for extracting the chemical from plant products (a coffee maker), but Western societies were not always so accepting of this drug.

The newest revision of the *Diagnostic and Statistical Manual of Mental Disorders* (DSM-5) includes caffeine withdrawal as a new disorder under Substance-Related and Addictive Disorders; this topic is discussed in more detail later in this chapter.

Coffee

Statistics Canada reports that coffee consumption increased from 96 litres per person in 1990 to 106 litres per person in 2009.[2] Daily coffee consumption varies across the country. Approximately 70% of adults in Quebec, 60% in Ontario, 67% in the Prairies, 61% in B.C., and 53% in the Atlantic region drink coffee daily.[3]

The majority of reports on the coffee-drinking habits of Canadians summarize statistics garnered from studies commissioned by the Coffee Association of Canada and information released by Statistics Canada. Some usage trends are presented in Figure 11.1. Differences among levels of coffee consumption exist among such factors as gender, location within Canada, and age. However, both the percentage of adults who are coffee drinkers and the quantity of coffee they consume have remained strikingly consistent over the past three years, with the largest growth at 13% between 2009 and 2010.

The words *caffeine* and *coffee* are both derived from the Arabic word *qahweh* (pronounced "kahveh" in Turkish). Legends have grown up around the discovery of coffee. An Ethiopian goat herder named Kaldi couldn't understand why his goats were bounding around the hillside so playfully. One day he followed them up the mountain and ate some of the red berries

Figure 11.1 Coffee Consumption Statistics from Canadian Coffee Drinking Studies, by Year, 2009–2014

The solid blue line represents the percentage of adults who drink coffee on a daily basis; this has remained consistent over the past four years. The large-dashed red line shows the percentage of coffee consumers who drink regular coffee, and the small-dashed green line shows the increase in the percentage of homes with a single-cup coffee maker. The authors thank Richard Patrick for contribution to this figure.

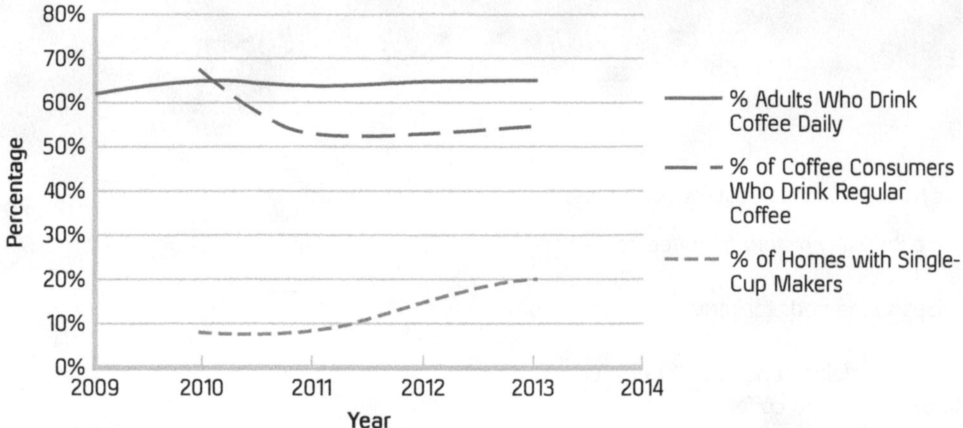

Sources: Coffee Consumption Statistics from Canadian Coffee Drinking Studies by Year, "Highlights—2010 Canadian Coffee Drinking Study," Coffee Association of Canada, accessed January 28, 2014, http://www.coffeeassoc.com/coffeeincanada.htm; "Canadian Coffee Drinking Study—2011 Highlights," Coffee Association of Canada, accessed January 28, 2014, http://www.coffeeassoc.com/coffee-in-canada/canadian-coffee-drinking-study-2011-highights/; "Wake Up and Smell the Coffee!" Coffee Association of Canada, accessed January 28, 2014, http://www.coffeeassoc.com/coffee-in-canada/wake-up-and-smell-the-coffee/; "Coffee . . . The Number One Beverage Choice for Adult Canadians," Coffee Association of Canada, accessed January 28, 2014, http://www.coffeeassoc.com/coffee-in-canada/coffee-the-number-one-beverage-choice-for-adult-canadians/.

the goats were munching. "The results were amazing. Kaldi became a happy goat herder. Whenever his goats danced, he danced and whirled and leaped and rolled about on the ground." Kaldi had taken the first human coffee trip! A holy man took in the scene, and "that night he danced with Kaldi and the goats." Whatever the actual origin of coffee use, the practice spread to Egypt and other Arabic countries by the fifteenth century, throughout the Middle East by the sixteenth century, and into Europe in the seventeenth century.

Coffee houses began appearing in England (1650) and France (1671), and a new era began. Coffee houses were all things to all people: a place to relax, to learn the news of the day, to seal bargains, and to plot. This last possibility made Charles II of England so nervous that he outlawed coffee houses, labelling them "hotbeds of seditious talk and slanderous attacks upon persons in high stations." In only 11 days the ruling was withdrawn, and the coffee houses developed into the "penny universities" of the early eighteenth century. For a penny a cup people could listen to and learn from most of the great literary and political figures of the period. Lloyds of London, an insurance house, started in Edward Lloyd's coffee house around 1700. Women in England argued against the use of coffee in a 1674 pamphlet titled "The Women's Petition Against Coffee, representing to public consideration the grand inconveniences accruing to their sex from the excessive use of the drying and

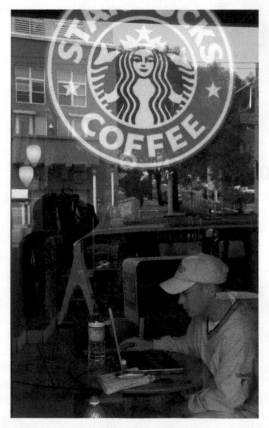

Younger coffee drinkers are a growing customer base for espresso bars and coffee houses.

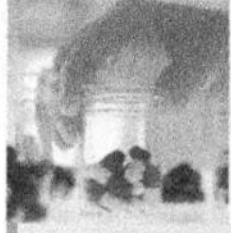

DRUGS IN THE MEDIA

Fair Trade Coffee

Fair trade is an organized social movement and a market-based approach to selling coffee that tries to help producers in developing countries work to better their trading conditions. The movement advocates for higher prices to be paid to producers and for higher social and environmental standards to be set for coffee companies. It focuses in particular on exports from developing countries to developed countries. When it was no longer possible for small-scale farmers to agree to the prices being offered by conglomerates, intermediaries, and large-scale companies, the fair trade movement began, subsidizing the prices to promote the growing of coffee as a method of self-sustenance.

Fair trade coffee companies are supported by Canadians: fair-trade-certified, organically cultivated coffee is abundant in the Canadian marketplace. Planet Bean Coffee in Guelph, Ontario, is one Canadian company that supports fair trade. The company Just Us! was founded in 1995 in Grand Pré, Nova Scotia, and originally sourced its coffee beans from Mexico.[5] Just Us! now buys fair trade organic coffee, tea, chocolate, and sugar from around the world. On April 17, 2007, Wolfville, Nova Scotia became Canada's first fair trade town.[6] Fair trade as a strategy for poverty alleviation and sustainable development has had a real impact on reducing poverty in developing countries.[7] Under fair trade arrangements, less money goes to intermediaries and more goes to the coffee grower.[5,6] The Canadian market for tea and coffee was almost $1.5 billion in 2008.[8]

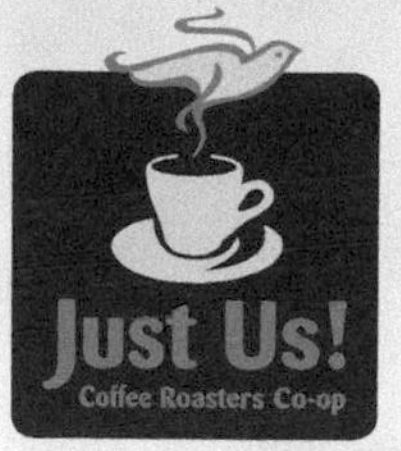

The authors thank Bafana Mashingaidze for his contribution to this section.

enfeebling liquor." The women claimed men used too much coffee, and as a result the men were as "unfruitful as those *Desarts* whence that unhappy *Berry* is said to be brought." The pamphlet continued:

> Our Countrymens pallates are become as *Fanatical* as their Brains; how else is't possible they should *Apostatize* from the good old primitive way of Ale-drinking, to run a *Whoreing* after such variety of distructive Foreign Liquors, to trifle away their time, scald their *Chops*, and spend their *Money*, all for a little *base, black, thick, nasty bitter stinking, nauseous* Puddle water.[4]

Some men probably sat long hours in one of the many coffee houses composing "The Men's Answer to the Women's Petition Against Coffee," which said in part:

> Why must innocent COFFEE be the object of your Spleen? That harmless and healing Liquor, which Indulgent Providence first sent amongst us. . . . Tis not this incomparable fettle Brain that shortens Natures standard, or makes us less Active in the Sports of Venus, and we wonder you should take these Exceptions.[4]

Across the Atlantic, coffee drinking increased in the English colonies, although tea was still preferred. Cheaper and more readily available than coffee, tea had everything, including, beginning in 1765, a tax of three pence on every half-kilogram that was imported.

The British Act that taxed tea helped fan the fire that lit the musket that fired the shot heard around the world. That story is better told in connection with tea, but the final outcome was that to be a tea drinker was to be a Tory, so coffee became the United States' national drink.

Coffee use expanded as the West was won, and per capita consumption steadily increased in the early 1900s. Some experts became worried about the increase, which some believed was caused by the widespread prohibition of alcohol.

But even after Prohibition went away, coffee consumption continued to rise. In 1946, annual per capita coffee consumption reached an all-time high of nine kilograms. The overall trend has been basically downhill since then, until the upsurge of interest in espresso and specialty coffees in Canada and the United States beginning in the late 1990s.

Some of the decrease in coffee consumption can be attributed to changing lifestyles. Sun and fun and convenient canned drinks seem to fit together, and soft drinks seem to go with fast food. In 1970, North Americans still drank more litres of coffee per capita than of any other nonalcoholic beverage product, but by 2007 they were consuming more than 190 litres of soft drinks and 110 litres of bottled water per person, compared with about 95 litres of coffee.[9]

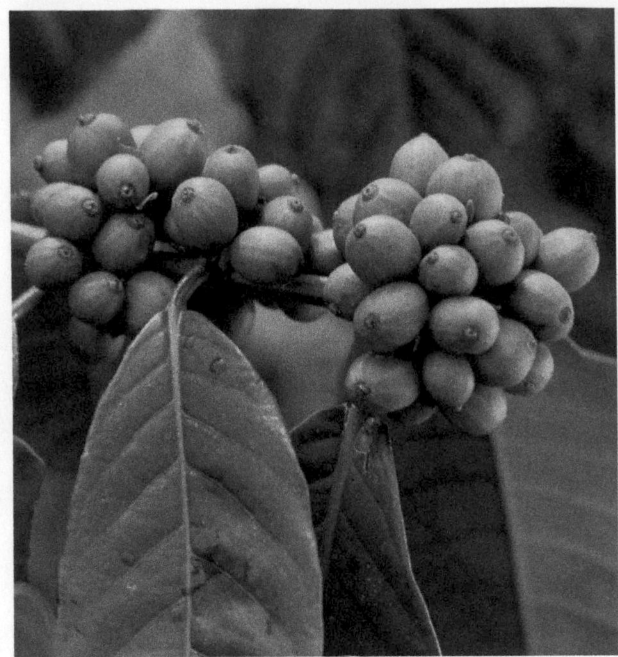

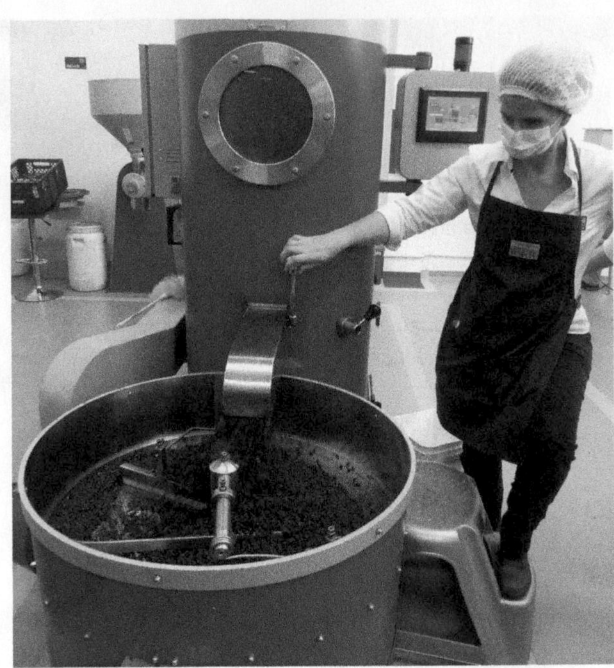

Green coffee beans are roasted to improve the colour and taste of the drink made from the beans.

If the U.S. national drink is not as national as it once was, neither is it as simple. Kaldi and his friends were content to simply munch on the coffee beans or put them in hot water. Somewhere in the dark past the Middle East discovered that roasting the green coffee bean improved the flavour, aroma, and colour of the drink made from the bean. For years, housewives, storekeepers, and coffee house owners bought the green bean, then roasted and ground it just before use. Commercial roasting started in 1790 in New York City, and the process gradually spread through North America. However, although the green bean can be stored indefinitely, the roasted bean deteriorates seriously within a month. Ground coffee can be maintained at its peak level in the home only for a week or two—and then only if it is in a closed container and refrigerated. Vacuum packing of ground coffee was introduced in 1900, a process that maintains the quality until the seal is broken.

Coffee growing spread worldwide when the Dutch began cultivation in the East Indies in 1696. Latin America had an ideal climate for coffee growing, and with the world's greatest coffee-drinking nation just up the road several thousand kilometres, it became the world's largest producer. Different varieties of the coffee tree and different growing and processing conditions provide many opportunities for varying the characteristics of coffee.

Although there are many bean-producing shrubs in the genus *Coffea,* virtually all coffee is made from two species: *Coffea arabica* and *Coffea robusta. Arabica* beans have a milder flavour, take longer to develop after planting, and require a near-tropical climate to grow properly. They are therefore more expensive and more desirable for most purposes. *Robusta* beans have a stronger, more bitter flavour and a higher caffeine content, and they are used primarily in less-expensive blends and to make instant coffee. In some countries, such as Colombia, only *arabica* beans are grown, whereas Brazil, the world's largest coffee producer, produces both kinds. In 2009 Brazil produced almost 2.5 times as much coffee as Vietnam, the second biggest coffee-growing country.[10] Colombia and Indonesia tied for third, followed by India and Ethiopia. You can see that coffee is now grown in tropical climates around the globe. As for imports, the European Union imported almost half of the available exports, followed by the United States, Japan, and Canada.[10]

Beginning in the early 1970s, health-conscious North Americans began to drink more decaffeinated coffee and less regular coffee. There are several ways of removing caffeine from the coffee bean. In the process used by most North American companies, the unroasted beans are soaked in an organic solvent, raising concerns about residues of the solvent remaining in the coffee. The most widely used solvent has been methylene chloride, and studies have shown that high doses of that solvent can cause cancer in laboratory mice. In 1985, the FDA banned the use of methylene

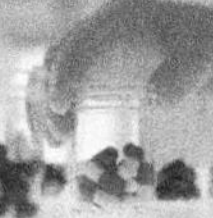

DRUGS IN THE MEDIA

Tim Hortons Coffee

The Tim Hortons franchise, Canada's largest coffee chain, captures 76% of the coffee market in Canada.[11] Tim Hortons was started by a Canadian hockey player, Tim Horton, and his partner, Jim Charade, and much of its marketing is targeted at a specific Canadian demographic: hockey parents. The company invests large amounts of money into its sponsorship of children's programs, especially hockey, and provides financial and education aid to employees. One long-running Tim Hortons commercial showed a parent taking a child to practice at 5 a.m. in the dead of winter, holding a steaming Timmy's coffee. The Tim Hortons brand has become a national cultural icon. An outlet was even set up near the Kandahar and Bagram airfields in Afghanistan.[12]

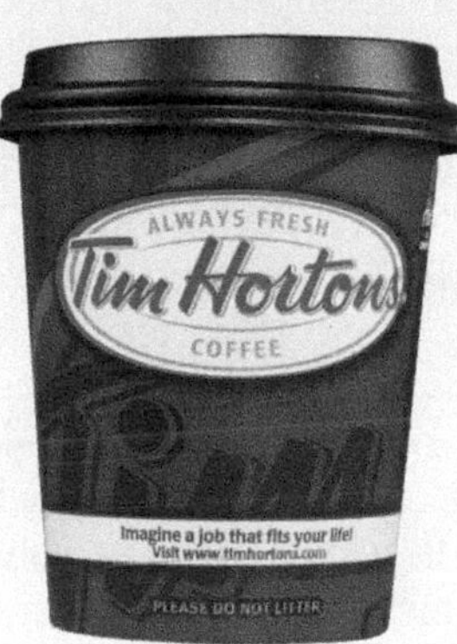

With the successful growth of Tim Hortons stores in Canada, which boast almost 3200 outlets with another 400 locations expected to open in the next year, the quintessential Canadian company has moved beyond its borders.[13] It has already opened more than 600 locations in the United States,[14] and its first store in the United Arab Emirates opened in Dubai in 2011.[15] Another 120 stores across the Persian Gulf region are expected in the next five years.[16] Figure 11.2 depicts the growth in Tim Hortons outlets, including international locations.

The authors thank Brian Grant for this article.

Figure 11.2 Growth of Tim Hortons Restaurants (includes international outlets)

Graph demonstrating the rise of the total number of Tim Hortons restaurants over time, including international outlets. According to data from June 30, 2013, Tim Hortons had 4304 establishments, 3468 of which were Canadian. Data obtained from Tim Hortons Web site. The authors thank Richard Patrick for contribution to this figure.

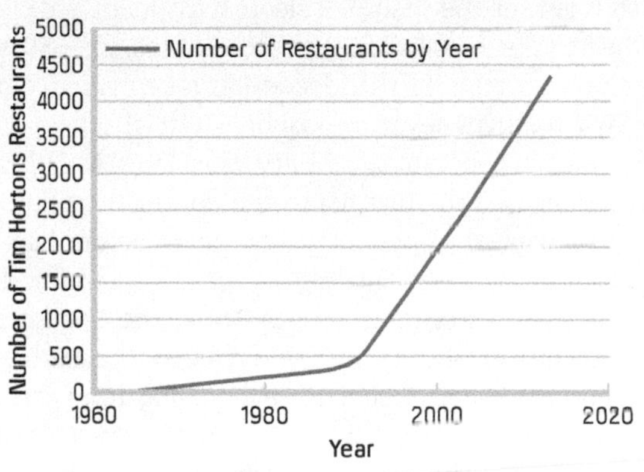

chloride in hairsprays, which can be inhaled during use, but allowed the solvent to be used in decaffeination as long as residues did not exceed 10 parts per million. Because the solvent residue evaporates during roasting, decaffeinated coffees contain considerably lower amounts than that, so the assumption is that the risk is minimal. The Swiss water process, which is not used on a large commercial scale in North America, removes more of the coffee's flavour. The caffeine that is taken out of the coffee is used mostly in soft drinks. One of the largest decaffeinating companies is owned by Coca-Cola.

Today's supermarket shelves are filled with an amazing variety of products derived from this simple bean: pure Colombian, French roast, decaf, half-caf, flavoured coffees, instants, mixes, and even cold coffee beverages. The competition for the consumer's coffee dollar has never been greater, it seems. North Americans are lining up in record numbers at espresso bars to buy cappuccinos, lattes, and other exotic-sounding mixtures of strong coffee, milk, and flavourings. The number of these specialty coffee shops in North America increased from fewer than 200 in 1989 to about 25 000 in 2010.[17] They are found in small towns, shopping malls, and on practically every corner in cities.

Tea

Tea and coffee are not like day and night, but their differences are reflected in the legends surrounding their origins. The bouncing goat herder of Arabia suggests that coffee is a boisterous, blue-collar drink. Tea is a different story: much softer, quieter, more delicate.

According to one legend, Daruma, the founder of Zen Buddhism, fell asleep one day while meditating. Resolving that it would never happen again, he cut off both eyelids. From the spot where his eyelids touched the earth grew a new plant. From its leaves a brew could be made that would keep a person awake. Appropriately, the tea tree, *Thea sinensis* (now classed as *Camellia sinensis*), is an evergreen, and *sinensis* is the Latin word for "Chinese."

The first report of tea that seems reliable is in a Chinese manuscript from around the middle of the fourth century, 350 CE, when it was primarily seen as a medicinal plant. The non-medical use of tea is suggested by a book written in the latter half of the eighth century (780 CE) on the cultivation of tea, but the real proof that it was in wide use in China is that a tax was levied on it in the same year. Before this time Buddhist monks had carried the cultivation and use of tea to Japan.

Europe had to wait eight centuries to savour the herb that was "good for tumors or abscesses that come from the head, or for ailments of the bladder . . . it quenches thirst. It lessens the desire for sleep. It gladdens and cheers the heart." The first European record of tea, in 1559, says, "One or two cups of this decoction taken on an empty stomach removes fever, headache, stomachache, pain in the side or in the joints. . . ." Fifty years later, in 1610, the Dutch delivered the first tea to the continent of Europe.

An event that occurred ten years before had tremendous impact on the history of the world and on present patterns of drug use. In 1600, the English East India Company was formed, and Queen Elizabeth gave the company a monopoly on everything from the east coast of Africa across the Pacific to the west coast of South America. The English East India Company concentrated on importing spices, so the first tea was taken to England by the Dutch. As the market for tea increased, the English East India Company expanded its imports of tea from China. Coffee had arrived first, so most tea was sold in coffee houses. Even as tea's use as a popular social drink expanded in Europe, there were some prophets of doom. A 1635 publication by a physician claimed that, at the very least, using tea would speed the death of those over 40 years old. The use of tea was not slowed, however, and by 1657 tea was being sold to the public in England. This was no more than ten years after the English had developed the present word for it: *tea*. Although spelled *tea*, it was pronounced "tay" until the nineteenth century. Before this period the Chinese name *ch'a* had been used, anglicized to either *chia* or *chaw*.

With the patrons of taverns off at coffee houses living it up with tea, coffee, and chocolate, tax revenues from alcoholic beverages declined. To offset this loss, coffee houses were licensed, and a tax of eight pence was levied on each gallon of tea and chocolate sold.

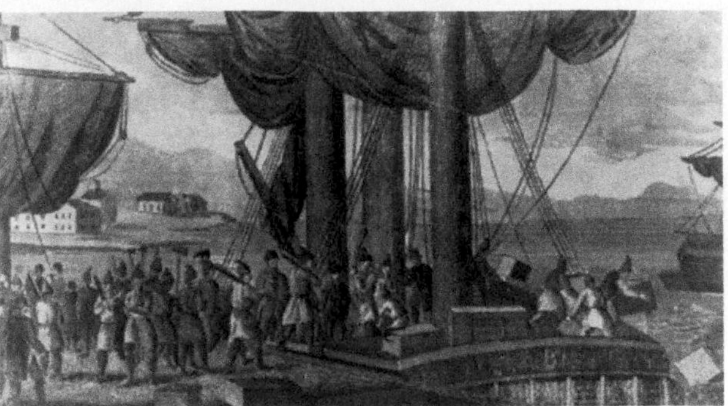

The Boston Tea Party contributed to the English preference for tea over coffee.

Britain banned Dutch imports of tea in 1669, which gave the English East India Company a monopoly. Profit from the China tea trade colonized India, brought about the Opium Wars between China and Britain, and induced the English to switch from coffee to tea. In the last half of the eighteenth century, the East India Company conducted a "Drink Tea" campaign unlike anything ever seen. Advertising, low cost on tea, and high taxes on alcohol made Britain a nation of tea drinkers.

The Canadian and American colonies, ever loyal to the king, had become big tea drinkers, which helped the king and the East India Company stay solvent. The Stamp Act of 1765, which included a tax on tea, changed everything in the United States. Even though the Stamp Act was repealed in 1766, it was replaced by the Trade and Revenue Act of 1767, which did the same thing. These measures made the colonists unhappy over paying taxes they had not helped formulate (taxation without representation), and in 1767 this resulted in a general boycott on the consumption of English tea. Coffee use increased, but the primary increase was in the smuggling of tea. In 1773 Parliament gave the East India Company the right to sell tea in the American colonies without paying the tea taxes. The company was also allowed to sell the tea through its own agents, thus eliminating the profits of the merchants in the colonies.

Several boatloads of this tea, which would be sold cheaper than any before, sailed toward various ports in the colonies. The American merchants, who would not have made any profit on this tea, were the primary ones who rebelled at the cheap tea. Some ships were turned away from port, but the end came with the 342 chests of tea that turned the Boston harbour into a teapot on the night of December 16, 1773.

The revolution in America and the colonists' rejection of tea helped tea sales in Great Britain—to be a tea drinker was to be loyal to the Crown. Although their use of coffee increases yearly and that of tea declines, the English are still tea drinkers. In Canada, the per capita consumption of tea was 79.4 litres in 2008, possibly because of the antioxidant properties of some teas.[18]

Tea starts its life on a three-metre bush high in the mountains of China, Sri Lanka, India, or Indonesia. Without pruning, the bush would grow into a five- to ten-metre tree, which would be difficult to pluck, as picking tea leaves is called. The pluckers select only the bud-leaf and the first two leaves at each new growth.

In one day a plucker will pluck enough leaves to make 4.5 kilograms of tea as sold in the grocery store. Plucking is done every six to ten days in warm weather as new growth develops on the many branches. The leaves are dried, rolled to crush the cells in the leaf, and placed in a cool, damp place for fermentation (oxidation) to occur. This oxidation turns the green leaves to a bright copper. Nonoxidized leaves are packaged and sold as green tea, sales of which have seen large increases in recent years. Oxidized tea is called black tea and accounts for about 98% of the tea North Americans consume. Oolong tea is greenish-brown, consisting of partially oxidized leaves.

MIND/BODY CONNECTION

Health Benefits of Tea

Tea is a very popular and commonly consumed beverage in Canada. There are many different types of tea, all with their own unique tastes and health benefits. Consuming tea is excellent for the human body because tea contains many helpful natural compounds including various amino acids and antioxidants flavonoids.

Black tea is the most common type of tea in both production and consumption. Black tea is made from the leaves of the plant *Camellia sinensis,* which is native to Asia but grown all over the world. The leaves are fermented (giving the tea its darker colour), dried, and then crushed. Black tea has the highest caffeine content among teas, with about 40 mg of caffeine per cup. Health benefits of black tea have been linked to lowering cholesterol, reducing the risk of stroke, and protecting the lungs from smoke damage.

Flavonoids are bioactive compounds that are thought to improve the body's health in many ways. They are found in the highest quantity in black tea, with slightly less in green tea (see Figure 11.3). Teas of all types can provide many health benefits as well as a healthy drink option. For any noticeable changes in health, tea must be consumed on a regular basis over a long period of time.[19]

Green tea, similar to black tea, is also made from the leaves of the *Camellia sinensis.* However, in the production of green tea the leaves are not fermented and this type does not contain caffeine. Green tea can help with the prevention of cancerous cells that cause illness. It also has high levels of antioxidants. Green tea is also commonly used for weight loss, and assists insulin in lowering blood sugar in diabetes.

Oolong tea is another type of tea made from the *Camellia sinensis* plant. It is less fermented than black tea but more so than green tea, and it also contains caffeine. In production the leaves are withered under the sun and then oxidized.

Figure 11.3 Flavonoid Content in Selected Beverages

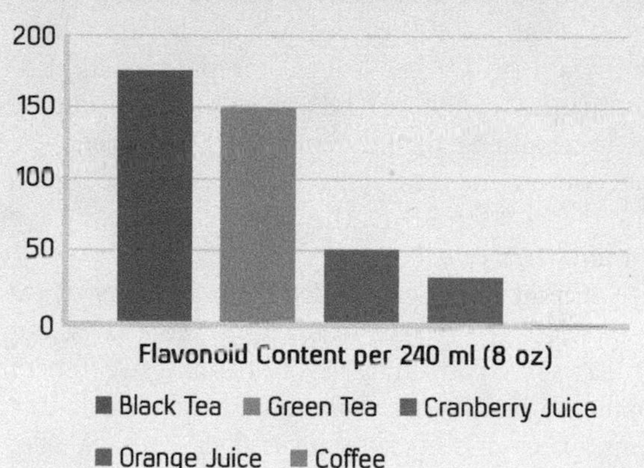

Source: USDA database for flavonoid content of selected foods (2007)

Oolong tea is commonly known for helping with weight loss by activating fat-burning enzymes in the body.

Red Rose is a Canadian brand of black tea called orange pekoe. It is produced in the same way that other black tea is made, except it uses different parts of the leaf. Orange pekoe tea is very high quality, made from only the best part of the tea leaf. Like other black teas, orange pekoe has higher caffeine content and a higher level of antioxidants than most teas. Because of its strength and caffeine content, black tea such as the Red Rose brand is commonly consumed to "wake up" the body.

The authors thank Emma Kearney for article contribution.

Sources: "Tea for Your Health," *Tea Association of Canada: Tea for Your Health, January 2014 Comments.* http://www.tea.ca/tea-health/tea-for-your-health-january-2014/; "List of Tea Types," *WikiTea,* http://tea.wikia.com/wiki/WikiTea; "6 Healthy Types of Tea," *Real Simple,* http://www.realsimple.com/health/nutrition-diet/healthy-eating/types-of-tea-00100000068566/index.html; Feature, Julie Edgar, "Types of Teas and Their Health Benefits," *WebMD,* http://www.webmd.com/diet/features/tea-types-and-their-health-benefits.

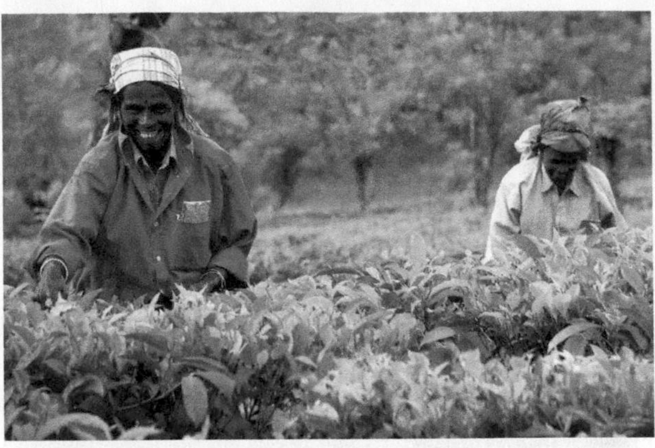

Most tea is grown in Sri Lanka, India, and Indonesia. The leaves are harvested by hand, with only the top few leaves of new growth harvested every six to ten days.

At equal weights, loose black tea contains a higher concentration of caffeine than do coffee beans. However, because about 400 cups of tea can be made from each kilogram of dry tea leaves, compared with 100 or 120 cups of coffee per kilogram, a typical cup of tea has less caffeine than a typical cup of coffee. The caffeine content of teas varies widely, depending on brand and the strength of the brew. Most teas have 40–60 milligrams of caffeine per cup.

The market has been flooded with a variety of tea products. Most tea is sold in tea bags these days, but instant teas, some containing flavourings and sweeteners, are popular for convenience. Flavoured teas—which contain mint, spices, or other substances along with tea—offer other options. The biggest boom in recent years has been in so-called herbal teas, which mostly contain no real "tea." These teas are made up of mixtures of other plant leaves and flowers for both flavour and colour and have become quite popular among people who avoid caffeine.

Although tea contains another chemical that derived its name from the tea plant, **theophylline** ("divine leaf") is present only in very small, nonpharmacological amounts in the beverage. Theophylline is very effective at relaxing the bronchial passages and is prescribed for use by asthmatics.

Chocolate

Now we come to the third legend, one concerning the origin of the third xanthine-containing plant. Long before Columbus landed on San Salvador, Quetzalcoatl, the Aztec god of the air, gave humans a gift from paradise: the chocolate tree. Linnaeus was to remember this legend when he named the cocoa tree *Theobroma*, "food of the gods." The Aztecs treated it as such, and the cacao bean was an important part of their economy, with the cacao bush being cultivated widely. Montezuma, emperor of Mexico in the early sixteenth century, is said to have consumed nothing other than 50 goblets of *chocolatl* every day. The *chocolatl*—from the Mayan words *choco* ("warm") and *latl* ("beverage")—was flavoured with vanilla but was far from the chocolate of today. It was a thick liquid, like honey, that was sometimes frothy and had to be eaten with a spoon.

Cortez introduced sugarcane plantations to Mexico in the early 1520s and supported the continued cultivation of the *Theobroma cacao* bush. When he returned to Spain in 1528, Cortez carried with him cakes of processed cocoa. The cakes were eaten, as well as being ground up and mixed with water for a drink. Although chocolate was introduced to Europe almost a century before coffee and tea, its use spread very slowly. Primarily this was because the Spanish kept the method of preparing chocolate from the cacao bean a secret until the early seventeenth century. When knowledge of the technique spread, so did the use of chocolate.

During the seventeenth century, chocolate drinking reached all parts of Europe, primarily among the wealthy. Maria Theresa, wife of France's Louis XIV, enjoyed hot chocolate, and this furthered its use among the wealthy

theophylline: a xanthine found in tea.

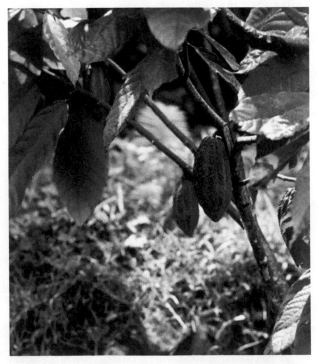

The genus of the chocolate (cacao) tree, *Theobroma*, is Latin for "food of the gods."

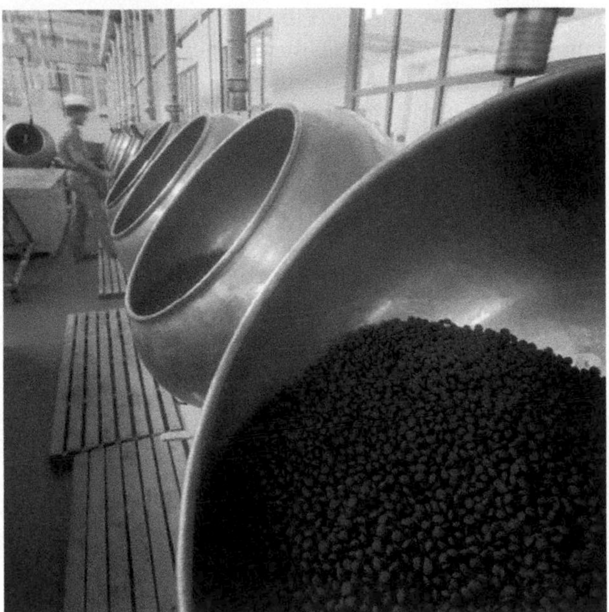

Chocolate candy is made by mixing cocoa butter, sugar, and chocolate powder.

and fashionable. Gradually it became more of a social drink, and by the 1650s chocolate houses were open in England, although usually chocolate was sold alongside coffee and tea in the established coffee houses.

In the early eighteenth century, health warnings were issued in England against the use of chocolate, but use expanded. Its use and importance are well reflected in a 1783 proposal in the U.S. Congress that the United States raise revenue by taxing chocolate as well as coffee, tea, liquor, sugar, molasses, and pepper.

Although the cultivation of chocolate never became a matter to fight over, it, too, has spread around the world. The New World plantations were almost destroyed by disease at the beginning of the eighteenth century, but cultivation had already begun in Asia, and today a large part of the crop comes from Africa.

Until 1828, all chocolate sold was a relatively indigestible substance obtained by grinding the cacao kernels after processing. The preparation had become more refined over the years, but it still followed the Aztec procedure of letting the pods dry in the sun, then roasting them before removing the husks to get to the kernel of the plant. The result of grinding the kernels is a thick liquid called chocolate liquor. This is baking chocolate. In 1828, a Dutch patent was issued for the manufacture of "chocolate powder" by removing about two thirds of the fat from the chocolate liquor.

The fat that was removed, cocoa butter, became important when someone found that, if it was mixed with sugar and some of the chocolate powder, it could easily be formed into slabs or bars. In 1847, the first chocolate bars appeared, but it was not until 1876 that the Swiss made their contribution to the chocolate industry by inventing milk chocolate, which was first sold under the Nestlé label. In Canada, milk chocolate today must contain at least 12% milk solids, although better grades contain almost twice that amount.

The unique xanthine in chocolate is **theobromine**. Its physiological actions closely parallel those of caffeine, but it is much less potent in its effects on the central nervous system. The average cup of cocoa contains about 200 milligrams of theobromine but only 4 milligrams of caffeine. Table 11.1 compares the caffeine contents of various forms of coffee, tea, and chocolate.

Health Canada recommends a daily caffeine intake of less than 400 milligram for healthy adults, the equivalent of three 237-millilitre (8-ounce) cups of coffee. Health Canada also recommends that women of reproductive age consume less than 300 milligrams of caffeine per day. Caffeine intake should be limited to less than 85 milligrams for children ages 10–12, less than 62.5 milligrams for children ages 7–9, and less than 45 milligrams for children ages 4–6. Adolescents ages 13–16 should consume no more than 2.5 milligrams per kilogram of body weight.[20] Canadian children consume approximately half the amount of caffeine (7 milligrams per day) that American children do (14 milligrams per day). The difference in consumption is due largely to higher intakes of carbonated soft drinks in the United States.[21]

Table 11.1 Caffeine in Foods and Drinks

	Amount of Caffeine (mg)
Coffee (200 mL)	
percolated	72–144
filter drip	108–180
instant	60–90
Tea (200 mL)	
weak	18–24
strong	78–108
Some varieties of soft drinks (one 355-mL can)	28–64
Chocolate bar (60 g)	
milk chocolate	3–20
dark chocolate	40–50

Source: Caffeine and Pregnancy. Public Health Agency of Canada, 2014. Reproduced with permission from the Minister of Health, 2014.

theobromine: a xanthine found in chocolate.

LO3 Other Sources of Caffeine

Coffee, tea, and chocolate are not the only sources of caffeine today. Others include soft drinks, so-called energy drinks, and some over-the-counter medications.

Soft Drinks

The early history of cola drinks is not shrouded in the mists that veil the origins of the other xanthine drinks, so there is no problem in selecting the correct legend. That's what the story of Coca-Cola is–a true legend in our time. From a green nerve tonic in 1886 in Atlanta, Georgia, that did not sell well at all, Coca-Cola has grown into "the real thing," providing "the pause that refreshes," selling almost 3 billion cases a year and operating in more than 200 countries.

Dr. J. C. Pemberton's green nerve tonic in the late nineteenth century contained caramel, fruit flavouring, phosphoric acid, caffeine, and a secret mixture called Merchandise No. 5. The unique character of Coca-Cola and its later imitators comes from a blend of fruit flavours that makes it impossible to identify any of its parts. An early ad for Coca-Cola suggested its varied uses:

> The "INTELLECTUAL BEVERAGE" and TEMPERANCE DRINK contains the valuable TONIC and NERVE STIMULANT properties of the Coca plant and Cola (or Kola) nuts, and makes not only a delicious, exhilarating, refreshing and invigorating Beverage, (dispensed from the soda water fountain or in other carbonated beverages), but a valuable Brain Tonic, and a cure for all nervous affections–SICK HEADACHE, NEURALGIA, HYSTERIA 8 MELANCHOLY.[22]

Coca-Cola was touted as "the new and popular fountain drink, containing the tonic properties of the wonderful coca plant and the famous cola nut." In 1903, the company admitted its beverage contained small amounts of cocaine, but soon after that it quietly removed all the cocaine; a government analysis of Coca-Cola in 1906 did not find any.

The name *Coca-Cola* was originally conceived to indicate the nature of its two ingredients with tonic properties: coca leaves and cola (kola) nuts. In 1909, the U.S. FDA seized a supply of Coca-Cola syrup and made two charges against the company. One was that the syrup was misbranded because it contained "no coca and little if any cola" and, second, that it contained an "added poisonous ingredient": caffeine.

Before a 1911 trial in Chattanooga, Tennessee, the company paid for research into the physiological effects of caffeine and, when all the information was in, the company won. The government appealed the decision. In 1916, the U.S. Supreme Court upheld the lower court by rejecting the charge of misbranding, stating that the company had repeatedly said that "certain extracts from the leaves of the coca shrub and the nut kernels of the cola tree were used for the purpose of obtaining a flavour" and that "the ingredients containing these extracts," with the cocaine eliminated, were called Merchandise No. 5. Today, coca leaves are imported by a pharmaceutical company in New Jersey. The cocaine is extracted for medical use and the decocainized leaves are shipped to the Coca-Cola plant in Atlanta, where Merchandise No. 5 is produced. A 1931 report indicated that Merchandise No. 5 contained an extract of three parts coca leaves and one part cola nuts, but to this day it remains a secret formula.

In 1981, the U.S. FDA changed its rules so that a cola no longer has to contain caffeine. If it does contain caffeine, it may not be more than 0.02%, which is 0.2 milligrams per millilitre, or a little less than 6 milligrams per ounce. Some consumer and scientist groups believe that all cola manufacturers should indicate on the label the amount of caffeine the beverage contains. This has not happened, even though soft drinks, as with other food products, must now list nutrition information, such as calories, fat, sodium, and protein content.

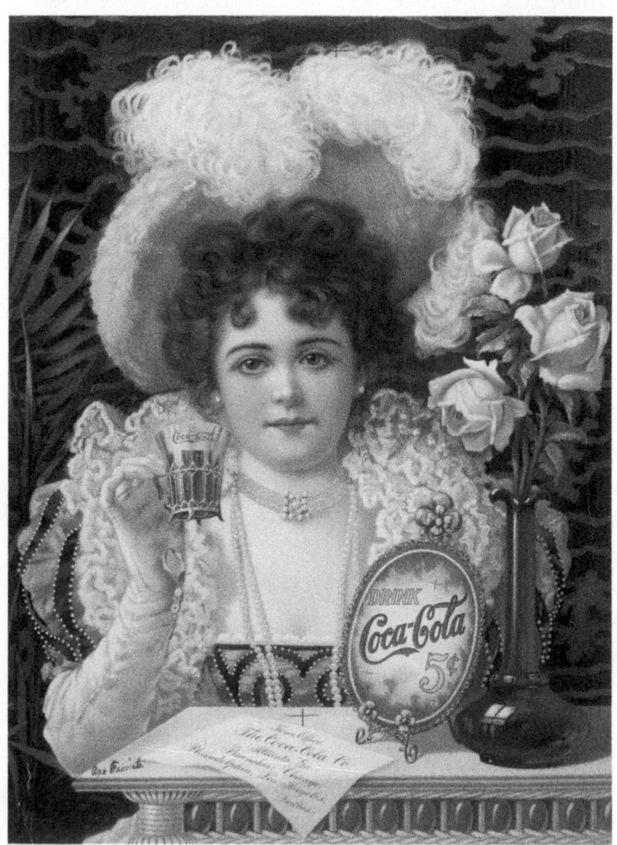

When introduced in the late nineteenth century, Coca-Cola was marketed as a tonic and named for two flavouring ingredients with tonic properties: coca leaves and cola (kola) nuts. The coca leaves used in Coca-Cola today have had the cocaine extracted.

Table 11.2 lists the caffeine content in a 355-millilitre (12-ounce) serving of popular soft drinks. Diet soft drinks, most now sweetened with aspartame, and caffeine-free colas are commanding a larger share of the market, but regular colas are still the single most popular type of soft drink. Health Canada originally prevented Pepsi–the maker of Mountain Dew–from adding caffeine to the formulation sold here a few years ago, though it remained in the drink sold in the United States. However, Mountain Dew has since changed the version they sell in Canada so that it is now identical to the U.S. version, with caffeine. The non-caffeinated form is no longer sold here at all. Drink companies have found a way to skirt those rules with guarana–its extract, guaranine, is really caffeine, just from a different plant.[23,24] Health Canada imposes strict regulations limiting caffeine but almost none on guaranine, despite caffeine levels in these energy drinks being potentially very high.[24]

As with beers and some other products, the modern marketing strategy seems to be for each company to try to offer products of every type and cover the market. Also as with beers, the large companies are buying up their competitors. In 2001, the Coca-Cola and PepsiCo companies represented more than 75% of total shipments. Coca-Cola Classic remains the most popular single brand, with almost 20% of the total market. Soft drinks have become increasingly popular. However, per capita consumption of soft drinks in Canada fell from 76.4 litres in 2007 to 73.2 litres in 2008.[18] Compare this with the 189 litres consumed per person each year. Some literature suggests that the pandemic of type 2 diabetes in North America is related to the use of soft drinks. Drinking one or two sugared soft drinks a day increased the risk of developing type 2 diabetes by 26%.[25]

Table 11.2 Caffeine in Popular Soft Drinks

Brand	Caffeine† (mg)
7-Up	0*
A&W Root Beer	0*
Sprite, regular or diet	0*
Mountain Dew, regular or diet	54 (20 oz = 90)
Diet Coke	47 (20 oz = 78)
Diet Coke Lime	47 (20 oz = 78)
Dr. Pepper	42 (20 oz = 68)
Dr. Pepper, diet	44 (20 oz = 68)
Pepsi	38 (20 oz = 63)
Diet Pepsi	36 (20 oz = 60)
Coca-Cola Classic	35 (20 oz = 58)
Coke Black Cherry Vanilla, regular or diet	35 (20 oz = 58)
Coke Lime	35 (20 oz = 58)
Coke Vanilla	35 (20 oz = 58)
Coke Zero	35 (20 oz = 58)
Barq's root beer, regular or diet	23 (20 oz = 38)

*These are examples of many soft drinks available that do not contain any caffeine.

†Per 12-ounce (355-millilitre) serving; 20 ounces = 590 millilitres

Source: Center for Science in the Public Interest (CSPInet.org).

"Energy" Drinks

Some consumers have always preferred to obtain their caffeine from soft drinks instead of from coffee. This led to the development and promotion of Jolt cola, the first energy drink, in 1985. Jolt had the maximum allowable caffeine content at almost 72 milligrams in a 355-millilitre (12-ounce) can. This might be a lot for a soft drink, but it isn't a great deal when compared with 320 milligrams in a 475-millilitre (16-ounce) cup of Starbucks coffee. In 2003 in Montreal, the energy drink Reload was launched, ranking first in sales in Quebec in the first week and third in Canada the same year. In September 2009, after 25 years in business, Jolt Co. Inc. filed for bankruptcy and its assets were sold.

Mountain Dew's hugely successful television marketing campaign links its product with heavy-metal music and extreme skiing, snowboarding, and similar high-energy activities. The parent company, PepsiCo, says on the Mountain Dew Web site that "Doing the 'Dew' is like no other soft drink experience because of its daring, high-energy, high-intensity, active, extreme citrus taste," but most of its users know its caffeine content in

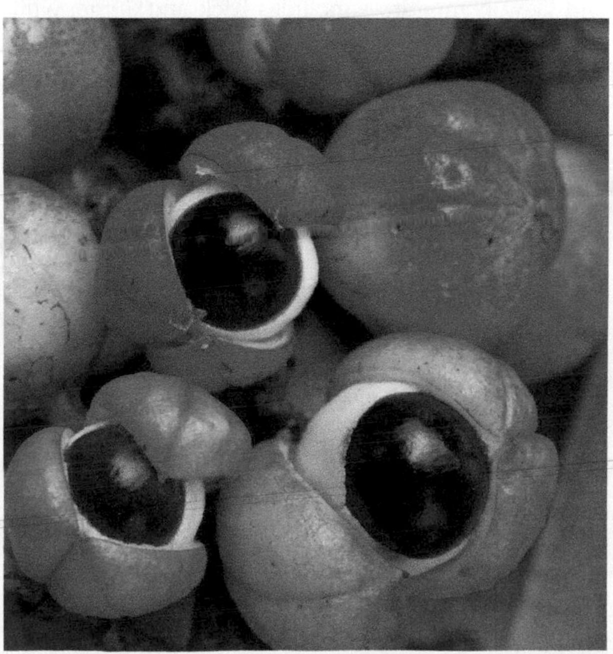

Guarana beans look similar to coffee beans.

the United States is higher than the major brands of colas (but still not high compared with brewed coffee). Then along came the Austrian sensation in a small can, Red Bull. Touted as an energy drink, the main active ingredient in this expensive drink is caffeine, at 80 milligrams per 245-millilitre (8.3-ounce) can (still less than a cup of coffee). The original marketers seemed to be aiming the product at people who exercise and want to "build" their bodies by including some ingredients found in dietary supplements sold to athletes, such as the amino acid taurine. Such products as Red Bull do appear to have unique properties. While both glucose and caffeine can improve particular aspects of cognitive performance and, with respect to caffeine, mood, evidence is mounting that when the sugar, caffeine, and taurine are considered together (but not separately), such drinks as Red Bull have statistically significant effects on a variety of psychological functions compared with placebo controls. The mixture has been found to exert positive synergistic effects on reaction time, attention, memory, and mood, including enhanced feelings of well-being and social extravertedness compared with placebo controls.[26,27,28]

Because Red Bull has also become a popular mixer for alcohol there have been some concerns that taurine might intensify alcohol's effect, but careful animal studies have found no interaction between taurine and the behavioural effects of alcohol.[29]

Much of the explosion in soft drink varieties has been aimed at this high-energy market. The hype has been pretty high energy, even if the products are nothing special, urging consumers to "feed the rush," or "blow your mind" using the drink. The list of Mountain Dew competitors includes Kick and Surge, while

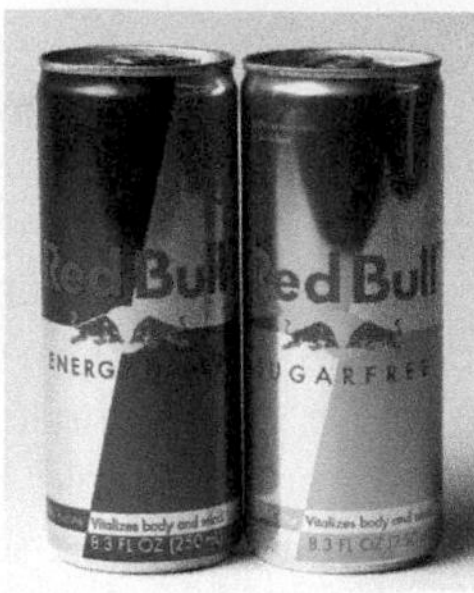
The main active ingredient in so-called energy drinks is caffeine.

Red Bull imitators have names like Stallion, Whoopass, Adrenaline Rush, Monster, and Rockstar.

Sobering Up It has long been thought that coffee can help a drinker to sober up, but little evidence supports the value of this. "Contrary to popular belief, drinking coffee will not help you to 'sober up' if you've had too much alcohol. The caffeine will make you more alert, but your co-ordination and concentration will still be impaired."[2] Caffeine will not lower blood-alcohol concentration, but it might arouse the drinker. As they say–put coffee in a sleepy drunk and you get a wide-awake drunk. This might be more dangerous than if the drunk had been left to sleep it off. There has been increasing evidence of interaction between caffeine-containing energy drinks and subjective reports of alcohol intoxication. One fairly recent study showed that caffeine could counteract some of the motor-impairing effects of alcohol but not others.[30] The striking finding in this study was that caffeine reduced subjective reports of intoxication, despite the persistence of alcohol-impairment.

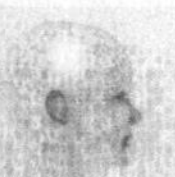

MIND/BODY CONNECTION

Energy Drink Consumption in Canadian Teens

Energy drinks have become popular among Canadian teens. Individuals consume energy drinks—which are suggested to provide optimal energy and alertness via caffeine and vitamins—to combat fatigue. Cognitive enhancement is suggested in the form of improvements to attention, wakefulness, memory, and concentration. Health Canada recommends no more than 400 mg of caffeine per day. Energy drinks are intended and properly advertised for adults as per Canadian regulations. However, more than 50% of adolescent students have reportedly consumed energy drink beverages within the past year in New Brunswick. There is also a strong relationship between energy drink consumption and alcohol use, with over 70% of middle and high school students who consume energy drinks reporting combining with alcohol. The consumption and availability of energy drinks is increasing. However, Health Canada recommends teens not drink energy drinks due to high levels of both caffeine and sugar, correlating with increased childhood obesity. Energy drinks comprise high levels of calories and lots of sugar, which influences the eating and drinking habits that lead to and affect obesity. In

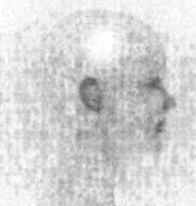

MIND/BODY CONNECTION

New Brunswick rates of obesity have been increasing, which poses a health concern among Canadians and especially in young adults. Figures 11.4, 11.5, and 11.6 provide some insight into energy drink usage among adolescents in New Brunswick.

The authors thank Kara Jenkins for article contribution.

Figure 11.4 Percentage of Adolescent Students Reporting Use of Caffeinated Energy Drinks in the Past 12 Months, by Frequency of Use, New Brunswick, 2012

Note: Data captured self-reports from a representative sample of students in grades 7, 9, 10 and 12. Don't know/no response = does not know what are caffeinated energy drinks/did not respond to the survey question.

Source: Office of the Chief Medical Officer of Health. (2013). Energy Drink Consumption Among Youth. New Brunswick Health Indicators. Issue 9; [PDF Document]. Retrieved from http://www2.gnb.ca/content/dam/gnb/Departments/h-s/pdf/en/Publications/Health%20Indicators%209_Energy%20drinks_Sept%202013.pdf

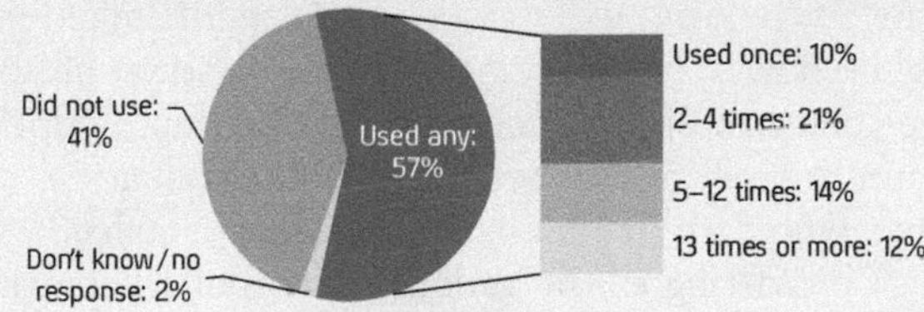

Figure 11.5 Percentage of Adolescent Students Using Caffeinated Energy Drinks in the Past 12 Months, by Health Region, New Brunswick, 2012

Note: Rates by health region not statistically different from the provincial average (57%; p<0.05). Data captured self-reports of consuming any caffeinated energy drinks in the past 12 months.

Source: Office of the Chief Medical Officer of Health. (2013). Energy Drink Consumption Among Youth. New Brunswick Health Indicators. Issue 9; [PDF Document]. Retrieved from http://www2.gnb.ca/content/dam/gnb/Departments/h-s/pdf/en/Publications/Health%20Indicators%209_Energy%20drinks_Sept%202013.pdf

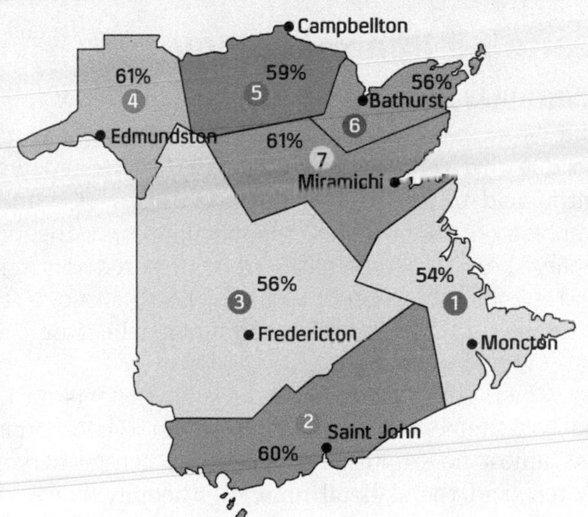

Figure 11.6 Rates of Energy Drink Consumption by Level of Alcohol Use, New Brunswick, 2012

Note: *statistically higher than the rate for students who did not use any alcohol (p<0.05). Occasional alcohol users refer to consuming beer, wine or hard liquor about once a month or less in the last 12 months. Frequent use refers to consuming alcohol on a weekly basis.

Source: Office of the Chief Medical Officer of Health. (2013). Energy Drink Consumption Among Youth. New Brunswick Health Indicators. Issue 9; [PDF Document]. Retrieved from http://www2.gnb.ca/content/dam/gnb/Departments/h-s/pdf/en/Publications/Health%20Indicators%209_Energy%20drinks_Sept%20 2013.pdf

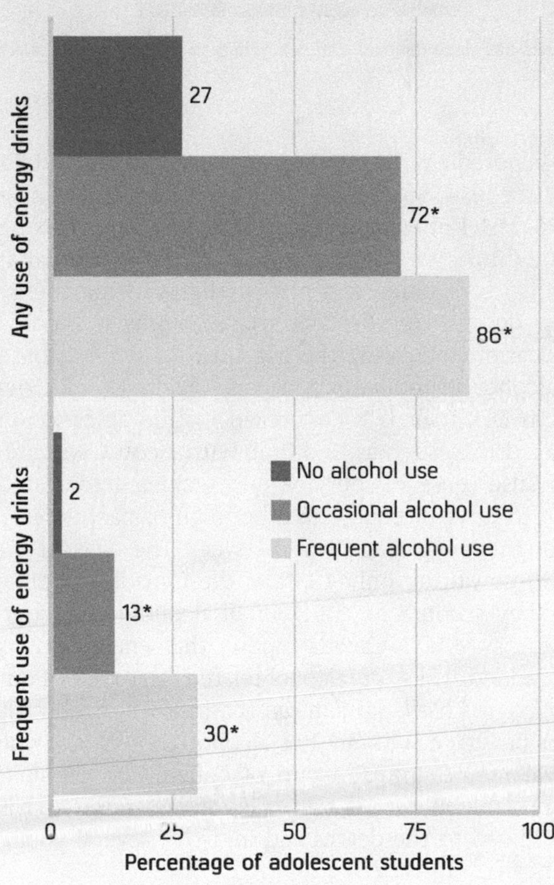

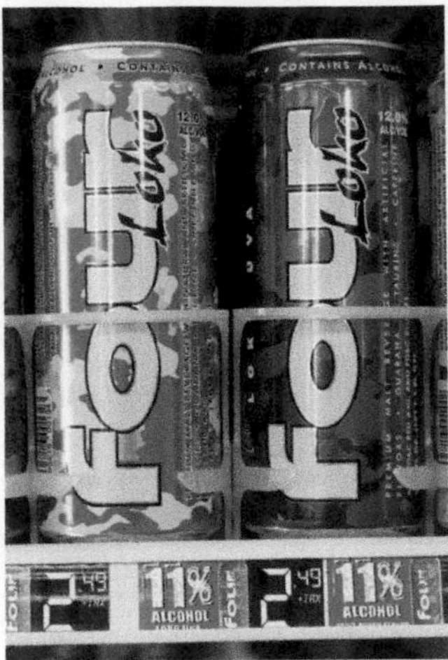

Four Loko has since removed caffeine from their product due to health fears.

Table 11.3 Caffeine Content of Nonprescription Drugs

Drug	Caffeine (mg)
Stimulants	
Kaizen Caffeine	200.0
Wake-Ups	100.0
Pep-Back Peak Performance	200.0
Analgesics	
Anacin	32.0
Excedrin	65.0
Midol	32.4
Diuretics	
Diurex (Ultra)	100.0

As noted earlier, the consumption of energy drinks is on the rise. In Canada, per capita consumption in 2006 was 1.1 litres, up from 0.8 litres in 2001.[31] Mixing energy drinks with alcohol has also become popular at Canadian bars, clubs, and parties. High-caffeine energy drinks desensitize the user to symptoms of alcohol intoxication, increasing the potential for alcohol abuse and alcohol-related harm. Mothers Against Drunk Driving (MADD) Canada is concerned that combination of energy drinks, such as Red Bull, with alcohol will create a false sense of sobriety, encouraging intoxicated youth to drive or engage in other high-risk activities.[32] Although young Canadians between the ages of 16 and 25 constitute only 13.7% of the Canadian population, they account for 32.1% of all alcohol-related traffic deaths. MADD Canada reports that energy drinks pose added risks of alcohol-related trauma.[32] Four Loko, coined *black out in a can* is a fruit-flavoured malt liquor beverage with an 11% alcohol content and the equivalent caffeine of a cup of coffee. The product, also available in Canada sold at 8% alcohol content, has been linked to the deaths and injury of several young Americans.[33,34]

Over-the-Counter Drugs

Few people realize that many nonprescription drugs also include caffeine, some in quite large amounts. Table 11.3 lists the caffeine content of some of these drugs. Presumably many people who buy "alertness tablets," such as Wake-Ups and Pep-Back Peak Performance, are aware that they are buying caffeine. But many buyers of such tablets as Excedrin might not realize how much caffeine they are getting. Imagine the condition of someone who took a nonprescription water-loss pill and a headache tablet containing caffeine, who then drank a couple of cups of coffee.

Considering all the various sources of caffeine, it is estimated that 80% of Canadians regularly use caffeine in some form, and that the average intake is 200–250 milligrams per day.[35] As with other psychoactive substances, this "average" takes in a wide range, with some users regularly consuming 1000 milligrams or more each day.

LO4, LO5, LO6, LO7

Caffeine Pharmacology

Xanthines are the oldest stimulants known. *Xanthine* is a Greek word meaning "yellow," the colour of the residue that remains after xanthines are heated with nitric acid until dry. The three xanthines of primary importance are caffeine, theophylline, and theobromine. These three chemicals are methylated xanthines and are closely related alkaloids. Most alkaloids are insoluble in water, but these are unique, because they are slightly water soluble.

These three xanthines have similar effects on the body. Caffeine has the greatest effect. Theobromine has almost no stimulant effect on the central nervous system and the skeletal muscles. Theophylline is the most potent, and caffeine the least potent, agent on the cardiovascular system. Caffeine, so named because

xanthines: the class of chemicals to which caffeine belongs.

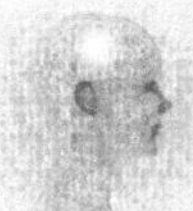

MIND/BODY CONNECTION

Alcohol and Energy Drinks

Despite warning labels and negative media attention, mixing alcohol and energy drinks has become increasingly popular. Youth and young adults are the biggest consumers of caffeinated alcoholic beverages. About one in five Canadian students say they have mixed alcohol with energy drinks. People can either purchase premixed caffeinated alcoholic beverages from a manufacturer, or the drinks can be hand-mixed by consumers themselves. Popular brands of premixed caffeinated alcoholic drinks are Rev and Rockstar. A trendy mixed caffeinated alcoholic beverage is a Jägerbomb, which is a shot of Jägermeister liquor with a can of Red Bull. Studies show that youth and young adults prefer hand-mixed drinks to premixed drinks. This puts them at a greater risk because normally hand-mixed drinks contain more caffeine than premixed ones do. The appeal to youth of mixing alcohol and energy drinks is that it masks the symptoms of intoxication and gives them more energy to stay up longer. Youth and young people who mix alcohol and energy drinks are more likely to engage in risky behaviour. This behaviour includes drinking and driving, getting in a car with a driver who has been drinking, perpetrating or being a victim of sexual assault, consuming increased quantities of alcohol, and alcohol poisoning. Health Canada has enforced labelling regulations for energy drinks requiring a statement that identifies the drink as a "high source of caffeine" and a statement "do not mix with alcohol."

A study by Mark Ashbridge of Dalhousie University in 2013 was done to determine how commonly alcohol is consumed together with energy drinks or in premixes sold in stores. In the study nationally representative data were used from 36 155 students who were in Grades 7 through 12 in 2010–2011. About 20% of the participants said they mix energy drinks with alcohol. Similar studies done in Canada, the United States, and Europe have had the same results. The provinces that had the highest percentage of respondents who said they drink alcoholic caffeinated beverages were Nova Scotia (26%) and British Columbia (26%); the lowest was Prince Edward Island (16%).

Sources: http://www.torys.com/Publications/Documents/Publication%20PDFs/FDR2011-9.pdf; http://www.hc-sc.gc.ca/ahc-asc/media/ftr-ati/_2010/2010_83-eng.php; http://www.cbc.ca/news/health/teens-mixing-alcohol-and-energy-drinks-a-growing-problem-1.137854; http://www.ccsa.ca/Eng/Priorities/Alcohol/Caffeinated-Alcoholic-Beverages-in-Canada/Pages/default.aspx; http://www.cmajopen.ca/content/1/1/E19.full

The authors thank Sara Casey for article contribution.

it was isolated from coffee in 1820, has been the most extensively studied and, unless otherwise indicated, is the drug under discussion here.

Time Course

In humans, the absorption of caffeine is rapid after oral intake; peak blood levels are reached 30 minutes after ingestion. Although maximal CNS effects are not reached for about two hours, the onset of effects can begin within half an hour after intake. The half-life of caffeine in humans is about three hours, and no more than 10% is excreted unchanged.

Cross-tolerance exists among the methylated xanthines; loss of tolerance can take more than two months of abstinence. The tolerance, however, is low grade, and by increasing the dose two to four times an effect can be obtained even in the tolerant individual. There is less tolerance to the CNS stimulation effect of caffeine than to most of its other effects. The direct action on the kidneys, to increase urine output, and the increase of salivary flow do show tolerance.

Dependence on caffeine is real (see the Taking Sides box). People who are not coffee drinkers or who have been drinking only decaffeinated coffee often report unpleasant effects (nervousness, anxiety) after being given caffeinated coffee, but those who regularly consume caffeine report mostly pleasant mood states after drinking coffee. Various experiments have reported on the reinforcing properties of caffeine in regular coffee drinkers; one of the most clear-cut allowed patients on a research ward to choose between two coded instant coffees, identical except that one contained caffeine. Participants had to choose at the beginning of each day which coffee they would drink for the rest of that day. People who had been drinking caffeine-containing coffee before this experiment almost always chose the caffeine-containing coffee.[36] Thus, the reinforcing effect of caffeine probably contributes to psychological dependence.

There has long been clear evidence of physical dependence on caffeine as well. The most reliable withdrawal sign is a headache, which occurs an average of 18–19 hours after the most recent caffeine intake.

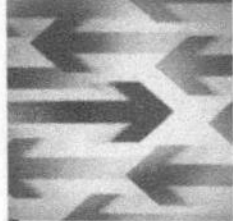

TAKING SIDES

Caffeine-Dependence Syndrome?

The American Psychiatric Association's DSM-IV-TR lists the criteria for substance abuse, substance dependence, substance withdrawal, and substance intoxication. The team that developed the revision did not include caffeine among the substances that would be considered to produce substance dependence. However, in 1994 a group of researchers reported the cases of 16 individuals who they considered to meet the general criteria for a DSM-IV-TR diagnosis of substance disorder.[37]

Of 99 subjects who responded to newspaper notices asking for volunteers who believed they were psychologically or physically dependent on caffeine, 27 were asked to undergo further testing, which included a psychiatric interview to assess caffeine dependence. Although the DSM-IV-TR requires that only three of seven criteria be met for a diagnosis of dependence, this study was more conservative in requiring three of the four most serious criteria (tolerance, withdrawal, persistent desire or efforts to cut down, and continued use despite knowledge of a persistent or recurrent problem caused by use). Sixteen of the 27 were diagnosed as having caffeine dependence by using these criteria. Of those 16, 11 agreed to participate in a double-blind caffeine withdrawal experiment. All were placed on a restricted diet during two two-day study periods and were given capsules to take at various times of the day to match their normal caffeine intake. During one of the two sessions, each volunteer was given caffeine, and during the other session the capsules contained a placebo. Neither the participants nor the interviewers were told on which session they were getting the caffeine. Withdrawal symptoms found during the placebo session included headaches, fatigue, decreased vigour, and increased depression scores. Several of the subjects were unable to go to or stay at work, went to bed several hours early, or needed their spouse to take over child care responsibilities.

A decision to accept caffeine-dependence syndrome as an official diagnosis would have several implications—some feel that it would trivialize the diagnosis for "serious" drug dependence or complicate questions of insurance payment for treatment of substance dependence. Others feel that this syndrome could be a serious dependence disorder for some coffee drinkers and deserves to be recognized as such.

Ozsungur and colleagues at the University of Toronto grouped 14 common caffeine withdrawal symptoms into three clusters they termed "fatigue and headache," "dysphoric mood," and "flu-like somatic symptoms" that occurred after abruptly stopped high levels of habitual caffeine consumption (>200 milligrams per day).[38] These withdrawal symptoms are strongest during the first two days of withdrawal, then decline over the next five or six days.[39] Strategies to eliminate withdrawal symptoms would be to slowly lessen caffeine intake over time.

As noted above, the DSM-5 removes the segregation between abuse and dependency diagnoses, replaced by a single term, Substance Use Disorder, with severity and course specifiers. Caffeine withdrawal syndrome had been provisional in the DSM-IV, and criteria for caffeine use disorder are included in the new DSM-5. Caffeine withdrawal symptoms include fatigue, headache, and difficulty focusing, and the condition is considered a mental disorder.[40] The following table provides a summary of the DSM-5 changes.[41]

DSM-IV-TR:	DSM-5:
305.90 Caffeine Intoxication	305.90 Caffeine Intoxication
292.89 Caffeine-Induced Anxiety Disorder	292.0 Caffeine Withdrawal
292.85 Caffeine-Induced Sleep Disorder	Other Caffeine-Induced Disorders
292.9 Caffeine-Induced Disorder Not Otherwise Specified	292.9 Unspecified Caffeine-Related Disorder

Mechanism of Action

For years no one really knew the mechanism whereby the methylxanthines had their effects on the central nervous system (CNS). In the early 1980s, evidence was presented that caffeine and the other xanthines block the brain's receptors for a substance known as **adenosine**, which is a neurotransmitter or neuromodulator. Adenosine normally acts in several areas of the brain to produce behavioural sedation by inhibiting the release of other neurotransmitters. Caffeine's stimulant action results from blocking adenosine receptors.[42] Caffeine works by preventing adenosine

adenosine: an inhibitory neurotransmitter through which caffeine acts.

DSM-5

Caffeine Intoxication

Diagnostic Criteria

A. Recent consumption of caffeine (typically a high dose well in excess of 250 mg)

B. Five (or more) of the following signs or symptoms developing during, or shortly after, caffeine use:
1. Restlessness
2. Nervousness
3. Excitement
4. Insomnia
5. Flushed face
6. Diuresis
7. Gastrointestinal disturbance
8. Muscle twitching
9. Rambling flow of thought or speech
10. Tachycardia or cardiac arrhythmia
11. Periods of inexhaustibility
12. Psychomotor agitation

C. The signs or symptoms in Criterion B cause clinically significant distress or impairment in social, occupational, or other important areas of functioning.

D. The signs or symptoms are not attributable to another medical condition and are not better explained by another mental disorder, including intoxication with another substance.

DSM-5

Caffeine Withdrawal Disorder

Diagnostic Criteria

A. Prolonged daily use of caffeine

B. Abrupt cessation of or reduction in caffeine use, followed within 24 hours by three or more of the following signs or symptoms:
1. Headache
2. Marked fatigue or drowsiness.
3. Dysphoric mood, depressed mood or irritability.
4. Difficulty concentrating.
5. Flu-like symptoms (nausea, vomiting, or muscle pain/stiffness).

C. The signs or symptoms in Criterion B cause clinically significant distress or impairment in social, occupational, or other important areas of functioning.

D. The signs or symptoms are not associated with the physiological effects of another medical condition (e.g. migraine, viral illness) and are not better explained by another mental disorder, including intoxication or withdrawal from another substance.

from binding to and activating the receptor. It binds to receptors but has no intrinsic effects by itself (see Figure 11.7). Caffeine is classified together with cocaine and amphetamines as a CNS stimulant. When caffeine reaches the brain, norepinephrine, a neurotransmitter that is associated with the so-called fight or flight stress response, is released. Caffeine also increases dopamine levels in the same way as amphetamine does, activating mesolimbic pathways involved in reward.[43] Dopamine is linked to the addictive properties of caffeine. Now that this mechanism is understood, it may lead to the development of new chemicals having similar but perhaps more potent effects.

Physiological Effects

"Coffee sets the blood in motion and stimulates the muscles; it accelerates the digestive processes, chases away sleep, and gives us the capacity to engage a little longer in the exercise of our intellects."[44] The

Figure 11.7 How Caffeine Works

Adenosine (A) decreases neuronal activity and dilates blood vessels, which increases oxygen flow in preparation for sleep. Caffeine (C) works as an adenosine antagonist, blocking adenosine from its receptors. Without adenosine, brain activity increases and results in increased alertness. Caffeine also constricts blood vessels, relieving headaches.

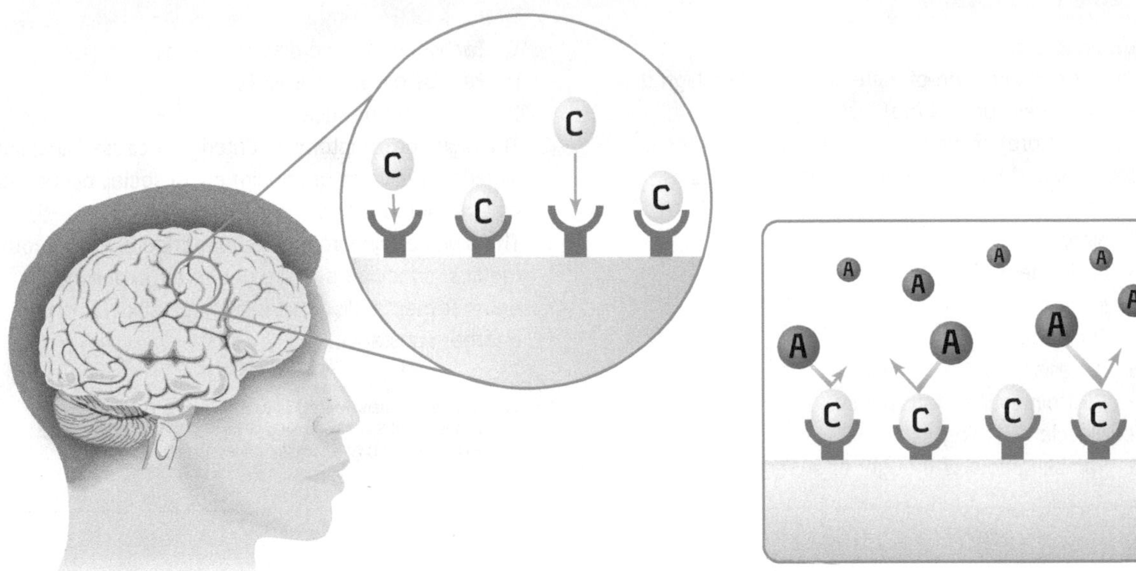

pharmacological effects on the CNS and the skeletal muscles are probably the basis for the wide use of caffeine-containing beverages. With two cups of coffee taken close together (about 200 milligrams of caffeine), the cortex is activated, an EEG shows an arousal pattern, and drowsiness and fatigue decrease. This CNS stimulation is also the basis for "coffee nerves," which can occur at low doses in sensitive individuals and in others when they have consumed large amounts of caffeine. In the absence of tolerance, even 200 milligrams will increase the time it takes to fall asleep and will cause sleep disturbances. Researchers at the University of Montreal conducted a double-blind cross-over experiment testing the effects of caffeine on sleep disruption in young and middle-aged subjects. The results showed that 200 milligrams of caffeine interrupted the ability to fall asleep, the time spent sleeping, and the quality of sleep relative to a placebo.[45] There is a strong relationship between the mood-elevating effect of caffeine and the extent to which it will keep the individual awake.

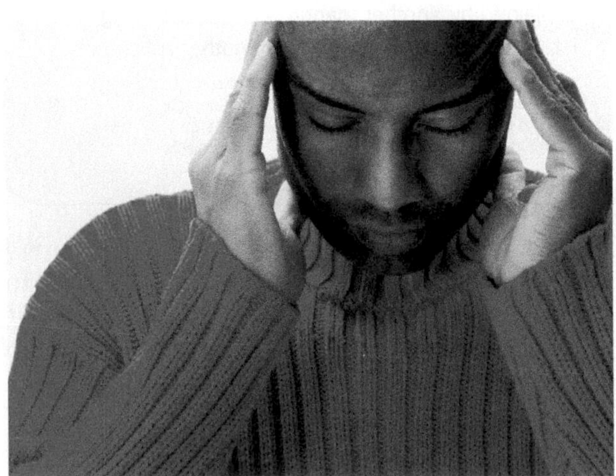

People can develop dependence on caffeine and experience withdrawal symptoms, such as headaches, if they discontinue caffeine intake.

Higher doses (about 500 milligrams) are needed to affect the autonomic centres of the brain, and heart rate, and respiration can increase at this dose. The direct effect on the cardiovascular system is in opposition to the effects mediated by the autonomic centres. Caffeine acts directly on the vascular muscles to cause dilation, whereas stimulation of the autonomic centres results in constriction of blood vessels. Usually dilation occurs, but in the brain the blood vessels are constricted, and this constriction might be the basis for caffeine's ability to reduce migraine headaches. A number of studies have demonstrated that regular coffee consumption reduces the risk for

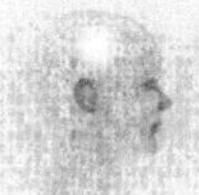

MIND/BODY CONNECTION

Caffeine and "Geek" Culture: Buying a Dream

Considerable mythology surrounds the supposed ability of caffeine to support sustained, high-level mental effort. For example, the famous mathematician Paul Erdos once said, "A mathematician is a device for turning coffee into theorems." This mythology of caffeine as brain fuel has been adopted by the so-called geek culture that grew so rapidly during the dot-com era of the late 1990s and remains strong among programmers, systems engineers, and those who identify with them. ThinkGeek.com, purveyors of all kinds of gadgets and supplies related to geek culture, sells an amazing variety of caffeine-based products in addition to coffee and tea, including candies, syrups, gum, and even ShowerShock, a caffeinated soap that is supposed to help you get going even before you get to the coffee cup. It is questionable whether or not this product, available in the United States and Canada, provides an effective delivery mechanism for caffeine.[46]

We have to ask whether those people who believe they can't work effectively without their coffee are more dependent on the caffeine or on the idea that caffeine helps them work harder or smarter. The evidence reviewed in this textbook indicates that once a person has developed a tolerance to higher levels of daily caffeine consumption, the caffeine probably does little good. However, stopping use at that point will likely lead to a lack of energy and headaches, interfering with work production.

In this competitive world, we'd all like to think that there's a magic substance that could give us intelligence and energy, and it's that mythical dream that helps sell everything from ShowerShock to Red Bull.

Parkinson's disease,[47] and higher intake of caffeinated coffee is associated with a further decreased risk for Parkinson's disease.[48] An inverse association also exists between higher coffee consumption and the risk for type 2 diabetes,[49,50] although the evidence for the sole benefits of antioxidants found in both caffeinated and decaffeinated coffee are mixed.[51,52] The opposing effects of caffeine make it very difficult to predict the results of normal (that is, less than 500 milligrams) caffeine intake. At higher levels, the heart rate increases, and continued use of large amounts of caffeine can produce an irregular heartbeat in some individuals. The basal metabolic rate might be increased slightly (10%) in chronic caffeine users, because 500 milligrams has frequently been shown to have this effect. This action probably combines with the stimulant effects on skeletal muscles to increase physical work output and decrease fatigue after the use of caffeine.

Behavioural Effects

The behavioural effects of caffeine depend on the difficulty of the task, the time of day, and to a great extent on how much caffeine the subject normally consumes.

Stimulation Low doses of caffeine (100 milligrams) are associated with increased activity in brain areas that support short-term memory and increased attention, concentration, and performance in short-term memory

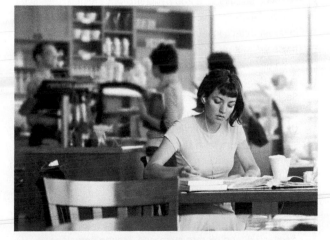

The primary behavioural effect of caffeine is stimulation, although high levels of caffeine consumption among postsecondary students have been associated with lower academic performance.

tasks.[53] When regular users of high amounts of caffeine (more than 300 milligrams per day, the equivalent of three cups of brewed coffee) were tested on a variety of study-related mental tasks without caffeine, they performed more poorly than did users of low amounts, perhaps because of withdrawal effects. Although their performance was improved after being given caffeine, they still performed more poorly on several of the tasks than did users of low amounts. It seems as though the beneficial short-term effects can be offset by the effects of tolerance and dependence in regular users.[54] High levels of caffeine consumption among postsecondary students have been associated with lower academic performance.[55]

There is considerable evidence that 200–300 milligrams of caffeine will partially offset fatigue-induced decrement in the performance of motor tasks. Like the amphetamines, but to a much smaller degree, caffeine prolongs the amount of time an individual can perform physically exhausting work.

Headache Caffeine's vasoconstrictive effects are considered to be responsible for the drug's ability to relieve migraine headaches. However, a study of nonmigraine headache pain found that caffeine reduced headache pain, even in individuals who normally consumed little or no caffeine (in other words, not only headaches resulting from caffeine withdrawal).[56] As for migraine headaches, Health Canada has allowed the relabelling of some analgesics that contain caffeine to focus on migraines. For example, Tylenol Ultra Relief Migraine Pain contains 65 milligrams of caffeine in each tablet.

Hyperactivity Many studies have looked at the effect of caffeine on the behaviour of children diagnosed with attention-deficit/hyperactivity disorder, and the results have been inconsistent. There is some indication that relatively high doses of caffeine may decrease hyperactivity, though not as well as methylphenidate.[57] The data available on the effects of caffeine on children are limited. Sleep loss is one effect of caffeine on children. Lost sleep in kids has been linked to emotional, learning, safety, and health problems. However, researchers really have no idea what 200–400 milligrams every day in a 5- to 13-year-old is going to do in the long term.[58]

MIND/BODY CONNECTION

Military Medicine

Caffeinating soldiers has benefits. Studies conducted by the Canadian and other international militaries showed that sleep-deprived soldiers with 200 milligrams of caffeine in their system had faster reaction times (just under a half-second faster) in target detection studies over a three-hour period than did those without caffeine. These studies also showed that the dose of caffeine increases firing accuracy and reaction time in target practice. A study done by the U.S. military on Navy Seals during intensive training showed a dose-dependent, task-dependent effect of caffeine on various reaction time tasks but no effect on rifle marksmanship.[59]

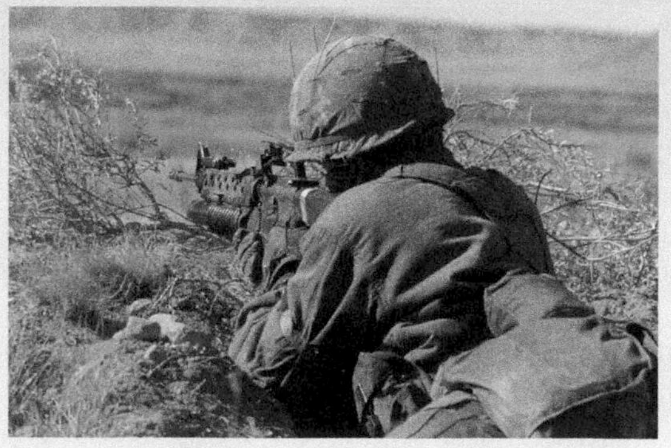

The military also tested a caffeinated gum for soldiers who were sleep deprived by having them perform a visual vigilance test. This test measures reaction time, false alarms, and hits on targets. Groups received either a placebo or 400 milligrams of caffeine. During the test period, soldiers' response time steadily decreased, false alarms decreased, and hit rate increased. Among non-sleep-deprived military volunteers, a moderate 200-milligram dose of caffeine significantly improved vigilance attending to a radar-screen-like display for two hours[60] and improved target detection speed without adversely affecting rifle-firing accuracy.[61,62]

The authors thank Brian Grant for this article.

Source: National Defence and the Canadian Forces. Retrieved from http://www.journal.dnd.ca/vo4/no4/military-meds-eng.asp

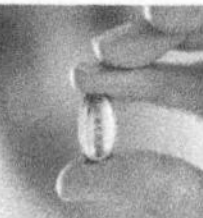

DRUGS IN DEPTH

Caffeine and Panic Attacks

Four caffeine-related syndromes are recognized in the DSM-IV-TR: caffeine intoxication, caffeine-induced anxiety disorder, caffeine-induced sleep disorder, and caffeine-related disorder not otherwise specified.[63] What's interesting about acute caffeine intoxication is that a threshold dose is specified: 250 milligrams. No other psychoactive substance in the DSM-IV-TR comes with a minimum dose to meet the diagnostic criteria. There are many ways to easily get 250 milligrams of caffeine in a single serving if a person is drinking some specialty coffees and energy drinks.

The National Institute of Mental Health (NIMH) has reported that caffeine can precipitate full-blown *panic attacks* in some people.[64] High levels of caffeine are able to block benzodiazepine receptors, which may underlie the anxiogenic effects of caffeine in inducing panic.[65] Panic attacks are not common but can be very debilitating for those who experience them. They consist of sudden, irrational feelings of doom, sometimes accompanied by choking, sweating, heart palpitations, and other symptoms.

In an experiment conducted at NIMH laboratories in Maryland, a group of people who had previously had panic attacks were given 480 milligrams of caffeine, equivalent to about five cups of brewed coffee. Panic attacks were precipitated in almost half of those people. In a group of 14 people who had never before experienced a panic attack, two had an attack after receiving 720 milligrams of caffeine.

The results are interesting from a scientific point of view not only because they reveal individual differences in susceptibility to panic but also because of the possible implications for an understanding of the biochemistry of panic disorders. The experiment may also have more immediate and practical implications in that, if a person does experience a panic attack, caffeine consumption should be looked at as a possible cause.

LO8 Causes for Concern

Because caffeine is probably the most widely used psychoactive drug in the world, it is understandable that it would elicit both good and bad reports. Although there is not yet clear evidence that moderate caffeine consumption is dangerous, the scientific literature has investigated the possible effects of caffeine in cancer, benign breast disease, reproduction, and heart disease. Part of the problem in knowing for certain about some of these things is that epidemiological research on caffeine consumption is difficult to do well, because of the many sources of caffeine and the variability of caffeine content in coffee. Coffee drinkers also tend to smoke more, for example, so the statistics have to correct for smoking behaviour.

Cancer

In the early 1980s, an increased risk of pancreatic cancers was reported among coffee drinkers. However, studies since then have criticized procedural flaws in that report and have found no evidence of such a link. The Canadian Cancer Society[66] and the 1984 American Cancer Society nutritional guidelines indicate there is no reason to consider caffeine a risk factor in human cancer. In a single case-control study conducted in Ontario of more than 5000 people from 1992 to 1994, coffee intake was inversely correlated with colon cancer–the more coffee a person drank, the lower was the risk.[67]

Pregnancy and Conception

Although studies in pregnant mice have indicated that large doses of caffeine can produce skeletal abnormalities in the pups, studies on humans have not found a relationship between caffeine and birth defects. However, studies do strongly suggest that consumption of more than 300 milligrams of caffeine per day by a woman can reduce her chances of becoming pregnant, increase the chances of spontaneous abortion (miscarriage), and slow the growth of the fetus so that the baby weighs less than normal at birth.[30] The most controversial of these findings has been the reported increase in spontaneous abortion, which is found in some studies but not in others. The best advice for a woman who wants to become pregnant, stay pregnant, and produce a strong, healthy baby is to avoid caffeine, alcohol, tobacco, and any other drug that is not absolutely necessary for her health.

Heart Disease

There are many reasons for believing that caffeine might increase the risk of heart attacks, including the fact that it increases heart rate and blood pressure. Until recently, about as many studies found no relationship between caffeine use and heart attacks as found such a relationship. One interesting report used an unusual approach. Rather than asking people who had just had heart attacks about their prior caffeine consumption and comparing them with people who were hospitalized for another ailment (the typical retrospective study), this study began in 1948 to track male medical students enrolled in the Johns Hopkins Medical School.[68] More than 1000 of these students were followed for 20 years or more after graduation and were periodically asked about various habits, including drinking, smoking, and coffee consumption. Thus, this was a prospective study, to see which of these habits might predict future health problems. Those who drank five or more cups per day were about 2.5 times as likely as non-coffee drinkers to have coronary heart disease.

However, there is also some evidence that consuming small amounts of coffee can actually reduce the risk of heart attack. Therefore, as with alcohol, the relationship between coffee drinking and this important health risk is complex. A recent review indicated that the *diterpines* that are present in brewed coffee may increase blood cholesterol levels. A high intake of coffee (seven cups per day) has been shown to increase total and LDL cholesterol,[49] and this effect combined with the increase in blood pressure produced by caffeine can raise the risk of heart attack. However, coffee also contains antioxidants, which might account for the apparent protective effect of small amounts of regular coffee use.[69]

caffeinism: a condition caused by an excessive intake of caffeine; characteristics include insomnia, restlessness, excitement, tachycardia (fast heart rate), tremors, and diuresis (increased urination).

Table 11.4 Main Symptoms of Caffeine Overdose

Central	**Visual**
irritability	seeing flashes
anxiety	**Auditory**
restlessness	ringing ears
confusion	**Skin**
delirium	increased sensitivity
headache	**Cardiovascular**
insomnia	increased heart rate
Muscular	irregular heartbeat
seizures	**Gastric**
trembling	abdominal pain
twitching	nausea
overextension	vomiting (possibly with blood)
Respiratory	**Systemic**
rapid breathing	dehydration
Urinary	fever
frequent urination	

The latest research, then, says that one or two cups of coffee per day are probably okay, but four or five (or more!) definitely increases the risk of heart attack. This is of special concern to those with other risk factors (e.g., smoking, family history of heart disease, obesity, high blood pressure, and high cholesterol levels).

Caffeinism

Caffeine is not terribly toxic, and overdose deaths are extremely rare. An estimated 10 grams (equivalent to 100 cups of coffee) would be required to cause death from caffeine taken by mouth. Death is produced by convulsions, which lead to respiratory arrest.

However, **caffeinism** (a condition caused by an excessive intake of caffeine) can cause a variety of unpleasant symptoms (see Table 11.4), and because of caffeine's domesticated social status, it might be overlooked as the cause. For example, nervousness, irritability, tremulousness, muscle twitching, insomnia, flushed appearance, and elevated temperature can all result from excessive caffeine use. A person can also have palpitations, heart arrhythmias, and gastrointestinal disturbances. In several cases in which serious disease has been suspected, the symptoms have miraculously improved when coffee was restricted.

Summary

- Coffee use began in the fifteenth century in Arabic countries and spread into Europe in the seventeenth century. Tea was also prevalent in Europe at this time. Chocolate was introduced to Europe almost a century before coffee and tea.
- The coffee, tea, and cacao plants contain caffeine, theophylline, and theobromide, all of which are xanthines.
- Caffeine is removed from the coffee bean most commonly by soaking the unroasted beans in an organic solvent. The Swiss water process, which is not used on a large commercial scale in North America, involves soaking the beans in water and removing the caffeine through a carbon filtering system.
- Energy drinks, such as Red Bull, have as much as 80 milligrams of caffeine in each 245-millilitre (8.3-ounces) can. That is less than a cup of coffee, which can have up to 180 milligrams of caffeine, and most colas, which have up to 64 milligrams of caffeine.
- Caffeine exerts a stimulating action in several brain regions by blocking inhibitory receptors for adenosine.
- In regular caffeine users, headache, fatigue, or depression can develop if caffeine use is stopped.
- Caffeine is capable of reversing the effects of fatigue on both mental and physical tasks, but it might not be able to improve the performance of a well-rested individual, particularly on complex tasks.
- Heavy caffeine use during pregnancy is associated with such problems as low birth weight, caffeine withdrawal symptoms in newborns, and spontaneous abortion.
- Daily use of large amounts of caffeine increases the risk of heart attack.
- Excessive caffeine consumption, referred to as caffeinism, can produce a panic reaction.

Review Questions

1. Rank the caffeine content of a cup of brewed coffee, a cup of tea, a chocolate bar, and a 355-millilitre (12-ounce) serving of Coca-Cola.
2. What are the differences among black tea, green tea, and oolong?
3. What are the two xanthines contained in tea and chocolate, besides caffeine?
4. What are the typical symptoms associated with caffeine withdrawal?
5. How does caffeine interact with adenosine receptors?
6. What are some of the physiological and behavioural effects of excessive caffeine consumption?
7. Describe the effects of caffeine on migraine headaches, caffeine-withdrawal headaches, and other headaches.
8. What is the relationship between caffeine and panic attacks?
9. What are three possible ways in which caffeine use by a woman might interfere with reproduction?

CHAPTER 12

NATURAL HEALTH PRODUCTS AND OVER-THE-COUNTER DRUGS

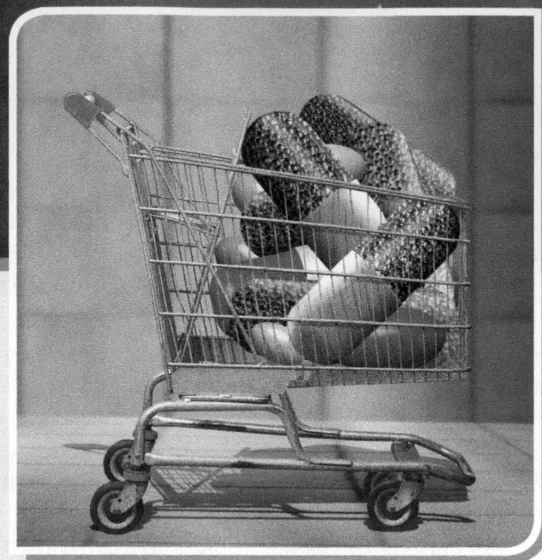

OBJECTIVES

When you have finished this chapter, you should be able to

- **LO1** Summarize the rationale behind the creation of the Natural Health Products Directorate.
- **LO2** List several natural health products with purported psychoactive effects.
- **LO3** Explain how improved labelling of over-the-counter drugs may lead to better safety and effectiveness.
- **LO4** Explain the rationale for the practice of keeping some over-the-counter drugs behind the counter.
- **LO5** Name the active ingredients permitted in licensed over-the-counter sleep aids.
- **LO6** Describe the benefits and dangers of Aspirin.
- **LO7** Name the three types of ingredients found in many over-the-counter cold and allergy drugs.
- **LO8** Describe the extent of dextromethorphan misuse by Canadian youth.

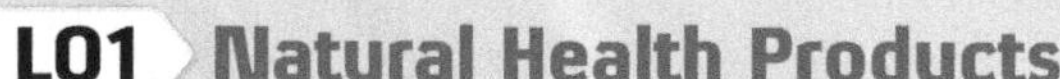

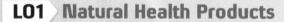

LO1 Natural Health Products

Health Canada is responsible for establishing standards for the safety and quality of all foods and drugs sold in this country. It exercises this mandate under the authority of the Food and Drugs Act (FDA) and pursues its regulatory mandate under the Food and Drug Regulations.[1] According to the FDA any substance "manufactured, sold or represented for use in the diagnosis, treatment, mitigation or prevention of a disease, disorder or abnormal physical state, or its symptoms, in human beings or animals" is a drug.[1] Foods are defined as any article manufactured, sold, or represented for use as food or drink for human beings.

In the 1990s, officials at Health Canada became concerned with the rapidly growing market in natural health products (NHPs). The term NHP is used to represent a variety of substances that are formulated, packaged, or promoted in a manner similar to drugs but that are classified and regulated as foods. These substances include vitamins and mineral supplements; herbal remedies (herb- and plant-based remedies); homeopathic medicines; traditional medicines, such as traditional Chinese and Ayurvedic medicines; probiotics; amino acids; and essential fatty acids. Growth in the public awareness of and demand for these products was fuelled by a number of factors, including (1) an increased interest in foods that can be used in prevention and as a treatment of illness, (2) a growing belief that NHPs are better than conventional (chemical) drugs, and (3) the emergence of aggressive multilevel marketing organizations that have become distributors of purported natural cures and preventions.

Health Canada's concerns lay in that fact that these natural products, while being promoted as therapeutic, were classified as foods. Recall from Chapter 3 that drug manufacturers have to demonstrate, before marketing a drug, that it is (1) *safe* when used as intended and (2) *effective* for its intended use. However, with foods, Health Canada is concerned only with ensuring their purity and safety, not their efficacy. As such, when NHPs were classified as foods, the manufacturers had to provide evidence that the product was pure and safe, but they were not required to provide proof of any health claims made. Furthermore, because these NHPs were not considered drugs, the manufacturers were exempt from providing information on potential contraindications, side effects, or toxicities associated with the use of their products.

To address these concerns the Government of Canada established a regulatory authority, the Natural Health Products Directorate (NHPD). Beginning in January 2004 all natural products with associated claims of health benefits became subject to the regulations of the NHPD. These regulations define NHPs as products manufactured, sold, or represented for use in (1) diagnosing, treating, mitigating, or preventing a disease, a disorder, or an abnormal physical state or its symptoms in humans; (2) restoring or correcting organic functions in humans; or (3) modifying organic functions in humans, such as modifying functions in a manner that maintains or promotes health. Through these regulations, NHPs must be as safe to use as over-the-counter (OTC) products (described below) and do not need a prescription to be sold. Perhaps most important is the requirement that health claims attributed to products must now be supported by evidence that confirms their safety and effectiveness. Evidence in support of health claims may include clinical trial data, references to published studies and pharmacopoeias, and traditional resources.

Often, no scientific evidence exists for an NHP. In these instances, traditional resources (evidence) may be used in support of an NHPD application (e.g., in the form of a traditional use claim). To constitute traditional use, an NHP must have a history of at least 50 consecutive years of use as a medicinal ingredient within a cultural belief system or healing paradigm (e.g., traditional Chinese medicine). This span was chosen because it represents two generations, thereby allowing possible reproductive side effects to be identified. Furthermore, when making a traditional use claim, the applicant must include references that support the recommended condition of use and that describe dose information and the method of preparation. For more information on what constitutes reputable references, visit Health Canada's Drug and Health Product Web site.

To be legally sold in Canada, NHPs must have a product licence and the Canadian sites that manufacture, package, label, and import these products must have site licences. To obtain a licence the manufacturer must submit to the NHPD detailed information on the product, including its active (medicinal) ingredients, source, potency, nonmedicinal ingredients, and recommended use. Furthermore, the manufacturer must meet labelling and packaging requirements and follow good manufacturing practices.

Once a product has been licensed, the manufacturer is granted market authorization by Health Canada. Licensed products will bear on their label an eight-digit product licence number preceded by the letters NPN (Natural Product Number) or, in the case of a homeopathic medicine, by the letters DIN-HM.

Today the NHPD provides Canadians with access to a wide range of NHPs that are purportedly safe, effective, and of high quality. This is especially important given that a recent national survey showed that 71% of Canadians regularly use NHPs, 38% of whom do so on a daily basis.[2] The most commonly used NHPs include vitamins (57%), *Echinacea* (15%), herbal remedies (11%), glucosamine (8%), and homeopathic medicine (5%).[2]

Despite attempts to protect Canadian consumers of NHPs, one recent study reminds us of the need for continued vigilance. In that study, conducted at the University of Guelph, researchers used DNA barcode technology to assess the quality and content of 44 commercially available herbal products from 12 companies. DNA barcoding, which uses a short sequence of DNA from a standard segment in plants, provides an accurate means to identify the authenticity and purity of purported species in herbal products. That study revealed "product substitutions" in 20/44 of the products tested. Furthermore, 10/12 companies had products with substitution, contamination, or fillers, some of which pose serious health risks to consumers.[3]

LO2 Some Natural Health Products Have Psychoactive Properties

Some common psychoactive NHPs include St. John's wort, S-adenosyl-L-methionine (SAMe), *ginkgo biloba*, caffeine, products for weight control, and sleep aids.

St. John's Wort

St. John's wort (botanical name *Hypericum perforatum*) has been used for centuries and was once known as "the devil's scourge" because it was supposed to prevent possession by demons. In recent years, its psychoactive uses have included the treatment of anxiety and depression. In Canada, St. John's wort is sold as an NHP and licensed for the recommended use "to relieve restlessness or nervousness and to help treat symptoms of sleep disorders." There is limited evidence

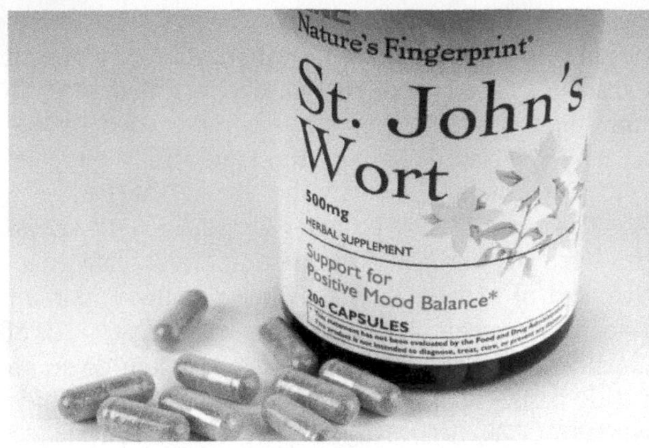

In Canada, the licensing of NHPs, such as St. John's wort, is regulated by the Natural Health Products Directorate. To obtain a licence, manufacturers must demonstrate their product's efficacy and safety.

on the effectiveness of St. John's wort in the treatment of anxiety, but several studies have indicated potential usefulness in treating depression. Available evidence, summarized in a recent systematic review of 29 clinical trials, suggests that hypericum extracts (1) are superior to placebo in patients with major depression, (2) are similarly effective as standard antidepressants, and (3) have fewer side effects than standard antidepressants.[4] Why do you think that the manufacturers of St. John's wort products do not claim "for relief of the symptoms of depression" as a recommended use? Health Canada has raised concerns about St. John's wort interacting with various prescription drugs (e.g., antiretroviral agents, oral contraceptives, digoxin, cyclosporine, warfarin, theophylline, and antiepilepsy drugs), so people using it should notify their physicians and pharmacists.[5]

SAMe

S-adenosyl-L-methionine is a naturally occurring substance found in the body. It is an active form of the amino acid methionine, and it acts as a "methyl donor" in a variety of biochemical pathways. (A methyl group consists of one carbon and three hydrogen atoms.) As long ago as the 1970s, SAMe was tested in Italy for its effectiveness as an antidepressant, and a recent summary analysis found that SAMe was more effective than a placebo and apparently no less effective than tricyclic antidepressants. In Canada, this NHP is licensed for the recommended use "to help support a healthy mood balance." Less research is available on SAMe for this use than for St. John's wort. Researchers continue to investigate the possibility that, by combining SAMe with prescription antidepressants, a more rapid remission of symptoms can be achieved.

Ginkgo Biloba

Extracts from the leaves of the *ginkgo biloba* tree have a long history of medical use in China. In Canada, *ginkgo* is regulated as an NHP and sold with the recommended uses "to improve memory and cognitive function. To enhance circulation. To help improve memory and cognitive function in adults." It is not clear which of the identified ingredients in *ginkgo* are the active agents, and it is not completely clear how effective it is for the variety of uses for which it has been proposed. The substance does reduce blood clotting, so it has been proposed as a blood thinner, which improves circulation. However, combining *ginkgo* with Aspirin, which also reduces clotting, could be dangerous. The most interesting suggestion is that *ginkgo biloba* extract might improve memory in people with Alzheimer's because of its presumed ability to increase blood circulation in the brain. Several studies have tested *ginkgo* in both normal and memory-impaired older adults. In a recent systematic review of 36 clinical trials, the authors concluded that *ginkgo biloba* appeared safe for use as a standalone drug. However, evidence supporting its predictable and clinically significant benefit for people with dementia or cognitive impairment was inconsistent and unreliable (most

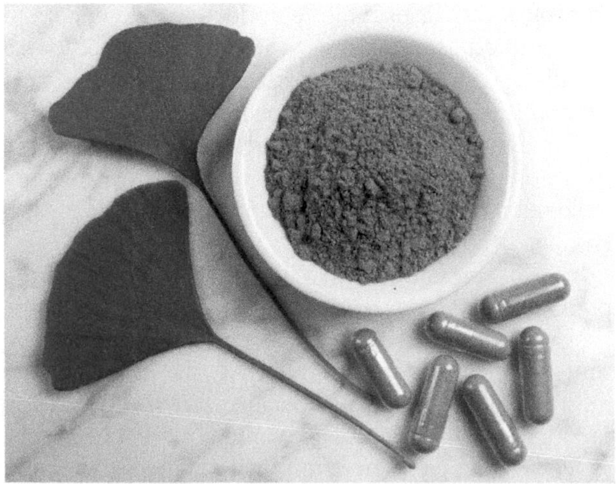

Evidence suggests that a compound in *ginkgo* acts as a blood thinner; it may be dangerous for people to take *ginkgo* supplements in combination with Aspirin or other drugs that also reduce clotting.

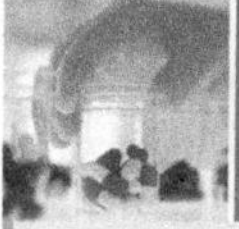

DRUGS IN THE MEDIA

Natural Male Enhancement?

Many Canadians purchase NHPs through U.S.-based Internet and mail-order sites. It is important to recognize that the U.S. Food and Drug Administration categorizes such products as dietary supplements and not as NHPs. This is an important distinction because under this category, they need to be pure and they need to be safe, but the manufacturer doesn't have to show to the Food and Drug Administration or to anyone else that they provide any benefit, either nutritionally or as a treatment for disease. Furthermore the amount of presumed active ingredient can vary according to the manufacturer's whims. In this environment the consumer needs to beware of products that are made to appear therapeutic but in fact are not.

Consider the following. In the United States, television ads for Enzyte or some other brands of "natural male enhancement" don't explain exactly what that means, but the not-so-subtle implication is that the guy who takes this is going to improve his sex life. Following on the success of prescription erectile-dysfunction drugs, such as Viagra and Cialis, the makers of these "male enhancement" pills are perhaps hoping that consumers will think that their products are nonprescription versions of the same thing. An unwary shopper might even confuse the term *enhancement* with *enlargement*. Enzyte's Web site[6] explains that the product will not alter the size or shape of the penis but that it contains a mixture of ingredients "designed to improve the quality of men's erections." Notice that it doesn't actually claim to be effective in doing so, only that it was designed to do that. The pills contain small amounts of several plant extracts, most notably *Tribulus terrestris, Panax ginseng,* and *ginkgo biloba*. Controlled clinical studies provide limited evidence that *ginseng* (widely available in many products) might be helpful in treating men with erectile dysfunction, though it is not clear what value this would have for men with otherwise normal penile function. The clinical results for *ginkgo* have been mixed, but the only controlled study showed no effect. Controlled clinical studies have not been done with *Tribulus terrestris,* which proponents claim will enhance the production of the steroid DHEA, a form of andosterone.[7] They've also added a small amount of *avena sativa* extract. This is the common oat plant from which oatmeal is made. The extract has been promoted as an aphrodisiac in several products but without scientific evidence. Finally, there is some *epimedium sagittatum,* called "horny goat weed." This has been used to enhance male sexual energy in traditional Chinese herbal medicine. It appears to dilate blood vessels, possibly lowering blood pressure. This is another plant derivative that is included in several products sold on the Internet as aphrodisiacs or treatments for erectile dysfunction. These Web sites include glowing anecdotal reports, but again no solid science backs up the effectiveness of this ingredient. In other words, the existing evidence would be far from enough to allow the U.S. Food and Drug Administration to approve Enzyte as a drug to treat any type of sexual dysfunction.

This is just one example of the kinds of products sold as *dietary supplements* in the United States. Again, these tablets and capsules are treated in the United States as foods, not drugs, and as such there is no requirement that the manufacturer demonstrate the effectiveness of the products. The label for Enzyte includes the standard disclaimer that "these statements have not been evaluated by the Food and Drug Administration." If you have questions about perceived claims made by a manufacturer, Health Canada's Licensed Natural Health Products Database[8] is an excellent source of information.

trials used unsatisfactory methods and were small).[9] Finally, it is interesting to note that studies using animal and cell culture models of stroke have recently demonstrated the ability of *ginkgo* extracts to protect neurons against oxidative stress.[10]

Caffeine

For many years caffeine was licensed and sold as an OTC drug (described below). It was labelled with the intended use "to temporarily restore mental alertness or wakefulness when experiencing fatigue or drowsiness." With the creation of the Natural Health Products Directorate in 2004, caffeine-based cerebral stimulants were transitioned from OTCs to NHPs. A number of cerebral stimulant NHPs are licensed for sale in Canada, including such brands as Wake-Ups, Full Throttle Blue Demon, and Peptime Energy Xtreme T. All these products contain between 100 and 200 milligrams of caffeine per dose. Although the packages look different and different companies make them, a smart consumer would choose among these products based on the price per milligram of caffeine–or buy a medium coffee (which contains 80 milligrams of caffeine), or get enough rest and save money. You can compare the amount of caffeine found in the various NHPs brands by visiting Canada's Licensed Natural Health Products Database.

A number of Canadian OTC products contain caffeine in doses similar to those in the cerebral stimulant NHPs. One example is Tylenol Ultra Relief, which contains 65 milligrams caffeine per capsule. The difference is that these products are not intended to be used as stimulants. Caffeine is there as an adjunct, enhancing the response to the active analgesic ingredient *acetaminophen.* To use Tylenol to temporarily restore mental alertness or wakefulness is inappropriate as it requires the unnecessary co-consumption of acetaminophen, which has been linked to liver disease (described below). See Chapter 11 for an in-depth discussion about caffeine.

Weight-Control Products

In Canada, no NHPs or OTCs are currently licensed for sale as weight-control products. Before 2001 products containing **phenylpropanolamine (PPA)**, a psychoactive drug of the amphetamine chemical class, were available and considered safe and effective anorexic agents. One popular appetite suppressant product, Ayds, enjoyed strong sales in Canada during the 1970s and 1980s. Ayds was sold in candy form, available in chocolate, chocolate mint, butterscotch, and caramel flavours. The active ingredient in this product was PPA.[11] As early as the 1980s, people began expressing concern about the safety of products containing PPA.[11] At the recommended dose for weight loss (75 milligrams), PPA had been shown to increase blood pressure. Subsequent reports that the product could lead to an increased risk of hemorrhagic stroke (bleeding into the brain, usually a result of elevated blood pressure) in women prompted Health Canada to issue a Public Health Advisory on the safety of PPA.[12] In May 2001, Health Canada requested that all drug companies discontinue marketing products containing PPA and that consumers not use any products containing it. Manufacturers and retailers responded quickly, and by late 2001 no products contained PPA.

One product historically misused in the quest of weight loss is ephedra (known in Chinese as *ma huang*). For a number of years, many Canadians used a combination of ephedra and caffeine to lose weight. Ephedra and caffeine were authorized for sale OTC in Canada as separate products, but they were not authorized to be sold or taken in combination. To get around this regulation, manufacturers, such as 4Ever Fit, sold ephedra and caffeine pills packaged in separate bottles but sold together in a convenience pack. The active ingredients of ephedra are the alkaloids ephedrine and pseudoephedrine. A number of studies have suggested that ephedra promotes modest, short-term weight loss, although there is no evidence that it is effective for long-term weight loss.[13] In January 2002, Health Canada issued a voluntary recall of all ephedra products containing more than 8 milligrams of ephedrine per dose; all combinations of ephedra with other stimulants, such as caffeine; and all ephedrine products marketed for weight-loss or bodybuilding indications, citing a serious risk to health.[14] This action was in response to emerging studies linking ephedra use to incidences of sudden cardiac death.[15] 4Ever Fit convenience packs were subsequently recalled from retail stores by the Canadian distributor.

With the creation of the NHPD, ephedra, like caffeine, was transitioned from OTC to NHP status. Today NHPs containing only ephedra (8 milligrams of ephedrine per dose) are licensed for sale, and the recommended use is "to relieve nasal congestion due to cold or hayfever."

In 2007, the U.S. Food and Drug Administration approved the OTC status of the drug Orlistat, which had been a prescription-only medicine called Xenical. Orlistat became the first weight-loss drug officially sanctioned by the U.S. government for OTC use. Orlistat's intended use is as an "anti-obesity agent" that works in the intestine, inhibiting an enzyme that breaks down dietary fats. Therefore, some of the fat that could have been absorbed is instead retained in the intestine and passed out in the feces. When given in conjunction with a restricted diet, Orlistat has been shown to help people lose some weight, but once the drug is stopped there is a tendency to gain back some of the lost weight. The major problem with using this drug is that the fats and oils that remain in the bowel can lead to loose, oily stools; frequent, urgent bowel movements that sometimes are hard to control; and flatulence. In Canada, Orlistat (sold as Xenical) is available only by prescription.

In recent years regulating authorities have reviewed and ruled against several other products that have been

phenylpropanolamine (PPA): until 2002, an active ingredient in OTC weight-control products in Canada and the United States.

proposed for weight control. None of these products has been demonstrated to be effective in weight loss, despite claims of "burning fat," causing "natural" weight loss, using an "Asian weight-loss secret," and so on.

Sleep Aids

While a number of OTC products for the management of insomnia exist, many Canadians prefer to use NHPs. Perhaps the best-known NHP sleep aid is melatonin, a hormone, which is licensed for the recommended use of "increasing the total sleep time (aspect of sleep quality) in people suffering from sleep restriction or altered sleep schedule, e.g. shift-work and jet lag." In humans, melatonin is an endogenous hormone produced by the pineal gland. Numerous studies have demonstrated its physiological role in the promotion and maintenance of sleep. For example, the circadian rhythm of endogenous melatonin release has been shown to be synchronized with the habitual hours of sleep. Furthermore, the daily onset of melatonin secretion is correlated with the onset of nocturnal sleepiness.[16] A recent meta-analysis of 19 studies concluded that exogenous melatonin treatment significantly decreased sleep onset latency, improved overall sleep quality, and increased total sleep time.[17] Numerous other NHPs, including valerian root, chamomile, and inhaled lavender essential oil, have been purported efficacious in the treatment of insomnia. Systematic reviews and meta-analysis of the current research literature have produced conflicting conclusions pertaining to the efficacy of these substances in treating insomnia. As such, evidence of their efficacy is weak and unsupportive. Larger scale studies with stronger methods and endpoints are warranted.[18,19,20]

LO3 Over-the-Counter Drugs

OTC drugs (also called nonprescription drugs) are medicines that may be sold directly to a consumer without a prescription from a health care professional. In other words, this category represents those drugs that are self-prescribed and self-administered for the relief of symptoms of self-diagnosed illnesses. A recent survey has indicated that self-treatment with OTC and NHPs is extremely common in Canada.[2,21] OTC drugs are regulated by Health Canada, through the FDA, ensuring that their ingredients are safe and effective when used without a physician's or pharmacist's input. The decision about whether a drug meets the criteria for an OTC drug is typically determined by evaluation of its active pharmaceutical ingredients (APIs), not the final products. By regulating APIs instead of specific drug formulations, Health Canada allows manufacturers freedom to formulate ingredients, or combinations of ingredients, into proprietary mixtures.

Canadians spend more than $3 billion a year on OTC products.[22] That's not as much as we spend on prescription drugs, alcohol, or cigarettes, but it's enough to keep several OTC drug manufacturers locked in fierce competition for those sales. The two biggest markets are for Aspirin-like analgesics and for cough, cold, and flu products. A quick trip to the drug store will reveal the multitude of brands.

Do we really need all these nonprescription tablets, capsules, liquids, and creams? The exact number of OTC products on the market is not known because they still come and go and change, but we do know that there are more than 100 000, and they contain fewer than 1000 total active ingredients.

How much of what we buy is based on advertising hype, and how much is based on sound decisions about our health? How are we as consumers to know the difference? We can figure this out in a few ways. (1) We can visit a neighbourhood drugstore and look at the lists of ingredients on a variety of medications for the same intended use (cough syrup, for example). You may be surprised to discover that all the competing brands contain much the same type and quantity of active ingredients. In some classes, there might be only one active ingredient, meaning that all competing brands are essentially identical. In reality, the differences among them often are in the long lists of other (inactive) ingredients (colourings, flavourings, etc.). (2) We can visit Health Canada's online Drug Product Database, which provides detailed descriptions of every OTC and prescription drug sold in Canada. You can compare the types and doses of active and inactive ingredients across all brands. Taking the time to appreciate the differences and similarities across OTC brands will help you make a good financial choice when purchasing such products.

Regulation of Over-the-Counter Products

Before a prescription or an OTC drug can be sold in Canada, the manufacturer must seek a Notice of Compliance (NOC) from Health Canada. As discussed in Chapter 3, Health Canada requires that all prescription and OTC drugs be evaluated for both safety and effectiveness.

Effectiveness means a reasonable expectation that in a significant proportion of the target population, the pharmacological effect of the drug, when used

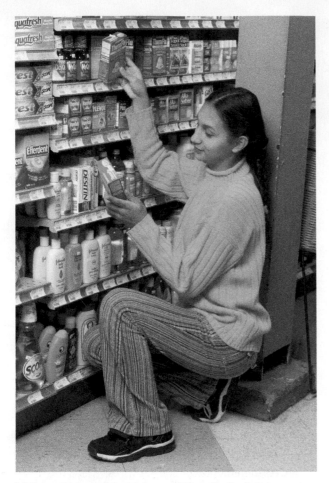

It is important to read the label on an OTC medication before purchasing.

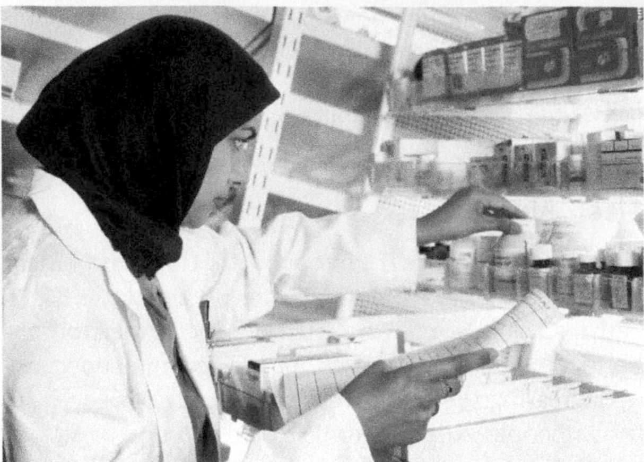
Should some over-the-counter drugs be kept behind the counter, where they can be dispensed only after a pharmacist has advised the consumer about safe use?

under adequate directions for use and warnings against unsafe use, will provide clinically significant relief of the type claimed.

Improved Labelling of Over-the-Counter Drugs

Both the safety and the effectiveness of OTC drugs depend greatly on consumers using them according to the directions and warnings on the label. To reduce confusion and make it more likely that consumers will be able to understand the labels, Health Canada has established uniform standards for labels, with minimum print size, required topics (active or medicinal ingredients, directions for use, etc.), and bold, bulleted headings indicating precautions and warnings. Language must be clear and concise, avoiding medical terminology (e.g., *pulmonary* replaced by *lung*). This approach to labelling has made it easier to compare products and their ingredients.

One area in need of development is the listing of nonmedicinal ingredients (NMIs) on the labels of OTC drugs. As part of the licensing process, manufacturers of drugs and NHPs must make evident to Health Canada all ingredients (medicinal and nonmedicinal) included in a drug. While the manufacturers of NHPs are required to list NMIs on their packaging labels, the manufacturers of drugs are not. This is of concern because many of the NMIs present in drugs can cause adverse reactions in individuals with sensitivities or allergies. This is not as great an issue with prescription drugs because with these products the physician and pharmacist, who have ready access to lists of NMIs in drugs, can counsel the consumer on potential risks. In a nonprescription environment, however, where consumers often self-select a drug product without the counsel of a physician or pharmacist, it is difficult for them to avoid consuming certain NMIs. The Government of Canada is working on an amendment to Canada's Food and Drug Regulations to require the identification of NMIs on the labels of OTC drugs for human use.[23] This is particularly timely given the growing list of drugs that are being shifted from prescription-only to OTC status in Canada (described below).

LO4 Over-the-Counter versus Prescription Drugs

In Canada, regulations pertaining to the prescribing, distribution, selling, and dispensing of drugs derive from the FDA and the Controlled Drugs and Substances Act (CDSA) (described in Chapter 3). Drugs approved for

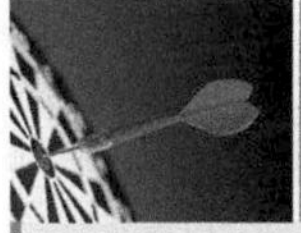

TARGETING PREVENTION

The Medicine Cabinet

The family medicine cabinet is often a treasure trove of old tablets, capsules, liquids, and lozenges. Start digging around and see how many different OTC drugs you can find in yours. How old do you think some of them are? If any of them have expiration dates, have the dates passed?

Because formulations change from year to year, there's a good chance the medicines you now have are not the same as the ones being sold in the drugstore. Write down the formulations for a few of your medicine cabinet drugs. Then go online to Health Canada's Drug Product Database[24] and compare them with the current formulation for the same brand of product. Do you wonder if some of the old ingredients were removed because Health Canada no longer considers them safe?

use are classified according to Canada's National Drug Scheduling System, which is maintained by the National Association of Pharmacy Regulatory Authorities (NAPRA). In this scheduling system, drugs are assigned to one of three categories called NAPRA Schedules. The schedule in which a drug is placed is determined by that drug's pharmacological and toxicological profile. The NAPRA Schedules include the following:

- Schedule I: Drugs that can be sold only with a prescription
- Schedule II: Drugs that can be sold without a prescription but must be kept behind the counter (described below)
- Schedule III: Drugs that can be sold without a prescription (OTC) and can be displayed in the pharmacy

Basically, a drug should be permitted for OTC sale unless because of potential toxicity or for other reasons (e.g., if it must be injected) it can be safely sold and used only under a prescription.

Sometimes the only difference between an OTC product and a prescription product is the greater amount of active ingredient in each dose. For example, Tylenol #1, which contains 8 milligrams of codeine, is a NAPRA Schedule II drug in Canada. However, Tylenol #3, which contains 30 milligrams of codeine, is a NAPRA Schedule I drug. More often, however, prescription drugs are chemicals that are unavailable OTC. In recent years there has been a push to deregulate many prescription drugs to OTC status. This movement has been driven by a number of forces, including (1) a growth in modern notions of individual responsibility and self-care, (2) pharmaceutical companies seeking increased sales, and (3) growing challenges in maintaining public and private prescription drug plans.[25]

antihistamine: the active ingredient in OTC sleep aids and cough and cold products.

Behind-the-Counter Nonprescription Drugs

In Canada, NAPRA Schedule II drugs can be sold without a prescription but must be kept behind the counter. Some examples of Schedule II drugs include EpiPens, Polysporin eye drops or eardrops, the strongest lice shampoos, and Tylenol #1. Schedule II drugs are kept behind the counter because although they are safe and effective when used as recommended, adverse events can occur. Controlling their dispension gives the pharmacist an opportunity to counsel patients about the drugs' proper use and precautions. Pharmacists are reimbursed for their time through dispensing fees that are established by the provinces and territories.

LO5 Sleep Aids

In the past, pharmacy shelves contained a number of OTC sedative or "calmative" preparations, like Compoz, which contained very small amounts of the acetylcholine receptor blocker *scopolamine* combined with the **antihistamine** methapyrilene. At the same time, sleep aids, such as Sleep-Eze and Sominex, contained just a bit more of the same two ingredients. The rationale for the scopolamine, particularly at these low doses, was under U.S. Food and Drug Administration investigation, but scopolamine had traditionally been included in many such medications in the past. Some antihistamines do produce a kind of sedated state and might produce drowsiness. Eventually methapyrilene was accepted as a sleep aid but scopolamine was rejected. For a while all these medications contained only methapyrilene. Then, in 1979 it was reported that methapyrilene caused cancer in laboratory animals, so it was no longer generally recognized as safe. Next came pyrilamine maleate, then doxylamine succinate, and then diphenhydramine–all antihistamines. If you bought the same brand from one year to the next, you would get a different formulation each time. But if you bought several different brands at the same time, you stood a good chance of getting the same formulation in all of them. Today in Canada, OTC sleep aids come in a variety of forms (tablet, capsule, caplet, powder, or elixir) that are recommended for the relief of occasional sleeplessness by persons who have difficulty falling asleep. The medicinal ingredients approved for OTC sleep aids include diphenhydramine hydrochloride (25 or 50 milligrams per dosage form) and diphenhydramine citrate (38 or 76 milligrams per dosage form). Diphenhydramine's sedating effects derive from the drug's ability to block the effects of histamine at H_1 receptor sites in the CNS. Some common OTC sleep aid brands include Nytol and Sleep-Eze D.

As we saw in Chapter 7, insomnia is perceived to be a bigger problem than it actually is for most people, and it is rare that medication is really required. Antihistamines can induce drowsiness, but not very quickly. If you do feel the need to use these to get you to sleep more rapidly, take them at least 20 minutes before retiring. Their sedative effects are potentiated by alcohol, so it is not a good idea to take them after drinking.

LO6 Analgesics

Pain is such a little word for such a big experience. Most people have experienced pain of varying intensities, from mild to moderate to severe to excruciating. Two major classes of drugs are used to reduce pain or the awareness of pain: anaesthetics and analgesics.

People and Pain

Anaesthetics (meaning "without sensibility") have this effect by reducing all types of sensation or by blocking consciousness completely. The local anaesthetics used in dentistry and the general anaesthetics used in major surgery are examples of this class of agent. The other major class, the analgesics (meaning "without pain"), are compounds that reduce pain selectively without causing a loss of other sensations. The analgesics are divided into two groups. Opioids (see Chapter 13) are one group of analgesics, but this chapter primarily discusses the OTC internal analgesics, such as Aspirin, acetaminophen, and ibuprofen.

Although pain itself is a complex psychological phenomenon, there have been attempts to classify different types of pain to develop a rational approach to its treatment. One classification divides pain into two types, depending on its place of origin. Visceral pain, such as intestinal cramps, arises from nonskeletal portions of the body; opioids are effective in reducing pain of this type. Somatic pain, arising from muscle or bone and typified by sprains, headaches, and arthritis, is reduced by salicylates (Aspirin) and related products.

Pain is unlike other sensations in many ways, mostly because of nonspecific factors. The experience of pain varies with personality, gender, and time of day and is increased with fatigue, anxiety, fear, boredom, and anticipation of more pain. Because pain is very susceptible to nonspecific factors, studies have shown that about 35% of people will receive satisfactory pain relief from a placebo.

Aspirin

More than 2400 years ago, the Greeks used extracts of willow and poplar bark in the treatment of pain, gout, and other illnesses. Aristotle commented on some of the clinical effects of similar preparations, and Galen made good use of these formulations. These remedies fell into disrepute, however, when St. Augustine declared that all diseases of Christians were the work of demons and thus a punishment from God. Aboriginal peoples, unhampered by this enlightened attitude, used a tea brewed from willow bark to reduce fever. This remedy was not rediscovered in Europe until about 200 years ago, when an Englishman, Reverend Edward Stone, prepared an extract of the bark and gave the same dose to 50 patients with varying illnesses and found the results to be "uniformly excellent." In the nineteenth century, the active ingredient in these preparations was isolated and identified as salicylic acid. In 1838, salicylic acid was synthesized, and in 1859 procedures were developed that made bulk production feasible. Salicylic acid and sodium salicylate were then used for many ills, especially arthritis.

In the giant Bayer Laboratories in Germany in the 1890s worked a chemist named Hoffmann. His father had a severe case of rheumatoid arthritis, and only salicylic acid seemed to help. The major difficulty then, as today, was that the drug caused great gastric discomfort. So great was the stomach upset and nausea that

Hoffmann's father frequently preferred the pain of the arthritis. Hoffmann studied the salicylates to see if he could find one with the same therapeutic effect as salicylic acid but without the side effects.

In 1898, he synthesized **acetylsalicylic acid** and tried it on his father, who reported relief from pain without stomach upset. The compound was tested, patented, and released for sale in 1899 as *Aspirin*. Aspirin is a trademark name derived from the name *acetyl* and *spiralic acid* (the old name for salicylic acid).

The two famous compounds that the Bayer Laboratories in Germany were instrumental in introducing to the world are rapidly transformed in the body to their original form after absorption. Both heroin and Aspirin were first synthesized in the Bayer Laboratories. Aspirin, either in the gastrointestinal tract or in the bloodstream, is converted to salicylic acid. Taken orally, Aspirin is a more potent analgesic than salicylic acid, because Aspirin irritates the stomach less and is thus absorbed more rapidly.

Aspirin was marketed for physicians and sold as a white powder in individual dosage packets, available only by prescription. It was immediately popular and the market became large enough that it was very soon being manufactured worldwide. In 1915, the 5-grain (325-milligram) white tablet stamped "Bayer" first appeared, and, for the first time, Aspirin became a nonprescription item. The Bayer Company was on its way. It had an effective drug that could be sold to the public and was known by one name—Aspirin—and the name was trademarked. Before February 1917, when the U.S. patent on Aspirin was to expire, Bayer started an advertising campaign to make it clear that there was only one Aspirin, and its first name was Bayer. Several companies started manufacturing and selling Aspirin as Aspirin, and Bayer sued. What happened after this is a long story, but Bayer lost its battle in the United States and Aspirin became a generic name there and in several other countries; however, it is still a trademark name in 80 other countries, including Canada.[26]

Therapeutic Use Aspirin is truly a magnificent drug. It is also a drug with some serious side effects. Aspirin has three effects that are the primary basis for its clinical use. It is an analgesic that effectively blocks somatic pain in the mild-to-moderate range. Aspirin is also **antipyretic**: it reduces fever. Last but not least, Aspirin is an **anti-inflammatory** agent: It reduces the swelling, inflammation, and soreness in an injured area. Its anti-inflammatory action is the basis for its extensive use in arthritis. It is difficult to find another drug that has this span of effects coupled with a relatively low toxicity. It does, however, have side effects that pose problems for some people.

Aspirin is absorbed readily from the stomach but even faster from the intestine. Thus, anything that delays movement of the Aspirin from the stomach should affect absorption time. The evidence is mixed on whether taking Aspirin with a meal, which delays emptying of the stomach, increases the time before onset of action. It should, however, reduce the stomach irritation that sometimes accompanies Aspirin use.

The *therapeutic* dose for Aspirin is generally considered to be in the range of 600–1000 milligrams. Most reports suggest that 300 milligrams is usually more effective than a placebo, whereas 600 milligrams is clearly even more effective. Many studies indicate that increasing the dose above that level does not increase Aspirin's analgesic action, but some research indicates that 1200 milligrams of Aspirin provides greater relief than 600 milligrams. The maximum pain relief is experienced about one hour after taking Aspirin, and the effect lasts for up to four hours.

At therapeutic doses, Aspirin has analgesic actions that are fairly specific. First, and in marked contrast to narcotic analgesics, Aspirin does not affect the impact of the anticipation of pain. It seems probable also that Aspirin has its primary effect on the ability to withstand continuing pain. This, no doubt, is the basis for much of the self-medication with Aspirin, because moderate, protracted pain is fairly common. Aspirin is especially effective against headache and musculoskeletal aches and pains, less effective for toothache and sore throat, and only slightly better than placebo in visceral pain, as well as in traumatic (acute) pain.

The antipyretic (fever-reducing) action of Aspirin does not lower temperature in an individual with normal body temperature. It has this effect only if the person has a fever. The mechanism by which Aspirin decreases body temperature is fairly well understood. It acts on the temperature-regulating area of the hypothalamus to increase heat loss through peripheral mechanisms. Heat loss is primarily increased by vasodilation of peripheral blood vessels and by increased perspiration. Heat production is not changed, but heat loss is facilitated so that body temperature can go down.

acetylsalicylic acid: the chemical known as Aspirin.

antipyretic: fever reducing.

anti-inflammatory: reducing swelling and inflammation.

More Aspirin has probably been used for its third major therapeutic use than for either of the other two. The anti-inflammatory action of the salicylates is the major basis for its use after muscle strains and in rheumatoid arthritis.

Most tablets, including Aspirin, develop a harder external shell the longer they sit. This hardening effect does not change the amount of the active ingredient, but it does make the active ingredient less effective because disintegration time is increased by the hard exterior coating. Along the same line, moisture and heat speed the decomposition of acetylsalicylic acid into two other compounds: salicylic acid, which causes gastric distress, and acetic acid–vinegar. When the smell of vinegar is strong in your Aspirin bottle, discard it.

Effects: Adverse and Otherwise *Aspirin increases bleeding time by inhibiting blood platelet aggregation.* This is not an insignificant effect. Two or three Aspirin tablets can double bleeding time, the time it takes for blood to clot, and the effect can last four to seven days. There's good and bad in the anticoagulant effect of Aspirin. Its use before surgery can help prevent blood clots from appearing in patients at high risk for clot formation. For many surgical patients, however, facilitation of blood clotting is desirable, and the general rule is no Aspirin for seven to ten days before surgery.

Aspirin will induce gastrointestinal bleeding in about 70% of normal subjects. In most cases, this is only about 5 millilitres per day, but that is five times the normal loss. In some people the blood loss can be great enough to cause anemia. The basis for this effect is not clear but is believed to be a direct eroding by the Aspirin tablets of the gastric mucosa. Aspirin can be deadly with severe stomach ulcers. For the rest of us, the rule is clear: Drink lots of water when you take Aspirin or, better yet, crush the tablets and drink them in orange juice or other liquid.

The anticoagulant effect of Aspirin has a potentially beneficial effect in preventing heart attacks and strokes. Either can be brought on by a blood clot becoming lodged in a narrowed or hardened blood vessel. Several studies have demonstrated that patients who are at high risk for these problems can help to prevent both strokes and heart attacks by taking a small dose of Aspirin daily. Many doctors are recommending that all their patients over a certain age begin taking low-dose Aspirin (81 milligrams is typical) regularly, even though the available research doesn't provide clear evidence for any benefit for low-risk patients.[27]

In the early 1980s, concern increased about the relationship of Aspirin use to *Reye's syndrome*, a rare disease (fewer than 20 cases per year in Canada). Almost all of the cases occur in people under the age of 20, usually after they have had a viral infection, such as influenza or chicken pox. The children begin vomiting continually; then they might become disoriented, undergo personality changes, shout, or become lethargic. Some enter comas, and some of those either die or suffer permanent brain damage. The overall mortality rate from Reye's syndrome is about 25%.

No one knows what causes Reye's, and it isn't believed to be caused by Aspirin. However, data suggest the disease is more likely to occur in children who have been given Aspirin during a preceding illness. In late 1984, the results of a U.S. Centers for Disease Control and Prevention pilot study were released, indicating that the use of Aspirin can increase the risk of Reye's syndrome as much as 25 times. In 1985, makers of all Aspirin products were asked to put warning labels on their packages. These labels recommend that you consult a physician before giving Aspirin to children or teenagers with chicken pox or flu.

In early 1986, it was reported that fewer parents in Michigan were giving Aspirin to children for colds and influenza, and the incidence of Reye's syndrome had also decreased in Michigan. The Michigan study lends further strength to the relationship between Aspirin use and Reye's syndrome. No one under the age of 20 should use Aspirin in treating chicken pox, influenza, or even what might be suspected to be a common cold.

Mechanism of Action Aspirin is now believed to have both a central and a peripheral analgesic effect. The central effect is not clear, but the peripheral effect is well on its way to being understood; it is now known that Aspirin modifies the *cause* of pain.

Prostaglandins are local hormones that are manufactured and released when cell membranes are distorted or damaged–that is, injured. The prostaglandins then act on the endings of the neurons that mediate pain in the injured areas. The prostaglandins sensitize the neurons to mechanical stimulation and to stimulation by two other local hormones, histamine and bradykinin, which are more slowly released from the damaged tissue. Aspirin blocks the synthesis of the prostaglandins by inhibiting two forms of the cyclooxygenase enzyme (COX-1 and COX-2).

The antipyretic action has also been spelled out: A specific prostaglandin acts on the anterior hypothalamus to decrease heat dissipation through the normal procedures of sweating and dilation of peripheral blood vessels. Aspirin blocks the synthesis of this prostaglandin in the anterior hypothalamus, and this is followed by increased heat loss.

Acetaminophen

There are two related analgesic compounds: *phenacetin* and **acetaminophen**. Phenacetin was sold for many years in combination with Aspirin and caffeine in the "APC" tablets that fought headache pain "three ways." Phenacetin has been around since 1887 and had long been suspected of causing kidney lesions and dysfunction.[28,29] In 1964, the Food and Drug Directorate of the Department of National Health and Welfare Canada (the predecessor to Health Canada) issued a warning for products containing phenacetin that limited their use to ten days because the phenacetin might damage the kidneys. Phenacetin was withdrawn from the Canadian market in June 1973.

The only real question is why all these drugs took so long to get off the market. Phenacetin was known to be rapidly converted to acetaminophen, which was the primary active agent. Acetaminophen is equipotent with Aspirin in its analgesic and antipyretic effects. Acetaminophen causes less gastric bleeding than Aspirin, but it is also less useful as an anti-inflammatory drug for arthritis.

acetaminophen: an Aspirin-like analgesic and antipyretic.

Acetaminophen has been marketed as an OTC analgesic since 1961, but it was the big advertising pushes in the 1970s for two brand-name products, Tylenol and Datril, that brought acetaminophen into the big time. Acetaminophen was advertised as having most of the good points of "that other pain reliever" and many fewer disadvantages. To a degree this is probably true: If only analgesia and fever reduction are desired, acetaminophen might be safer than Aspirin *as long as dosage limits are carefully observed.* Overuse of acetaminophen can cause serious liver disorders. Analysis of data collected by the Canadian Institute for Health Information (described in Chapter 2) has identified acetaminophen as the leading cause of overdose and acute liver failure in Canada.[30] In response to these findings Health Canada updated its labelling requirements for acetaminophen, requiring inclusion of the statements "taking more than the maximum daily dose may cause severe or possibly fatal liver damage" and "in case of overdose call a poison control centre or doctor immediately, even if you do not notice any signs or symptoms." This second statement reflects the fact

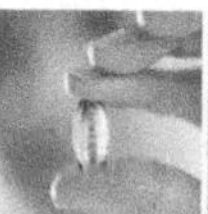

DRUGS IN DEPTH

The Vioxx Controversy

In 2004, the NSAID drug Vioxx, widely used as an anti-inflammatory drug by people with arthritis, was withdrawn from the worldwide market by its manufacturer Merck & Co. because the drug increased risk of heart attacks. As a selective COX-2 inhibitor, Vioxx produced only half as many gastric ulcers as the nonspecific inhibitors, such as Aspirin. COX-2 is not involved in regulating blood platelets, so gastrointestinal bleeding is much less than when COX-1 is also inhibited. Early studies indicated a somewhat higher rate of heart attacks in patients on Vioxx compared with nonselective COX inhibitors, but at first this was interpreted to mean that the nonselective inhibitors were protecting against clotting and therefore heart attacks, and Vioxx was simply not providing this preventive effect. But eventually it became clear that Vioxx actually increased the risk relative to placebo, and the drug was discontinued.

In 2002, Health Canada had issued an advisory about the increased risk of cardiovascular events related to the use of Vioxx. Their advisory was prompted by the results of a study entitled *VIGOR: Vioxx Gastrointestinal Outcomes Research.*[31,32] This advisory was followed by labelling changes to reflect the findings, specifically the inclusion of information that Vioxx should be used with caution in patients with a history of heart disease. The fact that it was the drug manufacturer and not Health Canada that initiated the withdrawal of Vioxx from the market has led to controversy about whether Health Canada had done its job, particularly enforcing the need for postmarketing studies and the reporting of adverse side effects. Health Canada is likely to make some organizational changes to strengthen its postmarketing research on newly introduced drugs.[33]

Table 12.1 Ingredients in OTC Analgesics (mg)

Brand	ASA	Acetaminophen	Ibuprofen	Naproxen	Caffeine	Other
Aleve	–	–	–	220	–	–
Anacin	325	–	–	–	32	–
Advil	–	–	200	–	–	pseudoephedrine hydrochloride (30 mg)
Bufferin	325	–	–	–	–	magnesium carbonate, calcium carbonate, magnesium oxide
Excedrin		500	–	–	65	–
Aspirin	325					
222	375				30	codeine (8 mg)
Tylenol #1		300			15	codeine (8 mg)

Source: Health Canada. *Drug Product Database Online Query*. 2011. Retrieved October 1, 2011, from http://webprod3.hc-sc.gc.ca/dpd-bdpp/index-eng.jsp.

that damage to the liver might not be noticed until 24 to 48 hours later, when the symptoms of impaired liver function finally emerge. You should remember that acetaminophen is not necessarily safer than Aspirin, especially if the recommended dose is exceeded.

Ibuprofen and Other NSAIDs

Since the discovery that Aspirin and similar drugs work by inhibiting the two COX enzymes, the drug companies have used that information to design new and sometimes more potent analgesics, which were introduced as prescription products. **Ibuprofen**, which originally was available only by prescription, is now found in more than 70 OTC analgesics products. In addition to its analgesic potency, ibuprofen is a potent anti-inflammatory and has received wide use in the treatment of arthritis. The most common side effects of ibuprofen are gastrointestinal: nausea, stomach pain, and cramping. There have been reports of fatal liver damage with overdoses of ibuprofen, so again it is wise not to exceed the recommended dose.

Ibuprofen was the first of several new drugs that are now collectively referred to as nonsteroidal anti-inflammatory drugs (**NSAIDs**). Naproxen is also available OTC under the brand name Aleve.

One product that luckily did not make the switch to OTC was vofecoxib (Vioxx), which as described in the Drugs in Depth box was pulled from the market in 2004.

Table 12.1 lists several OTC analgesics along with the amounts of each ingredient they contain. Health Canada has been discussing whether to exclude products that contain both Aspirin and acetaminophen. Products containing ibuprofen warn against combining them with Aspirin, because that mixture hasn't been thoroughly studied.

Products Containing Codeine

A number of OTC analgesic products in Canada contain the narcotic codeine (8 milligrams or less per tablet). Codeine is a weak pain reliever. When consumed it is converted by the body into morphine, which relieves pain.

Codeine preparations can be sold only at a pharmacy and are dispensed from behind the counter. Furthermore, codeine can be sold over the counter only when formulated with two or more non-narcotic active ingredients. These requirements have resulted in the prevalence of *co-codaprins*, drugs that contain acetylsalicylic acid, codeine, and caffeine, and similar combinations that use acetaminophen rather than acetylsalicylic acid. In these formulations caffeine serves as a stimulant to offset the sedative effects of codeine. Examples of OTC co-codaprin containing codeine include 222 and Tylenol #1. Formulations containing more than 8 milligrams of codeine are available by prescription only. Recently concerns have been raised

ibuprofen: an Aspirin-like analgesic and anti-inflammatory.

NSAIDs: nonsteroidal anti-inflammatory drugs, such as ibuprofen.

about the safety of codeine as an analgesic. Researchers citing advances in our understanding of its pharmacogenetics and emerging evidence that the narcotic can cause death even at conventional doses have prompted critical appraisal of its place in OTC medications.[34]

LO7 Cold and Allergy Products

Cold and allergy medications are popular OTC products.

The All-Too-Common Cold

There has to be something good about an illness that Charles Dickens could be lyrical about:

> *I am at this moment*
> *Deaf in the ears,*
> *Hoarse in the throat,*
> *Red in the nose,*
> *Green in the gills,*
> *Damp in the eyes,*
> *Twitchy in the joints,*
> *And fractious in temper*
> *From a most intolerable*
> *And oppressive cold.*[35]

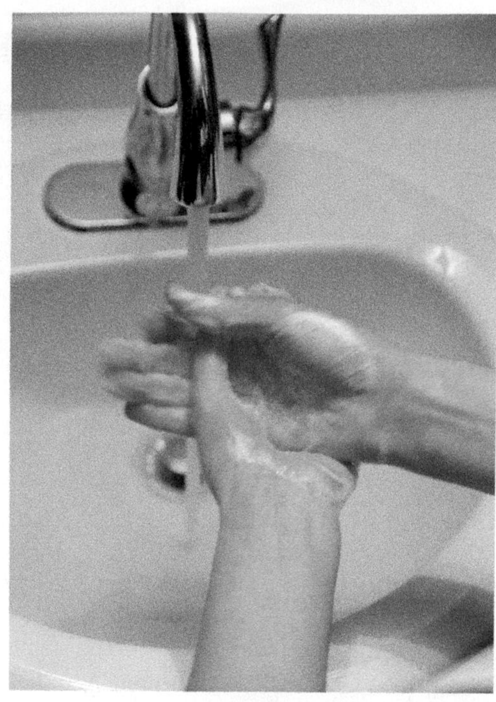

Frequent handwashing is a good strategy to reduce the risk of contracting a cold.

The common cold is caused by viruses: more than a hundred have been identified. But in 40–60% of individuals with colds, researchers cannot connect the infection to a specific virus. That makes it tough to find a cure. Two groups of viruses are known to be associated with colds–the *rhinoviruses* and the more recently identified *coronaviruses*. These viruses are clearly distinct from those that cause influenza, measles, and pneumonia. Success in developing vaccines against other diseases has made some experts optimistic about finding a vaccine for the common cold. Others are pessimistic because of the great variety of viruses and the fact that the rhinoviruses can apparently change their immunological reactivity very readily.

Viruses damage or kill the cells they attack. The rhinoviruses zero in on the upper respiratory tract, at first causing irritation, which can lead to reflex coughing and sneezing. Increased irritation inflames the tissue and is followed by soreness and swelling of the mucous membranes. As a defence against infection, the mucous membranes release considerable fluid, which causes the runny nose and the postnasal drip that irritates the throat.

Although the incubation period for a cold can be a week in some cases, the more common interval between infection and respiratory tract symptoms is two to four days. Before the onset of respiratory symptoms, the individual might just feel bad and develop joint aches and headaches. When fever does occur, it almost always develops early in the cold.

Most of us grew up believing that colds are passed by airborne particles jet-propelled usually through unobstructed sneezing. ("Cover your mouth! Cover your face!") The old folklore–and the scientists–had it only partially right. You need to know four things so you can avoid the cold viruses of others–and avoid reinfecting yourself:

1. Up to 100 times as many viruses are produced and shed from the nasal mucosa as from the throat.
2. There are few viruses in the saliva of a person with a cold, probably no viruses at all in about half of these individuals.
3. Dried viruses survive on dry skin and nonporous surfaces–plastic, wood, and so on–for more than three hours.
4. Most cold viruses enter the body through the nostrils and eyes.

Usually colds start by the fingers picking up viruses and then the individual rubs the eyes or picks the nose. In one study of adults with colds, 40% had viruses on their hands but only 8% expelled viruses in coughs or sneezes.[36] To avoid colds, wash your hands

Table 12.2 Ingredients (mg/tablet) in Selected Brand-Name OTC Cold and Allergy Products

Brand	Sympathomimetic	Antihistamine	Analgesic	Cough Suppressant
Benylin Cold and Sinus	5 phenylephrine		500 acetaminophen	
Dristan	5 phenylephrine HCl	2 chlorpheniramine maleate	325 acetaminophen	—
Tylenol Cold Daytime	30 phenylephrine HCl		325 acetaminophen	15 dextromethorphan
Theraflu Cold and Flu	10 phenylephrine HCl	20 chlorpheniramine maleate	325 acetaminophen	
Advil Cold and Sinus	30 pseudoephedrine HCl		200 Ibuprofen	

Source: Health Canada. *Drug Product Database Online Query*. 2011. Retrieved October 1, 2011, from http://webprod3.hc-sc.gc.ca/dpd-bdpp/index-eng.jsp.

frequently, and you may kiss but not hold hands with your cold-infected sweetheart. You don't have to worry about your pets—only humans and some apes are susceptible to colds.

The experimental animal of choice for studying colds has to be the human. In many studies with human volunteers, three types of findings seem to recur. First, not all who are directly exposed to a cold virus develop cold symptoms. In fact, only about 50% do. Second, in individuals with already existing antibodies to the virus, there might be only preliminary signs of a developing cold. These signs might last for a brief period (12–24 hours) and then disappear. Finally, it doesn't seem to matter whether people are subjected to "chilling" treatment (e.g., sitting in a draft in a wet bathing suit). *Being* cold has nothing to do with *catching* a cold.

Treatment of Cold Symptoms

There's no practical way to prevent colds and no way to cure the infection once it starts. So why do Canadians spend hundreds of millions each year on cold "remedies"? Apparently, it's in an effort to reduce those miserable symptoms described by Dickens. Cold symptoms are fairly complex, so most cold remedies have traditionally included several active ingredients, each aimed at a particular type of symptom. In some ways, the U.S. Food and Drug Administration's Cold, Cough, Allergy, Bronchodilator, and Antiasthmatic Advisory Review Panel probably had the most difficult job: multiple symptoms, many ingredients for each symptom, and rapid changes in scientific evidence during the time it studied these products. In the preliminary report, issued in 1976, the panel approved less than half of the 119 ingredients it reviewed. Modern cold remedies contain three common types of ingredients: *antihistamines*, for the temporary relief of runny nose and sneezing; *sympathomimetic nasal decongestants*, for the temporary relief of swollen membranes in the nasal passages; and *analgesic-antipyretics*, for the temporary relief of aches and pains and fever reduction. The most common antihistamine to be found in cold remedies is **chlorpheniramine maleate**; the most common nasal decongestant in cold remedies is now phenylephrine. The analgesic-antipyretic is usually acetaminophen.

Table 12.2 gives recent formulations for five popular OTC cold remedies in Canada. Note that one of them also contains the cough suppressant **dextromethorphan**, which is the most common active ingredient in OTC cough medicines.

One type of ingredient found in almost every cold remedy continues to come under attack. The U.S. Food and Drug Administration advisory panel had serious questions about the data supporting the effectiveness of antihistamines in treating colds. Although some studies have since reported that chlorpheniramine maleate is better than placebo at reducing runny noses, more recent controlled experiments have not found any benefit. A 1987 symposium of specialists concluded that "antihistamines do not have a place in the management of upper respiratory infection, though they continue to be useful for allergy." Still more studies have been done that question the effectiveness of antihistamines. They're still there.

chlorpheniramine maleate: a common antihistamine in cold products.

dextromethorphan: an OTC antitussive (cough control) ingredient.

In 2007 Health Canada issued a public advisory warning parents not to give OTC cough and cold products to children under two years of age. This advisory was prompted by reports to Health Canada of serious and potentially life-threatening adverse events, including unintentional overdose in that age group. The same advisory recommended that parents or caregivers also use caution if they choose to give cough and cold products to older children. The most critical parts of this include a reminder that these products do not cure nor shorten the duration of the cold and a caution to read the labels and follow the dosing directions carefully.

Allergy and Sinus Medications

There are other related products on your pharmacy shelves. In addition to the cough medicines, there are *allergy* relief pills, which rely mainly on an antihistamine, to slow down the runny nose. Sinus medicines use one of the sympathomimetic nasal decongestants (phenylephrine), often combined with an analgesic, to reduce swollen sinus passages and to treat sinus headache.

LO8 Choosing an OTC Product

By now you should be getting the idea that, thanks to Health Canada's decision to review ingredients rather than individual formulations, you as a consumer can now review and choose from among the great variety of products by knowing just a few ingredients and what they are intended to accomplish. Table 12.3 lists the six major active ingredients found in different combinations in OTC sleep aids, analgesics, and cold, cough, allergy, and sinus medications.

Do you want to treat your cold without buying a combination cold remedy? If you have aches and pains, take your favourite analgesic. For the vast majority of colds, the slight elevation in temperature should probably not be treated, because it is not dangerous and can even help fight the infection. Unless body temperature remains at 39°C or above or reaches 40.5°C, fever is not considered dangerous. If you have a runny nose, you might or might not get relief from an antihistamine. Generic chlorpheniramine maleate or a store-brand allergy tablet is an inexpensive source. These will probably give you a dry mouth and might produce some sedation or drowsiness (which, of course, is why some of the more sedating antihistamines are used in sleep aids). Do you have a stuffed-up nose? Pseudoephedrine nose drops will shrink swollen membranes for a time. Although oral sympathomimetics will work, nose drops are more effective. You can find these ingredients in sinus and allergy preparations. However, these sympathomimetics should be used cautiously. There is a rapid tolerance to their effects, and, if they are used repeatedly, a rebound stuffiness can develop when they are stopped. Do you have a cough? Dextromethorphan can be obtained in cough medications.

Why not buy all this in one tablet or capsule? That's a common approach. But why treat symptoms you don't have? During a cold, a runny nose might occur at one time, congestion at another, and coughing not at all. By using just the ingredients you need, when you need them, you might save money, and you will have the satisfaction of being a connoisseur of colds. Then again, given the state of research on the effectiveness of these "remedies," why buy them at all? It's easy for a skeptic to conclude that there's little or no real value in cold remedies. The experts say to rest and drink fluids. But when they actually have a cold, most people are less inclined to be skeptical and more inclined to be hopeful that something will help.

Table 12.3 Common OTC Ingredients

Ingredient	Action	Source
acetylsalicylic acid (ASA; Aspirin)	analgesic-antipyretic	headache remedies, arthritis formulas, cold and sinus remedies
acetaminophen	analgesic-antipyretic	headache remedies, cold and sinus remedies
chlorpheniramine maleate	antihistamine	cold remedies, allergy products
dextromethorphan	antitussive	cough suppressants, cold remedies
diphenhydramine	antihistamine	sleep aids, some cold remedies
phenylephrine	sympathomimetic	cold and sinus remedies

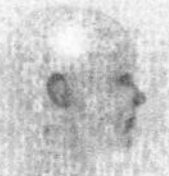

MIND/BODY CONNECTION

Abuse of OTC Dextromethorphan

High school and postsecondary students have been "getting high" with large doses of OTC cough suppressants containing dextromethorphan (DM). Possibly, students first discovered the effects, including visual and auditory hallucinations, of DM by drinking large quantities of Robitussin or similar cough syrups containing alcohol. However, the effects, including visual and auditory hallucinations, reported by those using 250 millilitres of Robitussin (up to 750 milligrams DM) could not be due to the less than 15 millilitres (one-half ounce) of alcohol in them.[37] The altered psychological state may last for several hours. The few cases reported in the literature and individual reports from postsecondary students indicate that habitual use (e.g., twice per week or more) is common.

DM has been the standard ingredient in OTC cough suppressants for many years and was originally developed as a nonopiate relative to codeine. DM is not an opioid-like narcotic, produces no pain relief, and does not produce an opioid-like abstinence syndrome. More recent evidence indicates that it may interact with a specific receptor from the opioid family known as the sigma receptor. This apparently safe and simple drug, which is contained in more than 200 OTC products, has more complicated effects when taken in the large doses by recreational users.

It's not clear how recent this phenomenon really is. The Swedish government restricted DM to prescription-only use in 1986 as a result of abuse of OTC preparations, and there were two later reports of DM-caused fatalities in Sweden. In Canada, this has remained a mostly underground activity, apparently spread by word of mouth.

A posting to the alt.psychoactives newsgroup on the Internet described a user's first DM experience, after taking 20 capsules of an OTC cough remedy (600 milligrams DM):

> 45 minutes worth of itching and for ten seconds it stopped. During one of the most weirdest and stupidest visions, I flew quickly over a mountain. As I did this in that second the itching seemed to go away and it seemed like I wasn't in my body anymore. I flew from one side of a rainbow to another. Then I was flying quickly towards the head of an ostrich and when I got close it only showed the silhouette of the head and I flew into the black nothingness. All that craziness in ten seconds made me laugh out loud as I tried to look at it all soberly. Then the itching came back into my body. No matter how hard I tried the itching never went away.

The itching feeling has been reported by others, along with nausea and other unpleasant side effects. Despite such unpleasantness, some users find it difficult to stop using DM once they have tried it a few times.

In 2013 the *Ontario Student Drug Use Health Survey* asked students (Grades 7–12) if they, during the past year, had used an OTC cough or cold medication containing DM to "get high." Some 9.7% of students reported they had. This estimate represents approximately 70 000 students in Ontario.[38] In a similar vein, the U.S. Substance Abuse and Mental Health Services Administration (SAMHSA) issued a press release based on results from the *National Survey of Drug Use and Health* reporting that more than 3 million adolescents and young adults reported having used OTC cough and cold medicines to get high at least once in their lifetime. In the United States, it was also pointed out that this rate of use is actually higher than the rate of use of methamphetamine in this age group.

Summary

- Since 2004 all NHPs have been required to be proven safe and effective before they can be sold in Canada.
- In creating the NHPD the Government of Canada established a mechanism to ensure Canadians receive access to a wide range of NHPs that are safe, effective, and of high quality.
- St. John's wort and SAMe have been proposed to treat depression.
- A drug can be sold over the counter only if Health Canada agrees it can be used safely when following the label directions.
- For a given category of OTC drug, most of the various brands all contain the same few ingredients.
- Natural health product stimulants are based on caffeine.

- OTC sleep aids are based on antihistamines.
- Ephedra has been proposed to promote modest, short-term weight loss. Caution is strongly recommended with its use as emerging studies have linked ephedra to sudden cardiac death.
- Health Canada has not approved any OTC or NHP weight-control medicines.
- Certain OTC drugs are kept behind the pharmacist's counter. This gives the pharmacist an opportunity to counsel patients about the drugs' proper use and precautions.
- Aspirin has anti-inflammatory, analgesic, and antipyretic actions. Because of its ability to increase bleeding time and induce gastrointestinal bleeding, Aspirin should be used with caution.
- Acetaminophen, ibuprofen, and other NSAIDs (nonsteroidal anti-inflammatories) have effects similar to those of Aspirin.
- Cold remedies usually contain an antihistamine (e.g., chlorpheniramine maleate), an analgesic (e.g., acetaminophen), and a decongestant (e.g., phenylephrine).
- An informed consumer can understand a large fraction of OTC medicines by knowing only six ingredients.

Review Questions

1. What are the main differences between drugs and NHPs?
2. What are the criteria for deciding whether a drug should be sold OTC or by prescription?
3. Why are some OTC drugs kept behind the counter?
4. What is the main ingredient found in OTC sleep aids?
5. What effect of Aspirin might be involved in its use to prevent heart attacks and strokes?
6. What are the differences in the therapeutic effects of acetaminophen and ibuprofen?
7. What is the most common route for a cold virus to enter a person's system?
8. Which cold symptoms are supposed to be relieved by chlorpheniramine maleate and which by phenylephrine?

SECTION

6

CHAPTER 13

Opioids

The opioids include some of the oldest and most useful medicines. Why did they also become one of the most important illicit drugs?

CHAPTER 14

Hallucinogens

Are some drugs really capable of enhancing intellectual experiences? Of producing madness?

CHAPTER 15

Cannabis

Why has a lowly and common weed become such an important symbol of the struggle between lifestyles?

CHAPTER 16

Performance-Enhancing Drugs

What improvements can athletes obtain by resorting to drugs? What are the associated dangers?

RESTRICTED DRUGS

The drugs discussed in this section include some of the most feared substances: heroin, LSD, and marijuana. More recently, the anabolic steroids used by some athletes have also become widely feared by the public, most of whom have no direct contact with the drugs. Along with the stimulants, cocaine, and amphetamines, these substances are commonly viewed as evil, "devil drugs."

CHAPTER 13

OPIOIDS

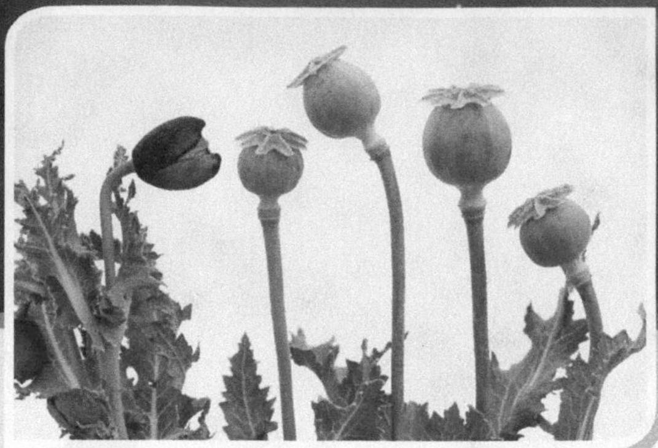

OBJECTIVES

When you have finished this chapter, you should be able to

- **LO1** List several historical uses for opium including early recreational uses of opium and its derivatives.
- **LO2** Describe the supply, distribution, and trafficking of opium and heroin in Canada.
- **LO3** Explain how the profile of the "typical" opioid abuser has changed in Canada.
- **LO4** Describe the pharmacokinetic properties and mechanism of action of the opioids.
- **LO5** Describe the current medical uses for opioids.
- **LO6** Discuss some of the concerns associated with the use of opioids.
- **LO7** Describe the key findings from Insite, Vancouver's supervised injection facility.

And soon they found themselves in the midst of a great meadow of poppies. Now it is well known that when there are many of these flowers together their odor is so powerful that anyone who breathes it falls asleep, and if the sleeper is not carried away from the scent of the flowers he sleeps on and on forever. But Dorothy did not know this, nor could she get away from the bright red flowers that were everywhere about; so presently her eyes grew heavy and she felt she must sit down to rest and to sleep. . . . Her eyes closed in spite of herself and she forgot where she was and fell among the poppies, fast asleep. . . . They carried the sleeping girl to a pretty spot beside the river, far enough from the poppy field to prevent her breathing any more of the poison of the flowers, and here they laid her gently on the soft grass and waited for the fresh breeze to waken her.[1]

opium: a raw plant substance containing morphine and codeine.

From the land of Oz to the streets of Vancouver, the poppy has caused much grief–and much joy. **Opium** is a unique substance. This juice from the plant *Papaver somniferum* has a history of medical use perhaps 6000 years long. Except for the past century and a half, opium has stood alone as the one agent from which physicians could obtain sure results. Compounds containing opium solved several of the recurring problems for medical science wherever used. Opium relieved pain and suffering magnificently. Just as important in the years gone by was its ability to reduce the diarrhea and subsequent dehydration caused by dysentery, which is still a leading cause of death in underdeveloped countries.

Parallel with the medical use of opium was its use as a deliverer of pleasure and relief from anxiety. Because of these effects, extensive recreational use of opium has also occurred throughout history. Through all those years, many of its users experienced dependence.

LO1 History of Opioids

Opium

The opium poppy is an annual plant that grows more than a metre high with large flowers about ten centimetres in diameter. The flowers can be white, pink, red, purple, or violet.

Opium is produced and available for collection for only a few days of the plant's life, between the time the petals drop and the seedpod matures. Today, as before, opium harvesters move through the fields in the early evening and use a sharp, clawed tool to make shallow cuts into, but not through, the unripe seedpods. During the night a white substance oozes from the cuts, oxidizes to a red-brown colour, and becomes gummy. In the morning the resinous substance is carefully scraped from the pod and collected in small balls. This raw opium forms the basis for the opium medicines that have been used throughout history and is the substance from which morphine is extracted and then heroin is derived.

Early History of Opium The most likely origin of opium is in a hot, dry, Middle Eastern country several millennia ago, when someone discovered that for seven to ten days of its yearlong life *Papaver somniferum* produced a substance that, when eaten, eased pain and suffering.

The importance and extent of use of the opium poppy in the early Egyptian and Greek cultures are still under debate, but in the Ebers Papyrus (circa 1500 BC) a remedy is mentioned "to prevent the excessive crying of children." Because a later Egyptian remedy for the same purpose clearly contained opium (as well as fly excrement), many writers report the first specific medical use of opium as dating from the Ebers Papyrus.

Opium was important in Greek medicine. Galen, the last of the great Greek physicians, emphasized caution in the use of opium but felt that it was almost a cure-all, saying that it

> resists poison and venomous bites, cures chronic headache, vertigo, deafness, epilepsy, apoplexy, dimness of sight, loss of voice, asthma, coughs of all kinds, spitting of blood, tightness of breath, colic, the iliac poison, jaundice, hardness of the spleen, stone, urinary complaints, fevers, dropsies, leprosies, the troubles to which women are subject, melancholy and all pestilences.[2]

Greek and Roman knowledge of opium use in medicine languished during the Dark Ages and thus had little influence on the world's use of opium for the next thousand years. The Arabic world, however, clutched opium to its breast. Because the Koran forbade the use of alcohol in any form, opium and hashish became the primary social drugs wherever the Islamic culture moved, and it did move. While Europe rested through the Dark Ages, the Arabian world reached out and made contact with India and China. Opium was one of the products they traded, but they also sold the seeds of the opium poppy, and cultivation began in these countries. By the tenth century AD, opium had been referred to in Chinese medical writings.

During this period when the Arabic civilization flourished, two Arabic physicians made substantial contributions to medicine and to the history of opium. Shortly after AD 1000, Biruni composed a pharmacology book. His descriptions of opium contained what some believe to be the first written description of **opioid** addiction.[3] In the same period the best-known Arabic physician, Avicenna, was using opium preparations very effectively and extensively in his medical practice. His writings, along with those of Galen, formed the basis of medical education in Europe as the Renaissance dawned, and thus the glories of opium were advanced. (Avicenna, a knowledgeable physician and a believer in the tenets of Islam, died as a result of drinking too much of a mixture of opium and wine.)

Early in the sixteenth century lived a European medical phenomenon. Paracelsus apparently was a successful clinician and accomplished some wondrous cures for the day. One of his secrets was an opium extract called laudanum. Paracelsus was one of the early Renaissance supporters of opium as a panacea and referred to it as the "stone of immortality."

Due to Paracelsus and his followers, awareness increased of the broad effectiveness of opium, and new opium preparations were developed in the sixteenth, seventeenth, and eighteenth centuries. One of these was laudanum as prepared by Dr. Thomas Sydenham, the father of English clinical medicine. Sydenham's general contributions to English medicine are so great that he has been called the English Hippocrates. He spoke more highly of opium than did Paracelsus, saying that "without opium the healing art would cease to exist." His laudanum contained two ounces of strained opium, one ounce of saffron, a dram of cinnamon, and a dram of cloves dissolved in one pint of Canary wine, taken in small quantities.

Writers and Opium: The Keys to Paradise Several famous English authors wrote about the joys of opium, including Elizabeth Barrett Browning and Samuel Taylor Coleridge. Coleridge's beautiful "Kubla Khan" is believed to have been conceived and partially composed in an opium reverie. But, perhaps the author who most enthusiastically articulated the powers of opium was Thomas De Quincey. In his 1821 book *Confessions of an English Opium-Eater*, De Quincey

opioid: a drug derived from opium (e.g., morphine and codeine) or a synthetic drug with opium-like effects (e.g., oxycodone).

meticulously describes both the pleasures and pains of regular opium use. Of the pleasures, he wrote:

> . . . my pains had vanished . . . here was the secret of happiness, about which philosophers had disputed for so many ages, at once discovered: happiness now might be bought for a penny, and carried in a waistcoat pocket: portable ecstasies might be had corked up in a pint-bottle . . . [4]

The effects of most psychoactive agents are not unidimensional. De Quincey discovered that opium was no exception. He detailed the pains of opium withdrawal and reported not being able to write for long periods of time due to his dependence on the drug. Even in the early nineteenth century, a period during which many contemporary observers tend to regard as one with few drug use moral strictures, De Quincey felt compelled to provide justification for his daily use of opium:

> True it is, that for nearly ten years I did occasionally take opium for the sake of the exquisite pleasure it gave me . . . It was not for the purpose of creating pleasure, but of mitigating pain in the severest degree, that I first began to use opium as an article of daily diet. In the twenty-eighth year of my age, a most painful affection of the stomach, which I had first experienced about ten years before, attached me in great strength.[4]

It seems that regular use of opium has a long history of being viewed unfavourably by certain members of society, and this view was prevalent even when De Quincey wrote about his opium experiences.

The Opium Wars Although opium and the opium poppy had been introduced to China well before the year AD 1000, there was only a moderate level of use there by a select, elite group. Tobacco smoking spread much more rapidly after its introduction. It is not clear when tobacco was introduced to the Chinese, but its use had spread and become so offensive that in 1644 the emperor forbade tobacco smoking in China. The edict did not last long (as is to be expected), but it was in part responsible for the increase in opium smoking.

Up to this period the smoking of tobacco and the eating of opium had existed side by side. The restriction on the use of tobacco and the population's appreciation of the pleasures of smoking led to the combining of opium and tobacco for smoking. Presumably the addition of opium took the edge off the craving for tobacco. The amount of tobacco used was gradually reduced and soon omitted. Although opium eating had never been very attractive to most Chinese, opium smoking spread rapidly, perhaps in part because smoking opium results in a rapid effect, compared with oral use.

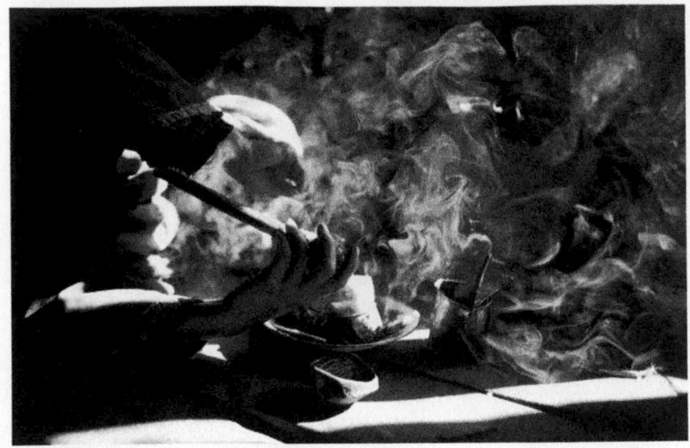

Smoking opium results in rapid effects.

In 1729, China's first law against opium smoking mandated that opium shop owners be strangled. Once opium for non-medical purposes was outlawed, it was necessary for the drug to be smuggled in from India, where poppy plantations were abundant. Smuggling opium was so profitable for everyone–the growers, the shippers, and the customs officers–that unofficial rules were gradually developed for the "game."[2] The background to the Opium Wars is lengthy and complex, but the following can help explain why the British went to war so they could continue pouring opium into China against the wishes of the Chinese national government.

Since before 1557, when the Portuguese were allowed to develop the small trading post of Macao, pressure had been increasing on the Chinese emperors to open up the country to trade with the "barbarians from the West." Not only the Portuguese but also the Dutch and the English repeatedly knocked on the closed door of China. Near the end of the seventeenth century the port of Canton was opened under very strict rules to foreigners. Tea was the major export, and the British shipped out huge amounts. There was little that the Chinese were interested in importing from the "barbarians," but opium could be smuggled so profitably that it soon became the primary import. The profit the British made from selling opium paid for the tea they shipped back to England.[5] In the early nineteenth century the government of India was actually the British East India Company. As such, it had a monopoly on opium, which was legal in India. However, smuggling it into China was not. The East India Company auctioned chests of opium cakes to private merchants, who gave the chests to selected British firms, which sold them for a commission to Chinese merchants. In this way the British were able to have the Chinese "smuggle" the opium into China. The number of chests of opium, each with about 120 pounds of smokeable opium, imported annually by China increased from 200 in 1729 to about 5000 at the century's end to 25 000 chests in 1838.

In 1839, the emperor of China made a fatal mistake—he sent an honest man to Canton to suppress the opium smuggling. Commissioner Lin demanded that the barbarians deliver all their opium supplies to him and subjected the dealers to confinement in their houses. After some haggling, the representative of the British government ordered the merchants to deliver the opium—20 000 chests worth about $6 million—which was then destroyed and everyone was set free. Pressures mounted, however, and an incident involving drunken American and British sailors killing a Chinese citizen started the Opium Wars in 1839. The British army arrived 10 months later, and in two years, largely by avoiding land battles and by using the superior artillery of the royal navy ships, they won a victory over a country of more than 350 million citizens. As victors, the British were given the island of Hong Kong, broad trading rights, and $6 million to reimburse the merchants whose opium had been destroyed.

The Chinese opium trade posed a great moral dilemma for Britain. The East India Company protested until its end that it was not smuggling opium into China, and technically it was not. From 1870 to 1893, motions in Parliament to end the extremely profitable opium commerce failed to pass but did cause a decline in the opium trade. In 1893, a moral protest against the trade was supported, but not until 1906 did the government support and pass a bill that eventually ended the opium trade in 1913.

Morphine

In 1806, Friedrich Sertürner published a report of more than 50 experiments, which clearly showed that he had isolated the primary active ingredient in opium. The active agent was 10 times as potent as opium. Sertürner named it *morphium* after Morpheus, the god of dreams. Use of the new agent developed slowly, but by 1831 the implications of his chemical work and the medical value of **morphine** had become so overwhelming that this pharmacist's assistant was given the French equivalent of the Nobel Prize. Later work into the mysteries of opium found more than 30 different alkaloids, with the second most important one being isolated in 1832 and named **codeine**, the Greek word for "poppy head."

The availability of a clinically useful, pure chemical of known potency is always capitalized on in medicine. The major increase in the use of morphine came as a result of two nondrug developments, one technological and one political. The technological development was the perfection of the hypodermic syringe in 1853 by Dr. Alexander Wood. This made it possible to deliver morphine directly into the blood or tissue rather than by the much slower process of eating opium or morphine and waiting for absorption to occur from the gastrointestinal tract. A further advantage of injecting morphine was thought to exist. Originally it was felt that morphine by injection would not produce the same degree of craving (hunger) for the drug as with oral use. This belief was later found to be false.

The political events that sped the drug of sleep and dreams into the veins of people worldwide were the American Civil War (1861–1865), the Prussian-Austrian War (1866), and the Franco-Prussian War (1870). Military medicine was, and to some extent still is, characterized by the dictum "first provide relief." Morphine given by injection worked rapidly and well, and it was administered regularly in large doses to many soldiers for the reduction of pain and relief from dysentery. The percentage of veterans returning from these wars who were dependent on morphine was high enough that the illness was later called "soldier's disease" or the "army disease."

Heroin

Toward the end of the nineteenth century, a small but important chemical transformation was made to the morphine molecule. In 1874, two acetyl groups were attached to morphine, yielding diacetylmorphine, which was given the brand name Heroin and placed on the market in 1898 by Bayer Laboratories. The chemical change was important because **heroin**

morphine: the primary active agent in opium.

codeine: the secondary active agent in opium.

heroin: diacetylmorphine, a potent derivative of morphine.

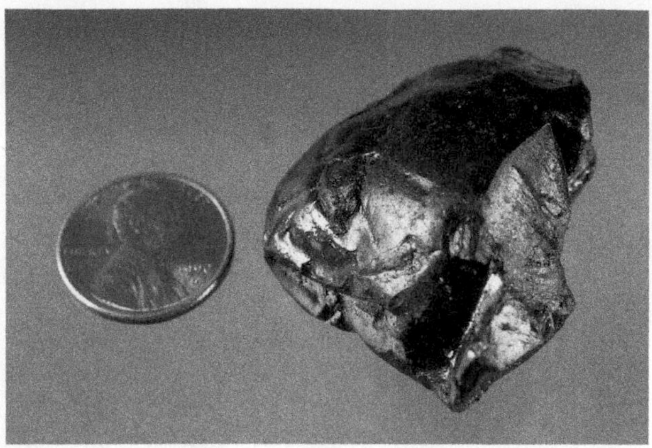

Raw opium is the substance from which morphine is extracted and then heroin is derived.

is about three times as potent as morphine. The pharmacology of heroin and morphine is identical, except that the two acetyl groups increase the lipid solubility of the heroin molecule, and thus the molecule enters the brain more rapidly. The additional groups are then detached, yielding morphine. Therefore, the effects of morphine and heroin are identical, except that heroin is believed to be more potent and acts faster.

Heroin was originally marketed as a non-addictive cough suppressant that would replace morphine and codeine.[6] It seemed to be the perfect drug, more potent yet less harmful. Although not introduced commercially until 1898, heroin had been studied, and many of its pharmacological actions had been reported in 1890.[7] In January 1900, a comprehensive review article concluded that tolerance and dependence on heroin were only minor problems.

> Habituation has been noted in a small percentage . . . of the cases. . . . All observers are agreed, however, that none of the patients suffer in any way from this habituation, and that none of the symptoms which are so characteristic of chronic morphinism have ever been observed. On the other hand, a large number of the reports refer to the fact that the same dose may be used for a long time without any habituation.[8]

The basis for the failure to find dependence probably was the fact that heroin was initially used as a

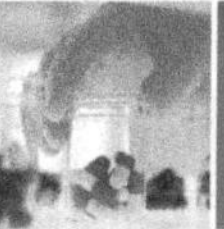

DRUGS IN THE MEDIA

The Rise and Fall of Heroin "Epidemics"

The term *epidemic* refers to a rapidly spreading outbreak of contagious disease or, by extension, to any rapid spread, growth, or development of a problem. Heroin use has always been restricted to a very small proportion of the population, and it would be an overstatement to say that heroin use has reached or will reach epidemic proportions, if by that we mean that the problem is widely prevalent. Nevertheless, there are periodic news reports about the most recent "heroin epidemic," amid speculation about its rapid spread.

What usually triggers these reports is the heroin-related death of a celebrity, the arrest of some young heroin users (seen as evidence that a new generation is being affected), or the spectacular seizure of a large drug shipment. Despite these scary news accounts, filled with lurid details and predictions of doom, the predicted epidemic never seems to materialize and fades from memory. Once the epidemic has been forgotten, the television and newspaper reporters are primed to warn us about the next epidemic a few years later.

Seizures of drugs, for example, are a notoriously poor way to measure drug use trends. Researchers estimate that authorities capture only about one-tenth of the drugs on the market, but sometimes they get lucky. The amount of drugs seized, however, doesn't answer the question of whether the seizure is a representative portion of a steady market, a growing portion of a shrinking market, or a smaller portion of a growing market.

Keep your eyes and ears open, and it won't be long before you read or hear a news report about an epidemic of heroin use in a part of Canada or in another country (such reports also have appeared in the United States, Ireland, Russia, the UK, and elsewhere). Does the report cite formal studies that help quantify the problem, or does it vaguely point to "ominous signs" of increasing drug use? These reports really attract attention—and increase sales and advertising revenue—so there's always a market for the stories. As we have seen before, most of this kind of illicit drug use is better viewed as occurring in localized areas, taking on more of the character of a fad than of an epidemic.

substitute for codeine, which meant oral doses of 3 to 5 mg used for brief periods of time. Slowly the situation changed, and a 1905 text, *Pharmacology and Therapeutics*, took a middle ground on heroin by saying that it "is stated not to give rise to habituation. A more extended knowledge of the drug, however, would seem to indicate that the latter assertion is not entirely correct."[9] In a few more years, everyone knew that heroin could produce a powerful dependence when injected in higher doses.

LO2 Opium and Heroin Supply, Distribution, and Trafficking in Canada

Poppies do not grow naturally in Canada. As such, poppies are illegally imported and distributed within Canada from South and Southwest Asia. Opium, the least potent member of the opiate family, is sold as a dark brown solid or powder that can be ingested, smoked, or injected. In addition to opium, the poppy also contains morphine and codeine. Canadian supply of opium and heroin comes primarily from South and Southwest Asia (e.g., Afghanistan, Pakistan, Iran, India, and Turkey), which have surpassed and replaced Southeast Asia (e.g., Myanmar, Thailand, and Laos) as the primary source of opium to the Canadian market. Global illicit opium poppy cultivation fell 15% in 2009, resulting in a 10% decrease in global opium production.[10] Opium powder is popular among young adults throughout Toronto and Vancouver, as at $1 per gram it provides a cheap and unconventional high.[11,12] Naturally occurring opium or synthetic and semi-synthetic opioids work as agonists or antagonists on the opioid receptor. A major source of illicit opioid use is available through prescription (see Table 13.1 for examples of naturally occurring, synthetic, and semi-synthetic opioids).

Table 13.1 Prescription Opioids in Canada by Type

Generic Name	Canadian Trade Name Examples	Type
Naturally Occurring		
morphine	MS Contin, MOS, others	agonist
codeine	Tylenol #2–#4, others	agonist
Semi-synthetics		
heroin	(Not medically available in Canada)	agonist
oxycodone	OxyContin	agonist
oxycodone-acetaminophen	Percocet, Endocet	agonist
oxycodone-ASA	Percodan	agonist
hydromorphone	Dilaudid	agonist
hydrocodone	Tussionex	agonist
Synthetics		
alfentanil	Alfenta	agonist
fentanyl	Abstral	agonist
methadone	Metadol	agonist
meperidine	Demerol	agonist
sufentanil	Sufenta	agonist
tramadol	Tramacet	agonist
buprenorphine with naloxone	Suboxone	agonist-antagonist
butorphanol	APO-Butorphanol	agonist-antagonist
nalbuphine	Nubain	agonist-antagonist
pentazocine	Talwin	agonist-antagonist
naloxone	Targin	antagonist
naltrexone	Revia	antagonist

LO3 The Changing Profile of Opioid Users

A core element of high-risk street drug use in North America is heroin use.[13] There has been substantial growth in prevalence rates of illicit opioid use in North America for decades. Prescription opioid analgesics (e.g., morphine, hydromorphone, oxycodone) and not heroin account for increased use. The OPICAN study (2001), a large multi-city study in Edmonton, Montreal, Quebec City, Toronto, Vancouver, Fredericton, and Saint John, captured these data. From 2001 through 2005, regular illicit opioid users reported decreased use of heroin and increased prescription opioid use. Table 13.2 outlines the distribution of heroin-only, prescription-opioid-only, and combined use amongst the different sites.

In the OPICAN–non-medicinal use of opioids (OPI) in Canada (CAN)–study, use of prescription opioid (PO) only was three times more prevalent than heroin (H) only and prescription opioid and heroin (PO&H) (304 versus 94 and 86, respectively), although Vancouver and Montreal had a high number of H-only users. PO are more readily accessible than H, and the stereotypical face of the addict has changed to include prescription drug use for non-medicinal or self-prescribing purposes. What accounts for this significant shift in illicit opioid use from the prototypic heroin addict to one using prescription opioids in Canada? One explanation is the substantial rise in medical use of prescription opioids and a marked rise in non-medical use of these drugs in Canada. In 2005, Canada ranked first in the world in per capita consumption of Dilaudid (hydromorphone), second for MS Contin (morphine) and OxyContin (oxycodone), and third for Vicodin (hydrocodone). The exact extent of the problem is unknown. There are indications that both medical and non-medical uses precipitate opioid dependence and overdose, with consequent morbidity and mortality according to the International Narcotics Control Board.[14–22]

In a similar vein, a percentage of illicit opioid users entering a methadone maintenance treatment at a large Toronto treatment clinic (1997–99) were currently using POs, either with or without concurrent heroin use.[23]

Fentanyl is approximately 100 times stronger than morphine. The fentanyl transdermal patch is a slow-release patch initially intended mainly to treat patients suffering cancer-related pain, who have built up a tolerance to other opioids. Illegal fentanyl was associated with more than 100 deaths in Alberta alone in 2014.[24]

Table 13.2 Distribution of Heroin-Only, Prescription Opioid-Only, and Combined Users by Site in Canada

Site	Heroin-Only (*n* = 94)		Prescription Opioid-Only (*n* = 304)		Heroin and Prescription Opioid (*n* = 86)	
	n	%	*n*	%	*n*	%
Edmonton	0	0	32	88.9	4	11.1
Fredericton	0	0	49	100.0	0	0
Montreal	33	48.5	10	14.7	25	36.8
Quebec City	0	0	31	88.6	4	11.4
Saint John	0	0	93	92.1	8	7.9
Toronto	1	0.9	83	75.5	26	23.6
Vancouver	60	70.6	6	7.1	19	22.4

Source: Fischer, B., and others. "Comparing Heroin Users and Prescription Opioid Users in a Canadian Multi-site Population of Illicit Opioid Users." *Drug and Alcohol Review* 27 (2008), pp. 625–32. Drug and Alcohol Review by AUSTRALIAN MEDICAL AND PROFESSIONAL SOCIETY ON ALC Reproduced with permission of TAYLOR & FRANCIS LTD in the format Republish in a book via Copyright Clearance Center.

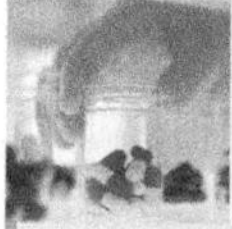

DRUGS IN THE MEDIA

CCENDU Drug Alerts and Bulletins: Increasing Availability of Counterfeit Oxycodone Tablets Containing Fentanyl

The Canadian Community Epidemiology Network on Drug Use (CCENDU) produces alerts and bulletins on drug use trends or topics of immediate concern. The reports use rapidly assembled information ranging from scientific literature to local observations by people directly serving local, high-risk populations.

This alert is to advise that counterfeit oxycodone (popular brand name OxyContin®) pills containing fentanyl have become increasingly available in several Canadian communities. The presence of fentanyl in these counterfeit pills increases the risk of overdose among people using them.

The pills resemble oxycodone tablets. Some are green and stamped with "CDN" on one side and the number 80 on the other. They are being referred to colloquially as "green monsters" or "green beans" in eastern Canada and "green jellies" or "street oxy" in Western Canada. While the green tablets appear to be more widely available, pills have also surfaced that are white with the number 10 stamped in place of the 80. We have reports of these pills appearing in Alberta and British Columbia in November–December 2013 and have recently received reports of large quantities available in St John's, Newfoundland (as of February 2014).

After verification with Health Canada's Drug Analysis Service (DAS), laboratory tests of seized counterfeit oxycodone tablets (different brands, sizes and colours) were most often found to contain fentanyl (89% of the time). Much less frequently tablets were found to contain Alprazolam or Ketamine as the active ingredient. Note that DAS only analyzes a subset of the substances seized by law enforcement agencies, which would also be a subset of the substances found on the illicit market.

Given the presence of fentanyl and other drugs in these counterfeit pills, individuals who believe they are using oxycodone are at greater risk of an accidental overdose.

Source: Reproduced with permission from the Canadian Centre on Substance Abuse (2014). Canadian Community Epidemiology on Drug Use. Retrieved on June 9, 2014 from http://www.ccsa.ca/Eng/collaboration/CCENDU/Pages/default.aspx

Prescription of opioids within the context of treatment of pain within the medical community has been identified as a contributing factor to opioid dependence and abuse in Canada and the United States compared with the rest of the world. The annual consumption of analgesic opioids increased substantially in Canada between 2001 and 2005, with oxycodone use increased by 230%, fentanyl by 159%, and morphine by 28%.[18,21]

Heroin use has for many years been restricted to a small fraction of any population studied. For example, only about 1% of adults reported ever having used heroin in their lifetimes, with 0.2% reporting use in the past year. These numbers have remained relatively stable for at least a decade, but this has not tempered periodic press reports indicating that the country is experiencing a heroin epidemic.

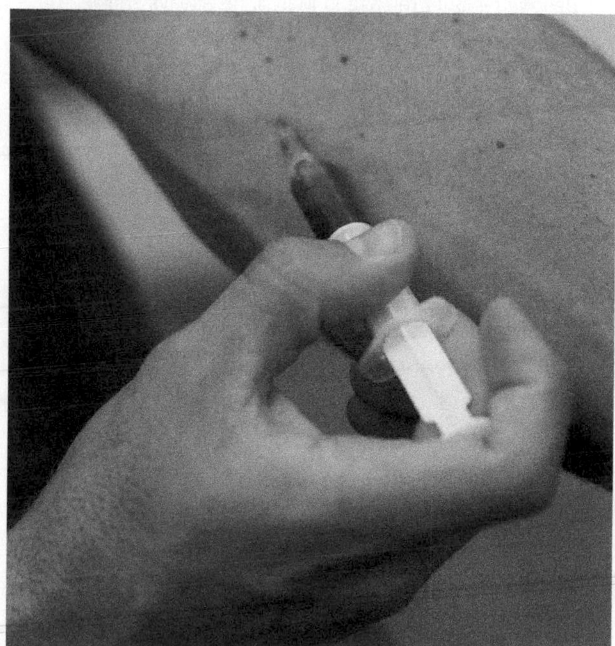

Although heroin dependence is often associated with intravenous use, dependence can occur via any route that produces behavioural or physiological effects.

Abuse of Prescription Opioids

The most popular prescription opioids are various brands of hydrocodone (e.g., Vicodin and Lortab) and oxycodone (OxyContin and Percocet). These are

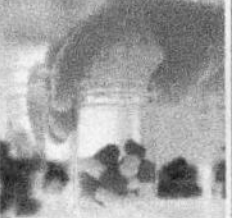

DRUGS IN THE MEDIA

Heroin (Alone) Is Not the Problem

Glee actor Cory Monteith was found dead in his hotel room on July 13, 2013, and the British Columbia coroner concluded that his death was the result of a toxic mixture of alcohol and heroin. The actor had an extensive history of drug use dating back to his teens, which he described as being out of control and that at that time he was "doing anything and everything, as much as possible."

After a stint in rehab at age 19, he went for more than a decade without apparent drug-related problems. Then, in March 2013, Monteith checked himself into a treatment program. He completed the program after about a month and seemed to be on the road to recovery at the time of his death.

For some observers, Monteith's death confirms the pernicious nature of illegal drug use and addiction that eventually ends in tragedy. Certainly, we've seen the gut-wrenching portrayals of heroin addicts agonizing, especially when experiencing withdrawal from the drug. This characterization, however, seems to be inconsistent with Monteith's behaviour and that of most heroin users. According to those close to him, he appeared to be healthy and showed no signs of a substance abuse problem. Despite his brief relapse in March, he always showed up on the set sober and was a model actor. Indeed, this description is more in line with the behaviour of most illegal drug users. Eighty percent or more use drugs without obvious problems.

Still others speculate that Monteith was more vulnerable to overdose after recently going through a detox program, because his body was no longer able to tolerate high doses of heroin. There is no evidence indicating he used high doses of heroin in the past or at the time of his death, making this conjecture less plausible. In addition, while it is theoretically possible to die from an overdose of heroin alone, in practical terms this is rare. Only about a quarter of the thousands of heroin-related deaths each year occur as a result of heroin alone. The vast majority of heroin-related deaths—a whopping 70% or more—are caused by combining heroin with another sedative, usually alcohol. Regrettably, Monteith, too, was a victim of this combination.

Several months later, on February 2, 2014, actor Philip Seymour Hoffman also died as a result of combining heroin with other drugs, including a benzodiazepine.

Given these observations, it seems that the focus on factors other than the heroin-sedative combination is distracting and irresponsible. Too often in these tragic cases some "experts" emphasize the failures of rehab, rather than providing the drug-using population with practical information that could prevent countless overdose deaths. We are potentially missing an important public health education opportunity to decrease drug-related accidents.

These horrible accidents, and the thousands of others that occur each year, could have been prevented if our public health education message clearly focused on the potential dangers associated with the heroin-sedative combination instead of being preoccupied with blaming rehab and vilifying heroin.

Each year there are hundreds of thousands of heroin users. This number has remained stable for decades: North Americans will always use heroin. To keep them safe, providing the best available public health information seems the responsible and ethical thing to do.

Source: Used with permission. Gabor Maté, M.D.

mostly taken orally but when used recreationally they are sometimes snorted or injected.

Recently, you may have seen or read news reports contending that prescription pain reliever use has now reached epidemic rates. Without any context, however, it can be difficult to determine whether past-month use of these drugs warrants our concern. When making this determination, you should know that over the past several years the prevalence of prescription opioids has remained relatively stable. Keep in mind also that past-month use could range from using only once to using on multiple occasions. Another question that you should probably ask is how do the rates of illicit prescription opioid use compare with other illicit drugs? Prescription opioid use far exceeds cocaine use but is markedly lower than marijuana use. What about toxicity? Are prescription opioids more likely to cause drug overdose compared with other drugs? In the most recent Drug Abuse Warning Network data, prescription opioids ranked

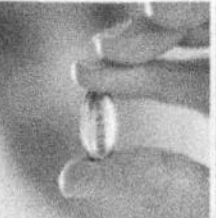

DRUGS IN DEPTH

Methadone Maintenance: A Failed Experiment?

Insite was a public health experiment. Insite is protected under Federal law, with the allowance of otherwise illegal drugs on the premises. Safe injection practices result in less HIV and less Hepatitis C which benefits all Canadians, not just the marginalized. The drugs that are brought into the facility are obtained on the street. This is what the RCMP should concentrate on, the availability of drugs. "The (federal) government supports needle exchange and rehab programs but so sternly opposes the existence of a facility where drug users can actually use the safe needles and be encouraged to enter rehab. The sticking point appears to be that, at Insite, drug users cannot be arrested and prosecuted."[25] "Allowing and/or encouraging people to inject heroin into their veins is not harm reduction, it is the opposite. . . . We believe it is a form of harm addition," Tony Clement said Tuesday in Mexico City, where he is attending the XVII International AIDS Conference.[25] The assumption is that harm reduction strategies cannot co-exist with the 'war on drugs', as the lines are blurred. Insite reports that patients have a better chance at change if they have a safe and clean place to go. Making the conjecture that a person registered with Insite will change, is just that, a conjecture.

Insite is described as an innovative and effective program for people with very serious illnesses. There are many assumptions being made about the programs, success and ability of Insite to take population health approaches and effectively intervene to improve the quality of care on an individual basis. An assumption that is being made is that interventions such as methadone are treatments for heroin addiction. It is not, but simply a maintenance program with the hopes that the person will never again touch another needle.[26] Yet it became increasingly apparent that methadone may in some cases simply be replacing one drug for another, being interchangeable. While no judgment may be appropriate in some cases, intervention strategies should be put in place to prevent relapse for others. It is not appropriate to generalize population health measures where individual treatment plans are needed. It is like taking a square peg and making it fit into a round hole. Insite and similar harm reduction strategies save some and fail others. Health care is not implemented in a one size fits all for the affluent, so why is it for marginalized individuals? That is a flaw of harm reduction strategies.

third among emergency room mentions and first among drug-associated deaths.

It is also important to note that most opioid overdoses occur in combination with a sedative such as alcohol. Nonetheless, concern about the relatively high rates of non-medical use of opioids and their potential for toxic consequences when misused has led Health Canada, the U.S. FDA, and drug manufacturers to take preventive measures. For example, opioid manufacturers are now required to prepare educational materials that physicians or prescribers can use when counselling patients about the risks and benefits of opioid use, while some opioid manufacturers have developed "abuse deterrent" formulations of their drug (e.g., the drug can't be dissolved in water and injected). The bottom line is that the use of prescription pain reliever has not dramatically increased in recent years, but there appears to be a real concern about the potential for toxicity when the drugs are misused. As is the case with many controlled substances, this situation requires balancing the need for continued access to these medications with measures to reduce their risks.

LO4 Pharmacology of Opioids

The pharmacological action of opioids within the body and brain includes their mechanism of action, chemical structure, and pharmacokinetic properties.

Chemical Characteristics

Raw opium contains about 10% morphine by weight and a smaller amount of codeine. The addition of two acetyl groups to the morphine molecule results in

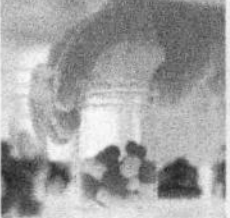

DRUGS IN THE MEDIA

Cottonland: A Community Overdoses on Oxycodone

When the last of Cape Breton's once thriving coal mines shut down in the late 1990s, the shrinking population of Glace Bay, Nova Scotia, faced chronic unemployment because of the collapse of the coal mining, fishing, and steel industries over the past decade. When 18 people died of drug-related overdoses, photojournalist Nancy Ackerman was sent by the *Toronto Star* to Glace Bay to investigate. The prescription medication related to the overdoses was OxyContin, which makes its manufacturer, Purdue Pharmaceutical, more than $1 billion annually. Ackerman decided to make a film, called *Cottonland,* about what she saw and heard. *Cottonland* can be ordered from the National Film Board of Canada (http://www.nfb.ca/film/cottonland/).

Purdue Pharma introduced OxyContin in 1995 and its active ingredient is oxycodone. In *Cottonland,* viewers learn that one 80-milligram OxyContin pill—known as a "green monster" in Glace Bay, contains as much oxycodone as 16 Percocets. As OxyContin came to market, doctors were already trending toward prescribing opioids for chronic pain. Purdue popularized its new drug with a widespread marketing campaign. As Cape Breton's mines were shutting down, OxyContin users discovered that simply crushing the pills ruined the time-release matrix, resulting in much more oxycodone reaching the bloodstream faster. Users then discovered that snorting crushed OxyContin produced a more intense high. Finally, crushing the pills, dissolving them in water, and injecting the mix produced the greatest euphoric effect.

In *Cottonland,* Ackerman interviews a number of people who were actively abusing OxyContin. One man, Eddie, was prescribed the drug for migraine headaches. He quickly became addicted and introduced his girlfriend, Mary, to the drug. Eddie agreed to narrate Ackerman's documentary film, and he provided an entry point into the lives of the people affected by opioid dependence. When Eddie made the decision to get treatment, he found that the closest withdrawal management program was five hours away in the city of Dartmouth. He ended up moving there, overcame his addiction and regained custody of his children. Mary also recovered from her addiction, and the family is now together again.

Cottonland guides us through a culture of despair. Audiences encounter a number of smart, self-aware individuals at different stages of dependency. Some have managed to enter into methadone maintenance treatment programs; others remain addicted to OxyContin. *Cottonland* does not absolve the addict of responsibility but it does illuminate the conditions under which the addict thrives. It also reminds us of the spiral of social ills that follow addiction as families break down and crime increases. The film raises many questions and then asks how an entire community falls into despair. What happens when the social order is weakened by forces beyond its control?

Sources: Based on Matthew McKinnon. 2006. *After the Coal Rush:* Cottonland *Examines the Perils of OxyContin Addiction.* Retrieved October 12, 2011, from http://www.cbc.ca/arts/film/cottonland.html; Herie, M., and W. Skinner. *Substance Abuse in Canada.* Toronto: Oxford University Press, 2010, p. 152; and Loreto, F. Review of *Cottonland.* 2007. Retrieved October 12, 2011, from http://umanitoba.ca/outreach/cm/vol13/no19/cottonland.html.

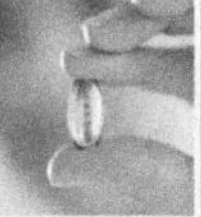

DRUGS IN DEPTH

Prescribing Pain Medications: Damned If You Do and Damned If You Don't

Chronic pain is a condition that can negatively impact an individual's quality of life, by disrupting sleep, employment, social functioning, and many other routine daily activities. In the U.S., approximately one-third of the population (or more than 90 million Americans) has symptoms of chronic pain. Opioids are the most effective medications in the treatment of chronic pain. But, periodic high-profile deaths of celebrities and reports of drugstore robberies reignite concerns about physicians overprescribing opioid pain medications. Many believe that physicians are too quick to distribute opioid medications to patients. Indeed, occasionally media headlines blare with stories about rogue physicians arrested for "pushing pills," that is, dispensing pain medications

continued

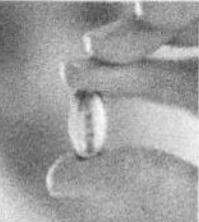

DRUGS IN DEPTH

Prescribing Pain Medications: Damned If You Do and Damned If You Don't

continued

indiscriminately for quick cash. There are also periodic stories of cunning patients who "doctor shop," deceiving physicians in order to obtain large amounts of opioid medications. The fact that most physicians want to do the right thing and are judicious in their prescribing of pain medications is frequently omitted from sensational accounts of the "drug pusher doctor."

This situation, coupled with the fact that pain is a subjective experience that can be difficult to rate externally, has placed pain management physicians in an awkward position. What's more, some patients may have developed tolerance to the medications and may require larger doses to alleviate their symptoms. Many responsible physicians attempting to adequately treat chronic pain patients have come under suspicion for running "pill mills." Some have even been prosecuted and convicted. The message seems clear: "Don't prescribe opioid pain medications but, if you absolutely have to, do so only in small doses." Of course, this could lead to charges of "grossly undertreating" patients' pain symptoms. In 1999, the Oregon Board of Medical Examiners disciplined Dr. Paul Bilder for precisely this reason. In several cases, Dr. Bilder was reluctant to give patients opioid medications, even though their symptoms clearly indicated that these medications were the most prudent course of action. As a result of physicians being sanctioned for both over- and underprescribing opioids, some feel that they are damned if they do and damned if they don't.

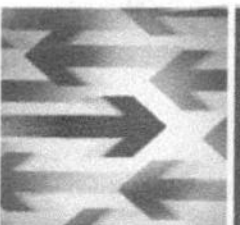

TAKING SIDES

Questioning the Status Quo: Exclusive Use of Opioids for Pain Management in Acute Care: Are We Creating an Impetus for Addiction?

"Pain is whatever the experiencing person says it is, existing whenever the experiencing person says it does."[27] This widely accepted definition was revolutionary in pain management and refers to the subjective nature of pain and its management. It dictates the patient's report of pain to be absolute. There are other methods of treating pain, although more time-consuming, than medical treatment. McCaffery's definition was primarily a response to a belief that pain was undertreated in health care. It did not dictate that opioid administration was the only means of treatment. Are we so encultured to popping a pill that we have we gone to the other extreme? Moreover, chronic administration of narcotics has been documented to exacerbate pain in some patients with or without established substance abuse/dependence.[28] Canadians are among the heaviest consumers of narcotics—the fourth highest per-capita use in the world.[29] In Canada, the predominant form of illicit opioid use (as compared to heroin) is the use of prescription opioids in varying forms originating from the Canadian medical system.[30] Twenty-one percent of Canadian respondents 15 years of age or older reported use of an opioid pain reliever within the past year, and 1.5% reported use to get high.[31,32] Even more problematic is that addiction often starts in hospital.[33]

Pesut and McDonald (2007) uphold that pain absolutely exists when the patient says it does but question whether it is whatever the patient says it is.[34] "Health care professionals, who are familiar with the medical history of an individual, along with the patient themselves, are best placed to determine the most appropriate treatment for an individual. Good communication is an essential risk management tool for all drugs, including opioids."[31] "Patients can be supported in their beliefs of pain while helping them to understand that the actual bodily disturbance may be less than what they believe. The experience of pain is no less real, but it may be appropriate to explore alternative explanations for the pain such as anxiety or suffering."[34] At the very least each situation and client deserve to be treated with respect and empathy as part of an interprofessional/interdisciplinary team during the continuum of use.

diacetylmorphine, or heroin (Figure 13.1). The acetyl groups allow heroin to penetrate the blood-brain barrier more readily, and heroin is therefore two to three times more potent than morphine.

Medicinal chemists have worked hard over the decades to produce compounds that would be effective painkillers, trying to separate the analgesic effect of the opioids from their dependence-producing effects. Although the two effects could not be separated, the research has resulted in a variety of opioids that are sold as pain relievers. Especially interesting among these is fentanyl, which is approximately a hundred times as potent as morphine. Fentanyl is used primarily in conjunction with surgical anaesthesia, although both fentanyl and some of its derivatives have also been manufactured illegally and sold on the streets.

In addition to the opioid analgesics, this search for new compounds led to the discovery of **opioid antagonists**, drugs that block the action of morphine, heroin, or other opioid agonists. The administration of a drug such as **naloxone** (Narcan) or *nalorphine* can save a person's life by reversing the depressed respiration resulting from an opioid overdose (see Taking Sides). If given to an individual who has been taking opioids and who has become physically dependent, these antagonists can precipitate an immediate withdrawal syndrome. Both naloxone and the longer-lasting *naltrexone* have been given to dependent individuals to prevent them from experiencing a high if they then use heroin. Table 13.3 summarizes the different pharmacokinetic properties of various opioids used in Canada.

opioid antagonists: drugs that can block the actions of opioids.

naloxone: an opioid antagonist.

enkephalins: morphine-like neurotransmitters found in the brain and adrenals.

Mechanism of Action

The finding that opioid receptors exist in the membrane of some neurons led to an obvious question: What are opioid receptors doing in the synapses of the brain—waiting for someone to extract the juice from a poppy? Scientists all over the world went to work, looking for a substance in the brain that could serve as the natural activator of these opioid receptors. Groups in England and Sweden succeeded in 1974: A pair of molecules, leu-enkephalin and met-enkephalin, were isolated from brain extracts. These **enkephalins** acted like morphine and were many times more potent. Next came the discovery of a

Figure 13.1 Narcotic Agents Isolated or Derived from Opium

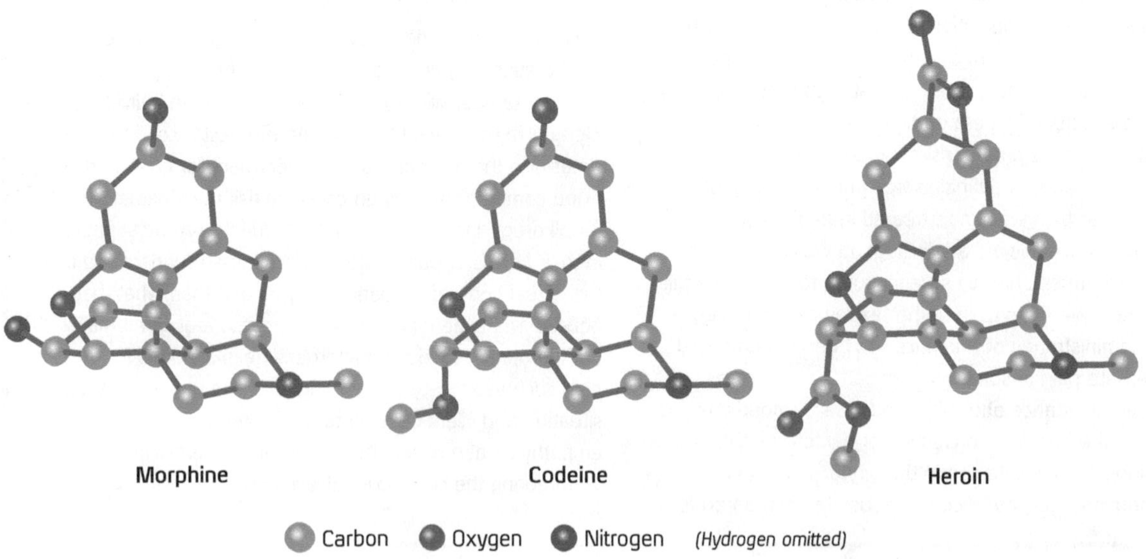

Table 13.3 Pharmacological Properties of Different Opioids Available in Canada

Generic Name	Trade Names	Routes of Administration*	Equivalent Dose (mg)†	Duration of Action (h)
Agonists				
alfentanil	Alfenta	intravenous	0.4–0.8	0.5–0.1
codeine	Various	oral	200	4–6
		injection	120	4–6
fentanyl	Duragesic, Fentanyl Citrate	transdermal	NA	NA
		injection	0.1–0.2	1–2
hydrocodone	Tussionex	oral	–	4–6
hydromorphone	Dilaudid	oral	4–6	>5
		injection	2	>5
methadone		oral	–	24–36
morphine	MS Contin, MOS, others	oral	30	4–5
		injection	10	4–5
oxycodone	Percodan, Percocet	oral	30	3–6
pethidine	Demerol	oral	300	2–4
		injection	75	2–4
sufentanil	Sufenta	intravenous	0.01–0.04	NA
tramadol	Tramacet	oral	NA	3–6
Agonists–Antagonists				
buprenorphine/naloxone	Suboxone	sublingual	NA	24
butorphanol	APO-Butorphanol	intranasal	2	3–4
nalbuphine	Nubain	subcutaneous	10	3–6
pentazocine	Talwin	oral	180	3–6
		injection	60	–
Antagonists				
naloxone	Targin	intravenous	NA	NA
naltrexone	Revia	oral	NA	NA

*Injection route (parenteral) may include subcutaneous, intramuscular, or intravenous; †Approximate equivalent dose (milligrams) compared with morphine 10 milligrams intramuscular; NA = not applicable.

Source: Adapted from the Canadian Pharmacists Association. *Compendium of Pharmaceuticals and Specialties*, 2010. Ottawa: Author, 2010.

group of **endorphins** (endogenous morphinelike substances) that are also found in brain tissue and have potent opioid effects. In addition to these two major types of endogenous opioids, dynorphins and other substances have some actions similar to those of morphine. These substances, as well as the natural and synthetic opioid drugs, have actions on at least three types of opioid receptors, the structures of which were discovered in the 1990s. Both mu and kappa opioid receptors play a role in pain perception, while the functions of the delta receptor are not as easily understood.[35] One of the most important sites of action may be the midbrain central gray, a region known to be involved in pain perception. However, there are many other sites of interaction between these systems and areas that relate to pain, and pain itself is a complex psychological and neurological phenomenon, so we cannot say that we understand completely how opioids act to reduce pain.

In addition to the presence of these endogenous opioids in the brain, large amounts of endorphins are released from the pituitary gland in response to

endorphins: morphine-like neurotransmitters found in the brain and pituitary gland.

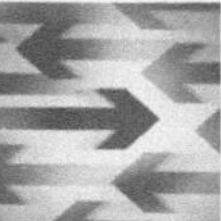

TAKING SIDES

Should Naloxone Be Made Available to Heroin Users?

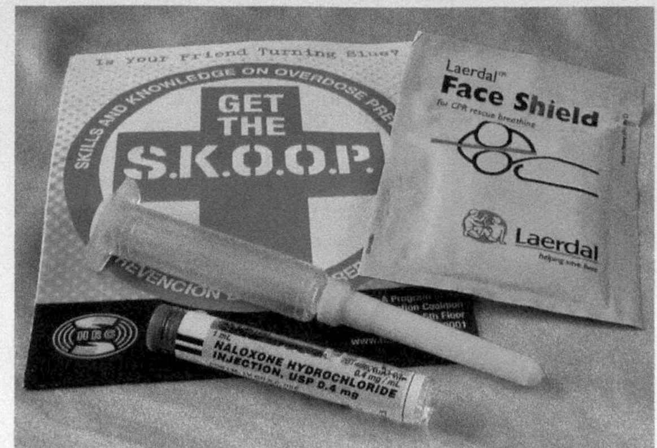

Each year hundreds of heroin users die from overdose. Most of these deaths occur in the presence of a drug-using mate, who may be reluctant to contact emergency medical services for fear of prosecution. Naloxone, a fast-acting opioid antagonist, can reverse opioid-induced respiratory depression and prevent death if given within minutes of an overdose. While naloxone has been used in hospital emergency departments for decades, it is not readily available to heroin users because it can be obtained only via a prescription. However, concern regarding the increased number of heroin-related overdose deaths has prompted health officials in several U.S. and Canadian cities, including Vancouver,[36] to initiate programs that would provide naloxone and rescue-breathing training to illicit drug users.

Despite reported reductions in the number of overdose deaths in areas where these programs exist, critics argue that by making heroin use less dangerous it sends a message that illicit drug use is condoned and will decrease the likelihood of heroin abusers seeking treatment. Proponents, however, view such programs as a form of harm reduction—that is, drug users will be kept alive until they are ready to enter treatment. What do you think?

stress. Also, enkephalins are released from the adrenal gland. The functions of these peptides circulating through the blood as hormones are not understood at this point. They could perhaps reduce pain by acting in the spinal cord, but they are unlikely to produce direct effects in the brain because they probably do not cross the blood-brain barrier. It has been speculated that long-distance runners experience a release of endorphins that might be responsible for the so-called runner's high. Unfortunately, the only evidence in support of this notion was measurements of blood levels of endorphins that seemed to be elevated in some, but not all, runners. These endorphins are presumably from the pituitary and might not be capable of producing a high. It is not known whether exercise alters *brain* levels of these substances.

LO5 Beneficial Uses

Opioids have defined medical uses, including pain relief, easing of intestinal disorders, and cough suppression.

Pain Relief

The major therapeutic indication for morphine and the other opioids is the reduction of pain. After the administration of an analgesic dose of morphine, some patients report that they are still aware of pain but that the pain is no longer aversive. The opioids seem to have their effect in part by diminishing the patient's awareness of and response to the aversive stimulus. Morphine primarily reduces the emotional response to pain (the suffering) and to some extent the knowledge of the pain stimulus.

The effect of opioids is relatively specific to pain. Fewer effects on mental and motor ability accompany analgesic doses of these agents than accompany equipotent doses of other analgesic and depressant drugs. Although one of the characteristics of these drugs is their ability to reduce pain without inducing sleep, drowsiness is not uncommon after a therapeutic dose. (In the user's vernacular, the patient is "on the nod.") The patient is readily awakened if sleeping, and dreams during the sleep period are frequent.

Intestinal Disorders

Opioids have long been valued for their effects on the gastrointestinal system. They quiet colic and save lives by counteracting diarrhea. In years past and today in many underdeveloped countries, contaminated food and water have resulted in severe intestinal infections (dysentery). Particularly in the young and the elderly, diarrhea and resulting dehydration can be a major cause of death.

Opioid drugs decrease the number of peristaltic contractions, which is the type of contraction responsible for moving food through the intestines. Considerable water is absorbed from the intestinal material; this fact, plus the decrease in peristaltic contractions, often results in constipation in patients taking the drugs for pain relief. This side effect is what has saved the lives of many dysentery victims. Although modern synthetic opioids are now sold for this purpose, old-fashioned paregoric, an opium solution, is still available for the symptomatic relief of diarrhea.

Cough Suppressants

The opioids also have the effect of decreasing activity in what advertisers refer to as the cough control centre in the medulla. Although coughing is often a useful way of clearing unwanted material from the respiratory passages, at times nonproductive coughing can itself become a problem. Since it was first purified from opium, codeine has been widely used for its **antitussive** properties and is still available in a number of prescription cough remedies. Nonprescription cough remedies contain dextromethorphan, an opioid analogue that is somewhat more selective in its antitussive effects. At high doses, dextromethorphan produces hallucinogenic effects through a different mechanism, by blocking one type of glutamate receptor.

Figure 13.2 Admissions to the CAMH Medical Withdrawal Management Service for Opioid Detoxification, 2000–2004

The number of admissions for opioid detoxification to the Centre for Addiction and Mental Health (CAMH) Medical Withdrawal Management Service increased over the five years (2000, $n = 78$; 2001, $n = 96$; 2002, $n = 120$; 2003, $n = 111$; and 2004, $n = 166$).

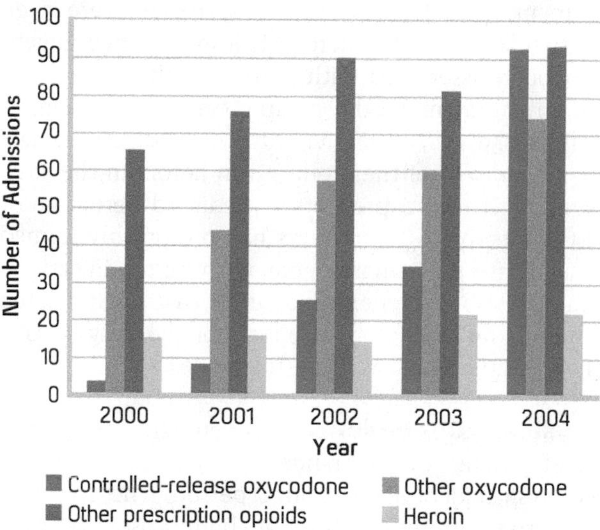

Source: Sproule, B., and others. "Changing Patterns in Opioid Addiction: Characterizing Users of OxyContin and Other Prescription Opioids." *Canadian Family Physician* 55 (2009), pp. 68, 69, 68.e1–69.e5. Copyright © The College of Family Physicians of Canada.

LO6 Causes for Concern

Despite their effectiveness as treatments for pain, intestinal disorder, and cough suppressants, opioid abuse, opioid dependence, and opioid toxicity are causes for concern. (See Figure 13.2 for data on admissions to a medical withdrawal management service.)

Dependence Potential

Tolerance Tolerance develops to most of the effects of the opioids, although with different effects tolerance can occur at different rates. If the drug is used chronically for pain relief, for example, it will probably be necessary to increase the dose to maintain a constant effect. The same is true for the euphoria sought by recreational users: Repeated use results in a decreased effect, which can be overcome by increasing the dose. Cross-tolerance exists among all the opioids. Tolerance to one reduces the effectiveness of each of the others. Siegel and others have shown that psychological processes can play an important role in the tolerance to opioids.[37] When a user repeatedly injects an opioid agonist, various physiological effects occur (changes in body temperature, intestinal motility, respiration rate, and so on). With repeated experience the dependent person might unconsciously learn to anticipate those effects and to counteract them. Animal experiments have shown that, after repeated morphine injections, a placebo injection produces changes in body

antitussive: a medication used to suppress or relieve coughing.

temperature opposite to those originally produced by morphine. Thus, some of the body's tolerance to opioids results from conditioned reflex responses to the stimuli associated with taking the drugs. To demonstrate how important these conditioned protective reflexes can become, Siegel and his colleagues injected rats with heroin every other day in a particular environment. After 15 such injections, the rats were given a much larger dose of heroin, half in the environment previously associated with heroin and half in a different environment. Of the group given the heroin injection in the different environment, most of the rats died. However, of the group given heroin in the environment that had previously predicted heroin, most of the rats lived.[38] Those rats had presumably learned to associate that environment with heroin injections, and conditioned reflexes occurred that counteracted some of the physiological effects of the drug. This is one example of behavioural tolerance.

Physical Dependence Concomitant with the development of tolerance is the establishment of physical dependence: in a person who has used the drug chronically and at high doses, as each dose begins to wear off, certain withdrawal symptoms begin to appear. These symptoms and their approximate timing after opioid use are listed in Table 13.4. This list of symptoms might have more personal meaning for you if you compare it to a case of the 24-hour, or intestinal, flu. Combine nausea and vomiting with diarrhea, aches, pains, and a general sense of misery, and you have a pretty good idea of what a moderate case of opioid withdrawal is like—rarely life-threatening, but most unpleasant. If an individual has been taking a large amount of the drug, then these symptoms can be much worse than those caused by 24-hour flu and can last at least twice as long. Note that **methadone**, a long-lasting synthetic opioid, produces withdrawal symptoms that are usually less severe and that appear later than with heroin but may last longer. Cross-dependence is seen among the opioids. No matter which of them was responsible for producing the initial dependence, withdrawal symptoms can be prevented by an appropriate dose of any opioid agonist. This is the basis for the use of methadone in treating heroin dependence, because substituting legal methadone prevents withdrawal symptoms for as much as a day.

methadone: a long-lasting synthetic opioid.

An interesting clue to the biochemical mechanism of withdrawal symptoms has been the finding that *clonidine*, an alpha-adrenergic agonist that is used to treat high blood pressure, can diminish the severity of withdrawal symptoms. Studies on brain tissue reveal that opioid receptors and alpha-adrenergic receptors are found together in some brain areas, including the norepinephrine-containing cells of the locus ceruleus.

Table 13.4 Sequence of Appearance of Some of the Abstinence Syndrome Symptoms

	Approximate Hours After Previous Dose	
Signs	**Heroin and Morphine**	**Methadone**
Craving for drugs, anxiety	6	24
Yawning, perspiration, running nose, teary eyes	14	34–48
Increase in above signs plus pupil dilation, goose bumps (piloerection), tremors (muscle twitches), hot and cold flashes, aching bones and muscles, loss of appetite	16	48–72
Increased intensity of above, plus insomnia; raised blood pressure; increased temperature, pulse rate, respiratory rate and depth; restlessness; nausea	24–36	
Increased intensity of above, plus curled-up position, vomiting, diarrhea, weight loss, spontaneous ejaculation or orgasm, hemoconcentration (an increase in the red blood cells in the blood), increased blood glucose	36–48	

Psychological Dependence That opioids produce psychological dependence is quite clear; in fact, experiments with opioids were what led to our current understanding of the importance of the reinforcing properties of drugs. Animals allowed to self-administer low doses of morphine or heroin intravenously will learn the required behaviours quickly and will perform them for prolonged periods, even if they have never experienced withdrawal symptoms. This is an example of what psychologists refer to as *positive reinforcement:* a behaviour is reliably followed by the presentation of a stimulus, leading to an increase in the probability of the behaviour and its eventual maintenance at a higher rate than before. Remember that the rapidity with which the reinforcing stimulus follows the behaviour is an important factor, which is why fewer experiences are needed with an opioid injected intravenously (fast acting) than with the same drug taken orally (delayed action).

Once physical dependence has developed and withdrawal symptoms are experienced, the conditions are set up for another behavioural mechanism, *negative reinforcement*. In this situation an act (drug taking) is followed by the *removal* of withdrawal symptoms, leading to further strengthening of the habit. In heroin dependence, the appearance of early withdrawal symptoms after only a few hours and their rapid alleviation by another injection typically leads to the development of a more robust dependence in many users. Remember, however, that heroin was prescribed in low doses and taken orally by many patients for several years during which it was believed not to produce dependence. Although heroin is more potent than morphine and may have a higher abuse potential because of its more rapid access to the brain, morphine taken intravenously is more likely to produce dependence than heroin taken orally.

Toxicity Potential

Both acute toxicity and chronic toxicity are possible with opioid use.

Acute Toxicity One specific effect of the opioids is to depress the respiratory centres in the brain, so that respiration slows and becomes shallow. This is perhaps the major side effect of the opioids and one of the most dangerous, because death resulting from respiratory depression can follow an excessive dose of these drugs. The basis for this effect is that the respiratory centres become less responsive to carbon dioxide levels in the blood. It is this effect that keeps opioids near the top of the list of mentioned drugs in DAWN coroners' reports. As discussed earlier, this respiratory depression is additive with the effects of alcohol or other sedative-hypnotics, and a large fraction of those who die from heroin overdose have elevated blood alcohol concentrations and might better be described as dying from a combination of heroin (or another opioid) and alcohol. Opioid overdose can be diagnosed on the basis of the *opioid triad:* coma, depressed respiration, and pinpoint pupils. Emergency medical treatment calls for the use of naloxone (Narcan), which antagonizes the opioid effects within a few minutes (see Targeting Prevention).

The behavioural consequences of having morphine like drugs in the brain are probably less dangerous.

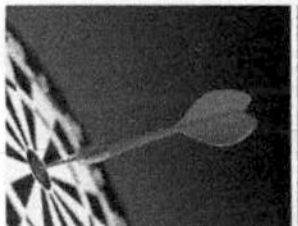

TARGETING PREVENTION

Take Home Naloxone: Backgrounder—Opioid Overdoses in BC

Opioid overdose is a public health issue in BC, contributing to significant mortality and morbidity. Provincewide in 2011, provisional data suggest over 275 deaths were attributed to illicit drug overdoses (96 in Fraser and 97 in Metro Vancouver regions). In 2011, the BC coroner's service reported a cluster of drug overdose deaths related to an increase in heroin potency. Prescription opioids contributed to over 70 deaths in 2009. Total overdose events are likely higher than what has been reported as overdose does not necessarily result in death. However the lack of oxygen to the brain during an overdose event can lead to lifelong harms.

Naloxone Can Prevent Opioid Morbidity and Mortality

Unintentional deaths from opioid overdose are preventable with overdose and naloxone education. Naloxone, or

continued

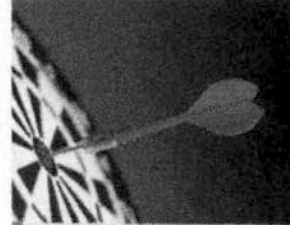

TARGETING PREVENTION

Take Home Naloxone: Backgrounder— Opioid Overdoses in BC

continued

Narcan®, has been used in emergency settings for over 40 years in Canada and is on the WHO List of Essential Medicines. The BC ambulance service administered naloxone 2367 times in 2011. It is a pure opioid antagonist which will quickly reverse life-threatening respiratory depression of opioids to restore breathing, usually in 2–5 minutes. Naloxone is not a controlled substance, it cannot be abused, and in the absence of narcotics has no pharmacologic activity. Research has shown having naloxone available does not increase risk taking behaviour. Naloxone is a safe drug with minimal side effects, even less than an epi-pen.

Naloxone Take-Home Programs in Canada and Around the World

Take Home Naloxone (THN) programs provide naloxone to people who use opioids (legally prescribed or illegally obtained) and are at risk of an overdose. It is not intended to replace emergency care or minimize the importance of calling 911. But because 85% of overdoses happen within the company of others, having naloxone offers the opportunity to save a life and reduce harms related to the overdose while waiting for the paramedics to arrive. Mathematical modelling in the U.S. has demonstrated that naloxone, in conjunction with overdose education, has a synergistic effect; having a greater effect on reducing overdose events than if provided individually.

Numerous programs already exist globally, including more than 180 programs in the U.S. BC's Overdose Prevention Program is modelled on the successes of such programs and combines education (prevention, identification, and response to overdose) with a Take Home Naloxone (THN) kit for individuals who are using opioids, thus individuals can reduce overdose risks and be prepared in the event of an opioid overdose.

The BC Pilot Program

Distribution of naloxone kits will be piloted through the BC Harm Reduction Program. In BC naloxone is a prescription-only medication (POM); therefore it must be prescribed to a specific individual with indications for personal use by a physician. BC has a unique challenge unlike other Canadian provinces that continue to utilize pre-written orders where a nurse can sign off on a prescription or medical directives are in place. In BC, training can be performed by a health care provider (i.e., nurse); however, a physician must prescribe the kit to a named patient. Resources to assist organizations wanting to address overdose in their community are available from our website at: www.towardtheheart.com

Considerations

Naloxone is relatively safe with minimal potential adverse effects. The only contraindication to naloxone is hypersensitivity. Naloxone may precipitate withdrawal in individuals with opioid dependency. Naloxone should be used with caution in patients with a history of seizures and cardiovascular disease. However, the harms associated with oxygen deprivation during an opioid overdose are likely far more serious. Naloxone only works to take the opioids out of an overdose scenario; individuals may have confounding medical factors and substances that need acute clinical care. Therefore medical professionals are the best individuals to deal with an overdose.

Calling 911 is an important component of the overdose response. Responders are taught to call 911 and stay with the individual for multiple reasons: to inform the person what has happened, to ensure that the person does not take more substances, to inform the medical response team of individual's current state, and to administer a second dose of naloxone if the overdose returns. The effect of naloxone begins to wear off after 30 minutes, therefore the overdose may return. This will depend if the drug taken has a long half-life (e.g., methadone), how much was consumed, the individual's metabolism (ability to break down the drugs) and other medical conditions.

Conclusion

Overdose and naloxone education programs are effective in communicating risks about substance use and will save lives. We believe there is a strong ethical responsibility to provide such services to individuals in BC who are at risk. We encourage people in BC affected by opioid overdose, physicians, policy makers, people who take opioids and their family members, and service providers, to identify ways they can reduce the occurrence and harmful consequences of opioid overdoses through education, and requesting and prescribing naloxone.

Source: Adapted from Toward the Heart (2014). A Project of the Provincial Harm Reduction Program. Retrieved June 2, 2014 from http://towardtheheart.com/naloxone/. Used with permission. BC Centre for Disease Control.

Those who inject heroin might nod off into a dream-filled sleep for a few minutes, and opium smokers are famous for their "pipe dreams." It is perhaps not surprising that individuals under the influence of opioids are likely to be less active and less alert than they otherwise would be. A clouding of consciousness makes mental work more difficult.

Opioid agonists also stimulate the brain area controlling nausea and vomiting, which are other frequent side effects. Nausea occurs in about half of ambulatory patients given a 15 mg dose of morphine. Also, nausea and vomiting are a common reaction to heroin among street users.

Chronic Toxicity Although early in the twentieth century many medical authorities believed that chronic opioid use weakened the user both mentally and physically, there is no scientific evidence that exposure to opioid drugs per se causes long-term damage to any tissue or organ system. Many street users do suffer from sores and abscesses at injection sites, but these can be attributed to the lack of sterile technique. Also, the practice of sharing needles can result in the spread of such blood-borne diseases as serum hepatitis and HIV. Again, this is a result not of the drug but of the technique used to inject it.

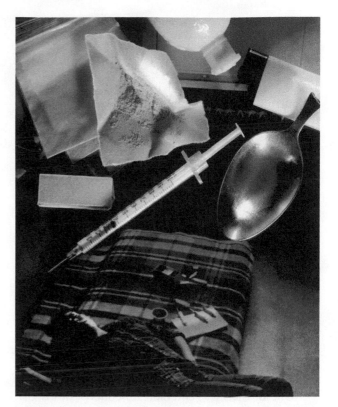

Supplies for shooting up heroin.

Patterns of Abuse

The Life of a Person Addicted to Heroin Only a glimpse of some of the mechanics of a heroin addict's life can be presented here. And it's important to emphasize here that the following presentation does not represent the typical heroin user, but it attempts to provide one view of heroin addiction. Withdrawal signs might begin about four hours after the previous use of the drug, but many users report that they begin to feel ill six to eight hours after the previous dose. That puts most heroin abusers on a schedule of three or four injections every day. Today's heroin user is not spending a lot of time nodding off in opium dens, as in the "good old days." When you have a very important appointment to keep every six to eight hours, every day of the week, every day of the year, you've got to hustle not to miss one of them. Remember, there are no vacations, no weekends off for the regular user, just 1200 to 1400 appointments per year to keep. And each one costs money. Heroin is frequently sold on the street in "dime" bags: $10 for a small plastic bag containing anybody's guess. The material in a $10 bag might have 3 mg or 30 mg. Of course, you might not get *any* heroin, and you can't complain to the Better Business Bureau. At any rate, your habit can cost you $30 to $100 a day.

The variability is a problem because of the possibility of an overdose. Heroin users should worry about an overdose with each new batch of drug used. A sophisticated user buying from a new or questionable source will initially try a much smaller than normal amount of the powder to evaluate its potency.

The most common form of heroin use by male users is to inject the drug intravenously–colloquially referred to as banging. A convenient site is the left forearm (for right-handed users), and frequent injection leaves the arm marked with scar tissue. If the larger veins of the arm collapse, then other body areas are used. Many beginning users start by "skin-popping"–subcutaneous injections. Skin-popping increases the danger of tetanus but decreases the risk of hepatitis compared with banging. Because of the lack of sterility, hepatitis, tetanus, and abscesses at the site of injection are not uncommon in street users who inject drugs.

If the user survives the perils of an overdose, escapes the dangers of contaminated equipment, and avoids being caught, there are still other dangers. Heroin is a potent analgesic, and its regular use can conceal the early symptoms of an illness, such as pneumonia. The user's lack of money for, or interest in, food can result in malnutrition. With low resistance from malnutrition and the symptoms of illness going unnoticed as a result of heroin use, the user may be more susceptible to serious disease.

If all these dangers are overcome, the user might continue to use opioids to an advanced age. Sometimes, however, the user who avoids illness, death, or arrest and who does not enter and stay in a rehabilitation program or withdraw him- or herself from the drug might no longer feel the need for the drug and gradually stop using it. This "maturing out" is probably what happens to a large number of heroin abusers.

Misconceptions and Preconceptions Most people have strongly held beliefs about heroin, derived from television, magazines, movies, and conversations. These individuals, including many professionals, have major misconceptions about non-medical use and misuse of opioids.

One of the most common misconceptions is that injecting heroin or morphine induces in everyone an intense pleasure unequalled by any other experience. Often it is described as similar to a whole-body orgasm that persists up to five or more minutes. Some users report that they try with every injection to re-experience the extreme euphoria of the first injection, but always have a lesser effect. However, studies, as well as clinical and street reports, show that some people experience nausea and discomfort after the initial intravenous administration of morphine or heroin. Despite this, some of these users persist and the discomfort decreases–that is, it shows tolerance more rapidly than the euphoric effects. Under these conditions the injections soon result primarily in pleasant effects. To maintain these pleasurable feelings, though, the dose level must gradually be increased if the drug is used on a regular basis.

Another misconception has to do with the development of withdrawal symptoms. The heroin user undergoing withdrawal without medication is always portrayed as being in excruciating pain, truly suffering. It depends. With a large habit, withdrawal without medication is truly subjective hell. The opioid abuse scene is changing too rapidly to be definite about today's user, but many street users use a low daily drug dose. For many such users, the withdrawal symptoms resemble a mild case of intestinal flu (cramps, diarrhea).

Perhaps the most common misconception about heroin is that, after one shot, you are hooked for life. None of the opioids, or any other drug, fits into that fantasized category. Becoming dependent takes time, perhaps weeks, and persistence on the part of the beginner. Regular use of the drug seems to be more important in establishing physical dependence than the size of the dose used. Becoming physically dependent is possible on a weekend, but it frequently requires a longer period, with three or four injections a day.

There are probably about one million opioid-dependent individuals in the United States. There may be two to three times as many heroin *chippers*–occasional users. Several reports have appeared on the characteristics of these occasional users, but no consistent differences, compared with opioid-dependent persons, have yet been found other than the pattern of use.

LO7 Research Studies and Pilots Addressing the Needs of Injection Drug Users in Canada

A number of research studies and service initiatives in Canada are designed to evaluate the needs of injection drug users.

"Drug use must be addressed as a public health issue across Canada."[39] In May 2003, the Government of Canada underscored its commitment to addressing the ongoing public health concern of substance abuse with its renewed Canada's Drug Strategy (CDS). The goal of the CDS was to significantly reduce the harm associated with alcohol and other drugs using a broad four-component approach that included education, prevention, harm reduction, and enforcement. The CDS initiative balances a population-based approach, with the goal of decreasing consumption and related risks, with harm-reduction measures that focus on reducing the risks and severity of adverse consequences arising from drug and alcohol use while not necessarily reducing consumption.[40,41] Harm-reduction strategies include supervised injection sites such as Insite in Vancouver's Downtown Eastside.

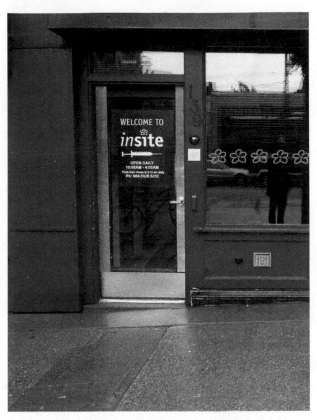

Insite: A unique entry point into Canadian health care services for drug users.

Insite: Vancouver's Supervised Injection Facility*

Insite was an experiment in population health, and as an experiment was granted exemption from drug enforcement laws (Section 56 of the Controlled Drugs and Substances Act), allowing the injection of illegal drugs on the premises. Insite does not provide the drugs. At first glance Insite may be thought to promote intravenous drug use, but closer inspection reveals Insite as a unique entry point into the Canadian health care system for marginalized populations, even if that means a clean needle or a safe place to inject. For every dollar spent, four dollars are saved. Clients are 33% more likely to get into detox if they are registered with Insite.[39,42]

*The authors thank Lindsay Leighton and Anne Brochu for contributions to this section.

Insite offers an opportunity for political action and health policy reform:

> Inequities in health and access to health care for marginalized groups have received limited attention in bioethics. People who are street involved such as those experiencing homelessness and drug use face multiple inequities in health and access to health care. Morbidity and mortality are significantly increased among those who are street involved. Incorporation of a harm reduction philosophy in health care has the potential to shift the moral context of health care delivery and enhance access to health care services. However, harm reduction with a primary focus on reducing the harms of drug use fails focus on the harms associated with the context of drug use such as homelessness, violence and poverty.[43]

Insite offers onsite detox services and housing services. Housing and poverty are social determinants of health that nurses can advocate for and against, respectively.[44] The role of the nurse is both as a health care service provider and as an educator. Nursing staff educate drug users who use the facility on a number of issues related to injection health and safety, as discussed in more detail below. Insite saves lives.[45]

An Attempt to Deal with Injection Drug Users

Supervised injection sites began to gain recognition in the 1980s in reaction to growing incidents of public injecting, drug overdoses, and sharing syringes. For decades now, drug use by route of IV injection has been highly correlated with the disease. Through the sharing of needles, injection drug users (IDU) account for a large portion of people affected by hepatitis C, HIV, or AIDS.[46] Innovative strategies needed to be developed in order to control for the increasing rate of IDU who have been diagnosed with either HIV or AIDS. There are currently approximately 65 recognized supervised injection facilities (SIF) in eight different countries around the world.[47] Although the number of SIFs has grown steadily over the last 30 years, their establishment is still a hotly debated topic among citizens and government officials.

Insite, the first SIF in North America, was created in the Downtown Eastside of Vancouver and opened in September 2003.[48] Insite is able to operate under an exemption to the Controlled Drugs and Substances Act, which allows the facility to operate despite the presence of illegal drugs. Medically supervised SIFs allow injection drug users to safely inject pre-obtained illicit drugs, to reduce the impacts of drug use on the public health system.[45] The exemption was awarded based on the idea that research would be done at Insite to determine its effectiveness. The Downtown Eastside area is the location of well-documented overdose and infectious disease epidemics among its estimated 5000 injection drug users.[48,49] At present, 26 research studies have validated the effectiveness of the Insite SIF operations.[50] Two court decisions have supported the notion of SIFs as health care services appropriate for caring for persons who use drugs. Despite these findings, the Conservative federal government of Canada has appealed these decisions in an effort to shut down Insite; however, these attempts have been unsuccessful and the facility continues to provide health care services through professionals who work without contravention of the law.[50]

An essential part of the research component connected with Insite is an onsite database that is used to track activities and health-related events at the facility. Each SIF user is registered anonymously and provides basic demographic information.[45] This allows each event at the site to be tracked back to particular visitors. These records also include details about all overdoses and interventions that occur at Insite.[49]

One of the components of the Insite program includes safer injection education. Nursing staff educate drug users who use the facility on a number of issues related to injection health and safety. Some of the topics most frequently discussed and/or demonstrated include being shown how to find a vein and/or tie off properly; being shown how to heat the solution to dissolve solid constituents and filter properly; being shown how to inject safely; and receiving information about safer injecting.[51] A principal reason for launching SIFs like Insite is to lessen the occurrence of overdose, through education, clean facilities, and the provision of emergency response in the event of an overdose.[49] Insite also provides health care, counselling, treatment, and referrals to external health and social services.[46]

Relationship between SIF Participation and Drug Use Behaviours Benefits of the Insite SIF seem to stem from two distinct sources. One is the direct availability of clean injecting equipment, and the other is the indirect change in behaviours among injection drug users.[48] Of the 336 overdoses that happened onsite during one particular 18-month study, 89% involved only one injection; of these, 71% involved heroin, 13% involved cocaine, 10% involved speedballs (cocaine + heroin), 2% involved morphine, 1.7% involved Dilaudid, 1.4% involved crack, and 0.7% involved methadone. Instances that included two successive injections during the same visit accounted for 11% of the overdoses.[45]

Although these numbers represent a smaller proportion of overdoses than are seen outside of Insite, a fair number still occur, and medical staff must be prepared to respond. The most frequently seen indicators of overdose included depressed respiration, limp body, facial discolouring, and failing to respond to pain stimulus.[49] The most common medical interventions to overdoses at the SIF included oxygen administration, calling an ambulance (28% included transfer to a hospital), and naloxone hydrochloride administration. No overdoses resulted in fatalities.[47,49] A number of factors have been identified as predictors of time to first overdose at the SIF. These include fewer years injecting, being female, engaging in daily heroin use, being a binge drug user, having a history of overdose, and involvement in the sex trade.[49] One of the mandates at Insite is to provide visitors with safe injection education. Predictors associated with those who are likely to receive this information included being female, having difficulty accessing syringes, engaging in public injection, syringe borrowing and lending, requiring assistance with the injection, being a binge drug user, participation in an addiction treatment program, involvement in the sex trade, and use of Insite for more than 75% of all injections.[51] The results from these various research studies illustrate how SIFs can help manage injection drug overdoses, and reduce fatalities associated with injection drug use through direct response to overdoses and indirect education that has the potential to change the behaviours of drug users.[45] Further evaluations confirmed that the primary objectives of reducing public injecting, syringe sharing, overdose risk, and increasing access to treatment were met, along with the potentially more controversial goal of showing that SIFs like Insite do not encourage drug use or increase crime.[47,48]

Accessibility and Available Resources Insite offers visitors the chance to anonymously take advantage of the resources available onsite. These resources include a clean environment, sterile equipment, medical supervision over 12 injection booths, education, addiction treatment services, and referrals to other social and health agencies. Visitors are free to make use of any or all of these resources during hours of operation, currently between 10 a.m. and 4 a.m., which aims to maximize the time available for safer injections. Insite was not developed as an independent facility, but rather is part of a continuum of care for people struggling with substance abuse, specifically targeted at those who are not well supported or connected to health care services.[52] Participation as a visitor to Insite is the first step in dealing with addiction for many users. Located above Insite is a partnered program known as Onsite, which is capable of caring for 12 clients who are ready to begin detox and withdrawal management. Following treatment at Onsite, clients can then be assisted through the transition into housing and continuing community support as they reintegrate into the community.[52]

Statistics from Insite show that in 2009 alone, 5446 individuals made use of resources at the SIF, resulting in a total of 276 178 visits over the course of the year. An average of 702 visits were made each day, resulting in an average of 491 daily injections. Almost 2500 clinical treatments were provided and over 6000 referrals were made.[52] Since it opened in 2003, Insite has had more than 1.5 million visits, and 12 000 clients are currently registered at the SIF.[52] Approximately half of these clients are not ready for addiction treatment as other factors in their lives currently take precedence, such as stabilizing a chaotic lifestyle, or requiring other medical interventions.[52] For these visitors Insite can help foster positive attachment to the overall health care system, which enhances the opportunity to provide other services like care for wound infections, TB, and inoculations for flu and pneumonia, and increases the likelihood of taking HIV/AIDS medications if needed.[52] Injection drug users who visit Insite are more likely to enter a detox program than users who do not make use of the SIF, and that number increases further for users who visit Insite weekly and speak with an addiction counsellor.[52] Twenty percent of Insite clients have accessed detox services, which is noteworthy as this population is least likely to access care.[52]

Cost-Benefit Analysis As limited resources for public health care must be distributed based on some form of economic efficiency, Andresen and Boyd (2010) conducted a detailed cost-benefit analysis for the operation of Insite using data from 2007.[48] The number of new HIV infections and deaths prevented was calculated using mathematical modelling and secondary data, and the cost of illness and death prevented was calculated and then compared to the cost to run the SIF. The annual costs for a number of factors were calculated and included in the cost-benefit analysis. Examples of these figures included operational cost ($1.5 million), individual HIV infection treatment ($150 000), and the loss to society for each new HIV infection ($500 000) and fatal overdose ($660 000). By combining HIV and fatal overdoses the number of potential deaths prevented by Insite was 2.87, as well as 35 prevented new HIV infections each year. The cost-benefit analysis showed an average benefit-to-cost ratio of 5.12 (range from 3.0–8.04), indicating a positive economic return.[48] Benefit-to-cost ratios for other conventional drug interventions have, on average, not been shown to be superior to Insite in cost savings to the public health sector (i.e., drug treatment programs 1.33–4.34, drug courts 1.74–6.32, and voluntary drug treatment in prison 1.79–5.74). In a study conducted by Pinkerton (2010), it was found that cases of HIV disease among Vancouver's IDU users would rise from 179.3 to 262.8, which is a difference of 83.5 infections each year.[46] The cost difference between prevention and treatment is 17.3 million to treat, whereas the cost to run Insite each year is $3 million. This will save Health Canada and the government millions of dollars in the long run.

Increased Drug Use? Many people fear that having such facilities can lead to increased drug use, relapse, reduced rates of cessation among current users, and higher rates of binge use. Kerr et al. (2006) conducted a study to see if such a place actually increased the rates of relapse, reduction in cessation among current users as well as whether there were any increases in binge use. This study looked at data from a year before the Insite facility had opened and one year following its opening. The results indicated that there were no significant differences in relapse, cessation of current users, and increases in binge use due to having such a facility.[45]

Canadian Reaction Topics such as needle exchange programs, supervised injection facilities, and safe injection education remain controversial, and are bound to elicit reactions from people who involve themselves in these issues. In general the Canadian public is currently fairly supportive of Insite and opposed to moves by the Conservative government to close the program[53] (see Table 13.5). Just under half (43%) of Canadians support the operation of Insite, whereas just under a quarter (24%) oppose the facility. Similar numbers were found when Canadians were asked their opinion on the federal government's decision to appeal to the Supreme Court of Canada in an effort to shut down Insite (40% disagreed and 27% agreed). Despite the intensity of

Table 13.5 Canadians Are Supportive of Insite and Oppose Moves to Shut It Down

Insite

As you may know, a facility known as Insite has operated in Vancouver since 2003. Insite is the first legal supervised injection site in North America. From what you have seen, read or heard about Insite, do you support or oppose its operation?

		Region					
	Total	**BC**	**AB**	**MB/SK**	**ON**	**QC**	**ATL**
Support	43%	68%	33%	37%	39%	41%	43%
Oppose	24%	30%	36%	28%	21%	23%	16%
Not Sure	33%	2%	31%	35%	40%	36%	42%

Insite

In January, the BC Court of Appeal rejected an appeal launched by the federal government and allowed Insite to remain open. The federal government has appealed to the Supreme Court of Canada in an effort to shut down Insite. From what you have seen, read or heard, do you agree or disagree with the government's decision?

		Region					
	Total	**BC**	**AB**	**MB/SK**	**ON**	**QC**	**ATL**
Agree	27%	36%	41%	28%	22%	25%	27%
Disagree	40%	58%	26%	42%	40%	36%	34%
Not sure	33%	6%	33%	30%	38%	39%	39%

Source: Angus Reid Public Opinion. *Canadians Are Supportive of Insite and Oppose Moves to Shut It Down.* Findings from opinion poll conducted July 23 to July 24, 2010, pp. 1–6.

support for Insite, some misconceptions about the SIF are yet to be overcome. Twenty-six percent of Canadians mistakenly believe that Insite actually provides drugs to people who use the facility, including 30% of British Columbians.[53]

Dr. Evan Wood, an independent Insite researcher, recently spoke to the government's attempt to close the SIF, stating that "There's just a huge discordance between scientific evidence and policy . . . Despite all the scientific evidence that shows Insite reduces the spread of HIV, reduces overdose deaths, saves taxpayer dollars, helps get people into addiction treatment, a lot of money is being spent on lawyers trying to close the program."[54]

North American Opiate Medication Initiative (NAOMI)

In Canada approximately 75 000 to 125 000 people are injection drug users, notably cocaine and heroin. Intravenous heroin use prevails in Vancouver and Montreal despite wide availability of the prescription opioids hydromorphone and morphine.[55]

Clinical evidence indicates abstinence-oriented therapies are not effective in the treatment of opioid dependency. The most effective treatment currently available is opioid agonist substitution therapy, with the illicit substance replaced with a legal substitution under close medical monitoring. The most commonly accepted substitution is oral methadone maintenance treatment utilizing best practices guidelines.[56]

Study to Assess Long-Term Opioid Maintenance Effectiveness (SALOME)

Results from NAOMI indicated that injectable diacetylmorphine maintenance was more effective than orally administered methadone maintenance both in reducing attrition and reducing the use of illicit drugs. However, it was concluded that diacetylmorphine maintenance therapy should be delivered in settings where prompt medical intervention is available because of a risk of overdoses and seizures. The Study to Assess Long-Term Opioid Maintenance Effectiveness (SALOME) clinical trial followed to test the hypothesis that hydromorphone (Dilaudid) is as good as diacetylmorphine for intravenous heroin replacement. This trial is still ongoing and will provide chronic addicts at a private Vancouver clinic with heroin or hydromorphone.[57] The NAOMI and SALOME projects are the only heroin maintenance programs to take place in North America.

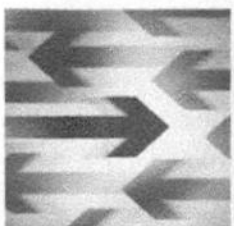

TAKING SIDES

B.C. Addicts Get Injunction to Continue Using Prescription Heroin

A group of addicts in Vancouver who were part of a clinical trial examining the use of prescription heroin have won a temporary injunction that will allow them to continue accessing the drug at least until a court challenge is heard. The ruling, issued Thursday by a B.C. Supreme Court judge, is the second time in recent months that courts have interfered with Ottawa's attempt to rein in the medical use of otherwise illegal drugs. Five people filed a lawsuit last fall alleging the federal government had violated their charter rights by denying access to prescription heroin to treat their addictions

Those patients received the heroin during a clinical trial, but once they left the trial last year, their doctors asked for approval under a special Health Canada program to continue prescribing the drug. Health Canada initially granted the approvals, but Health Minister Rona Ambrose quickly introduced new regulations to stop such approvals. The patients who were approved have not received any more prescription heroin and subsequent applications have been rejected.

A B.C. Supreme Court judge issued an injunction exempting the patients from the updated regulations until the case goes to trial, likely next year. Joseph Arvay, a lawyer who is representing the patients, said the federal government's decision was not based on scientific research that has shown prescription heroin is an effective treatment for patients suffering from severe addiction.

"What was fundamentally wrong with the minister's decision is failing to understand that heroin treatment is a treatment, and it's not just providing the addicts with a drug of their choice," Arvay told a news conference Thursday. "It (prescription heroin treatment) gives them an entry into the health-care system that they don't otherwise have. They're dealt with by social workers and psychologists, and people help them to deal with all the ramifications of their addictions."

The plaintiffs in the case all took part in clinical trials conducted by Providence Health Care, which operates St. Paul's Hospital in downtown Vancouver and is also involved in the lawsuit. The first trial, the North American Opiate Medication Initiative, or NAOMI, took place in Vancouver and Montreal between 2005 and 2008. It compared the effectiveness of pharmaceutical-grade heroin, known as diacetylmorphine, and oral methadone. Two of the plaintiffs were NAOMI participants. The Study to Assess Long-term Opioid Maintenance Effectiveness, or SALOME, began in 2011. The study is comparing the effectiveness of hydromorphone, a synthetic drug approved for use to control pain, and pharmaceutical heroin in treating severe addiction. All five plaintiffs took part, exiting the program last year.

Doctors applied to Health Canada for special permission to prescribe heroin to 21 former study participants, including the five plaintiffs. The updated regulations weren't retroactive, but the patients who were already approved still could not get the prescription heroin because the supplier didn't want to distribute the drug to the patients until the legal questions were cleared up. Arvay said the injunction means all patients who have participated in the clinical trials can now apply to Health Canada for special access if their doctors believe prescription heroin will benefit them.

Health Canada said it plans to study the injunction before deciding how to respond. "Dangerous drugs like heroin have a significant impact on Canadian families and their communities," said an email statement from department spokesman Sean Upton. "We will continue to support drug treatment and recovery programs that work to get Canadians off drugs in a safe way."

Do you agree with the decision of the B.C. Supreme Court?

Source: Adapted from CTV News (2014). B.C. Addicts Get Injunction to Continue Using Prescription Heroin. James Keller. The Canadian Press. Retrieved May 22, 2014 from http://www.ctvnews.ca/canada/b-c-addicts-get-injunction-to-continue-using-prescription-heroin-1.1844160

Summary

- Opium was used in its raw form for centuries, both medicinally and for pleasure.
- Opium had significant influences on medicine, literature, and world politics through the 1800s.
- Various synthetic opioids are now available along with the natural products of the opium poppy. These drugs all act at opioid receptors in the brain.
- Opioid receptors are normally acted on by the naturally occurring opioid-like products of the nervous system and endocrine glands, endorphins and enkephalins.
- The opioid overdose triad consists of coma, depressed respiration, and pinpoint pupils. Death occurs because breathing ceases.
- Combining opioids with sedatives can increase the likelihood of respiratory depression.
- Harm reduction strategies include safe injection sites such as Insite.

Review Questions

1. What two chemicals are extracted from the opium poppy?
2. What was the significance of De Quincey's writing about opium eating?
3. What were the approximate dates and who were the combatants in the Opium Wars?
4. How is it possible that heroin was at first sold as a non-addicting pain reliever?
5. What is the effect of a narcotic antagonist on someone who has developed a physical dependence on opioids?
6. What are the enkephalins and endorphins, and how do they relate to plant-derived opioids such as morphine?
7. Explain why taking opioids in combination with sedatives is not advised.

CHAPTER 14
HALLUCINOGENS

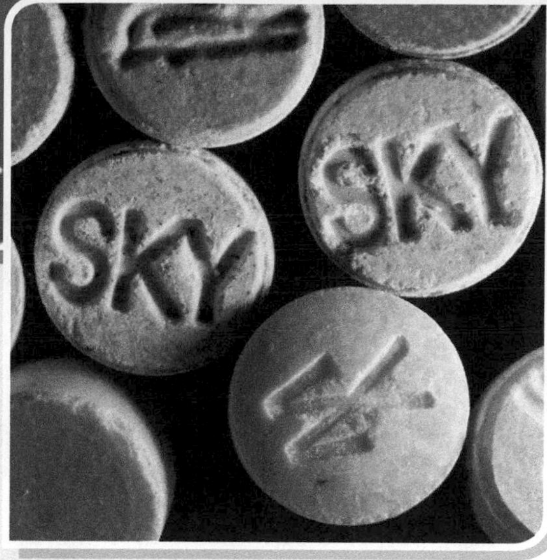

OBJECTIVES

When you have finished this chapter, you should be able to

- **LO1** Explain why plants with psychoactive effects have been used in religious practices all over the world.
- **LO2** Define the meaning of the term *psychotomimetic drugs.*
- **LO3** Define the term *phantastica* and recognize several examples of indole and catechol hallucinogens.
- **LO4** Discuss the early research and evidence on LSD for use in interrogation and in psychotherapy.
- **LO5** Identify the chemical relationship among DOM, MDA, and MDMA.
- **LO6** Explain what is meant by the term *deliriants.*
- **LO7** Explain how anticholinergic hallucinogens act in the brain.
- **LO8** Describe the major active ingredient and some history of use for anticholinergic hallucinogens including *Amanita muscaria* and *Salvia divinorum.*

From the soft, quiet beauty of the sacred *Psilocybe* mushroom to the angry, mottled appearance of the toxic *Amanita,* from the mountains of Mexico to the bays of Newfoundland, from before history to the twenty-first century, humans have searched for the perfect aphrodisiac, for spiritual experiences, and for other worlds. The plants have been there to help; plants have evolved to produce chemicals that alter the biochemistry of animals. If they make us feel sick, we are unlikely to eat them again, and if they kill us, we are certain not to eat them again. But humans long ago learned to "tame" some of these plants, to use them in just the right ways and in just the right amounts to alter perceptions and emotions without too many unpleasant consequences.

LO1 Animism and Religion

Animism, the belief that animals, plants, rocks, streams, and so on derive their special characteristics from a spirit contained within the object, is a common theme in most of the world's religions. Plants that are able to alter our perception of the world and of ourselves fit right into such a view. If the plant contains a spirit, then eating the plant transfers that spirit to the person who eats it, and the spirit of the plant can speak to the consumer, make that person feel the plant's joy, or provide special powers or insights.

In early societies, certain individuals became specialists in the ways of these plants, learning when to harvest them and how much to use under what circumstances. These traditions were passed down from one generation to another, and colourful stories were used to teach the principles to apprentices. Our modern term for these individuals is *shaman, medicine man,* or *medicine woman* because of their knowledge of drug-containing plants. But because they also were the experts on obtaining power from the spirit world, their function in early societies had as much to do with the origins of religion as with the origins of modern medicine. These plants and their psychoactive effects were probably important reasons for the development of spiritual and religious traditions and folklore in many societies all over the world.[1]

animism: the belief that objects attain certain characteristics because of spirits.

LO2 Terminology and Types

The issue of what to call this group of drugs is an old one. The first reference to this group was made in 1924 by Lewis Lewin (1850–1929), a medical doctor and toxicologist of the University of Berlin. Working to categorize psychoactive drugs, Lewin referred to them as a class of **phantastica**, drugs that can create in our minds a world of fantasy. Peyote, psilocybin, and LSD all produce this type of effect. In the 1960s, these drugs were described by enthusiastic users as allowing them to see into their own minds, and the term **psychedelic** ("mind-viewing") was widely used. It was Humphrey Osmond, a British psychiatrist working in Saskatchewan, who proposed the term *psychedelic* to refer to the wide range of effects caused by this group of drugs. To promote the use of his term, Osmond composed the rhyme "To fathom Hell or soar angelic, just take a pinch of psychedelic." The term itself implies a beneficial, visionary type of effect, and considerable disagreement exists over whether such effects are really beneficial. Because the drugs are capable of producing hallucinations and some altered sense of reality, a state that could be called psychotic, they have also been referred to as **psychotomimetic** drugs. This term implies that the drugs produce dangerous effects and a form of mental disorder, which is also a controversial conclusion.

More recently, proponents have popularized newer terms, such as *entheogen* and *entactogen*, to describe these substances. For example, *entheogen* is used to describe substances (e.g., sacred mushrooms) that are thought to create spiritual or religious experiences, whereas *entactogen*, meaning "to produce a touching within," is used to describe substances, such as MDMA, that are said to enhance feelings of empathy.

Is there a descriptive and unbiased term that will allow us to categorize the drugs and then to examine their effects without prejudice? One thing common to these drugs is some tendency to produce hallucinations, so we will refer to them by the name *hallucinogens*.

phantastica: drugs that create a world of fantasy.

psychedelic: "mind-viewing."

psychotomimetic: mimicking psychosis.

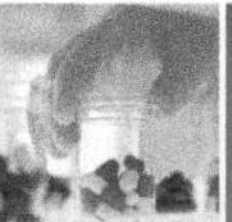

DRUGS IN THE MEDIA

The Psychedelic '60s: Reflections in Film, Music, and Literature

In a peculiar interaction between a new drug phenomenon (experimenting with perception-altering drugs, such as LSD) and a time of many radical changes in society (the civil rights movement, the war in Vietnam, the British invasion of popular music led by the Beatles), a cultural mixture was formed that we now call "the psychedelic '60s" (which for most people probably coincided with the decade 1965 to 1975). All you need to do is to look at popular films from that time or at photographs of relatives to see the influence on hairstyles and clothing. But what was psychedelic about this period, and was it in fact important or interesting from a cultural or an artistic perspective?

We can see the transition in the music of the Beatles. Their early work sounded a lot like mainstream rock and roll, but a visit to India and experimentation with various drugs changed the way they sounded, dressed, and talked. And they in turn influenced many others.

What other writers, artists, and musicians are associated with this phenomenon? The Grateful Dead and Jefferson Airplane may have started it all in music, and Ken Kesey may have started it all in literature, but no popular figure could ignore the influence. Perhaps its most obvious presentation can be seen by looking at album covers, the cardboard jackets that contained the long-playing record albums of the era. To say that the art form of these music-album covers flowered during that period would be both a pun and an understatement.

The University of Virginia library supports an online virtual exhibition called The Psychedelic '60s: Literary Tradition and Social Change. Search for it in your Web browser to read about the music, the social protests, the literature, and the big events that shaped the period, and you can view enough psychedelic art to satisfy anyone's curiosity.

LO3, LO4, LO5 Phantastica

Although we will call all these drugs hallucinogens, important differences exist among them. They can be classified according to their chemical structures, their known pharmacological properties, how much loss of awareness occurs under their influence, and how dangerous they are. The first types we will review are the classical phantastica. They are capable of altering perceptions while allowing the person to remain in communication with the present world. The individual under the influence of these drugs will often be aware of both the fantasy world and the real world at the same time, might talk avidly about what is being experienced, and will be able to remember much of it later. These drugs can be seen as having more purely hallucinogenic effects in that they do not produce much acute physiological toxicity—that is, there is relatively little danger of dying from an overdose of LSD, psilocybin, or mescaline. The two major classes of phantastica, the indole and catechol hallucinogens, are grouped according to their chemical structures.

Indole Hallucinogens

The basic structure of the neurotransmitter serotonin is referred to as an **indole** nucleus. Figure 14.1 illustrates that the hallucinogens LSD and psilocybin also contain this structure. For that reason and the fact that some other chemicals with this structure have similar hallucinogenic effects, we refer to one group of the phantastica as the indoles.

d-Lysergic Acid Diethylamide (LSD) The most potent and notorious of the hallucinogens, and the one that brought these drugs into the public eye in the 1960s, is not found in nature. Although there are naturally occurring compounds that resemble the indole d-lysergic acid diethylamide (LSD), their identity as hallucinogens was not known until after the discovery of LSD.

indole: a particular chemical structure found in serotonin and LSD.

Figure 14.1 Indole Hallucinogens

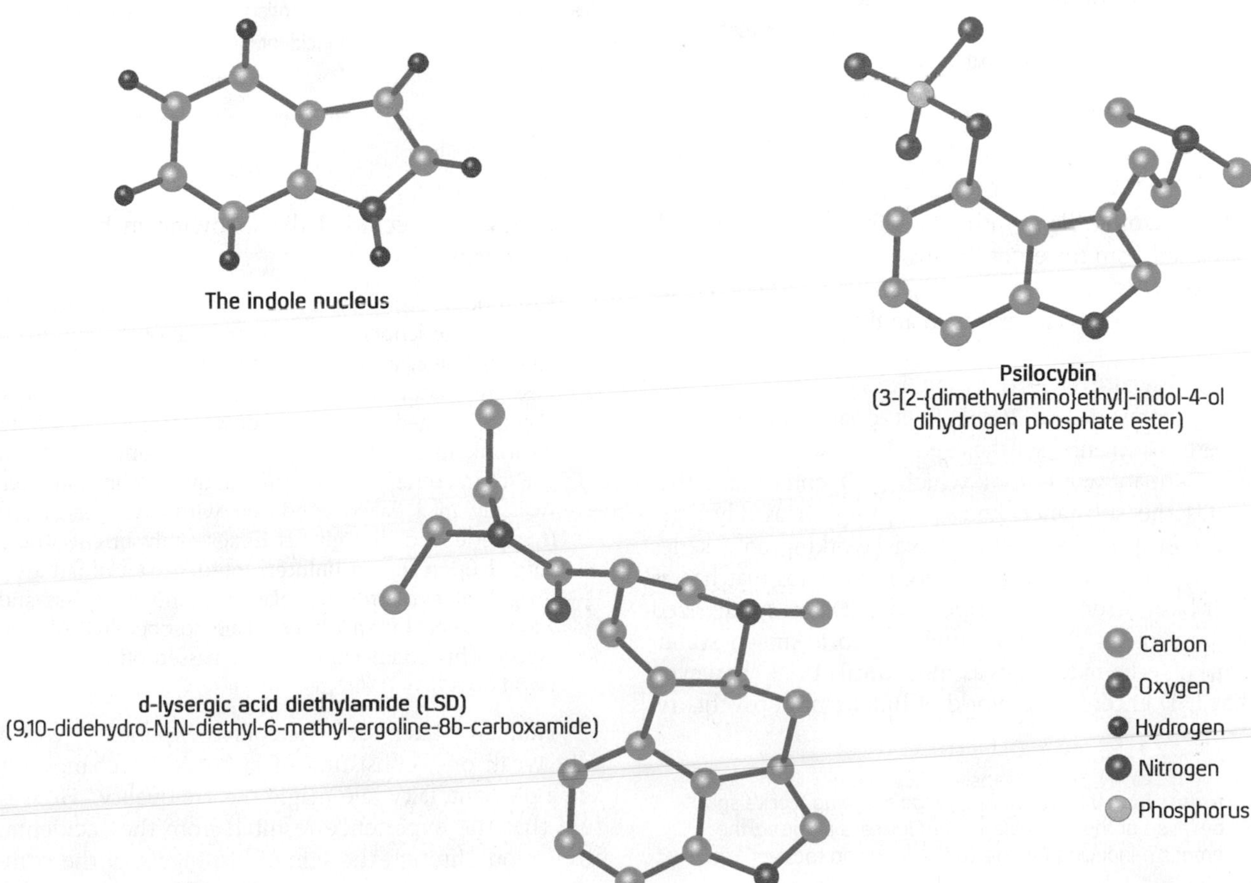

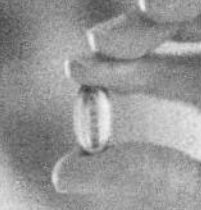

DRUGS IN DEPTH

Saint Anthony's Fire: Ergotism

Grain that has been infected with the ergot fungus is readily identified and is usually destroyed. During periods of famine, however, the grain might be used in making bread. In France between 945 and 1600 CE, at least 20 outbreaks of ergotism, also known as *Saint Anthony's fire,* occurred. The illness results from eating infected bread, and although the cause of the illness was established before 1700, only symptomatic treatment exists even today. There are two forms of the disease. In one, tingling sensations in the skin and muscle spasms develop into convulsions, insomnia, and various disturbances of consciousness and thinking. In the other form, gangrenous ergotism, the limbs become swollen and inflamed, with the individual experiencing "violent burning pains" before the affected part becomes numb. Sometimes the disease moves rapidly, with less than 24 hours between the first sign and the development of gangrene. Gangrene develops because the ergot causes a contraction of the blood vessels, cutting off blood flow to the extremities.

During the twelfth century, ergotism became associated with Saint Anthony, although the reason for this is not completely clear. It might be that the hospital for the treatment of ergotism was built near the shrine of Saint Anthony because he had suffered from a minor attack of ergotism. Others believe the illness was called Saint Anthony's fire because those who made the pilgrimage to Egypt, where Saint Anthony had lived, were cured. Those who journeyed to Egypt and those who entered the hospital did lose their symptoms, probably as a result of a diet that did not include ergot-infected rye.

Two interesting articles discussed a possible link between convulsive ergotism and the Salem witch trials of 1692, in which 20 people were executed. The first article built a very strong case that (1) the original symptoms exhibited by the "possessed" eight girls were similar to those seen in convulsive ergotism and (2) the conditions were right for the growth of the ergot fungus on the rye that was the staple cereal.[2] The second article constructed an equally convincing case that ergotism could not have been involved and that the "possession" was psychological.[3] We will never know for sure, but there are enough similarities and lingering doubts that ergotism seems to remain a possible basis for the Salem incident.

LSD was originally synthesized from **ergot** alkaloids extracted from the ergot fungus *Claviceps purpurea*. This mould occasionally grows on grain, especially rye, and eating infected grain results in an illness called *ergotism*.

LSD Discovery and Early Research In the Sandoz Laboratories in Basel, Switzerland, in 1938, Dr. Albert Hofmann synthesized ***l****yserg****s****aure****d****iethylamid*, the German word from which LSD comes and that names the substance known in English as d-lysergic acid diethylamide. Hofmann was working on a series of compounds derived from ergot alkaloids that had as their basic structure lysergic acid. LSD was synthesized because of its chemical similarity to a known stimulant, nikethamide. It was not until 1943, however, that LSD entered the world of biochemical psychiatry, when Hofmann recorded the following in his laboratory notebook:

> Last Friday, April 16, 1943, I was forced to stop my work in the laboratory in the middle of the afternoon and go home, as I was seized by a peculiar restlessness associated with a sensation of mild dizziness. Having reached home, I lay down and sank in a kind of drunkenness which was not unpleasant and which was characterized by extreme activity of imagination. As I lay in a dazed condition with my eyes closed (I experienced daylight as disagreeably bright) there surged upon me an uninterrupted stream of fantastic images of extraordinary plasticity and vividness and accompanied by an intense, kaleidoscope-like play of colors. This condition gradually passed off after about two hours.[4]

Hofmann later said, "The first experience was a very weak one, consisting of rather small changes. It had a pleasant, fairy tale–magic theatre quality." He was sure that the experience resulted from the accidental absorption, through the skin of his fingers, of the compound with which he was working. The next Monday

ergot: from the French word *argo* meaning "cock's spur," because of the resemblance of *Claviceps purpurea*, the ergotism-inducing fungus, to the spurs on roosters' legs.

morning Hofmann prepared what he thought was a very small amount of LSD, 0.25 milligrams, and made the following record in his notebook:

> April 19, 1943: Preparation of an 0.5% aqueous solution of d-lysergic acid diethylamide tartrate.
> 4:20 P.M.: 0.5 cc (0.25 mg LSD) ingested orally. The solution is tasteless.
> 4:50 P.M.: no trace of any effect.
> 5:00 P.M.: slight dizziness, unrest, difficulty in concentration, visual disturbances, marked desire to laugh.

At this point the laboratory notes are discontinued:

> The last words could only be written with great difficulty. I asked my laboratory assistant to accompany me home as I believed that my condition would be a repetition of the disturbance of the previous Friday. While we were still cycling home, however, it became clear that the symptoms were much stronger than the first time. I had great difficulty in speaking coherently, my field of vision swayed before me, and objects appeared distorted like images in curved mirrors. I had the impression of being unable to move from the spot, although my assistant told me afterwards that we had cycled at a good pace.
>
> Six hours after ingestion of the LSD-25 my condition had already improved considerably. Only the visual disturbances were still pronounced. Everything seemed to sway and the proportions were distorted like the reflections in the surface of moving water. Moreover, all objects appeared in unpleasant, constantly changing colors, the predominant shades being sickly green and blue. When I closed my eyes, an unending series of colorful, very realistic and fantastic images surged in upon me. A remarkable feature was the manner in which all acoustic perceptions (e.g., the noise of a passing car) were transformed into optical effects, every sound causing a corresponding collared hallucination constantly changing in shape and color like pictures in a kaleidoscope. At about 1 o'clock I fell asleep and awakened the next morning somewhat tired but otherwise feeling perfectly well.[4]

The amount Albert Hofmann took orally is five to eight times the normal effective dose, and it was the potency of the drug that attracted attention to it. Mescaline had long been known to cause strange experiences, alter consciousness, and lead to a particularly vivid kaleidoscope of colours, but it takes 4000 times as much mescaline as LSD. LSD is usually active when only 0.05 milligrams (50 micrograms) is taken, and in some people a dose of 0.03 milligrams is effective.

The first report on LSD in the scientific literature came from Zurich in 1947. In 1953, Sandoz applied to the U.S. Food and Drug Administration to study LSD as an investigational new drug. Between 1953 and 1966, Sandoz distributed large quantities of LSD to qualified scientists throughout the world. Most of this legal LSD was used in biochemical and animal behaviour research.

Besides an interest in trying to develop "model psychoses" in animals and humans so that treatments could be developed, the major thrust of LSD research had to do with its alleged ability to access the "subconscious mind." This notion probably derived from the dreamlike quality of the reports of LSD experiences and the long-held psychoanalytic view that dreams represent subconscious thoughts trying to express themselves. Thus, LSD was widely used as an adjunct to psychotherapy. When a psychiatrist felt that a patient had reached a roadblock and was unable to dredge up repressed memories and motives, LSD might be used for its psychedelic (mind-viewing) properties. Thus, LSD took over as a modern truth serum, replacing sodium pentothal and scopolamine. Whether LSD actually helped these patients in the long run or only seemed helpful to the psychiatrists who believed in it is still being debated.

Two other potentially therapeutic uses for LSD were investigated. For various theoretical reasons it was believed that LSD might be a good treatment for alcohol dependence, and initial reports of its effectiveness were quite positive (see the Mind/Body Connection box). Later it was hoped that LSD would allow people with terminal cancer to achieve a greater understanding of their own mortality. Thus, many such patients were allowed to explore their feelings while under the influence of this fantasy-producing agent. In April 1966, the Sandoz Pharmaceutical Company recalled the LSD it had distributed and withdrew its sponsorship for work with LSD. Large quantities of illegally manufactured LSD of uncertain purity were being used in the street, and Sandoz decided to give the responsibility for the legal distribution of LSD to the federal government.

Scientific study of the hallucinogens declined in the 1970s. A 1974 report by a U.S. National Institute of Mental Health (NIMH) research task force on hallucinogenic research stated:

> Virtually every psychological test has been used to study persons under the influence of LSD or other such halucinogens, but the research has contributed little to our understanding of the bizarre and potent effects of this drug.[5]

Partly as a reality-oriented response to this type of evaluation and partly because of the dead ends, the NIMH stopped its in-house LSD research on humans in 1968 and stopped funding university human research on LSD in 1974. The U.S. National Cancer Institute and the National Institute on Alcohol Abuse and

Alcoholism stopped supporting psychedelic research in 1975 because it was deemed to be nonproductive. Most of the LSD research since that time has been conducted on animals in an effort to better understand the mechanism of action at a neural level. Today, roughly 40 years later, a new wave of studies on hallucinogens, primarily psilocybin, is creating renewed interests in the clinical potential of psychedelics. Proposed clinical benefits of hallucinogenic compounds include reducing anxiety in people with cancer, supporting withdrawal from psychoactive substances, and improving the lives of persons with mood disorders.[6,7,8] It is too early to tell which way the story will turn, but the next few years are sure to make interesting viewing.

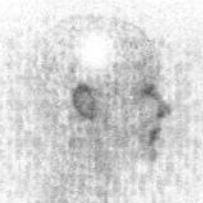

MIND/BODY CONNECTION

Canadian Pioneers in the Use of LSD: Unravelling the Mechanisms that Underlie Mental Illness and Alcoholism

The use of LSD in the treatment of mental illness and alcoholism was pioneered in Saskatchewan, where a socialist government, elected in 1944, had introduced innovative health care reform and significant support for research. Many medical researchers were lured to the province and granted a high degree of professional autonomy within a supportive, innovative, risk-taking research environment. Humphry Osmond, a British-trained psychiatrist, was one of the people who came to Saskatchewan. Osmond had been working on the relationship between mescaline and hallucinations, and he theorized that schizophrenia might be the result of an error in adrenalin metabolism that caused the body to produce a mescaline-like substance. It was here that Osmond met Saskatchewan-born psychiatrist Abram Hoffer, an agricultural chemist, who shared Osmond's belief that biochemical imbalances caused mental illness.[9,10,11,12]

Osmond and Hoffer began their research with mescaline, but since LSD was more readily available and potent, they decided to use it instead. At first they tested the drug on themselves and characterized their experiences. In time, they tested LSD on family and friends, health care workers, students, and mental health committee members at the Regina Chamber of Commerce. Their research catalogued the intense but usually pleasurable hallucinations, effects of LSD punctuated by profound feelings of spirituality, even among nonbelievers, as well as struggles with time perception and difficulties organizing and communicating thoughts.

Osmond and Hoffer were struck by the similarities between these LSD experiences and autobiographical experiences of mental illness. In time, they gave LSD to individuals in remission from active symptoms of schizophrenia and asked them to compare the experience of LSD and their illness. These observations led Hoffer and Osmond, along with Duncan Blewett (the founding chair of the University of Saskatchewan psychology department), to propose that schizophrenia was a biochemical imbalance. Unfortunately, their work received little recognition outside the Saskatchewan community and soon fell to the wayside.[9,10,11,12]

A great deal of Osmond and Hoffer's therapeutic LSD work (psychedelic treatment) focused on alcoholism. Osmond, Hoffer, and Blewett believed that LSD served as an excellent treatment tool given its ability to effect personal transformation, particularly spiritual growth. Blewett supported their theory, proposing that LSD was effective in treating alcoholism because it permitted patients to look within themselves. They treated hundreds of patients with LSD and their work with LSD was supported by the local Alcoholics Anonymous, which also emphasized the significance of spiritual growth. But by the late 1960s, it became difficult to continue their research because of widespread LSD use by young people, the growing black market for the drug, and the media portrayal of the dangers of LSD.

Osmond left Saskatchewan in the early 1960s, and Hoffer resigned in 1967, but by then he was investigating vitamin treatments.[13] Critics have since rejected their experiments because the researchers didn't use randomization and controls. Nevertheless, the work they began in Saskatchewan contributed to the theory of alcoholism as a biochemical disease that can be treated. In a study published in the *British Journal of Psychiatry* in 1970 researchers at the University of Saskatchewan conducted a randomized control trial to determine the efficacy of LSD in the treatment of alcoholism and a variety of other mental disorders, including obsessive-compulsive reaction, anxiety, phobia, hysteria, and neurosis. In that study subjects were randomly assigned to either a control group that did not receive any LSD or a treatment group receiving LSD as part of their treatment. Although no therapeutic benefit were reported, patients in the LSD treatment group were more likely to report having good health overall.[14,15]

Secret Army/CIA Research with LSD The unveiling of CIA/Army human research programs in the United States that used hallucinogens began with a June 1975 report by the Rockefeller Commission on the CIA. Through this report it was identified that a 43-year-old biochemist, Frank Olson, had committed suicide on November 28, 1953, less than two weeks after CIA agents had secretly slipped LSD into his after-dinner drink. This drug had caused a panic reaction in Dr. Olson, and he was taken to New York City for psychiatric treatment. After his suicide, his family was told only that he had jumped or fallen from his tenth-storey hotel room in Manhattan. In 1975, when the LSD link was uncovered, President Ford apologized to the Olson family at the White House and said the incident was "inexcusable and unforgivable . . . a horrible episode in American history."[16]

The Army's interest in, and human experiments with, the use of psychedelics for warfare and for interrogation of prisoners and spies was not hidden. It was open knowledge in the scientific and military communities that such research was conducted at Edgewood Arsenal in Maryland, where Dr. Olson had been given the LSD-laced beverage, and at several major universities in the United States.

It was easy to see how the military and intelligence agencies got involved in this work. "American military and intelligence officials watched men with glazed eyes pouring out rambling confessions at the Communist purge trials in Eastern Europe after World War II, and for the first time they began to worry about the threat of mind-bending drugs as weapons."[17] They worried enough to repeatedly contact Dr. Hofmann about the feasibility of large-scale production of LSD,[18] and the CIA considered buying 10 kilograms in 1953 for $240 000. We can all be pleased that they decided against the purchase, which would have provided 100 million doses.

As the information kept pouring out of government files from 1975 to 1976, it became clear that the Army sponsored research on 585 soldiers and 900 civilians between 1956 and 1967 had been poorly conducted. The Army and some of the university scientists had violated many of the ethical codes established as a result of the Nuremberg war crimes trials after World War II. Three failures were especially blatant. Many of the volunteers were not really volunteers, many of the participants could not quit an experiment if they wanted to, and the participants were not told the nature of the experiment.

The CIA was not without its conspirators in unethical LSD research. Throughout the 1950s and 1960s the Canadian government funded research, in collaboration with the CIA, in mind control and behaviour modification. This research was led by psychiatrist Dr. Donald Ewen Cameron and was part of a larger CIA program called Project MK-ULTRA. A component of Project MK-ULTRA had included the investigation of the effects of LSD on U.S. prison inmates and patients of Canadian and U.S. psychiatric hospitals. This work was done without their consent.[19]

Donald Cameron pioneered clinical research into psychic driving, a treatment that he believed could erase harmful memories and rebuild people's psyches without defect. This research had intrigued the CIA who recruited him to experiment in mind control in 1950. Between 1950 and 1964 Cameron conducted a range of experiments at the Allen Memorial Institute at McGill University. In some of these experiments, patients were subjected to experimental treatments that included electroshock therapy and LSD. Much of this work was done without the permission or consent of patients. Cameron's experiments were typically carried out on patients who had entered the institute for such problems as anxiety disorders and postpartum depression. Many of his patients suffered permanently from his actions and in 1988 nine Canadians treated at the Allen Memorial Institute were compensated by the CIA for their suffering. Similarly the Canadian government compensated 77 former patients of the institute. Recent allegations have suggested that Cameron's work eventually contributed to the KUBARK (cryptonym for the CIA) Counterintelligence Interrogation manual. Critics of Cameron's work claim that his contributions to the MK-ULTRA project were not about mind control but about the creation of a system for extracting information from resistant sources. In other words, torture.[20] Dr. Cameron died in 1967.

Other atrocities were also noted. CIA agents were accused of secretly placing LSD into the drinks of unsuspecting civilians in the United States and abroad. The inspector general of the Army issued an extensive report that criticized almost every aspect of the Army's involvement with human LSD research: its conception, execution, and productivity.[21] These events highlight the potential dangers of administering powerful psychoactive drugs to individuals without their knowledge. Under such conditions, the likelihood of precipitating negative effects increases.

Recreational Use of LSD The story starts in the summer of 1960 in Mexico, where for the first time a psychologist named Timothy Leary used magic mushrooms containing psilocybin. As he later said, he

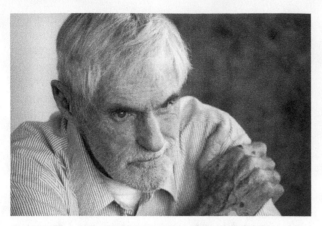

Timothy Leary was a well-known early proponent of the use of LSD.

realized then that the old Timothy Leary was dead; the "Timothy Leary game" was over. Working at Harvard University, Leary collaborated with Dr. Richard Alpert and discussed the meaning and implication of this new world with Aldous Huxley.

During the 1960–1961 school year, Leary and Alpert began a series of experiments on Harvard graduate students using pure psilocybin, which they had obtained through a physician. Leary's original work was apparently done under proper scientific controls and with a physician in attendance because drugs were used. The use of a physician was later eliminated, and then other controls were dropped. Leary believed strongly that the experimenter should use the drug along with the subject, in order to be able to communicate with the subject. This practice removes the experimenter from the role of objective observer and calls into question the scientific value of the research.

Leary's drug taking in the role of experimenter and the apparent abandonment of a scientific approach were questioned by Harvard authorities and other scientists. Some of the major issues were that no physician was present when drugs were administered, undergraduates were used in drug experiments, and drug sessions were conducted outside the laboratory in Leary's home and at other places off campus. As a result of many factors, Alpert and Leary were dismissed from their academic positions in the spring of 1963.[22]

All was reasonably quiet in 1964 and 1965. Alpert, now known as Baba Ram Dass, separated from Leary and lectured on the West Coast, whereas Leary settled at an estate in Millbrook, New York, which was owned by a wealthy supporter of Leary's beliefs. In 1964, Leary announced that drugs were not necessary to rise above and go beyond the ego. He reiterated this again in 1966 after he was arrested for possession of marijuana at the Millbrook estate.

Also in 1966, Leary started his religion, the League of Spiritual Discovery, with LSD as the sacrament. The league got off to a slow start, and Leary's home base at Millbrook was under attack around the same time. The concern was that Leary would attract "drug addicts to Millbrook. When their money runs out, they will murder, rob and steal, to secure funds with which to satisfy their craving."[23]

Leary was the guru of the age, but his sacrament was already being secularized. Increasing numbers of young people were responding to the motto of the League for Spiritual Discovery: "Turn on, tune in, and drop out." Leary phrased it meaningfully:

> Turning on correctly means to understand the many levels that are brought into focus; it takes years of discipline, training, and discipleship. To turn on a street corner is a waste. To tune in means you must harness rigorously what you are learning. . . .
>
> To drop out is the oldest message that spiritual teachers have passed on. You can get only by giving up.[24]

These were noble words, perhaps, but street-corner turn-ons were becoming more frequent. A combination of many things increased the use of hallucinogens, and especially LSD, during the early and mid-1960s. LSD's promise of new sensations (which were delivered), of potent aphrodisiac effects (which were not forthcoming), of feelings of kinship with a friendly peer group (which occurred) spread the drug rapidly.

In the summer of 1966, delegates to the annual convention of the American Medical Association passed a resolution urging greater controls on hallucinogens. They were a little uptight, as was the nation; in part, the resolution stated that

> These drugs can produce uncontrollable violence, overwhelming panic . . . or attempted suicide or homicide, and can result, among the unstable or those with preexisting neurosis or psychosis, in severe illness demanding protracted stays in mental hospitals.[25]

LSD use appears to have peaked in 1967 and 1968, after which it tapered off. Several factors probably contributed to this decline, including widely publicized "bad trips," prolonged psychotic reactions, worries about possible chromosome damage, self-injurious behaviour, and "flashbacks." Concerned, many people began to avoid hallucinogens, whereas others shunned the synthetic LSD for the natural experiences produced by psilocybin or mescaline (actually, into the mid-1970s, these natural substances were in short supply, and most street samples of either psilocybin or mescaline contained primarily LSD or PCP).

After a series of arrests on drug charges, Timothy Leary was sent to a minimum-security prison in 1969, from which he escaped in 1970. After wandering around the world for a couple of years, he surrendered and was sent back to prison. Before his release in 1976, he stated that he was "totally rehabilitated" and would "never, under any circumstances, advocate the use of LSD or any drug." Touring college campuses on the lecture circuit in the early 1980s, Leary talked about "how to use drugs without abusing them."[26]

In Canada, concerns about the possible long-term effects of LSD led to the creation of laws aimed at restricting its use. The sale, possession for the purpose of selling, and distribution of LSD became punishable by law in 1962. Today its use is strictly prohibited under Schedule III of Canada's Controlled Drugs and Substances Act. Despite restrictions the illicit use of LSD and other hallucinogenic drugs remains high, especially among younger Canadians, although it has been declining. For Ontario students (in grades 7-12) reports of past-year use of LSD, mescaline, and ecstasy saw significant decline over the past decade. Between 2001 and 2011 the use of LSD decreased from 4.8% to 2.1%; use of mescaline dropped from 11.1% to 3.5%; and use of ecstasy dropped from 6% to 3.3%.[27] Interestingly, the decline in use of many of these compounds corresponds to an increase in the perception of social disapproval and of risk with trying such drugs.

Surveys of Canadian university students have also demonstrated decreases in past-year hallucinogen use. For example, the past-year prevalence of mescaline and psilocybin use declined between 1998 and 2004, from 8.2% to 5.7 %. LSD use also decreased from 1.8% in 1998 to less than 1% in 2004. The use of ecstasy remained the same at 2.4%.[28] In 2013, the *National College Health Assessment–Student Health Survey* examined drug use patterns of students at 32 postsecondary Canadian institutions. This study determined the past lifetime use of LSD, ecstasy, and club drugs (GHP, ketamine, rohypnol, collectively) to be 5.7%, 8.8%, and 2.4%, respectively. Furthermore, students' past 30-day use of LSD, ecstasy, and club drugs (GHP, ketamine, rohypnol, collectively) was 0.6%, 1.4%, and 0.3%, respectively.[29]

Recent usage rates among Ontario students (grades 7-12) are presented in Table 14.1, while usage rates for Canadians 15 years of age and older are presented in Table 14.2.

LSD Pharmacology LSD is odourless, colourless, tasteless, and one of the most potent psychochemicals known. Remember the pharmacological meaning of *potent;* it takes little LSD to produce effects. A drug can be highly potent and yet not produce much in the way

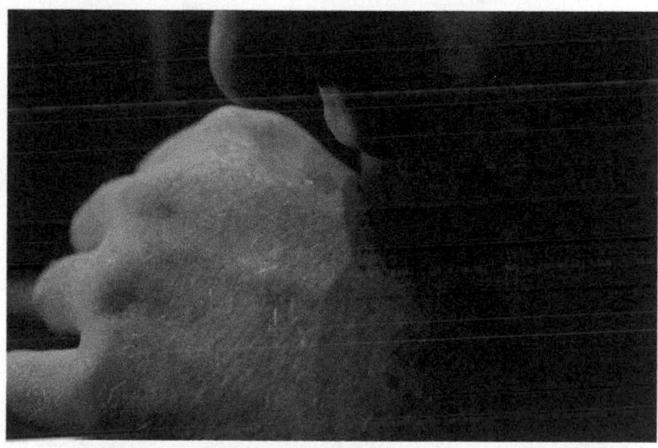

A very small dose of LSD has powerful effects. Liquid LSD solution may be taken orally; it is often applied to blotter paper divided into squares containing single doses.

Table 14.1 Percentage Reporting Past-Year Hallucinogen Drug Use, 2011 OSDUHS (Grades 7–12)

Drug	Total Use (%)	Males (%)	Females (%)	Grade 7 (%)	Grade 8 (%)	Grade 9 (%)	Grade 10 (%)	Grade 11 (%)	Grade 12 (%)
Salvia divinorum	3.7	5.1	2.1	s	s	3.1	5.0	5.2	6.2
Ecstasy (MDMA)	3.3	3.5	3.2	s	s	s	2.7	7.9	4.6
Hallucinogens other than LSD, PCP (e.g., psilocybin and mescaline)	3.8	5.8	2.6	s	1.1	1.6	3.5	8.0	6.3
Ketamine	0.9	1.4	s	s	s	s	s	s	s

Note: s = estimate suppressed because of high sampling variability.

Source: Adapted from, Paglia-Boak, A., Adlaf, E.M., Mann, R.E. (2011). *Drug Use among Ontario Students, 1977–2011: Detailed OSDHUS findings.* (CAMH Research Document Series No. 32). Toronto, ON: Centre for Addiction and Mental Health.

Table 14.2 Lifetime Prevalence of Drug Use, Canadians aged 15+, 2004, 2012

Report of Use	Lifetime Use (%)	
	2004	2012
Drug		
Hallucinogens (PCP or LSD, not salvia)	11.4	12.5
Males	16	16.6
Females	7.1	8.6
Ecstasy	4.1	4.4
Males	5.2	5.6
Females	3.0	3.2
Salvia	n/a	1.8
Males	n/a	2.9[Q]
Females	n/a	0.7[Q]

Note: n/a indicates data not available. [Q] Estimate qualified due to high sampling variability: interpret with caution.

Sources: Adlaf, E. M., P. Begin, and E. Sawka, eds. *Canadian Addiction Survey (CAS): A National Survey of Canadians' Use of Alcohol and Other Drugs, Prevalence of Use and Related Harms: Detailed Report.* Ottawa: Canadian Centre on Substance Abuse, 2005. Health Canada. *Canadian Alcohol and Drug Use Monitoring Survey 2012.* 2012. Retrieved October 29, 2013, from http://www.hc-sc.gc.ca/hc-ps/drugs-drogues/cadums-esccad-eng.php

of effects. For example, LSD has never been definitely linked to even one human overdose death. In rats, reliable behavioural effects can be produced by 0.04 milligrams/kilogram, whereas the LD_{50} is about 16 milligram/kilogram, 400 times the behaviourally effective dose.

Absorption from the gastrointestinal tract is rapid, and most humans take LSD through the mouth. At all post-ingestion times, the brain contains less LSD than any of the other organs in the body, so it is not selectively taken up by the brain. Half of the LSD in the blood is metabolized every three hours, so blood levels decrease fairly rapidly. LSD is metabolized in the liver and excreted as 2-oxy-lysergic acid diethylamide, which is inactive.

Tolerance develops rapidly, with repeated daily doses becoming ineffective in three to four days. Recovery is equally rapid, so weekly use of the same dose of LSD is possible. Cross-tolerance has been shown among LSD, mescaline, and psilocybin, and the psychological effects of each can be blocked with chlorpromazine. Physical dependence on LSD or on any of the hallucinogens has not been shown.

LSD is a sympathomimetic agent, and the autonomic signs are some of the first to appear after LSD is taken. Typical symptoms are dilated pupils, elevated temperature and blood pressure, and an increase in salivation.

The fact that the indole structure of LSD resembles that of serotonin led first to the idea that LSD works by acting at serotonin receptors. Mescaline and other catechol hallucinogens have chemical structures more similar to the neurotransmitters dopamine and norepinephrine than to serotonin. However, they have psychological effects that are very similar to those of LSD. Rats trained to press one lever after an injection of LSD and another lever after a saline (placebo) injection will respond on the LSD lever if given other indole or catechol hallucinogens, but not if given PCP, anticholinergics, stimulants, sedatives, or opiates.[30] Thus, the highly specific "LSD stimulus" in a rat appears to be similar to the stimuli produced by other indole and catechol hallucinogens.

Whereas most of the behavioural effects of LSD and the catechol hallucinogens can be blocked by drugs that act as serotonin-receptor antagonists, others cannot. Add to this that there are several subtypes of serotonin receptors, some of which are excitatory and others inhibitory, and that LSD can act as either an agonist or an antagonist at different serotonin receptors and you can begin to see how complicated this issue becomes. The best evidence seems to indicate that LSD and other hallucinogens, including mescaline and psilocybin, act by stimulating the serotonin 2A subtype of receptors. Among a large group of hallucinogenic chemicals, there is a high correlation between their potency in binding to this type of receptor from rat brains and their potency in producing hallucinogenic effects in humans.[31]

The LSD Experience Regardless of the chemical mechanism, most scientists feel that the most important effect is the modification of perception, particularly of visual images. Some of the experiences reported, especially after low doses, might best be described as illusions, or perceptual distortions, in which an object that is in fact present is seen in a distorted form (brighter than normal, moving, in multiple images). Siegel, who conducted laboratory research on the visual images reported after the ingestion of various drugs, reported that some images can be seen with eyes open or closed and thus are hallucinations rather than illusions.[32] One stage of such hallucinogen-induced imagery consists of form-constants: lattices, honeycomb or chessboard designs, cobwebs, tunnels, alley or cone shapes, and spiral figures. These shapes are generally combined with intense colours and brightness. At another stage, complex images, such as landscapes, remembered faces, or objects, might be combined with the form-constants (e.g., a face might be seen "through" a honeycomb lattice, or multiple images of the face might appear in a honeycomb configuration). Siegel suggested that the perceptual processing mechanisms might be activated at the same time as the sensory inputs are either reduced or impaired, thus allowing vivid perception of images that come from inside, rather than outside, the brain.

Besides changes in visual perception, users also report an altered sense of time, changes in the perception of their own body (perhaps indicating a reduction in somatic sensory input), and some alterations of auditory input. A particularly interesting phenomenon is that of **synesthesia**, a "mixing of senses," in which sounds might appear as visual images (as reported by Dr. Hofmann on the first-ever LSD trip), or the visual picture might alter in rhythm with music.

Altered perception is combined with enhanced emotionality, perhaps related to the arousal of the sympathetic branch of the autonomic nervous system. Thus, a person might interpret the images as exceptionally beautiful or awe-inspiring because of an enhanced tendency to react with intense emotion. Alternatively, an object appearing to break apart or move away from or toward the perceiver might be reacted to with intense sadness or fear. This fear can result in a pounding heart and rapid, shallow breathing, which further frightens the tripper and can lead to a full-blown panic reaction.

Part of the wonder of these agents is that they do not give repeat performances. Even though each trip differs, the general type of experience and the sequence of experiences are reasonably well delineated. When an effective dose (30–100 micrograms) is taken orally, the trip will last six to nine hours. It can be greatly attenuated at any time through the administration of chlorpromazine intramuscularly.

The initial effects noticed are autonomic responses, which develop gradually over the first 20 minutes. The individual might feel dizzy or hot and cold; the mouth might be dry. These effects diminish and, in addition, are less and less the focus of attention as alteration in sensations, perceptions, and mood begin to develop over the following 30–40 minutes. In one study, after the initial autonomic effects, the sequence of events over the next 20–50 minutes consisted of mood changes, abnormal body sensation, decrease in sensory impression, abnormal colour perception, space and time disorders, and visual hallucinations. One visual effect was described beautifully:

> The guide asked me how I felt, and I responded, "Good." As I muttered the word "Good," I could see it form visually in the air. It was pink and fluffy like a cloud. The word looked "Good" in its appearance and so it had to be "Good." The word and the thing I was trying to express were one, and "Good" was floating around in the air.[33]

About one hour after taking LSD the intoxication is in full bloom, but it is not until near the end of the second hour that changes occur in the perception of the self. Usually these changes centre on a depersonalization. The individual might feel that the sensations he or she experiences are not from the body or that he or she has no body. Body distortions are common, the sort of thing suggested by the comment of one user: "I felt as if my left big toe were going to vomit!" Not unusual is a loss of self-awareness and loss of control of behaviour.

Two frequent types of overall reactions in this stage have been characterized as "expansive" and "constricted." In the expansive reaction (a good trip) the individual can become excited and grandiose and feel that he or she is uncovering secrets of the universe or profundities previously locked within. Feelings of creativity are not uncommon: "If I only had the time, I could write the truly great American novel." The other end of the continuum is the constricted reaction, in which the user shows little movement and frequently becomes paranoid and exhibits feelings of persecution. The prototype individual in this situation is huddled in a corner, fearful that some harm will come to him or her or that the person is being threatened by some aspect of the hallucinations. As the drug effect diminishes, normal psychological controls of sensations, perceptions, and mood return.

Adverse Reactions The adverse reactions to LSD ingestion have been repeatedly emphasized in the popular and scientific literature. Because there is no way of knowing how much illegal LSD is being used or how pure the LSD is that people are taking, there is no possibility of determining the true incidence of adverse reactions to LSD. Adverse reactions to the street use of what is thought to be LSD can result from many factors. Drugs obtained on the street frequently are not what they are claimed to be—in purity, chemical composition, or quantity.

A 1960 study surveyed most of the legal U.S. investigators studying LSD and mescaline effects in humans. Data were collected on 25 000 administrations of the drug to about 5000 individuals. Doses ranged from 25 to 1500 micrograms of LSD and from 200 to 1200 milligrams of mescaline. In some cases the drug was used in patients undergoing therapy; in other cases the drug was taken in an experimental situation to study the effects of the drug. Only LSD and mescaline used under professional supervision were surveyed.

synesthesia: a sensation that normally occurs in one sense modality occurs when another modality is stimulated (e.g., hearing colours or seeing sounds).

A 1964 article, "The LSD Controversy," stated:

> It would seem that the incidence statistics better support a statement that the drug is exceptionally safe rather than dangerous. Although no statistics have been compiled for the dangers of psychological therapies, we would not be surprised if the incidence of adverse reactions, such as psychotic or depressive episodes and suicide attempts, were at least as high or higher in any comparable group of psychiatric patients exposed to any active form of therapy.[34]

But it then went on to say:

> It is also important to distinguish between the proper use of this drug in therapeutic or experimental settings and its indiscriminate use and abuse by thrill seekers, "lunatic fringe," and drug addicts. More dangers seem likely for the unstable character who takes the drug for "kicks," curiosity, or to escape reality and responsibility than someone taking the drug for therapeutic reasons under strict medical aegis and supervision.

Panic Reactions One type of adverse reaction that can develop during the drug-induced experience is the panic reaction, which is typified in the following case history:

> A 21-year-old woman was admitted to the hospital along with her lover. He had had a number of LSD experiences and had convinced her to take it to make her less constrained sexually. About half an hour after ingestion of approximately 200 micrograms, she noticed that the bricks in the wall began to go in and out and that light affected her strangely. She became frightened when she realized that she was unable to distinguish her body from the chair she was sitting on or from her lover's body. Her fear became more marked after she thought that she would not get back into herself. At the time of admission she was hyperactive and laughed inappropriately. Stream of talk was illogical and affect labile. Two days later, this reaction had ceased. However, she was still afraid of the drug and convinced that she would not take it again because of her frightening experience.[35]

Flashbacks More than any other reaction, the recurrence of symptoms weeks or months after an individual has taken LSD brings up thoughts of brain damage and permanent biochemical changes. Flashbacks consist of the recurrence of certain aspects of the drug experience after a period of normalcy and in the absence of any drug use. The frequency and duration of these flashbacks are quite variable and seem to be unpredictable. They are most frequent just before going to sleep, while driving, and in periods of psychological stress. They seem to diminish in frequency and intensity with time if the individual stops using psychoactive drugs.

The term *flashback* was replaced in the DSM-5 by the more formal term *hallucinogen persisting perception disorder*. An individual receiving this diagnosis has not used the drug recently but has re-experienced one or more of the perceptual symptoms experienced while intoxicated, such as geometric hallucinations, false perceptions of movement, flashes of colour, intensified colour, trails of images of moving objects, and so on. Because these experiences are rare and unpredictable, and vary so much from one person to another, it has been very difficult to develop any kind of scientific understanding of either the cause of the delayed experiences or of the best treatment to reduce or prevent them.[36]

Beliefs about LSD LSD is truly a legend in its own time—actually, there are many legends. People probably have more ideas about what LSD does and does not do than they have about any other drug.

- *Creativity*. One of the most widely occurring beliefs is that these hallucinogenic agents increase creativity or release creativity that our inhibitions keep bottled inside us. Several experiments have attempted to study the effects of LSD on creativity, but there is no good evidence that the drug increases it. In one laboratory study using LSD at doses of 0.0025 or 0.01 milligrams/kilogram of body weight, "the authors concluded that the administration of LSD-25 to a relatively unselected group of people for the purpose of enhancing their creative ability is not likely to be successful."[37] A double-blind, placebo-controlled study found that psilocybin made remote mental associations more available, which might enhance creativity. However, the research volunteers were less able to focus on their tasks under the influence of psilocybin.[38]
- *Therapy*. Another belief is that LSD has therapeutic usefulness, particularly in the treatment of alcohol dependence, even though reports of results with LSD in alcohol treatment gradually changed from glowing and enthusiastic to cautious and disappointing. One well-controlled study compared the effectiveness of one dose of 0.6 milligrams of LSD with 60 milligrams of dextroamphetamine in reducing drinking. No additional therapy, physical or psychological, was used. The authors found that "LSD produced slightly better results early, but after six months the results were alike for both treatment groups."[39] Some investigators reported considerable success with LSD in reducing the

pain and depression of patients with terminal cancer. The LSD experiences were part of a several-day program involving extensive verbal interaction between the therapist and patient. Although not successful in every case, the LSD therapy was followed by a reduction in the use of narcotics, "less worry about the future," and "the appearance of a positive mood state." The authors concluded that they had a treatment that "may be highly promising for patients facing fatal illness if implemented in the context of brief, intensive, and highly specialized psychotherapy catalyzed by a psychedelic drug such as LSD." However, federally funded research of this type ended in the 1970s, as noted earlier, when a scientific peer review by NIMH concluded that "research on the therapeutic use of LSD has shown that it is not a generally useful therapeutic drug as an adjunct to a routine psychotherapeutic approach or as a treatment in and of itself."[40]

Psilocybin The magic mushrooms of Mexico have a long history of religious and ceremonial use. These plants, as well as peyote, dropped from Western sight (but not from use by indigenous peoples) for 300 years after the Spanish conquered the Aztecs and systematically destroyed their writings and teachings. The mushrooms were particularly suppressed. The name *teonanacatl* can be translated as "God's flesh" or as "sacred mushroom," and either name was very offensive to the Spanish priests.

It was not until the late 1930s that it was clearly shown that these mushrooms were still being used by indigenous groups in southern Mexico, and the first of many species was identified. The real breakthrough came in 1955. During that year a New York banker turned ethnobotanist and his wife established rapport with a group still using mushrooms in religious ceremonies. Gordon Wasson became the first outsider to participate in the ceremony and to eat of the magic mushroom. He wrote of his experiences in a 1957 *Life* magazine article, spreading knowledge of the mushrooms and their psychoactive properties and religious uses.

The most well-known psychoactive mushroom is *Psilocybe mexicana*. The primary active agent in this mushroom is **psilocybin**, an indole that the discoverer of LSD, Albert Hofmann, isolated in 1958 and later synthesized. Psilocybin is a prodrug that is readily dephosphorylated after ingestion. The removal of the phosphate group results in the creation of the psychologically active compound psilocin.[41]

Another psilocybin-containing mushroom, *Psilocybe semilanceata,* is the most common in nature and

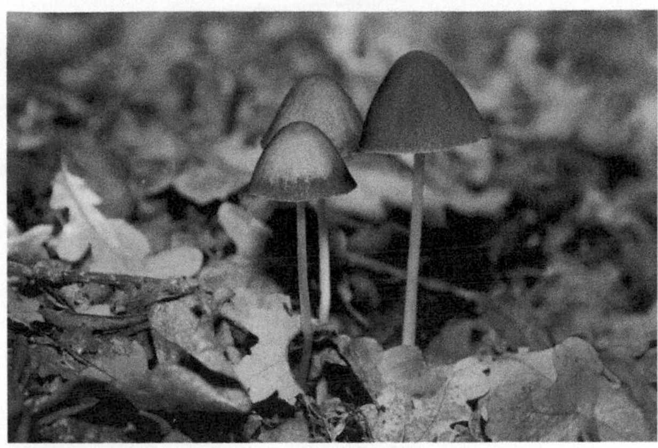

The primary active ingredient in so-called magic mushrooms is psilocybin, an indole hallucinogen.

the most potent. This psychedelic mushroom, commonly known as the liberty cap, grows in fields, grassy meadows, and similar habitats. It is widely distributed in cool temperate and subarctic regions of the Northern Hemisphere. In Canada it is found throughout the Atlantic provinces and in British Columbia.[42] Another psilocybin-containing mushroom, *Psilocybe cubensis,* grows on cow dung along the U.S. Gulf Coast. Aside from the obvious questions about eating something found on manure, identifying the correct psilocybin-containing mushrooms in the field can be tricky. Most *Psilocybe* species are described as "little brown mushrooms," and there are several toxic look-alikes.

The dried mushrooms are 0.2%–0.5% psilocybin. The hallucinogenic effects of psilocybin are quite similar to those of LSD and the catechol hallucinogen mescaline, and cross-tolerance exists among these three agents.

The psychoactive effects are clearly related to the amount used, with up to 4 milligrams yielding a pleasant experience, relaxation, and some body sensations. Higher doses cause considerable perceptual and body-image changes, with hallucinations in some individuals. Accompanying these psychic changes are dose-related sympathetic arousal symptoms. There is some evidence that psilocybin has its central nervous system (CNS) effects only after it has been changed in the body to psilocin. Psilocin is present in the mushroom only in trace amounts but is about 1.5 times as potent as psilocybin. Perhaps the greater CNS effect of psilocin is the result of its higher lipid solubility.

In 1963, as part of his Ph.D. requirements, Walter Pahnke conducted the classic "Good Friday Experiment,"

psilocybin: the active chemical in *Psilocybe* mushrooms.

in which the ability of psilocybin to induce meaningful religious experiences was investigated.[43] Twenty Christian theological seminary students were assigned to two groups: one group received psilocybin (30 milligrams); the other, nicotinic acid (200 milligrams) as a placebo. Following drug administration, the students attended a Good Friday religious service. Psilocybin occasioned a mystical experience, whereas nicotinic acid did not. However, an important methodological concern associated with the Pahnke study was that participants were explicitly told that they would receive psilocybin, and it was conducted in a group setting. These features compromised blinding procedures and undoubtedly influenced the findings.

More recently, Roland Griffiths and colleagues used rigorous double-blind clinical pharmacology methods to investigate both the acute (seven hours) and the longer-term (two months) mood-altering and psychological effects of psilocybin (30 milligrams) relative to methylphenidate (40 milligrams, the active placebo).[6,44] They found that psilocybin acutely increased mystical experience; two months later, research participants "rated the psilocybin experience as having substantial personal meaning and spiritual significance and attributed to the experience sustained positive changes in attitudes and behavior." These findings replicated and extended Pahnke's results, and raised questions about why so few studies evaluating the effects of hallucinogens in human volunteers have appeared in literature in the past half century (see Taking Sides).

With access to some spores of the mushroom and proper growing conditions, a person can cultivate *Psilocybe* in a closet. Although occasionally a major mushroom producer is discovered, most of the production seems to be on a local, amateur basis. Young people might obtain a few "shrooms" to consume at a party, usually in small quantities and in combination with alcoholic beverages. Under such circumstances it is difficult to tell how much of an effect is produced by the mushrooms and how much by the social situation and the alcohol. In Canada, spores, such as *Psilocybe cubensis,* can be readily purchased from suppliers over the Internet. Mushroom spore kits are legal and are sold

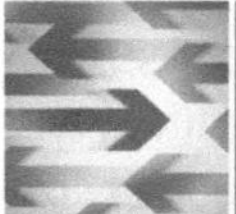

TAKING SIDES

Do You Think the Federal Government Should Fund Hallucinogen Research?

Findings from a recent study indicate that psilocybin produces positive mystical experiences, which may last at least two months.[44] This may not be a surprise to anyone who remembers the 1960s, but the study by Roland Griffiths and colleagues at Johns Hopkins University represents one of the few rigorous investigations in the past 40 years.[6] In response to widespread hallucinogen misuse and poorly conducted studies of these compounds both in Canada and the United States, laws were enacted and federal funding was terminated, virtually ending clinical research on this class of drugs for more than four decades. As a result, from a modern clinical scientific perspective, relatively little is known about psilocybin and other hallucinogens.

Proponents of this type of research suggest that understanding how psilocybin-induced mystical and altered consciousness states arise in the brain would inform us about basic neurobiology and have therapeutic implications, for example, delineation of molecular mechanisms underlying mystical religious experiences

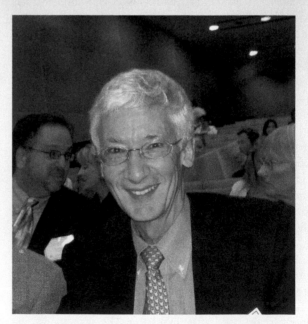

Roland Griffiths, of Johns Hopkins University, was the lead author on the landmark study evaluating the effects of psilocybin in humans.

continued

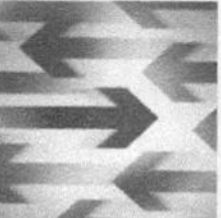

TAKING SIDES

Do You Think the Federal Government Should Fund Hallucinogen Research?

continued

and amelioration of pain and suffering of people with terminal illness. In an unprecedented editorial in the journal *Psychopharmacology,* where the Griffiths et al. study was published, Dr. Harriet de Wit remarked, "It is time for psychopharmacologists . . . to consider the entire scope of human experience and behaviour as legitimate targets for systematic and ethical scientific investigation. Griffiths et al. set an excellent example for such a venture."

Critics, conversely, are less enthusiastic about the study and results. They point out that the positive findings might increase experimentation with these drugs by young people. Moreover, in response to the Griffiths et al. study, Dr. Nora Volkow, director of the U.S. National Institute on Drug Abuse (NIDA), released a statement underscoring the risks of hallucinogen use. Dr. Volkow also noted, "Psilocybin can trigger psychosis in susceptible individuals and . . . its adverse effects are well known." Some have interpreted this as an indication that governments will not fund clinical research investigating the effects of hallucinogens, although many currently spend hundreds of millions of dollars each year supporting research on other psychoactive drugs, including alcohol, cocaine, heroin, marijuana, and methamphetamine. Do you think that governments should fund this type of research?

openly, as possession of the spores themselves is not illegal. However psilocybin and psilocin are illegal to possess and sell as they are listed as Schedule III drugs in Canada's Controlled Drugs and Substances Act.

Morning Glories and Hawaiian Baby Woodroses Of the psychoactive agents used freely in Mexico in the sixteenth century, *ololiuqui*, seeds of the morning glory plant *Rivea corymbosa*, perhaps had the greatest religious significance. These seeds tie America to Europe even today. When Albert Hofmann analyzed the seeds of the morning glory, he found several active alkaloids as well as d-lysergic acid amide, which is about one-tenth as active as LSD. The presence of d-lysergic acid amide is quite amazing (to botany majors) because before this discovery in 1960, lysergic acid had been found only in much more primitive groups of plants, such as the ergot fungus.[45]

The recreational use of seeds from *Argyreia nervosa*, commonly known as Hawaiian baby woodrose, has also been reported.[46] These seeds contain higher levels of d-lysergic acid amide than morning glories. However, recreational use of these seeds often has adverse effects, probably because the fuzzy outer coating contains toxic cyanogenic glycosides (which can make a person sick).

DMT Dimethyltryptamine (DMT) has never been widely used in Canada, although it has a long, if not noble, history. On a worldwide basis, DMT is one of the most important naturally occurring hallucinogenic compounds, and it occurs in many plants and in trace amounts in humans and other mammals, where it is derived from the essential amino acid tryptophan during normal metabolism. DMT is the active agent in Cohoba snuff, which is used by some South American and Caribbean indigenous people in hunting rituals. It was first synthesized in 1931 by Canadian chemist Richard Manske. Its discovery as the active ingredient in Cohoba led to examination of its psychoactive properties in 1956.

DMT is normally ineffective when taken orally and is usually snuffed, smoked, or taken by injection. The effective intramuscular dose is about 1 milligram/kilogram of body weight. Intravenously, hallucinogenic effects are seen within two minutes after doses of 0.2 milligrams/kilogram or more and last for less than 30 minutes. The freebase form of DMT can be smoked by adding the crystals to some type of plant, and 20–40 milligrams is the usual dose. The effect is brief, no matter how it is used. Well-controlled human studies have demonstrated that DMT is unique among classic hallucinogens in that tolerance does not develop to its psychological effects.[47] DMT is illegal to possess and sell. It is listed as a Schedule III drug in Canada's Controlled Drugs and Substances Act.

Ayahuasca The word *ayahuasca* is from the Quechuan language of the Amazon region, and it means "vine of the soul." The term is used both for the vine *Banisteriopsis caapi* and for the medicinal/divinatory brew made from it. The brew is a traditional South American preparation most commonly combining the

Banisteriopsis vine, which contains harmaline, with leaves of *Psychotria viridis*, which contains DMT. DMT is normally broken down quickly in the body by the enzyme monoamine oxidase (MAO). This means that, when DMT is taken orally, it is not usually effective. However, harmaline inhibits MAO (see Chapter 8 for a description of MAO inhibitors as antidepressants). Thus, neither plant alone has psychoactive properties, but together they are used by South American tribes as a psychoactive religious sacrament.[48] Doesn't it make you wonder how this combination was discovered before knowledge existed about these chemicals and how they work? Curiosity seekers from North America and Europe have been travelling to the Amazon to experience the effects of ayahuasca, often describing dramatic psychological effects.

Other Tryptamines There have been reports of a couple of "new" hallucinogenic drugs on the rave scene: 5-methoxy DIPT (known as "foxy methoxy") and alpha-methyltryptamine (AMT). Both may be taken orally. As of 2007, these substances were not specifically listed as controlled substances, but they are chemical analogues of DMT, so sellers can still be prosecuted.

Catechol Hallucinogens

The second group of phantastica, although having psychological effects quite similar to those of the indole types, is based on a different structure, that of the catechol nucleus. That nucleus forms the basic structure of the catecholamine neurotransmitters: norepinephrine and dopamine. Figure 14.2 shows the catechol

Figure 14.2 Catechol Hallucinogens

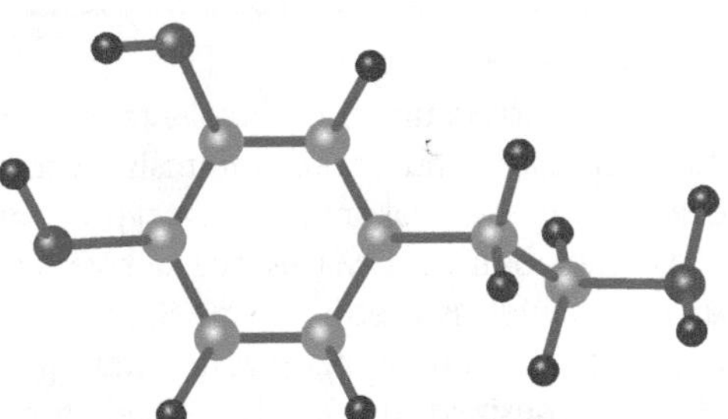

The basic catecholamine structure (dopamine)

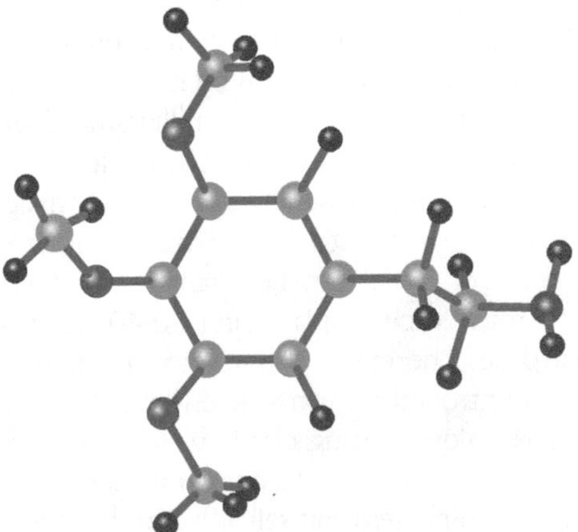

3,4,5-trimethoxyphenylethylamine (mescaline)

Carbon
Oxygen
Hydrogen
Nitrogen

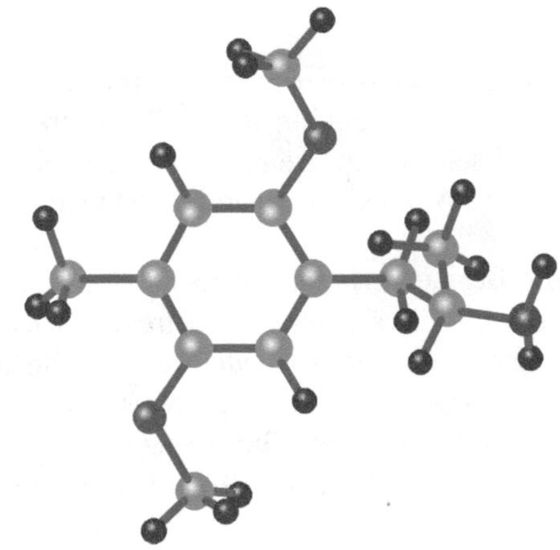

2',5'-dimethoxy-4'-methylamphetamine (DOM)

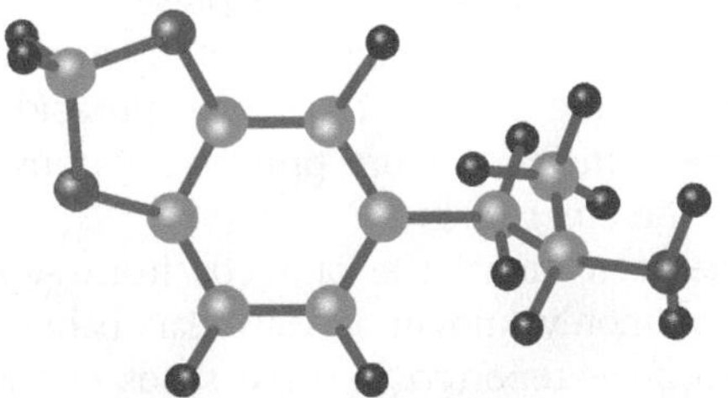

3,4-methylenedioxyamphetamine (MDA)

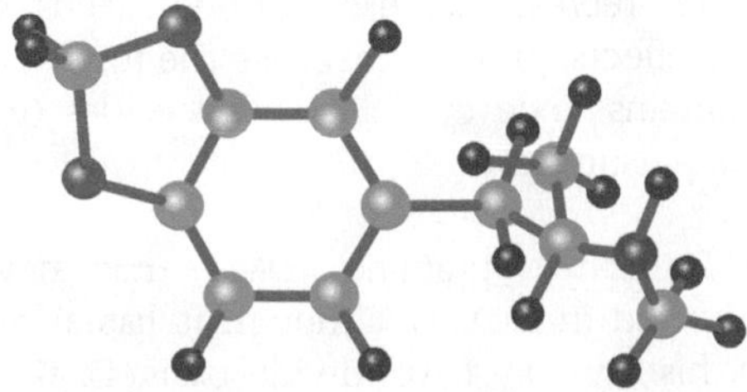

3,4-methylenedioxymethamphetamine (MDMA)

structure and the structures of some catechol hallucinogens. Look for the catechol nucleus in each of the hallucinogens, and then compare these structures with the structure of the amphetamines and other stimulants shown in Chapter 6.

Mescaline **Peyote** (from the Aztec *peyotl*) is a small, spineless, carrot-shaped cactus, *Lophophora williamsii*, which grows wild in the Rio Grande Valley and the Southwest. It is mostly subterranean, and only the greyish-green pincushion-like top appears above ground. In pre-Columbian times, the Aztec, Huichol, and other Mexican indigenous people ate the plant ceremonially in either the dried or the green state, producing psychological effects lasting an entire day.

Only the part of the cactus that is above ground is easily edible, but the entire plant is psychoactive. This upper portion, or crown, is sliced into disks and dried. These slices, known as "mescal buttons," remain psychoactive indefinitely and are the source of the drug between the yearly harvests. The indigenous peoples' journey in November and December to harvest the peyote is an elaborate ceremony, sometimes taking almost a month and a half. When the mescal buttons are to be used, they are soaked in the mouth until soft, then formed by hand into a bolus and swallowed.

Mescal buttons should not be confused with mescal beans—or with mescal liquor, which is distilled from the fermentation of the agave cactus and is the starting point for making tequila. Mescal buttons are slices of the peyote cactus and contain **mescaline** as the primary active agent. Mescal beans, however, are dark red seeds from the shrub *Sophora secundiflora*. These seeds, once used as the basis of a vision-seeking cult, contain a highly toxic alkaloid, cytisine, the effects of which resemble those of nicotine, causing nausea, convulsions, hallucinations, and occasionally death from respiratory failure. The mescal bean has a long history, and there is some evidence that use of the bean diminished when the safer peyote became available in the southwestern United States. In the transition from a mescal bean to a mescal button, some tribes experienced a period in which a mixture of peyote and mescal seeds was concocted and consumed. These factors contributed to considerable confusion in the early (and some recent) literature.[45]

Although evidence shows that the use of peyote had moved north into the United States as early as 1760, it was not until the late nineteenth century that a peyote cult was widely established among the Aboriginal Americans of the plains. From that time to the present, Aboriginal American missionaries have spread the peyote religion to almost a quarter of a million Aboriginal North Americans. The Native American Church was first chartered in Oklahoma in 1918 with the purpose of defending the beliefs and practices of peyotists. It is an amalgamation of Christianity and traditional beliefs and practices of the Aboriginal Americans, with peyote use incorporated into its ceremonies. The Church became international in 1954 with the establishment of the Native American Church of Canada. Peyotism continues to be an important religious practice among many Aboriginal Americans. Peyote is also used in other ways because Aboriginal Americans attribute spiritual power to the peyote plant. As such, peyote is believed to be helpful, along with prayers and modern medicines, in curing illnesses. It is also worn as an amulet, much as some Christians wear a Saint Christopher's medal, to protect the wearer from harm.

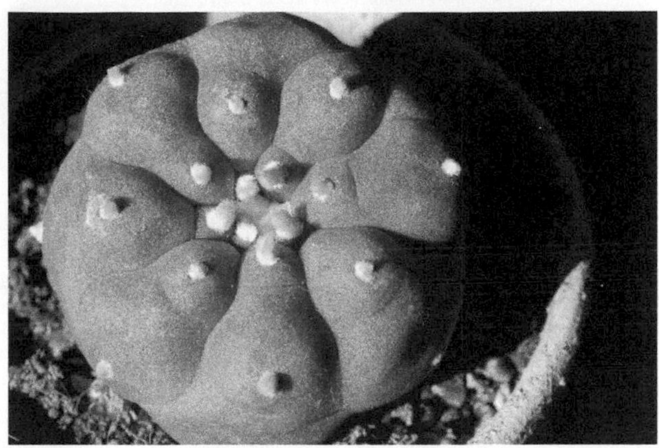

Only the top of the peyote cactus appears above ground, but the entire plant is psychoactive.

In 1955, Humphrey Osmond, who had long been interested in the use and effects of peyote, participated in a Native American Church ceremony with members of the Red Pheasant Band (Saskatchewan) and during which he ingested peyote. His experience did not replicate those reported historically, but after taking approximately 100 seeds he passed into what he described as a state of listlessness, accompanied by increased visual sensitivity and followed by a prolonged period of relaxed well-being. Osmond published the details of the ceremony and his conjecture as to the meaning of the experience to his hosts in *Tomorrow* magazine in the spring of 1961.[49]

peyote: a type of hallucinogenic cactus.

mescaline: the active chemical in the peyote cactus.

For many years the use of peyote as a sacrament by the Native American Church was protected in the United States by the constitutional guarantee of freedom of religion. That protection had inspired Timothy Leary to attempt a similar exclusion for LSD in his newly founded 1960s League of Spiritual Discovery. However, in 1990 the U.S. Supreme Court ruled that the State of Oregon could prosecute its citizens for using peyote, and the freedom of religion argument was not allowed. A large group of religious and civil liberties organizations asked the court to reconsider its decision, but it declined to do so. The two defendants in the case were Aboriginal Americans and members of the Native American Church. Federal law and many state laws specifically exclude sacramental peyote use, and the court pointed out that Oregon could exclude such use, too. Other states have not moved to outlaw religious use of peyote. Although mescaline is listed as a Schedule III drug in Canada's Controlled Drugs and Substances Act, peyote is specifically exempt.

San Pedro Cactus Another mescaline-containing cactus, *Trichocereus pachanoi,* whose common name is the San Pedro cactus, is native to the Andes Mountains of Peru and Ecuador and has been used for thousands of years as a religious sacrament.[50] The San Pedro is a large, multibranched cactus, often growing to heights of three to five metres. Its mescaline content is less than that of peyote, and its recreational use more often results in adverse side effects than in the desired hallucinogenic experience.

Discovery and Early Research on Mescaline

Near the end of the nineteenth century, Arthur Heffter isolated several alkaloids from peyote and showed that mescaline was the primary agent for the visual effects induced by peyote. Mescaline was synthesized in 1918, and most experiments on the psychoactive and behavioural effects since then have used synthesized mescaline. More than 30 psychoactive alkaloids have now been identified in peyote, but mescaline does seem to be the agent responsible for the vivid colours and other visual effects. The fact that mescaline is not equivalent to peyote is not always made clear in the literature.

One of the early investigators of the effects of peyote was Dr. Weir Mitchell, who used an extract of peyote and reported, in part,

> The display which for an enchanted two hours followed was such as I find it hopeless to describe in language which shall convey to others the beauty and splendour of what I saw. Stars, delicate floating films of color, then an abrupt rush of countless points of white light swept across the field of view, as if the unseen millions of the Milky Way were to flow in a sparkling river before my eyes . . . zigzag lines of very bright colors . . . the wonderful loveliness of swelling clouds of more vivid colors gone before I could name them.[51]

Another early experimenter was Havelock Ellis. Interestingly, he took his peyote on Good Friday in 1897, 65 years before the Good Friday experiment with psilocybin. His experience is described in detail in a 1902 article titled "Mescal: A Study of a Divine Plant" in *Popular Science Monthly,* but a brief quotation gives the essence of the experience:

> On the whole, if I had to describe the visions in one word, I should say that they were living arabesques. There was generally a certain incomplete tendency to symmetry, the effect being somewhat as if the underlying mechanism consisted of a large number of polished facets acting as mirrors. It constantly happened that the same image was repeated over a large part of the field, though this holds good mainly of the forms, for in the colors there would still remain all sorts of delicious varieties. Thus at a moment when uniformly jewelled flowers seemed to be springing up and extending all over the field of vision, the flowers still showed every variety of delicate tone and tint.[52]

Not every individual wants every educational opportunity. William James, surprisingly, was one who did not. He wrote to his brother Henry: "I ate one but three days ago, was violently sick for twenty-four hours, and had no other symptoms whatever except that and the *Katzenjammer* (hangover) the following day. I will take the visions on trust." Even Dr. Weir Mitchell, who had the effect previously recorded, said, "These shows are expensive. . . . The experience, however, was worth one such headache and indigestion but was not worth a second."

Even if you get by without too much nausea and physical discomfort, which Aboriginal Americans also report, all might not go well. Huxley, whose 1954 book *The Doors of Perception,*[53] which chronicles a mescaline trip Huxley took in the spring of 1953, made him a guru in this area, admitted, "Along with the happily transfigured majority of mescaline takers there is a minority that finds in the drug only hell and purgatory." It is reported that Aboriginal people sometimes wished for bad trips when taking this or other plants. By meeting their personal demons, they hoped to conquer them and remove problems from their lives.

Pharmacology of Mescaline Mescaline is readily absorbed if taken orally, but it poorly passes the blood-brain barrier (which explains the high doses required).

There is a maximal concentration of the drug in the brain after 30–120 minutes. About half of it is removed from the body in six hours, and there is evidence that some mescaline persists in the brain for up to ten hours. Similar to the indole hallucinogens, the effects obtained with low doses, about 3 milligrams/kilogram of body weight, are primarily euphoric, whereas doses in the range of 5 milligrams/kilogram give rise to a full set of hallucinations. Most of the mescaline is excreted unchanged in the urine, and the metabolites identified thus far are not psychoactive.

A dose that is psychoactive in humans causes pupil dilation, pulse rate and blood pressure increases, and an elevation in body temperature. All these effects are similar to those induced by LSD, psilocybin, and most other alkaloid hallucinogens. There are other signs of CNS stimulation, such as EEG arousal, after mescaline intake. In rats the LD_{50} is about 370 milligrams/kilogram of body weight, 10–30 times the dose that causes behavioural effects. Death results from convulsions and respiratory arrest. Tolerance develops more slowly to mescaline than to LSD, and there is cross-tolerance between them. As with LSD, mescaline intoxication can be blocked with chlorpromazine.

Although mescaline and the other catechol hallucinogens have a structure that resembles the catecholamine neurotransmitters, they act indirectly on the serotonin 2A receptor.

Amphetamine Derivatives A large group of synthetic hallucinogens is chemically related to the amphetamines. However, most of these drugs have little amphetamine-like stimulant activity. Thanks to certain chemical substitutions on the ring part of the catechol nucleus, these drugs are more mescaline-like (refer to Figure 14.2).

DOM (STP) DOM is 2,5-dimethoxy-4-methylamphetamine. In the 1960s and 1970s, DOM was called STP, and street talk was that the initials stood for serenity, tranquillity, and peace. Its actions and effects are similar to those of mescaline and LSD, with a total dose of 1–3 milligrams yielding euphoria and 3–5 milligrams a six- to eight-hour hallucinogenic period. This makes DOM about a hundred times as potent as mescaline but only one-thirtieth as potent as LSD.

MDA and Others In addition to DOM, many other amphetamine derivatives have been synthesized and shown to have hallucinogenic properties. Most of these have effects very similar to those of DOM and mescaline, as well as LSD and the indole types. There is some indication that one type of derivative, MDA (refer to Figure 14.2), has effects that are subjectively somewhat different. MDA, which is somewhat more potent than mescaline, has seen some recreational use through illicit manufacture. Because of the variety of possible hallucinogenic amphetamine derivatives and because most of these chemicals are not specifically listed as controlled substances, illicit drug makers were drawn to this group of chemicals in the production of various designer drugs to be sold on the street as hallucinogens.

MDMA One of the amphetamine derivatives–MDMA–received special attention in 1976 when it was included in Canada's Food and Drugs Act as a restricted drug. Today MDMA, along with DOM and STP, are listed as Schedule III drugs under Canada's Controlled Drugs and Substances Act. In the United States the Drug Enforcement Agency first proposed scheduling MDMA as a controlled substance in July 1984. Although there had been some recreational use of MDMA, a number of psychiatrists testified against the scheduling of MDMA. They insisted that it was not a true hallucinogen and that it had a special ability to promote empathy, thus aiding the psychoanalytic process.[54] MDMA is colloquially known as ecstasy or XTC, but MDMA and ecstasy are not the same drug, although the terms are used somewhat interchangeably. MDMA is pure, while ecstasy can be likened to a "salami of drugs," which supposedly but not always includes MDMA.

There is some evidence supporting this claim of increased empathy. In one study, 100 people completed detailed questionnaires describing the effects of their previous use of MDMA.[55] Although such retrospective reports are less reliable than reports obtained

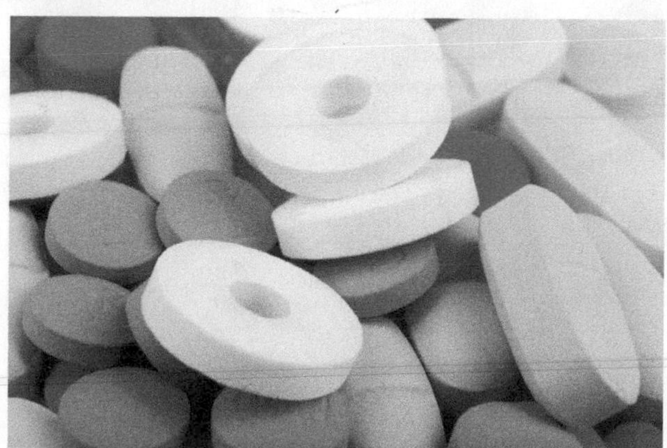

Some evidence suggests that ecstasy may be neurotoxic, affecting serotonin neurons in the brain.

Table 14.3 Adverse Effects Triggered by Ecstasy after Moderate Consumption or Repeated Doses and the Neurotransmitters Most Likely to Be Involved

Types of Use	Adverse Effects
Low doses	Palpitations,[*] hypertension,[*] loss of appetite,[‖] trismus,[*,†] bruxism,[*,†] nausea,[*] headache,[*] insomnia,[*] tremors,[*] sweating,[*] vomiting,[†] ataxy,[‖] nystagmus,[‖] visual hallucinations[†]
High doses	Palpitations,[*] hypertension,[*] hypotension,[*] arrhythmia,[*] hyperthermia,[†] increase in muscle tone,[†] visual hallucinations,[†] hepatotoxicity,[‖] acute kidney failure,[†] disseminated intravascular coagulation,[†] rhabdomyoiysis,[†] toxic hepatitis,[‖] panic,[‡] death[*,†]
Residual effects	Insomnia,[*] muscle pain,[†] fatigue[§]
Chronic effects	Fatigue,[§] depression,[§] nausea,[†] anxiety and panic attacks,[†] insomnia,[*] psychosis,[‡] weight loss,[*,†] irritability[‡]

* noradrenergic effects,
† serotoninergic stimulation,
‡ serotoninergic deficiency,
§ noradrenergic and serotoninergic deficiency,
‖ unknown

Source: Chart II: Adverse Effects Triggered by Ecstasy after Moderate Consumption or Repeated Doses and the Neurotransmitters most Likely to Be Involved. Adapted from Ferigolo et al. EXCERPTED FROM Moro, E. T., A. A. F. Ferraz, and N. S. P. Módolo. "Anesthesia and the Ecstasy User." *Revista Brasileira de Anestesiologia* 56 (2006), pp. 183–188. Retrieved October 4, 2011, from http://www.scielo.br/scielo.php?pid=S0034-70942006000200010&script=sci_arttext&tlng=en.

during or immediately after the experience, a remarkably common report (90% of the individuals) was that they experienced a heightened sense of "closeness" with other people. Like other amphetamines, MDMA increases euphoria, sociability, blood pressure, and heart rate (described in Table 14.3).[56] Although several people reported that objects seemed more "luminescent," very few reported actual visual hallucinations.

Anecdotal reports suggest that ecstasy users report substantially more negative or depressed mood states in the days immediately following its administration.

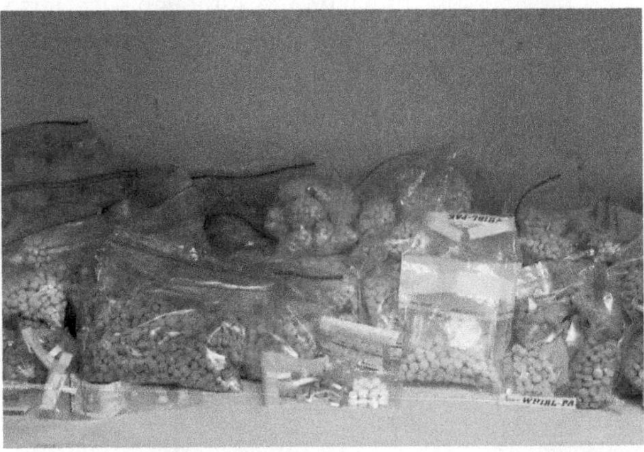

There are harms associated with ecstasy use. Police warn that ecstasy disrupts the body's regulation of temperature, blood pressure, and heart rate, which may cause sudden death.[57] Production of ecstasy has risen dramatically in Canada in recent years, with Canada replacing the Netherlands and Belgium as the primary source for the U.S. market.

Colloquially, this phenomenon is frequently referred to as "Suicide Tuesday." Some have speculated that initially ecstasy administration causes a substantial release of serotonin, followed by a marked reduction of the neurotransmitter, lasting several hours to days after the last dose. Because serotonin plays a major role in mood regulation, this produces the depressed mood state reported by ecstasy users in the days following drug use. However, there is no hard evidence to support this.

Another frequently mentioned potential negative consequence of MDMA is damage to brain cells. Several investigators have shown that large doses of MDMA given to laboratory animals can destroy serotonin neurons, but the relevance of this and related findings for human recreational use is unclear (see the Drugs in Depth box). Recreational users of the drug perform similarly to their education and age-matched counterparts on cognitive tests and do not typically use doses as large as those used in animal experiments. However, this does not suggest that the drug should be used recreationally. As a Schedule III drug in Canada, the recreational use of MDMA is strictly prohibited. Despite this status, the 2012 *Canadian Alcohol and Drug Use Monitoring Survey* has identified ecstasy as the third most commonly used illicit drug in Canada. In that year an estimated 0.6% of the population 15 years of age and older reported having used ecstasy in the previous 12 months. As described in Chapter 1, although the use of ecstasy in the general population is low, its use by students (grades 7–12) is considerably higher (3.3%).[27] Furthermore, ecstasy is the most sought after and widely available controlled synthetic substance in the Canadian illicit drug market. Since 2005, Canada has been recognized as a global MDMA source consequential to the development of large-scale production by organized crime.[58]

2-CB and 2-C-T7 It has happened before and it will happen again: as governments work to limit access to one drug, another arrives to fill the gap. In this case, two drugs have arrived to share the rave scene with MDMA: 4-bromo-2,5-dimethoxyphenethylamine (known as 2-CB) and 4-propylthio-2,5-dimethoxyphenethylamine (2-C-T7). As phenylethylamines, both are chemical cousins to the amphetamine series of hallucinogens. Along with the recently popularized tryptamine derivatives MTA and "foxy methoxy," a confusing array of chemicals is being made available to "ravers," who may find themselves trying unknown amounts of unfamiliar drugs more often than they'd like.

LO6, LO7, LO8 Deliriants

If the indole and catechol hallucinogens are grouped together as phantastica with all having similar effects and acting primarily through the serotonin 2A receptor, then how do we classify all the remaining hallucinogens? We have chosen the term *deliriants*, implying that the drugs to follow have somewhat more of a tendency to produce mental confusion and a loss of touch with reality. The drugs we describe next represent a variety of effects and act through different brain mechanisms, so it is perhaps better to think of each type by itself rather than as belonging to a group with common effects.

PCP

In the 1950s, Parke, Davis & Company investigated a series of drugs in the search for an efficient intravenous anaesthetic. On the basis of animal studies, the company selected 1-(1-phenylcyclohexyl) piperidine hydrochloride (PCP, generic name *phencyclidine*) for testing in humans. The studies on monkeys had indicated that **PCP** was a good analgesic but did not produce good muscle relaxation or sleep. Instead, the animals showed a sort of "dissociation" from what was happening: "During the operation the animal had its eyes open and looked about unconcernedly." In 1958, the first report was published on the use of PCP (Sernyl) for surgical anaesthesia in humans. Sernyl produced good analgesia without depressing blood circulation or respiration and did not produce irregularities in heartbeat. Loss of sensation occurred within two or three minutes of beginning the intravenous infusion, after about 10 milligrams of the drug had been delivered. The patients later had no memory of the procedure, did not remember being spoken to, and remembered no pain. Compared with existing anaesthetics, which tend to depress both respiration and circulation through general depression of the CNS, this type of "dissociative" anaesthetic seemed to be quite safe. However, the psychological reactions to the drug were unpredictable.

During administration of the drug, a few patients became very excited, and a different anaesthetic had to be used. Several patients were "unmanageable" as they emerged from the anaesthetic, exhibiting severely manic behaviour. This and later reports indicated that many people given anaesthetic doses of Sernyl reported changes in body perception and hallucinations, and about 15% of the patients experienced a "prolonged confusional psychosis," lasting up to four days after the drug was given. This period of confusion was characterized by feelings of unreality, depersonalization, persecution, depression, and intense anxiety.

News of this new hallucinogen soon reached Dr. Luby, a psychiatrist, who began testing it in both normal and schizophrenic subjects.[59] All the subjects reported changes in perception of their own bodies, with one normal subject saying, "my arm feels like a twenty-mile pole with a pin at the end." Another said, "I am a small . . . not human . . . just a block of something in a great big laboratory." There were a number of reports of floating, flying, dizziness, and alternate contraction and expansion of body size. All subjects also showed a thought disorder. Some made up new words, uttered strings of unrelated words, or repeated words or simple phrases. Also, all became increasingly drowsy and apathetic. At times a subject would appear to be asleep but when asked a direct question would respond. When asked, "Can you hear me?" subjects often responded, "No." The majority became either angry or uncooperative. Many of the normal subjects said they felt as if they were drunk from alcohol. All subjects displayed diminished pain, touch, and position sense, and all showed nystagmus (rapid oscillations of the eyes) and a slapping, ataxic walk. Luby and his colleagues felt that PCP was different from LSD or mescaline in

PCP: phencyclidine; originally developed as an anaesthetic; has hallucinogenic properties.

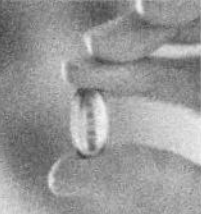

DRUGS IN DEPTH

Extrapolating Findings from Animals to Humans: What You Need to Know

"The amount of the drug Ecstasy that some recreational users take in a single night may cause permanent brain damage and lead to symptoms like those of Parkinson's disease," read an article published in *The New York Times* on September 27, 2002. This and similar statements were based on assertions made in a scientific paper that had just appeared in the highly respected and influential journal *Science*.[60] George Ricaurte and his team of researchers gave nonhuman primates three doses of MDMA over the course of six hours, and then a couple of weeks later evaluated neuroanatomical and neurochemical alterations. They found extensive damage to dopamine and serotonin neurons and reduced levels of these neurotransmitters in the brain.

The finding that MDMA damaged brain cells was not new. Several studies documented the neurotoxic effects of MDMA in laboratory animals.[61] The majority of these studies, however, had used dosing regimens that were much larger and longer than those used by recreational MDMA users. Studies that use laboratory animals, for instance, typically administer MDMA via routes other than oral and in doses greater than 5 milligrams/kilogram twice a day for four or more consecutive days. By contrast, human recreational drug users almost always administer the drug orally and typically do not exceed 2–4 milligrams/kilogram in only one evening.

What made Ricaurte and colleagues' results intriguing was that the doses of MDMA used and the pattern of drug administration were claimed to be comparable to those used by recreational human users. The researchers injected MDMA at a dosage of 2 milligrams/kilogram, three times, at three-hour intervals, for a total dose of 6 milligrams/kilogram. As noted above, even this dosing regimen does not exactly correspond with those typically used by humans. Importantly, the route of drug administration is a critical determinant of neurochemical consequences (e.g., toxicity) because these effects depend on the rate of rise of drug concentrations and the maximum brain concentrations achieved. Recall from Chapter 5 that drugs administered by injection result in a more rapid onset of effects and greater brain concentrations. Furthermore, potential toxicity is decreased when a drug is self-administered compared with experimenter-administered.[62] Thus, these two factors increased the likelihood of observing toxicity in the Ricaurte study.

Nevertheless, the study findings generated a wave of controversy. Critics argued that the total dose given to the animals far exceeded doses taken by humans and that the kind of brain damage observed has never been found in humans. They also noted that 20% of the animals died following MDMA administrations, whereas human mortality is rare. Supporters, in contrast, took the findings as evidence that MDMA is a highly toxic drug that should not be taken even once.

But in an embarrassing turn of events, Ricaurte and colleagues were forced to retract their paper one year after its publication because they discovered that methamphetamine had been mistakenly given, rather than MDMA.[63] This was deduced after several unsuccessful attempts by the researchers to replicate their original findings. It is noteworthy that those negative data were never published and the retraction did not receive much attention. This suggests that there is a bias toward publishing positive results (i.e., demonstration of MDMA-induced neurotoxicity). A similar situation has been noted regarding antidepressant medications (see Chapter 8). Even so, these events raise important questions about drug-induced neurotoxicity observed in laboratory animals and the relevancy of such findings for the human drug users.

Unfortunately, uneven (and sometimes sensationalized) reports about drug-induced toxicity can be discouraging to students. As a result, some may reject all related information from scientific sources. Whom should you believe? How do you determine which dataset is more compelling? In your attempt to understand research investigating drug-induced toxicity, you should ask a few simple questions: (1) What was the drug dosing regimen used, and is it similar to regimens used by humans? (2) What was the route of drug administration used and do humans use the drug in this manner? (3) Was the drug self-administered or administered by the experimenter? (4) Because the development of tolerance can be protective against some types of toxicity, like human drug-taking behaviour, were the animals administered escalating doses before receiving a larger dose? All these factors potentially affect neurochemical findings and should be considered when making extrapolations about data collected in laboratory animals to humans.

that there were few reports of intense visual experiences and many more reports of body image changes. The disorganized thinking, suspiciousness, and lack of cooperation made the PCP state resemble schizophrenia much more than the LSD state.

Thus, by 1960, PCP had been characterized as an excellent anaesthetic for monkeys, a medically safe but psychologically troublesome anaesthetic for humans, and a hallucinogen different from LSD and mescaline, with profound effects on body perception. Parke, Davis withdrew Sernyl as an investigational drug for humans in 1965 and in 1967 licensed another company to sell Sernylan as an animal anaesthetic. It was primarily used with primates, in both research laboratories and zoos. Also, because of its rapid action and wide safety margin, Sernylan was used in syringe bullets to immobilize stray, wild, or dangerous zoo animals. Because of the popular term *tranquillizer gun* for this use, PCP became popularly, and inaccurately, known as an animal "tranquillizer."

Other PCP-Like Drugs: Ketamine, Dextromethorphan, and Nitrous Oxide Even though Sernyl was never marketed for human use, a related chemical from the same series was marketed as a dissociative anaesthetic. Ketamine hydrochloride (Ketalar) has been in continued human use for more than 30 years. Although ketamine has more depressant effects than PCP and fewer prolonged reactions, clinical reports indicate that emergence reactions occur in about 12% of patients. These reactions include hallucinations and delirium, sometimes accompanied by confusion and irrational behaviour. In 2005, widespread reports of ketamine abuse and its notoriety as a party drug (called Special K, or K) prompted the Government of Canada to list ketamine as a Schedule I drug under the Controlled Drugs and Substances Act.

Like PCP and ketamine, two more common substances are also capable of causing dissociative effects, perhaps by blocking NMDA-type glutamate receptors in the brain. Nitrous oxide (laughing gas, Chapter 7) and dextromethorphan, an over-the-counter cough suppressant (Chapter 12) can, at very high doses, produce dissociative-type hallucinations similar to those produced by PCP. It has been reported that the combination of nitrous oxide and ketamine, sometimes used for general anaesthesia, produces synergistic neurotoxic effects in animals.[64] In 2011 approximately 6.9% of Ontario students (Grades 7–12) reported using over-the-counter cough/cold medication that contains dextromethorphan to "get high"; this represents

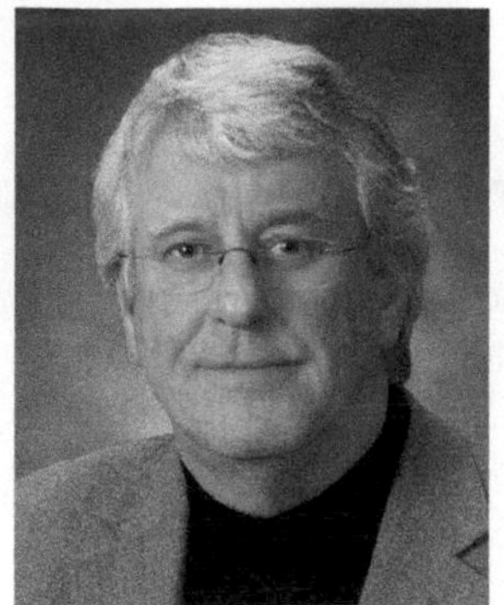

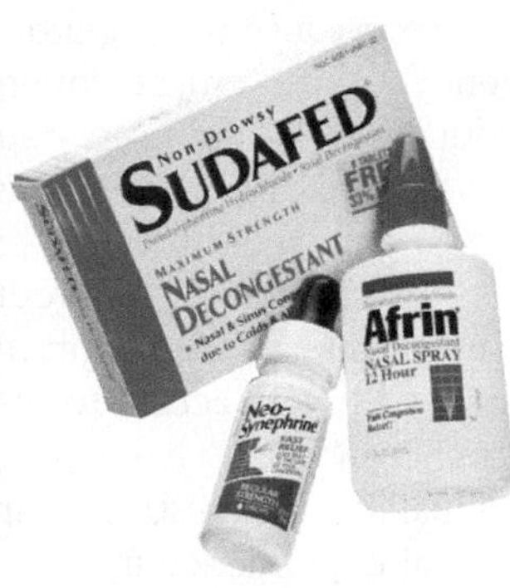

B.C.'s provincial health officer, Dr. Perry Kendall, says cough and cold medicines pose a real health risk when used incorrectly. The abuse of over-the-counter cough medicines, many containing dextromethorphan, is a continuing problem among youth.

approximately 68 600 students in Ontario. Males were significantly more likely to use over-the-counter cough/cold medications to get high than females.[27] Unfortunately, at doses required to get high, there is evidence of pathological changes to neurons in the cerebral cortex of animals.

Recreational Use of PCP In late 1967, workers at the Haight-Ashbury Medical Clinic obtained samples of a substance being distributed as the "Peace Pill." The drug was analyzed and determined to be PCP, and its identity and dangers were publicized in the community in December 1967. By the next year, it was reported that this drug had enjoyed only brief popularity and then disappeared. It appeared briefly in New York in 1968 as "hog" and at other times as "trank." Into the early 1970s, PCP was apparently regarded as pretty much a "garbage" drug by street people. In the early 1970s, PCP crystals were sometimes sprinkled onto oregano, parsley, or alfalfa and sold to unsuspecting youngsters as marijuana. In this form, it became known as **angel dust**. Because PCP can be made inexpensively and relatively easily by amateur chemists, when it is available it usually doesn't cost much. Eventually, the rapid and potent effects of angel dust made it a desired substance in its own right. Joints made with PCP sometimes contained marijuana, sometimes another plant substances, and were known as "killer joints" or "sherms" (because they hit the user like a Sherman tank). In the late 1970s, PCP use was the most

angel dust: the street name for PCP sprinkled on plant material.

common cause of drug-induced visits to hospital emergency rooms in many communities, and in some neighbourhoods young users could be seen "moonwalking" down the street (taking very high, careful, and slow steps) on any Saturday night.

The dependence-producing properties of PCP have also been studied in monkeys, which will press a lever to obtain access to the drug.[65] This is in contrast to LSD and other hallucinogens, which do not support animal self-administration and do not produce psychological dependence in most users.

Because some PCP users have been reported to behave violently, there is a question as to whether PCP tends to promote violence directly or whether violence is a side effect of the suspicion and anaesthesia produced by the drug. Most users do not report feeling violent and feel so uncoordinated that they can't imagine starting a fight. However, police who have tried to arrest PCP users have had trouble subduing them because many of the commonly used arrest techniques rely on restraining holds that result in pain if the arrestee resists. Because the PCP user is anaesthetised, these restraint techniques are less effective. Manual restraint by more than one officer might be required to arrest some PCP users, although this might not be much different from the problem of arresting an alcohol-intoxicated person who is "feeling no pain."

That PCP users might not feel pain has resulted in some gruesome legends about users biting or cutting off their own fingers and so forth. Like earlier stories about LSD users blinding themselves by staring at the sun, these legends cannot be substantiated and most likely have not really occurred. One oft-repeated story probably falls into the category of police folklore. Every cop knows for a fact the story about the PCP user who was so violent, had such superhuman strength, and was so insensitive to pain that he was shot 28 times (or a similar large number of times) before he fell. Although everyone "knows" that this happened, no one can tell you exactly when or where. One might dismiss such folklore as harmless, unless it contributes to such events as the shooting, six times at close range, of an unarmed, naked, 35-year-old biochemist who was trying to climb the street sign outside his laboratory. This story really did happen, on August 4, 1977, during the height of PCP use in the United States. The lethal shots were fired by a Los Angeles police officer. The coroner's office reported that the victim's blood did contain traces of a drug similar to PCP.[66] Several years later, Los Angeles police officers involved in the widely publicized videotaped beating of Rodney King said during their trial that they used such force because they believed King might have been "dusted"–under the influence of PCP. The use of PCP by youth has decreased over the past decade. In 2009 its use dropped to 0.8% among Ontario high school students (grades 7-12).[27]

The mechanism of PCP's action on the brain was a mystery for several years. Today it is known to possess a range of CNS actions, including the inhibition of voltage-dependent sodium and potassium ion channels, and ligand-gated nicotinic, acetylcholine, and N-methyl-D-aspartate (NMDA) glutamate ion channel. Despite its rich pharmacology, the neuropsychiatric profile of PCP, observed at clinically relevant doses, is believed to be mediated by noncompetitive antagonism of the CNS NMDA receptors.[67]

Anticholinergic Hallucinogens

The potato family contains all the naturally occurring agents to be discussed in this section. Three of the genera–*Atropa, Hyoscyamus,* and *Mandragora*–have a single species of importance and were primarily restricted to Europe. The fourth genus, *Datura,* is worldwide and has many species containing the active agents.

The family of plants in which all these genera are found is *Solanaceae,* "herbs of consolation," and three pharmacologically active alkaloids are responsible for the effects of these plants. *Atropine,* which is dl-hyoscyamine, scopolamine, or l-hyoscine, and l-hyoscyamine are all potent central and peripheral cholinergic blocking agents. These drugs occupy the acetylcholine receptor site but do not activate it; thus, their effect is primarily to block muscarinic cholinergic neurons, including the parasympathetic system.

These agents have potent peripheral and central effects, and some of the psychological responses to these drugs are probably a reaction to peripheral changes. These alkaloids block the production of mucus in the nose and throat. They also prevent salivation, so the mouth becomes uncommonly dry, and perspiration stops. Temperature can increase to fever levels (43°C has been reported in infants with atropine poisoning), and heart rate can show a 50-beat-per-minute increase with atropine. Even at moderate doses these chemicals cause considerable dilation of the pupils of the eyes, with a resulting inability to focus on nearby objects. With large enough doses, a behavioural pattern develops that resembles toxic psychosis; there is delirium, mental confusion, loss of attention, drowsiness, and loss of memory for recent events. These two characteristics–a clouding of consciousness and no memory for the period of intoxication–plus the absence of vivid sensory effects separate these drugs from the indole and catechol hallucinogens. The anticholinergics are the original *deliriants.*

Belladonna Atropine, which was isolated in 1831, is the active ingredient in the deadly nightshade, *Atropa belladonna.* The name of the plant reflects two of its major uses in the Middle Ages and before. The genus name reflects its use as a poison. Deadly nightshade was one of the plants used extensively by both professional and amateur poisoners; 14 of its berries contain enough of the alkaloid to cause death.

Belladonna, the species name, meaning "beautiful woman," comes from the use of the extract of this plant to dilate the pupils of the eyes. Interestingly, ancient Roman and Egyptian women knew something that science did not learn until more recently. In the 1950s, it was demonstrated, by using pairs of photographs identical except for the amount of pupil dilation, that most people judge the girl with the more dilated eyes to be prettier.

Of more interest here than pretty girls or poisoned men is the sensation of flying reported by some users of belladonna. The origin of this story goes back at least to the Middle Ages in Europe, and in particular to descriptions of witches and witchcraft. Every early society for which we have any history has a tradition of people with special knowledge of useful plants. In Europe, the people who were consulted for their special arcane knowledge of plant potions were most often women, and their traditions are kept alive in our modern concept of "witches." Among the rich folklore about witches are several accounts from the 1400s describing "flying ointments" (e.g., *The Book of the Sacred Magic of Abremelin the Mage,* 1458), and one ingredient often included in these ointments was deadly nightshade. The notion is that this ointment was spread on the body or on a stick, or "staffe," which was straddled. This is certainly the origin of our notion that witches flew about on broomsticks, though in many accounts it seems that the sticks were used more as phallic symbols and were perhaps ridden in a different manner. What is actually known about witches and witchcraft of that era is confused considerably by what was written about witches by Catholic priests during the Inquisition.

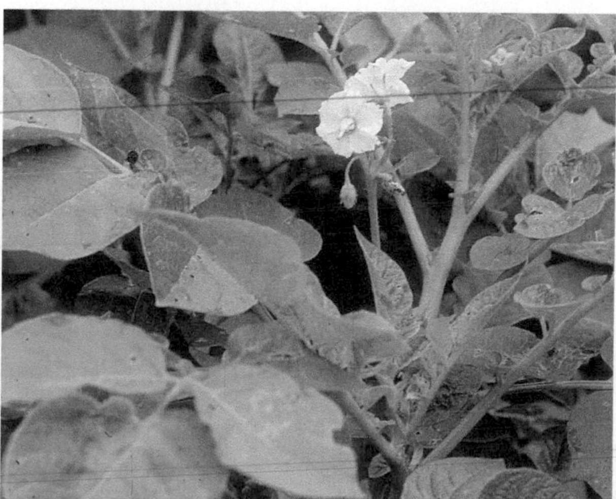

Belladonna, or deadly nightshade, is a poisonous plant that contains an anticholinergic hallucinogen.

During the Middle Ages, all such pagan rituals were considered to be heresy, and practitioners were tortured and killed. Admissions by witches that they "flew" long distances to celebrate Black Mass were extracted during torture and were likely to have reflected the beliefs of the inquisitors more than the history of the person being tortured. Some incredibly lurid accounts of the practices of witches associated drugs, sex, and human sacrifice. Similar lurid accounts linking other drugs (marijuana, LSD, cocaine) to sexual abandon and criminal violence have appeared during more recent years, also promoted by those protecting the established order. The facts are usually not as exciting. Anticholinergics can make people feel light-headed, and in conjunction with the power of suggestion a person might get the *sensation* of floating, or flying, but it's not a realistic way to get from Halifax to Penticton.

Mandrake The *mandrake* plant (*Mandragora officinarum*) contains all three alkaloids. Although many drugs can be traced to the Bible, it is particularly important to do so with mandrake because its close association with love and lovemaking has persisted from Genesis to recent times:

> In the time of wheat-harvest Reuben went out and found some mandrakes in the open country and brought them to his mother Leah. Then Rachel asked Leah for some of her son's mandrakes, but Leah said, "Is it so small a thing to have taken away my husband, that you should take my son's mandrakes as well?" But Rachel said, "Very well, let him sleep with you tonight in exchange for your son's mandrakes." So when Jacob came in from the country in the evening, Leah went out to meet him and said, "You are to sleep with me tonight; I have hired you with my son's mandrakes." That night he slept with her.[68]

The mandrake root is forked and, if you have a vivid imagination, resembles a human body. The root contains the psychoactive agents and was endowed with all sorts of magical and medical properties. The association with the human form is alluded to in Shakespeare's Juliet's farewell speech: "And shrieks like mandrakes torn out of the earth, That living mortals hearing them run mad."

Datura The distribution of the many *Datura* species is worldwide, but they all contain the three alkaloids under discussion–atropine, scopolamine, and hyoscyamine–in varying amounts. Almost as extensive as the distribution are its uses and its history. Although it is not clear when the Chinese first used *Datura metel* as a medicine to treat colds and nervous disorders, the plant was important enough to become associated with Buddha:

> The Chinese valued this drug far back into ancient times. A comparatively recent Chinese medical text, published in 1590, reported that "when Buddha preaches a sermon, the heavens bedew the petals of this plant with rain drops."[69]

Halfway around the world 2500 years before the Chinese text, virgins sat in the temple to Apollo in Delphi and, probably under the influence of *Datura,* mumbled sounds that holy men interpreted as predictions that always came true. Engraved on the temple at Delphi were the words "Know thyself."

Datura is associated with the worship of Shiva in India, where it has long been recognized as an ingredient in love potions and has been known as "deceiver" and "foolmaker." In Asia the practice of mixing the crushed seeds of *Datura metel* in tobacco, cannabis, and food persists even today.

One interesting use of *Datura stramonium,* which is native and grows wild in the eastern United States, was devised by the Algonquin Peoples. They used the plant to solve the problem of the adolescent search for identity:

> The youths are confined for long periods, given " . . . no other substance but the infusion or decoction of some poisonous, intoxicating roots . . ." and "they became stark, staring mad, in which raving condition they were kept eighteen or twenty days." These poor creatures drink so much of that water of Lethe that they perfectly lose the remembrance of all former things, even of their parents, their treasure, and their language. When the doctors find that they have drunk sufficiently of the wysoccan . . . they gradually restore them to their senses again. . . . Thus they unlive their former lives and commence men by forgetting that they ever have been boys.[69]

The same plant is now called Jamestown weed, or jimsonweed, as a result of an incident in the seventeenth century. This was recorded for history in the book *The History and Present State of Virginia,* published first in 1705 by Robert Beverly[70]:

> The *James-Town* Weed (which resembles the Thorny Apple of *Peru,* and I take to be the Plant so call'd) is supposed to be one of the greatest Coolers in the World. This being an early Plant, was gather'd very young for a boil'd Salad, by some of the Soldiers sent thither, to pacifie the Troubles of *Bacon;* and some of them eat plentifully of it, the Effect of which was a very pleasant Comedy; for they turn'd natural Fools upon it for several Days.

Although there has been some recent abuse of jimsonweed, the unpleasant and dangerous side effects of this plant limit its recreational use.

Synthetic Anticholinergics Anticholinergic drugs were once used to treat Parkinson's disease (before the introduction of L-dopa) and are still widely used to treat the pseudoparkinsonism produced by antipsychotic drugs (see Chapter 8). Particularly in older people there is concern about inadvertently producing an "anticholinergic syndrome," characterized by excessive dry mouth, elevated temperature, delusions, and hallucinations. Anticholinergic drugs, such as trihexyphenidyl (PMS Trihexyphenidyl) and benztropine (APO-Benztropine), have only rarely been abused for their delirium-producing properties.

Amanita Muscaria

The *Amanita muscaria* mushroom is also called "fly agaric," probably because of what it does to flies. It doesn't kill them, but when they suck its juice, it puts them into a stupor for two to three hours. It is one of the common poisonous mushrooms found in forests in many parts of the world. The older literature suggests that eating five to ten Amanita mushrooms results in severe effects of intoxication, such as muscular twitching, leading to twitches of limbs and raving drunkenness, with agitation and vivid hallucinations. Later follow many hours of partial paralysis with sleep and dreams.

When the ancient Aryan invaders swept down from the north into India 3500 years ago, they took soma, itself considered a deity. The cult of Soma ruled India's religion and culture for many years–the poems of the Rig Veda celebrate the sacramental use of this substance. It has only been within the past 30 years that scholars have discovered and agreed on the identity of soma as Amanita.[1]

The suggestion has been made that the ambrosia ("food of the gods") mentioned in the secret rites

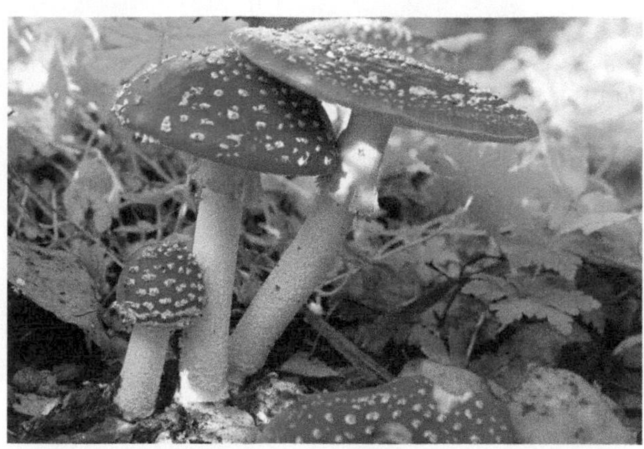

The red and white-speckled mushroom *Amanita muscaria* played a major role in the early history of Indo-European and Central American religions.

of the god Dionysius in Greece was a solution of the Amanita mushroom. And based on paintings representing the "tree of life" found in ancient European cave paintings, it has been suggested that *Amanita muscaria* use formed a basis for the cult that originated about 2000 years ago and today calls itself Christianity.[71]

Until the Russians introduced them to alcohol, many of the isolated nomadic tribes of Siberia had no intoxicant but Amanita:

> Use of the *Amanita* mushroom by Siberian tribes continues today largely free from social control of any sort. Use of the drug has a Shamanist aspect, and forms the basis for orgiastic communal indulgences. Since the drug can induce murderous rages in addition to more moderate hallucinogenic experiences, serious injuries frequently result.[72]

In the frozen northland, these mushrooms are expensive; sometimes several reindeer are exchanged for an effective number of the mushrooms. During the long winter months they might be worth the price. While the mushrooms themselves are not reusable

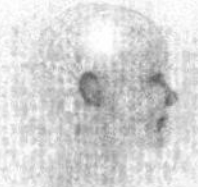

MIND/BODY CONNECTION

Living in the Flow

During the 1960s, the spirit of kinship with a peer group helped fuel the spread of LSD. More recently, the feeling of making intense emotional connections seems to have helped spread a "rave" subculture in Canada, the United States, and elsewhere. This scene, known for its all-night dance parties featuring techno tunes and the drug ecstasy, has had a dedicated following since the early 1990s. It's not, however, just about the music or the drugs, according to those in the rave community. It's about being in the moment, having a brief conversation with a stranger who affects you, having an emotional internal experience.

What really makes people glad to be alive? What are the inner experiences that make life worthwhile? It's easier to talk about dancing than it is to describe a moment of mystical union with the universe. Joy can find us and lift us in moments of ordinary connection, though, and the opening we feel to life is not unlike that experienced through a spiritual quest or mystical practice. The elation comes when we know we belong—to another, to ourselves, to the mystery that is larger than ourselves.

In our society, celebrations and relaxation often involve moving away from the emotion, numbing ourselves with alcohol or drugs. Dance and music are exceptions to this, but too often we are simply spectators in our lives. Sometimes we discount the small joys in daily living. Sometimes we spoil the good by focusing on the less than perfect or seemingly incompatible. Perhaps we don't want to be let down, so we anticipate disappointment rather than expect success and happiness.

Can you think of a time when joy came unexpectedly and caught you off guard? Maybe it was a sudden realization that made you smile. Perhaps it was something you didn't even know you were looking for. Chances are it was a moment when you felt so alive that, ironically, you forgot yourself. Mihaly Csikszentmihalyi, a leading researcher in positive psychology at the University of Chicago, has devoted his life's work to studying what makes people happy, satisfied, and fulfilled. Csikszentmihalyi describes "flow" as a state of consciousness so focused that you are totally absorbed in an activity and lose track of time. It is a state of complete engagement with life in which you feel strong, alert, in effortless control, unselfconscious, and at the peak of your abilities. Examples of when you might experience flow include after completing a hard task, when feeling the wind in your hair during a walk on the beach, during yoga or sex, and when seeing your child respond to your smile for the first time.

What activities usually make you feel happy and completely engaged? During the next week, be aware of and record what activities give you this feeling of deep enjoyment. Then try to build some of these activities into your daily routine to improve the spiritual and emotional quality of your life.

(once eaten, they're gone), the hallucinogen is excreted unchanged in the urine. When the effect begins to wear off, "midway in the party the cry of 'pass the pot' goes out."[73] The active ingredient can be reused four or five times in this way.

There is evidence that Amanita was also used as a holy plant by several tribal groups in the Americas, from Alaska and the Great Lakes to Mexico and Central America. In several of the legends, its origin is associated with thunder and lightning.[1]

For many years the active agent in this mushroom was thought to be *muscarine* (for which the muscarinic cholinergic receptors were named). This substance activates the same type of acetylcholine receptor that is blocked by the anticholinergics. However, pharmacological studies with other cholinergic agonists did not produce similar psychoactive effects. Next, attention focused on *bufotenin*, an indole that is found in high concentrations in the skins of toads. However, the hallucinogenic properties of bufotenin have been in doubt, and Amanita species contain only small amounts of it. In the mid-1960s, meaningful amounts of two chemicals were found: ibotenic acid and muscimol.

The effects of Amanita ingestion are not similar to those of other hallucinogens, and that helped confuse the picture with regard to the mechanism. Muscimol can act as an agonist at GABA receptors, which are inhibitory and found throughout the CNS. Muscimol is more potent than ibotenic acid, and drying of the mushroom, which is usually done by those who use it, promotes the transformation of ibotenic acid to muscimol. Muscimol has been given to humans, resulting in confusion, disorientation in time and place, sensory disturbances, muscle twitching, weariness, fatigue, and sleep.[45]

Amanita muscaria and other related poisonous mushrooms are found in North America, and they are a particularly dangerous type of plant with which to experiment.

Salvia Divinorum

Salvia divinorum, a member of the mint family, is known by its botanical name, which is translated as "diviner's sage." Other names for *Salvia divinorum* include "mystic sage" and "magic mint." It has been used for centuries by the Mazatec people of Oaxaca, Mexico, for shamanistic purposes, and more recently some young people in Mexico have smoked it as a substitute for marijuana. The traditional methods of using the plant include chewing the leaves, drinking a tea made from the crushed leaves, or smoking the dried leaves. The resulting hallucinatory effect is reported to last for up to an hour.[74] *Salvia divinorum* has emerged as a substance of interest worldwide. People in North America and Europe have cultivated the plant for the past several years and use it as a legal hallucinogen. Table 14.4 summarizes the effects of *Salvia divinorum*. Salvia is not currently listed as a controlled substance in Canada, but selling it is illegal, since any natural health product needs an NPN or DIN-HM to be sold legally. So far, salvia has not been approved for sale in Canada and remains illegal for consumption in many U.S. states.

The plant was identified in 1962 by Wasson and Hoffman, and the active component, salvinorin A, was identified in 1982. It is a psychotropic diterpene that produces hallucinations. Salvinorin A is nearly as potent as LSD, in that an effective human dose may be as little as 200 micrograms when smoked. It was reported in 1994 that salvinorin A is a highly selective, naturally occurring agonist of the kappa opioid receptor. The kappa receptor exists in both the spinal cord and the brain; however, the mechanism by which its stimulation produces hallucinations is not known. Thus, this drug represents a newly discovered type of chemical structure and a unique pharmacological effect, which is stimulating research to develop new, related compounds.[75,76]

Table 14.4 Summary of the Effects of *Salvia Divinorum*

Psychological	Systemic
increased self-confidence	feeling of warmth or cold
feeling like someone or something else	**Eyes**
	increased tear production
increased or decreased concentration	**Heart**
	increased heart rate
surroundings seeming unreal	**Respiratory**
increased insight	yawning
calmness	**Muscular**
spiritual experiences	lack of coordination
weird thoughts	**Skin**
floating feeling	chills or gooseflesh
racing thoughts	increased sweating
light-headedness	**Urinary**
euphoria	increased urine production
difficulty sleeping	
irritability	
anxiety	
drowsiness	
dizziness	

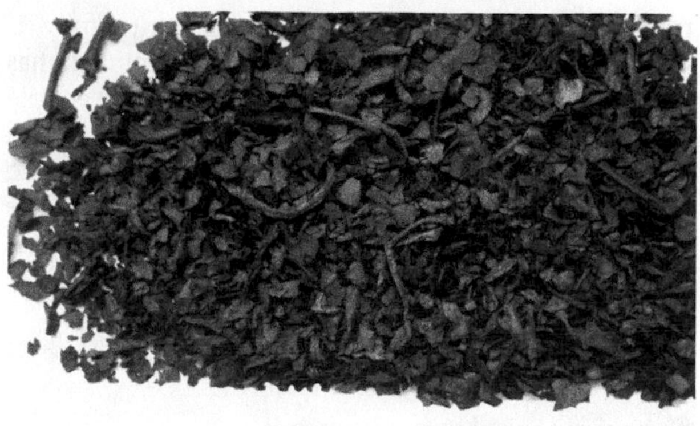

Salvia divinorum is also known as diviner's sage.

An estimated 1.6% of Canadians ages 15 years and older report that they had used salvia in their lifetime. Salvia appears to be a substance that is tried largely by youth (15–24 years of age), with a 6.5% prevalence of lifetime use, which was statistically significantly higher than that reported by persons 25 years of age and older (0.6%).[29] Several features of *Salvia divinorum* make it attractive to young users: (1) the plant material is readily available in stores and over the Internet in Canada; (2) a variety of online sources correctly point out that *Salvia divinorum* does not appear in urine drug screens; and (3) Internet instructions on *Salvia divinorum*'s use repeatedly emphasize its safety. Collectively the apparent safety, lack of detectability, and ease of access of *Salvia divinorum* make it a desirable hallucinogen for adolescents and youth.

With *Salvia divinorum* use, hallucinations occur quite rapidly. The hallucinogenic effects are typically brief, lasting one to two hours, and include synesthesia and confusion. Reports of acute or chronic toxicity have not been provided, although individuals may be susceptible to trauma through lack of insight when under the influence. Furthermore, the number of reports in the literature evaluating tolerance or withdrawal from the effects of salvinorin A are limited.

Recently *Salvia divinorum* has received much attention generated in part by the appearance of a number of popular YouTube videos demonstrating its use. Highly publicized examples of its use have no doubt influenced public opinion on the safety of this herb. In 2011 Health Canada posted notice of its intention to ban *Salvia divinorum* and its active ingredient, salvinorin A. It is proposing to add both to the Controlled Drugs and Substances Act, which would make it illegal to produce, possess, traffic, import, or export the substances. Do you think Health Canada's actions were based on evidence?

Summary

- Hallucinogenic plants have been used for centuries, not only as medicines but also for spiritual and recreational purposes to promote states of detachment from reality and to precipitate mystical insight.
- LSD, a synthetic hallucinogen, alters perceptual processes and enhances emotionality, so that the real world is seen differently and is responded to with great emotion.
- Other chemicals that contain the indole nucleus, such as psilocybin (from the Mexican mushroom), have effects similar to those of LSD.
- Phantastica alters perception while allowing the user to remain in communication with the present world.
- Compared with phantastica, deliriants produce more mental confusion, greater clouding of consciousness, and a loss of touch with reality.
- Indole hallucinogens are drugs that have the indole structure also found in the neurotransmitter serotonin. Examples include LSD and psilocybin.
- Mescaline, from the peyote cactus, and synthetic derivatives of the amphetamines represent the catechol hallucinogens. They have psychological effects quite similar to those of the indole types.
- LSD is not found in nature but synthesized from alkaloids extracted from the ergot fungus *Claviceps purpurea*.
- LSD was synthesized by Dr. Albert Hofmann of Sandoz Laboratories in Switzerland. In psychotherapy, LSD helped patients bring up repressed memories and emotions. In the 1950s the army and CIA used LSD for interrogation of prisoners and spies, believing the drug would reveal the captives' hidden motives.
- Hallucinogen persisting perception disorder is a disorder characterized by a continual presence of visual disturbances (flashbacks) that resemble

those generated by ingestion of hallucinogenic substances weeks or months previously.

- The primary active ingredient of magic mushrooms of Mexico is psilocybin, which has a long history of religious and ceremonial use.
- *Ololiuqui*, the seeds of the morning glory plant, contain several active alkaloids resembling LSD and have been used as psychoactive agents since the sixteenth century.
- Mescaline is the primary active ingredient of peyote and San Pedro cactus, used in the traditional beliefs and practices of Aboriginal peoples.
- *Ayahuasca* means "vine of the soul" a term used both for the vine *Banisteriopsis caapi* and for the medicinal or divinatory brew made from it. The brew contains harmaline, with leaves of *Psychotria viridis*, which contains DMT. Together DMT and harmaline inhibit monoamine oxidase, have psychoactive properties, and are used by South American peoples as a psychoactive religious sacrament.
- DOM, MDA, and MDMA are a group of synthetic hallucinogens chemically related to amphetamine.
- PCP, or angel dust, produces more changes in body perception and fewer visual effects than LSD.
- Anticholinergics are found in many plants throughout the world and have been used not only recreationally, medically, and spiritually but also as poisons. Anticholinergics block the acetylcholine receptor and with large enough doses to cause delirium, mental confusion, loss of attention, drowsiness, and loss of memory for recent events.
- *Amanita muscaria* mushrooms cause severe effects of intoxication, such as twitches of limbs and raving drunkenness, with agitation and vivid hallucinations.
- *Salvia divinorum*, a member of the mint family, is often called mystic sage and magic mint. It has been used for centuries by the Mazatec people of Oaxaca, Mexico, for shamanistic purposes, and more recently some young people in Mexico have smoked it as a substitute for marijuana. The active component, salvinorin A, is a psychotropic diterpene that produces hallucinations similar to LSD.

Review Questions

1. What are the distinctions among phantastica, deliriants, psychedelics, psychotomimetics, entheogens, and hallucinogens?
2. What is the precise relationship between ergotism and LSD?
3. Why was LSD used in psychoanalysis in the 1950s and 1960s? How does this relate to its proposed use by the CIA?
4. Describe the dependence potential of LSD in terms of tolerance, physical dependence, and psychological dependence.
5. What is the diagnostic term for flashbacks?
6. What is the active agent in the "magic mushrooms" of Canada, and is it an indole or a catechol?
7. Besides the psychological effects, what other effects are reliably produced by peyote?
8. Which of the hallucinogenic plants was most associated with witchcraft?
9. What can be concluded from the evidence regarding the neurotoxic effects of MDMA?
10. Which hallucinogen acts as an agonist at kappa opiate receptors?

CHAPTER 15

CANNABIS

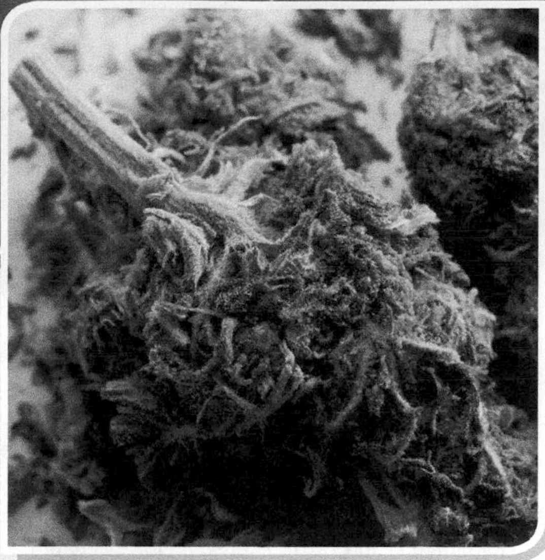

OBJECTIVES

When you have finished this chapter, you should be able to

- **LO1** Explain the relationship between marijuana and cannabis.
- **LO2** Describe the different preparations of cannabis and their THC concentrations.
- **LO3** Describe the use of cannabis throughout history.
- **LO4** Describe the supply, distribution, and trafficking of marijuana, hashish, and hash oil in Canada.
- **LO5** Discuss the prevalence of cannabis use in Canada.
- **LO6** Describe the pharmacological properties of cannabis.
- **LO7** Describe medical conditions for which marijuana has demonstrated effectiveness.
- **LO8** Describe the causes of concern associated with the use of cannabis.

Marijuana has meant many things to many people for a very long time. As such, it is difficult to describe it from a single perspective. This difficulty stems, at least in part, from the fact that marijuana has complex psychoactive properties. In the scientific literature and anecdotally it is purported to produce some pain relief, some sedative-like effects, and, in large doses, hallucinogenic effects. Thus, many of its users treat it as a depressant; it has been called a narcotic (for both pharmacological and political reasons); and it is often included among descriptions of hallucinogenic plants. When used as most people use it the effects of marijuana are quite unique and this makes it challenging to classify it among the other psychoactive drugs. Therefore, like most authors, we present marijuana as a unique substance.

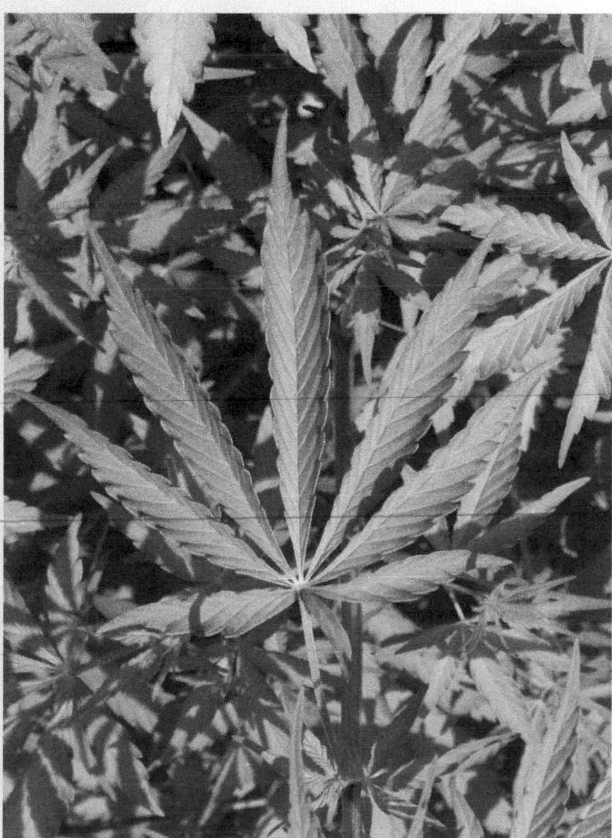

A leaf of the *Cannabis* (marijuana) plant.

LO1 *Cannabis*, the Plant

Marijuana (or *marihuana;* both spellings are correct) is a preparation of leafy material from the **Cannabis** plant that is smoked. The question is which *Cannabis* plant,

Cannabis: the genus of plant known as marijuana.

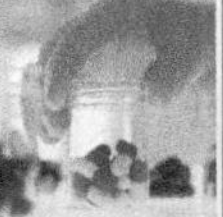

DRUGS IN THE MEDIA

Health Canada Statement: Changes to the Reporting Requirements in the MMPR

Health Canada does not endorse the use of marijuana and is taking the necessary steps to protect public safety while providing reasonable access to marijuana for medical purposes, as ordered by the Courts. The program introduced in 2001 under the *Marihuana Medical Access Regulations* was open to serious abuse and had unintended consequences for public health, safety and security, as a result of allowing individuals to produce marijuana in their homes. The *Marihuana for Medical Purposes Regulations,* which came into force in June 2013, strengthen the safety of Canadian communities, while making sure that Canadians who are authorized, have access to marijuana grown under secure and sanitary conditions.

As of April 1, 2014, producing marijuana in a home or private dwelling will be illegal. As of that date the only legal source of marijuana will be produced under secure and quality-controlled conditions by licensed producers. Licensed producers will have to comply with strict regulatory requirements to demonstrate security and quality.

Possession and use of marijuana remains illegal in Canada unless authorized under the regulations with the support of a doctor or nurse practitioner.

Recently, the Government of Canada amended the *Marihuana for Medical Purposes Regulations* to require participants of the Marihuana Medical Access Program to provide written notice to Health Canada by April 30, 2014, stating that they no longer possess marijuana (dried marijuana, plants or seeds) obtained under the old program. Those that were authorized to grow marijuana must also attest that they have discontinued production. Participants are also required to confirm the amount of marijuana and number of plants destroyed, if any.

If participants do not comply with the requirement to notify Health Canada, the Department will notify law enforcement. The Department will also continue to cooperate with police and provide information needed to protect public safety, as appropriate.

Source: Adapted from Health Canada (2014). Drugs and Health Products. Medical Use of Marihuana. Statement: Changes to the Reporting Requirements in the *Marihuana for Medical Purposes Regulations*. Retrieved from http://www.hc-sc.gc.ca/dhp-mps/marihuana/changesmmpr-changementsrmfm-eng.php on March 17, 2014.

because botanical debate continues over whether one, three, or more species of *Cannabis* exist. In previous years, this issue spurred legal arguments because the laws mentioned only *Cannabis sativa*. Does that include all marijuana or not? The evidence is strong that three separate species exist. *Cannabis sativa* originated in Asia but now grows worldwide and primarily has been used for its fibres, from which hemp rope and other items are made. This is the species that grows as a weed in the United States and Canada. *Cannabis indica* is grown for its psychoactive resins and is cultivated in many areas of the world, including backyards in Canada and the United States. The third species, *Cannabis ruderalis,* grows primarily in Russia and not at all in North America. The plant Linnaeus named *C. sativa* in 1753 is what is still known as *C. sativa.*[1]

THC: delta-9-tetrahydrocannabinol, the most psychoactive chemical in marijuana, hashish, and hash oil.

C. sativa that is cultivated for use as hemp grows as a lanky plant up to 5.5 metres high. *C. indica* plants cultivated for their psychoactive effects are more compact and usually only 1 metre tall. The psychoactive potency results from an interaction between genetics and environmental conditions. Plants of different species grown under identical conditions produce different amounts of psychoactive material, and the same plants vary in potency from year to year, depending on the amount of sunshine, warm weather, and moisture.

LO2 Cannabis Preparations

The primary psychoactive agent, delta-9-tetrahydrocannabinol (**THC**), is concentrated in the resin of the *Cannabis* plant; most of the resin is in the flowering tops, less is in the leaves, and little is in the fibrous stalks. The psychoactive potency of a cannabis preparation depends on the amount of resin present and therefore varies depending on the part of the plant used.[1] India has produced three traditional cannabis

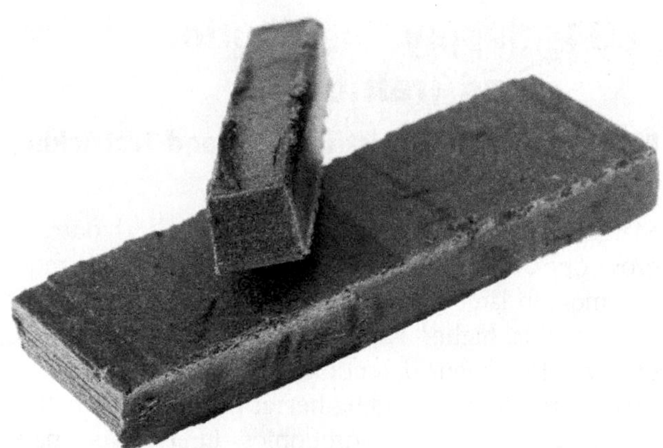

Hashish, concentrated resin from the *Cannabis* plant, is becoming more widespread in Canada but is relatively rare in the United States.

preparations that roughly correspond to those available in Canada. The most potent of these is called *charas,* and it consists of pure resin that has been carefully removed from the surface of leaves and stems. **Hashish**, or *hasheesh,* is a substance widely known around the world and in its purest form is pure resin, like charas. It may be less pure, depending on how carefully the resin has been separated from the plant material. In 2009, the quantity of hash products seized in Canada (9907 kilograms) was almost six times the amount seized in 2008 (1660 kilograms).[2]

The second most potent preparation is traditionally called *ganja* in India, and it consists of the dried flowering tops of plants with pistillate flowers (female plants). The male plants are removed from the fields before the female plants can become pollinated and put their energy into seed production. This increases the potency of the female plants and produces high-grade marijuana known as **sinsemilla** (from the Spanish *sin semilla,* "without seeds").

The weakest form is traditionally called *bhang* in India. Bhang is made from the remainder of the plant, after the top has been picked. These remnants are dried and ground into a powder that can then be mixed into drinks or candies.[1] This type of preparation is rare in Canada, but it is similar to our low-grade marijuana, which consists of the leaves of a plant and perhaps even components of the *sativa* plant. Some of this low-grade marijuana contains less than 1% THC.

Manually scraping exuded resin off the plant to make hashish is a tedious process, and more efficient methods for separating the resin exist. Products of these processes are referred to as "red oil of cannabis," or *hash oil.* These products vary widely in their potency but can contain more than 50% THC.

LO3 History of Cannabis

Documented use of cannabis goes back as far as the third millennium BCE.

Early History

The earliest reference to cannabis is in a pharmacy book written in 2737 BCE by Chinese emperor Shen Nung. Referring to the euphoriant effects of cannabis, he called it the "Liberator of Sin." He recommended it for some medical uses, including "female weakness, gout, rheumatism, malaria, beriberi, constipation and absent-mindedness." Social use of the plant had spread to the Muslim world and North Africa by 1000 CE. In this period in the eastern Mediterranean area, a legend developed around a religious cult that committed murder for political reasons. The cult was called "hashishiyya," from which our word *assassin* developed. In 1299, Marco Polo told the story he had heard of this group and its leader. It was a marvellous tale and had all the ingredients necessary for a story to survive through the ages: intrigue, murder, sex, the use of drugs, and mysterious lands. The story of this group and its activities has been told in many ways over the years, and Boccaccio's *Decameron* contains one story based on it. Stories of this cult, combined with the frequent reference to the power and wonderment of hashish in *The Arabian Nights,* were widely circulated in Europe over the years.

The Nineteenth Century: Romantic Literature and the New Science of Psychology

By the start of the nineteenth century, world commerce and travel was expanding. Exciting reports from travellers of the seventeenth and eighteenth centuries introduced new cultural practices and ideas to Europeans. Exploration of Asia and the Middle East had revealed exotic spices, as well as the stimulants coffee and tea. Europe was ready for another new sensation and got it. The returning veteran, as usual, gets part of the blame for introducing what Europe was ready to receive:

> Napoleon's campaign to Egypt at the beginning of the nineteenth century increased the Romantic's acquaintance with hashish and caused them to associate it with

hashish: concentrated resin from the *Cannabis* plant.

sinsemilla: "without seeds"; high-grade or more potent marijuana.

> the Near East. . . . Napoleon was forced to give an order forbidding all French soldiers to indulge in hashish. Some of the soldiers brought the habit to France, however, as did many other Frenchmen who worked for the government or traveled in the Near East.[3]

By the 1830s and 1840s, everyone who was anyone was using, thinking about using, or decrying the use of mind-tickling agents such as opium and hashish. One of the earliest (1844) popular accounts of the use of hashish is in *The Count of Monte Cristo* by Alexander Dumas. The story includes a reference to the assassin's tale and contains statements about the characteristics of the drug that still sound contemporary. During the 1840s, a group of artists and writers gathered monthly at the Hotel Pimodan in Paris's Latin Quarter to use drugs. This group became famous because one of the participants, Gautier, wrote a book, *Le Club de Hachischins,* which described their activities. From this group have come some of the best literary descriptions of hashish intoxication. These French Romantics, like the Impressionist painters of a later period, were searching for new experiences, new sources of creativity from within, and new ways of seeing the world outside. A few of the regulars were well-known writers, including Baudelaire, Gautier, and Dumas.

Baudelaire used hashish and was an astute observer of its effects in himself and in others. In his book *Artificial Paradises,* he echoed what Dumas had written about the kind of effect to expect from hashish:

> The intoxication will be nothing but one immense dream, thanks to intensity of color and the rapidity of conceptions; but it will always preserve the particular tonality of the individual. . . . The dream will certainly reflect its dreamer. He is only the same man grown larger . . . sophisticate and ingenu . . . will find nothing miraculous, absolutely nothing but the natural to an extreme.[4]

History of Cannabis Policy in Canada

Beginning with the passage of the Opium Act of 1908, Canada has followed a stern prohibitionist line to control illicit drug use.[5] For much of the twentieth century, Canada's illicit drug policies and laws were heavily influenced by law enforcement interests and seen as one of the most punitive drug control systems in the world.[6] Chapter 3 provides broad discussion pertaining to the history of drug regulation in Canada with specific reference to the evolution of laws and policies related to marijuana.

LO4 Supply, Distribution, and Trafficking

Marijuana Supply, Distribution, and Trafficking in Canada

Marijuana is cultivated in both indoor and outdoor grow operations in Canada. Indoor cultivation is more common, in large part due to our climate, and ensures larger yields, higher THC levels, and better avoidance of law enforcement detection. Advances in indoor cultivation methods, including better growing techniques and equipment (e.g., hydroponics, LED lights), have contributed to higher THC levels.[2]

In 2009 the Royal Canadian Mounted Police published a study entitled *Report on the Illicit Drug Situation in Canada.*[2] This report showed that the amount of marijuana produced in Canada exceeded domestic demand and that organized crime groups were producing it for export to other countries, most notably the United States. In fact, the U.S. National Drug Intelligence Center has identified Canada as a source country for high-grade marijuana.

Illicit marijuana cultivation is known to take place in all Canadian provinces and territories, however production predominantly occurs in British Columbia, Ontario, and Quebec. In 2009, Canadian law enforcement agencies seized 34 391 kilograms of marijuana and 1 845 734 marijuana plants. While the majority of marijuana seized was domestically produced, Jamaica,

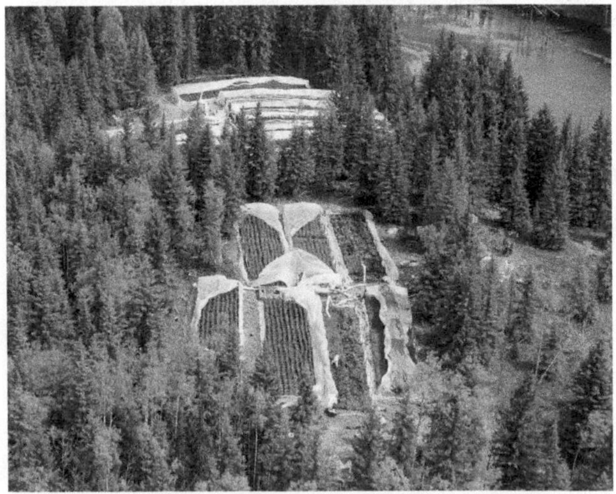

An example of an outdoor marijuana grow operation.

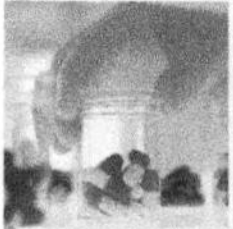

DRUGS IN THE MEDIA

Grow-Ops Worth $17 Million Busted in Calgary Area

Police have broken up nine grow-ops in the Calgary area and seized more than $17 million worth of marijuana, officials said on Thursday. Officers seized more than 13 500 plants and 44 kilograms of harvested marijuana, along with growing equipment. The operations were set up by two organized crime groups working in collaboration, officials said.

More than 80 criminal charges have been laid against nine people, said officials with Alberta Law Enforcement Response Team's (ALERT) Green Team South, which ran an 18-month investigation leading up the bust. Two of the grow-ops were in Okotoks, one in Strathmore and the rest were in Calgary. Some of the homes had been rented by people posing as legitimate families. After using false names and counterfeit identification on the rental agreement, the suspects then converted the properties to grow-ops, police said.

"This investigation confirmed that most large marihuana grow operations are connected to organized crime," said Staff Sgt. Tom Hanson. "Nearly all of the properties had dangerously compromised electrical and natural gas utilities, exemplifying the hazards inherent in many grow operations we dismantle." Two grow-ops dismantled in rural Alberta in 2010 are also believed to be connected to these two groups, police said.

Source: Used with permission of the CBC. CBC News (2011). Grow-Ops Worth $17 Million Busted in Calgary Area. Retrieved from http://www.cbc.ca/news/canada/calgary/story/2011/07/14/calgary-grow-bust.html

the United States, the Netherlands, and Thailand were also source countries for marijuana consumed in Canada. Shipments of marijuana destined for Canada were typically smuggled through air cargo or passenger flights arriving primarily at Toronto Pearson International Airport.

Hashish and Hash Oil Supply, Distribution, and Trafficking in Canada

Hash and hash oil smuggled into Canada originates predominantly from South Asia (e.g., Afghanistan and Pakistan), the Middle East (e.g., Lebanon), Africa (e.g., Morocco, South Africa, Mozambique, and Kenya), and the Caribbean (e.g., Jamaica). In the past, multi-metric-ton shipments of hash have been transported to Canada aboard *motherships* (vessels whose sole purpose is for the transport of drugs) or concealed in marine containers aboard commercial transport vessels. Commercial airlines have been used to smuggle smaller amounts of hash through either air freight or *drug mules*.[2]

For many years, Morocco was reportedly the largest supplier of hash to the world market. The United Nations Office on Drugs and Crime estimated that, in 2008, Morocco produced 877 metric tons of hash. However, a 2009 *Afghanistan Cannabis Survey* indicated that Afghanistan was emerging as one of the world's top hash producers with exports between 1500 and 3500 metric tons.

Pakistan is one of the main source countries of hash used in Canada. Of the 9907 kilograms of hash seized in 2009, approximately 40% originated from Pakistan. In that same year Canada's second major source of hash was Afghanistan, oftentimes transited through South Africa. The majority of hash product seized in 2009 arrived in Canada via marine shipments to the ports of Montreal and Halifax. However, the majority of actual seizures occurred at Toronto Pearson International Airport. Finally, for decades Jamaica had been Canada's primary supplier of hash oil. In 2009, 68% of all hash oil seized originated in Jamaica.

LO5 Prevalence Rates of Cannabis Use

The *Canadian Alcohol and Drug Use Monitoring Survey* (CADUMS), described in Chapter 1, is an ongoing general population survey of alcohol and illicit drug use among Canadians ages 15 years and older. Table 15.1 shows data describing the prevalence of past-year cannabis use, an estimate of lifetime use, and the age of initiation for use among Canadians in 2012.[7] Table 15.2

Table 15.1 Canadian Alcohol and Drug Use Monitoring Survey, Prevalence Rates of Cannabis Use by Sex and Age, 2012

	Overall	Males	Females	15–24 Years	25+ Years
N	11 090	4386	6704	687	10 403
Cannabis past-year use	10.2 9.1–11.4	13.7 11.8–15.6	7.0* 5.7–8.2	20.3 15.9–24.6	8.4† 7.3–9.5
Cannabis lifetime use	41.5 39.8–43.3	47.9 45.1–50.7	35.5* 33.4–37.7	34.8 29.5–40.1	42.8† 41.0–44.6
Age of initiation	18.6 18.4–18.9	18.5 18.1–18.8	18.8 18.5–19.1	16.1 15.8–16.4	19.0† 18.7–19.3

Notes: Prevalence rates are expressed as a percentage (%) with the corresponding 95% confidence interval.
* Indicates significant differences between males and females, $p < .05$.
† Indicates significant differences between youth ages 15–24 and adults ages 25 +, $p < .05$.

Table 15.2 Canadian Alcohol and Drug Use Monitoring Survey, Cannabis Use by Province, 2012

	Canada	NL	PE	NS	NB	QC	ON	MB	SK	AB	BC
N	11 090	1008	1008	1009	1009	1008	1011	1009	1010	1009	2009
Cannabis past-year use	10.2	11.0	10.6	12.1	8.5	9.0	9.1	13.2	10.2	11.4	13.8
Cannabis lifetime use	41.5	38.7	40.9	42.4	36.4	40.6	39.4	38.5	42.5	44.3	48.7

Note: Prevalence rates are expressed as a percentage (%).

illustrates cannabis use by province in 2012. Data presented in Table 15.3 allow the comparison of lifetime use, past-year use, and age of initiation, according to age and gender, across the years 2004 and 2012. For example, there was an increase in past-year cannabis use among adults aged 25 years and older, from 6.7% in 2011 to 8.4% in 2012. However, no change from 2011 among youth aged 15 to 24 years was observed. On the other hand, the prevalence of past-year cannabis use among among youth 15 to 24 years old (20.3%) remained higher than in adults 25 years of age and older (8.4%). Youths initiated use of cannabis at an older age in 2012 than in 2011 (16.1 versus 15.6 years), and the prevalence of past-year cannabis use in 2012 was lower than in 2004 among males (13.7% versus 18.2%), females (7.0% versus 10.2%), and youth aged 15 to 24 years (20.3% versus 37.0%). It is interesting to note that the prevalence of lifetime use among adults aged 25 years and older did not change between 2004 and 2012.

Table 15.2 shows that the provincial prevalence of past-year cannabis use ranged from 8.5% in New Brunswick to 13.8% in British Columbia. Each province's past-year cannabis prevalence was compared with the average prevalence for the nine remaining provinces. Of these, only British Columbia shows higher than average prevalence.

Table 15.3 illustrates changes in cannabis use between CAS 2004 and CADUMS 2008-2012 by age and gender. There were statistically significant decreases in past-year cannabis use over the five years by gender and within age categories.

What Canadian Youth Think about Cannabis

We have seen above and throughout this textbook that cannabis is one of the most commonly used illicit drugs among Canadian youth 15 to 24 years of age.[7] A recent cross-Canada study of student drug and

Table 15.3 Changes in Cannabis Use between CAS 2004 and CADUMS 2008–2012, by Age and Gender

	CAS	CADUMS					CAS	CADUMS				
	2004	2008	2009	2010	2011	2012	2004	2008	2009	2010	2011	2012
	Cannabis Use (%) by Age											
	15–24 years of age						**25 years of age+**					
N	2085	1443	955	3989	671	687	11 519	15 197	12 079	9626	9405	10 403
Cannabis lifetime	61.4	52.9*	42.9**	41.7(*)	34.0^‡	34.8†	41.8	42.1	42.3	41.4	40.4	42.8
Cannabis—past year	37.0	32.7	26.3**	25.1(*)	21.6^	20.3†	10.0	7.3*	7.6**	7.9	6.7^	8.4#
Age of initiation (years)	15.6	15.5	15.6	15.7	15.6	16.1#	19.7	19.2	19.3	18.9(*)	19.3	19.0
	Cannabis Use (%) by Gender											
	Males						**Females**					
N	5721	6583	5260	5980	4247	4386	8188	10 057	7822	7635	5829	6704
Cannabis—lifetime	50.1	49.3	48.0	48.8	45.5	47.9	39.2	38.8	37.2	34.5(*)	33.6^	35.5
Cannabis—past year	18.2	14.4*	14.2**	14.6(*)	12.2^	13.7†	10.2	8.6	7.2**	7.1(*)	6.2^	7.0†
Age of initiation (years)	18.8	18.5	18.7	18.4	18.6	18.5	18.7	18.4	18.7	18.4	19.0‡	18.8

N = sample size
* Indicates the difference between 2008 and 2004 is statistically significant.
** Indicates the difference between 2009 and 2004 is statistically significant.
(*) Indicates the difference between 2010 and 2004 is statistically significant.
^ Indicates the difference between 2011 and 2004 is statistically significant.
† Indicates the difference between 2012 and 2004 is statistically significant.
‡ Indicates the difference between 2011 and 2010 is statistically significant.
# Indicates the difference between 2012 and 2011 is statistically significant.

alcohol use determined that youths' past-year use of cannabis was three times higher than that of adults aged 25 years and older (21.6% vs. 6.7%). Furthermore, in some Canadian jurisdictions up to 50% of grade 12 students reported consuming cannabis within the last year.[8]

Despite the prevalence of cannabis use among Canadian youth, little is known about how they perceive the drug or what influences their decisions to use it. The Canadian Centre on Substance Abuse (CCSA) conducted a study to examine youth perceptions and decisions.[9] A total of 76 youth between the ages of 14 and 19 recruited from cities across Canada including Toronto, Moncton, Halifax, Salmon Arm, and Vancouver participated in 12 focus groups. It is important to note that this sample should not be considered representative of Canadian youth. Sixty-two percent of participants were male. Sixty-two percent of interviewed youth had used cannabis in the past, and approximately half indicated they had used it within the last 24 hours. Several key themes derived from this study are explored in the following sections. Even though this study of Canadian youth is based on a small sample size, the findings highlight the convolution surrounding the use of cannabis. Canadian youth appear puzzled with what they perceive as the current diverse messaging they are given about cannabis.

Influences for Smoking and Not Smoking Cannabis Peer pressure, social connectedness to peers, and the drug's perceived availability and popularity were all identified as factors associated with youths' decisions to use, or not to use, cannabis. Youth held a common belief that "everyone smokes weed" and that not using cannabis is abnormal. Alternatively, concerns pertaining to health risks, poor academic performance, and negative impacts on family relationships were factors associated with youths' decisions to abstain from using cannabis.

Perceived Positive and Negative Effects of Cannabis Use In general, youth perceived more positive effects than negative ones. Included among the positive effects of marijuana use was the ability to help one focus, relax, sleep, be less violent, and be

Table 15.4 Global Estimates of Illicit Drug Users by Region, 2011 (est. millions in past year)

Region	Cannabis	Opiates	Cocaine	Amphetamines	Ecstasy
Africa	27.7–52.8	0.7–2.9	1.0–2.7	1.6–5.2	0.4–1.9
Americas	38.2–40.0	2.3–2.4	8.7–9.1	4.8–5.9	3.0–3.3
Asia	31.5–64.6	6.5–12.5	0.4–2.3	4.4–40.0	2.4–15.6
Europe	29.4–30.0	3.3–3.8	4.6–5.0	2.5–3.2	3.9–4.1
Oceanic	2.1–3.4	0.1–0.2	0.3–0.4	0.5–0.6	0.8–0.9
Global	128.9–190.8	12.8–21.9	15.1–19.4	13.7–52.9	10.5–25.8

Source: Adapted from the United Nations Office on Drugs and Crime. *World Drug Report*. 2010. Retrieved March 12, 2011, from http://www.unodc.org/documents/wdr/WDR_2010/World_Drug_Report_2010_lo-res.pdf.

more creative. Some youth also reported the belief that cannabis could "purify one's system" or cure cancer. Perceived negative effects of the drug's use included developing a dependency, losing focus, becoming lazy, developing lung and heart conditions, and increasing criminality. It was interesting to note that the study participants perceived cannabis to affect each person differently, and negative effects, including long-term changes in chronic users, were attributed to the individual and not cannabis itself.

Perception That Cannabis Is Natural and Safe, and Not a Drug Many Canadian youth stated that cannabis was not a drug, for reasons including the belief that it was natural, safe, and non-addictive. Youth stated that, unlike harder drugs, cannabis could reduce violent tendencies and would not change the user's perception of reality. Overall they felt cannabis was much safer than alcohol and tobacco.

Cannabis and Driving As described above, many youth believe that cannabis is safe. Their opinions on driving under the influence of cannabis were varied, however. Some believed that cannabis makes people better drivers by increasing their focus, while others saw driving under its influence as dangerous and constituting impaired driving. It was interesting to discover that even those opposed to driving under the influence of cannabis believed it to be not as dangerous as drunk driving.

Legality of Cannabis Participants were uncertain about the legality of cannabis. Some felt cannabis was legal depending on age and the amount in one's possession. Lack of clarity pertaining to the legality of medical marijuana may have, in part, contributed to the confusion.

Worldwide Use of Cannabis

Cannabis is the most widely consumed illicit drug in the world. As shown in Table 15.4, the United Nations Office on Drugs and Crime estimates that between 155 million and 250 million people (3.5% to 5.7% of the population ages 15–64) used an illicit substance at least once in 2008. Cannabis users are the largest number of illicit drug users (129 million–190 million people) worldwide. Global annual cannabis use prevalence is estimated between 2.9% and 4.3% of the population ages 15–64. Amphetamine-group substances rank as the second most commonly used drug, followed by cocaine and opiates. Estimates of illicit drug use are often derived from household and school surveys, raising concern over the accuracy of the estimates. Furthermore, a lack of data, particularly for Africa, some parts of Asia, and the Pacific Islands, has limited our ability to gain a truly worldwide perspective on illicit drug use.

Compassion Clubs

Compassion clubs (also known as cannabis clubs or buyers' clubs) are organizations where Canadians can purchase a variety of strains of cannabis and other cannabis products. These clubs vary in size and organizational structure, with some being well established. Although these clubs are self-regulated, there are no federal standards under which they operate to produce and distribute marijuana. Typically, membership in these clubs involves filling out a form and having a physician sign it and provide a letter regarding the individual's health diagnosis and requirement for marijuana for the condition.[10] However, even with such documentation, Health Canada, under the Marihuana for Medical Purposes Regulations (MMPR), does not

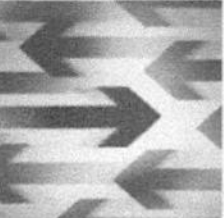

TAKING SIDES

Bring the Prince of Pot, Marc Emery, Back to Canada to Serve His Time, Say 3 MPs

The fight to have the U.S.-imprisoned Marc Emery, aka the Prince of Pot, transferred to Canada for the remainder of his prison sentence was taken to Parliament Hill Tuesday where members of parliament joined his wife, Jodie Emery, in a public call for his return. NDP deputy leader Libby Davies, Liberal public safety critic Wayne Easter and Green MP Elizabeth May all spoke out at the morning press conference, held to encourage federal safety minister Steven Blaney to sign the required paperwork for Emery's transfer home. While Jodie described the conference as a success in that it garnered a considerable amount of attention, she was dismayed with the response to the event reportedly offered by the minister's office.

"Unfortunately, it seems Minister Blaney's office commented on this press conference by saying they are disappointed that the opposition wants to continue to promote the drug trade," she said from Ottawa. "Of course, this is not what it is about. This is about Canadian citizenship. I don't know if that kind of hints towards either a rejection or just being ignored, but it doesn't sound like they are interested in taking action to help." A *Province* request for an official comment from the minister's office on the matter was not returned.

Marc Emery, a well-known pot activist and successful businessman, was extradited to the U.S. in 2010 and sentenced to a five-year prison term, to be served in a Mississippi jail, for selling marijuana seeds to U.S. customers through his Vancouver hemp shop. After initially denying his request for a transfer, U.S. authorities approved the move last July, and Jodie has since been pressuring Ottawa to offer its approval. Davies, who has been involved in the case since the beginning, said she was also disturbed by the very "political" comments that reportedly came from the minister's office. "This press conference is not about the war on drugs, it is about a Canadian, who has been cleared by U.S. to return home," said Davies. "I think it is better for Mr. Emery and his family to be here."

Jodie said the support offered from the members of parliament in attendance Tuesday shows that "Marc is clearly not a criminal" and that he is a "well-respected, highly-regarded Canadian" who has both the public's support and that of the political establishment. "It shows that he is someone who deserves to come home," she said, adding that even Ottawa doesn't approve his transfer, Marc will be eligible for release in July 2014. "They kick him out of the U.S. [at that date] and he will begin his trip home," she said. "So next August for sure, right after our anniversary, he will be home."

Source: Cassidy Olivier, *The Province*. (2013). "Bring the Prince of Pot, Marc Emery, Back to Canada to Serve His Time, Say 3 MPs." October 29, 2013. Retrieved from http://www.cannabisculture.com/content/2013/10/31/Bring-Prince-Pot-Marc-Emery-Back-Canada-Serve-His-Time-Say-3-MPs on January 22, 2014.

license or permit organizations like compassion clubs to possess, produce, or distribute marijuana for medicinal purposes. Purchasing marijuana from compassion clubs contradicts the regulations of the Controlled Drugs and Substances Act, meaning that individuals who purchase marijuana through these clubs can be subject to law enforcement measures. Additionally, compassion clubs operate outside of Canadian laws, making them a law enforcement issue.[11,12]

LO6 Pharmacology

Cannabinoid Chemicals

The chemistry of the *Cannabis* plant is quite complex, and the isolation and extraction of the active ingredient are difficult even today. There are more than 400 chemicals in marijuana, but only 66 of them are unique to the *Cannabis* plant—these are called cannabinoids. One of them, delta-9-tetrahydrocannabinol (THC), was isolated and synthesized in 1964 and is clearly the most pharmacologically active. Structures of some of these chemicals are shown in Figure 15.1. The major active metabolite in the body of THC is 11-hydroxy-delta-9-THC.

Absorption, Distribution, and Elimination

When smoked, THC is rapidly absorbed into the blood and distributed first to the brain, then redistributed to the rest of the body, so that within 30 minutes much is gone from the brain. The peak psychological and cardiovascular effects occur together, usually within 5–10 minutes. The THC remaining in the blood has a half-life

Figure 15.1 Delta-9-THC, the Most Psychoactive Substance Found in Cannabis, and Anandamide, Isolated from Brain Tissue

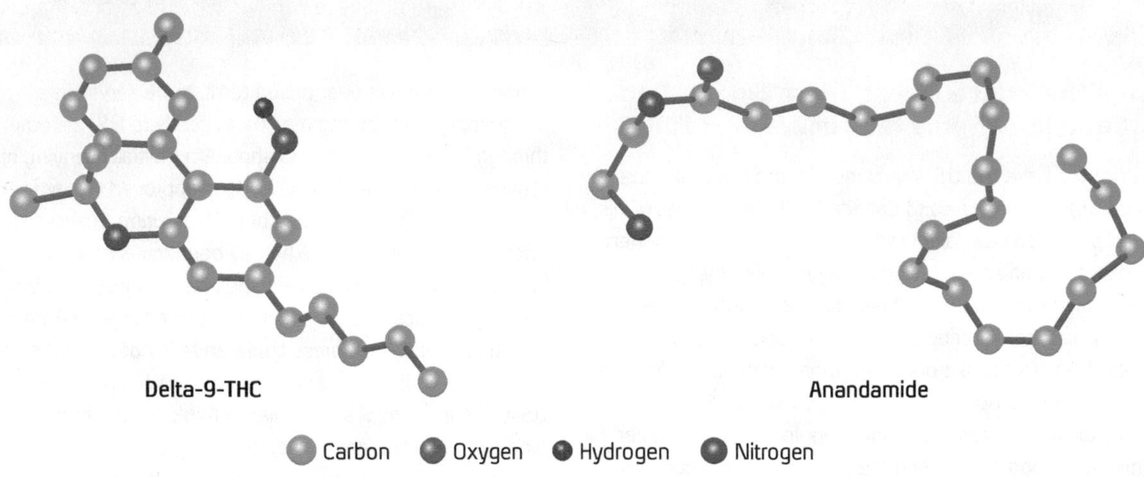

of about 19 hours, but metabolites (of which there are at least 45), primarily 11-hydroxy-delta-9-THC, are formed in the liver and have a half-life of 50 hours. After one week, 25%–30% of the THC and its metabolites might still remain in the body. Complete elimination of a large dose of THC and its metabolites might take two or three weeks. THC taken orally is slowly absorbed, and the liver transforms it to 11-hydroxy-delta-9-THC; therefore, much less THC reaches the brain after oral ingestion, and it takes much longer for it to have psychological and cardiovascular effects. The peak effects following oral ingestion usually occur at about 90 minutes.

The high lipid solubility of THC means that it (like its metabolites) is selectively taken up and stored in fatty tissue to be released slowly. Excretion is primarily through the feces. All of this has two important implications: (1) there is no easy way to monitor (in urine or blood) THC or metabolite levels and relate them to behavioural and physiological effects, as can be done with alcohol, and (2) the long-lasting, steady, low concentration of THC and its metabolites on the brain and other organs might have effects not yet determined.

Mechanism of Action

Scientists searched for years for a key to help them unlock the mystery of marijuana's action on the central nervous system. The identification and purification of THC was a necessary step. A significant breakthrough was made by researchers in 1988 when they developed a technique to identify and measure highly specific and selective binding sites for THC and related compounds in rat brains. One result was the development and testing of more potent marijuana analogues. Another result was the 1992 discovery of a natural substance produced in the body that has marijuana-like effects when administered to animals. This endogenous substance (shown in Figure 15.1) is called **anandamide** (*ananda* is sanskrit for "bliss").[13]

> **anandamide:** a chemical isolated from brain tissue that has marijuana-like properties.

THC and other cannabinoids are known to bind to two receptors, designated CB_1 and CB_2.[14] There are substantial differences in the structures of these two receptors and their anatomical distribution in the body. CB_2 receptors are found mainly outside the brain in immune cells, suggesting that cannabinoids may play a role in the modulation of the immune response. CB_1 receptors are found throughout the body, but primarily in the brain (see Figure 15.2). These receptors are much more abundant than receptors for morphine and heroin,[11] suggesting that the potential actions of cannabinoids are widespread. The locations of CB_1 receptors in the brain also may provide some clues about their functions. For example, the highest density of CB_1 receptors has been found in cells of the basal ganglia; its primary components include the caudate nucleus, putamen, and globus pallidus. Cells of the basal ganglia are involved in coordinating body movements. Other regions that also contain a larger number of CB_1 receptors include the *cerebellum*, which coordinates fine body movements; the *hippocampus*, which

Figure 15.2 Marijuana's Effects on the Brain

When marijuana, hashish, or hash oil is ingested, the psychoactive ingredient in these preparations, delta-9-THC, produces its effects through the activation of or binding to cannabinoid receptors (CB_1) in the brain. These CB_1 receptors are widely distributed throughout the brain but are found especially in areas responsible for the regulation of movement, coordination, learning and memory, and higher cognitive functions.

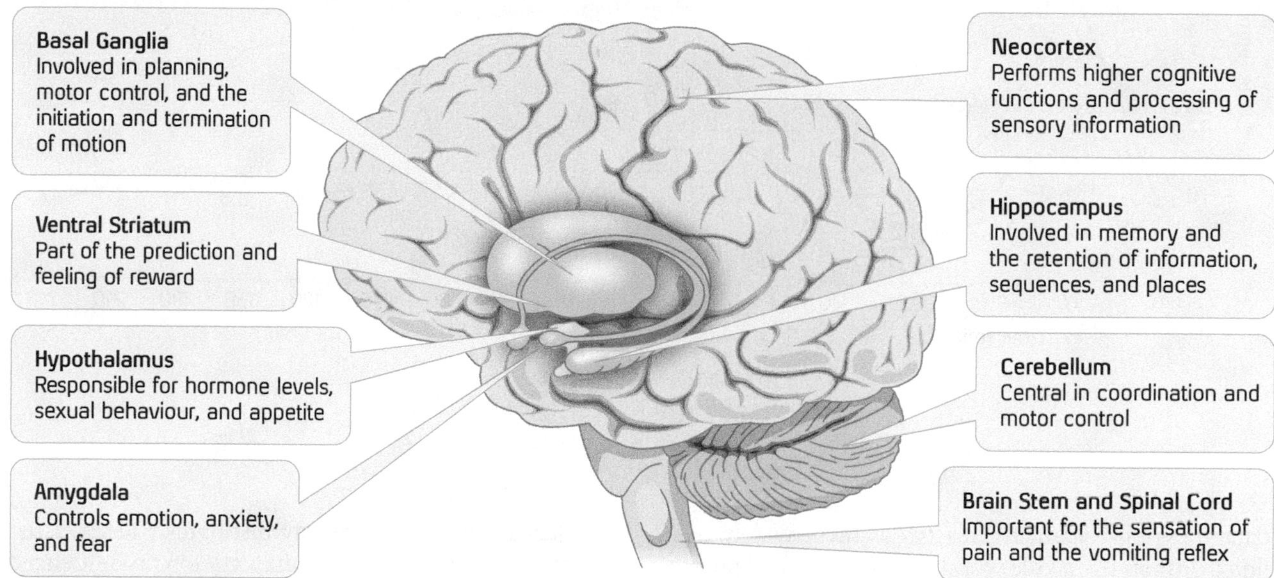
Basal Ganglia
Involved in planning, motor control, and the initiation and termination of motion
Ventral Striatum
Part of the prediction and feeling of reward
Hypothalamus
Responsible for hormone levels, sexual behaviour, and appetite
Amygdala
Controls emotion, anxiety, and fear
Neocortex
Performs higher cognitive functions and processing of sensory information
Hippocampus
Involved in memory and the retention of information, sequences, and places
Cerebellum
Central in coordination and motor control
Brain Stem and Spinal Cord
Important for the sensation of pain and the vomiting reflex

is involved in aspects of memory storage; the *cerebral cortex*, which regulates the integration of higher cognitive functions; and the *nucleus accumbens*, which is involved in reward.

Physiological Effects

One of the most consistent acute physiological effects of both smoked marijuana and oral THC is an increase in heart rate. Figure 15.3 shows that both smoked marijuana and oral THC increase the heart rate of marijuana smokers in a dose-dependent fashion (i.e., larger THC doses produce larger heart rate elevations).[15,16] While the peak effects produced by smoking marijuana containing 4% THC are similar to 20 milligrams oral THC, the drug's time course of action is different. Peak heart-rate elevations produced by smoked marijuana occur within 10 minutes and return to baseline levels after about 90 minutes, whereas peak heart-rate elevations produced by oral THC do not occur until 90 minutes following ingestion and remain elevated for at least four hours after drug administration. The effect of cannabis-based drugs on blood pressure is more variable, with some studies reporting slight increases and others reporting no effect. Concern has been raised that smoking marijuana might have permanent deleterious effects on the cardiovascular system, but there is no evidence to indicate that marijuana-related cardiovascular effects are associated with serious health problems for most young, healthy users.[17] Patients with hypertension, cerebrovascular disease, and coronary atherosclerosis, however, should probably avoid smoking marijuana or ingesting THC because of the drug's effects on heart rate. Other consistent acute effects of smoked marijuana are reddening of the eyes and dryness of the mouth and throat. Except for bronchodilation, acute exposure to marijuana has little effect on breathing as measured by conventional pulmonary tests. Heavy marijuana smoking over a much longer period could lead to clinically significant and less readily reversible impairment of pulmonary function.

Behavioural Effects

Self-administration While physiological effects produced by cannabis-based drugs provide important information, the behaviour of most interest for the assessment of abuse potential is drug taking. Until recently, cannabinoids were not shown to maintain self-administration in laboratory animals, suggesting that the abuse potential of cannabis-based drugs was minimal. This seemed inconsistent with epidemiological

Figure 15.3 The Time Course for Heart Rate after Smoking Marijuana (left) and Ingesting Oral THC (right)

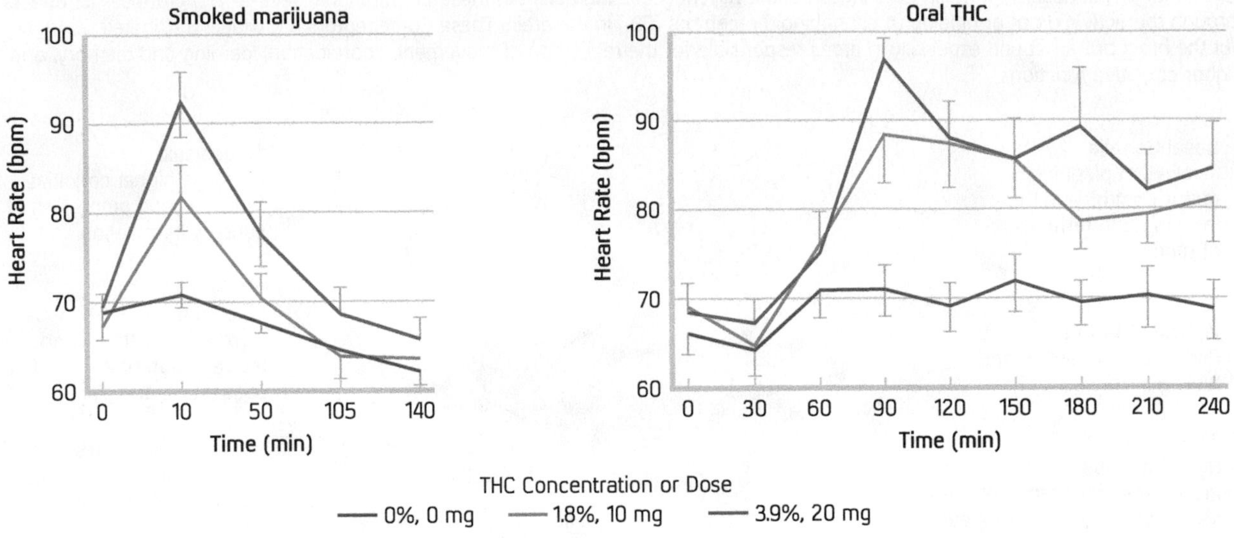

data showing that marijuana is the most widely used illicit drug in the world[18] and that a substantial proportion of North Americans seek treatment for marijuana abuse and dependence each year.[19] Findings from recent studies, however, demonstrate clearly that rats and squirrel monkeys will consistently self-administer cannabinoids.[20] The success of recent attempts to obtain reliable self-administration in laboratory animals has been attributed to intravenously injecting THC doses more rapidly than had been previously tried.

Several laboratory studies have shown that marijuana produces robust self-administration by human marijuana smokers and that marijuana self-administration is related to the THC content of the cigarettes. That is, marijuana cigarettes containing a higher concentration of THC are preferred to those containing a lower THC concentration.[21] These findings not only confirm the abuse potential of smoked marijuana but also suggest that THC administered alone (e.g., oral administration of THC capsules) might have abuse potential. In a recent study, experienced marijuana smokers were given repeated opportunities to self-administer oral THC capsules or to receive $2. Several important findings from that study are worth mentioning. Participants selected (1) money on more occasions than the capsules, (2) more drug-containing capsules than placebo, and (3) more THC capsules during social and recreational periods than in periods that were not social and recreational. These observations indicate that oral THC's abuse potential is modest at best, experienced marijuana smokers can readily distinguish THC-related effects, and cannabis self-administration is influenced by social factors.[16]

Subjective Effects Some have argued that before novice marijuana smokers are able to experience marijuana-associated positive subjective effects (e.g., euphoria, stoned), they must go through a process by which they learn to recognize and interpret the psychoactive effects produced by smoked marijuana.[22] While this position remains open for debate, the subjective effects on experienced marijuana smokers have been well characterized. In general, experienced smokers report increased ratings of euphoria, "high," mellowness, hunger, and stimulation after smoking marijuana. These effects peak within 5–10 minutes and last for about two hours; they are usually THC-concentration dependent (i.e., the magnitude of the effects is increased with increasing THC concentrations). Subjective effects reported by infrequent smokers are similar but more intense because these individuals are less tolerant to marijuana-associated effects. Also, at higher THC concentrations some infrequent smokers may report negative effects, such as mild paranoia and hallucination. As seen with heart rate, peak subjective effects of oral THC are similar to those produced by smoked marijuana except that the time course of the effects is different. Peak subjective effects occur about 90 minutes following oral ingestion and can last for several hours. An important factor in determining whether a drug is likely to be abused

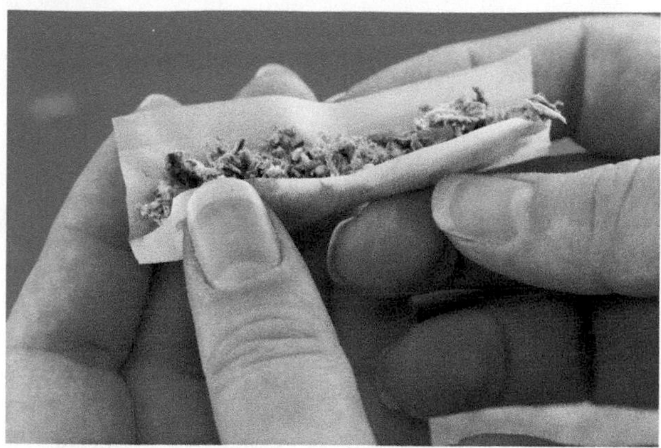

Experienced marijuana smokers report euphoria, "high," hunger, and mellowness after smoking; the magnitude of the effects depends on the THC concentration.

is the rapidity of the onset of its effects. The more rapidly a drug's effects are experienced, the more likely it will be abused. This might be why the abuse potential of oral THC is limited.

While an earlier study demonstrated that relatively less-experienced marijuana smokers reported being intoxicated after smoking a placebo cigarette, more recent studies demonstrate that regular marijuana smokers are not so readily duped. Placebo cigarettes were made by extracting the THC and other cannabinoids from marijuana—the cigarettes looked and smelled like regular marijuana cigarettes. In these studies, participants "sampled" marijuana cigarettes (containing placebo or different THC concentrations) and alternative reinforcers (e.g., money or snack food), and subsequently were given an option to choose. Participants selected cigarettes containing THC on more than 75% of choice opportunities compared with only about 40% when placebo cigarettes were available.[23] Furthermore, subjective effects produced by the placebo cigarette were identical to baseline levels, whereas subjective effects produced by cigarettes containing THC were significantly elevated.

Cognitive Effects The effect of marijuana on cognitive performance has received a great deal of attention in the popular press and the scientific literature for many years with little resolution. Unfortunately, many discussions on this topic add to the confusion because they fail to differentiate between the direct (acute) effects and long-term (chronic) effects of marijuana. They also fail to consider the marijuana use history of the user. Following acute administration of smoked marijuana to infrequent marijuana smokers, cognitive performance is disrupted temporarily in several domains:

- The amount of time that is required to complete cognitive tasks increases (*slowed cognitive processing*)
- Performance on immediate recall tasks decreases (*impaired short-term memory*)
- Premature responding increases (*impaired inhibitory control*)
- Performance on tracking tasks decreases (*loss of sustained concentration or vigilance*)
- Performance on tasks requiring participants to reproduce computer-generated patterns is disrupted (*impaired visuospatial processing*)

The acute effects of marijuana on the performance of frequent smokers are less dramatic, leading some to hypothesize that regular marijuana smokers are tolerant to many marijuana-related cognitive effects.[16] Some negative cognitive effects, however, have been reported. For example, slowing of cognitive performance is a consistent finding, even in regular users. This effect may have significant behavioural consequences under circumstances requiring complex operations that must be accomplished in a limited period, such as certain workplace tasks and the operation of machinery and automobiles.

It is also difficult to make definitive statements about *long-term* cognitive effects of marijuana use because of divergent findings and interpretations. More general conclusions, however, are possible. Based on the available evidence, it appears that following a sufficient period of abstinence (greater than one month), regular marijuana use produces minimal effects on cognition as measured by standard neuropsychological tests.[24] The reader is cautioned, though, because as the number of better-controlled studies increase, the current conclusions about the long-term effects of marijuana on cognition may change.

Today, it is almost impossible to review the cognitive effects of marijuana without a discussion of brain-imaging findings. Recent studies have combined cognitive testing and brain-imaging techniques to examine differences in cognitive performance and brain activation between marijuana users and nonusers. One study used positron emission tomography (PET) and an executive function task to investigate brain activation and cognition in a group of control subjects and frequent marijuana smokers who had been abstinent for 25 days.[25] The researchers found increased activity in the hippocampus and decreased activity in the left anterior cingulate and left lateral prefrontal cortex among marijuana users compared to control subjects. Despite these differential brain activations, there were no differences between marijuana users and nonusers on cognitive performance. Others have reported similar findings.[26,27] These observations highlight at least two important points: (1) subtle brain activation differences may have little impact on behaviour; and (2) it is advised to first carefully examine the major behaviour of interest–cognitive performance. Otherwise, researchers may conduct neuroimaging studies with limited or no behavioural correlates, and they (and the public) may be enticed to draw inappropriate conclusions about the neural basis of cognition. The take-home message is that there has been no scientific study demonstrating meaningful brain differences between marijuana users and controls.

Appetite We've all heard about someone smoking marijuana and then getting a case of the "munchies," a marked increase in food intake. Data from a large number of studies clearly demonstrate that marijuana and oral THC significantly increase food intake. These findings provided the basis for at least one clinical use of cannabis-based drugs–appetite stimulation (see the section "Medical Uses of Cannabis"). A related question that has received less scientific attention is, Why aren't most chronic marijuana users overweight? Some have speculated that tolerance develops to the food intake-enhancing effect of cannabis-based drugs, but no empirical data support this view. The bottom line is that the average weight of chronic marijuana users is not known because there have been no studies addressing this issue. The average chronic marijuana user may indeed be overweight. Or it could be that most marijuana use occurs during youth (this is certainly supported by data from national surveys), when people and their metabolism are most active.

Talking Another consistent behavioural effect of marijuana is on verbal behaviour (talking). Stimulant drugs, such as amphetamines, have been shown to increase verbal interactions, as have moderate doses of alcohol. Marijuana appears to be different. Several researchers have reported that while nonverbal social interactions are increased following marijuana smoking, verbal exchanges are dramatically decreased.[28]

dronabinol: the generic name for prescription THC in oil in a gelatin capsule.

Marinol: the brand name for dronabinol.

LO7 Medical Uses of Cannabis in Canada

A number of cannabis-based medicines are approved for use in Canada. The oral form of synthetic THC, **dronabinol** (2.5, 5, or 10 milligrams, dissolved in sesame oil, in capsules) is marketed in Canada and the United States as **Marinol®**. It is indicated for the treatment of severe nausea and vomiting associated with cancer chemotherapy and for AIDS-related anorexia associated with weight loss. Sativex®, made by Bayer, is a buccal spray containing delta-9-THC 27 milligrams/millilitre and cannabidiol 25 milligrams/millilitre. It is marketed in Canada as an adjunctive treatment for the symptomatic relief of neuropathic pain in adults with multiple sclerosis and as an adjunctive analgesic in adults with advanced cancer who experience moderate to severe pain during the highest tolerated dose of strong opioid therapy for persistent background pain. Cesamet® (nabilone), made by Lilly, is a synthetic cannabinoid with purported antiemetic properties. It has been found to be of value in the management of some patients with nausea and vomiting associated with cancer chemotherapy. While there are many anecdotal reports of the therapeutic value of smoked marijuana, scientific studies supporting the safety and efficacy of marijuana for therapeutic claims are generally inconclusive. For a comprehensive review of the pharmacology of cannabis-based medications and current clinical studies pertaining to their purported uses we recommend the Health Canada document *Information for Health Care Professionals: Cannabis (Marihuana, Marijuana) and the Cannabinoids*.[29] The following sections provide synopses of the information, collected by Health Canada, pertaining to the clinical use and effectiveness of cannabis.

Nausea and Vomiting

Chemotherapy-induced nausea and vomiting (CINV) is one of the most common adverse events associated with cancer treatment. It is also considered one of the most distressing side effects. Although CINV is generally well controlled with conventional pharmacological therapies for some people, acute, delayed, and anticipatory nausea is not well controlled. In some of these cases the use of cannabis/cannabinoids has been reported to provide a measure of relief. The activation of cannabinoid CB_1 and CB_2 receptors, identified in areas of the brain stem associated with emetogenic control, may underlie in these purported effects. However, it has been theorized that cannabinoids may exert their antiemetic action through more than one mechanism including antagonism of 5-HT_3 receptors. It is important to note that while clinical trials of the effects of smoked cannabis on CINV have been performed, none have been peer reviewed. The use of cannabinoids is currently considered a fourth-line adjunctive therapy in CINV when conventional antiemetic therapies have failed. More research is required to determine if combination therapy provides added benefits above those observed with newer standard treatments.

Wasting Syndrome in AIDS and Cancer

The ability of cannabis to increase appetite has been reported anecdotally for decades. Today both epidemiological and controlled laboratory studies suggest that exposure to marijuana, whether by inhalation or oral ingestion of THC-containing capsules, correlates positively with an increase in food consumption, caloric intake, and body weight. Furthermore, scientific evidence suggests a physiological role for the endocannabinoid system in modulating appetite, food intake, and energy metabolism.

Appetite Stimulation and Weight Gain in People with AIDS Because of marijuana's capacity to stimulate appetite and food intake it can be used clinically, when deemed beneficial, to promote weight gain. One indication for its use is HIV-associated muscle wasting and weight loss. Marinol®, an oral synthetic form of THC, is approved for use in Canada for AIDS-related anorexia associated with weight loss.

Appetite Stimulation and Weight Gain in People with Cancer Anorexia is one of the more troublesome symptoms associated with cancer. More than half of patients with advanced cancer experience a lack of appetite or weight loss. The effects of smoking marijuana on appetite and weight gain in patients with cancer cachexia have not been studied. The results from trials with oral THC (dronabinol) or oral cannabis extract are mixed. Cancer cachexia is not an approved indication for Marinol in Canada. However, the Marihuana for Medical Purposes Regulations allow the use of dried marijuana in the context of anorexia, cachexia, and weight loss associated with cancer in patients who have either not benefited from, or would not be considered to benefit from, conventional treatments.

Anorexia Nervosa The endocannabinoid system has been implicated in appetite regulation and is suspected to play a role in eating disorders, such as anorexia nervosa. However, little evidence exists to support the use of marijuana to treat anorexia nervosa, and the British Medical Association and the Institute of Medicine have both concluded that cannabis is unlikely to be effective in patients with anorexia nervosa.

Multiple Sclerosis and Amyotrophic Lateral Sclerosis

Anecdotal reports propose that marijuana can reduce spasticity in people who have multiple sclerosis (MS), amyotrophic lateral sclerosis (ALS), or a spinal cord injury when other medications are ineffective or produce undesirable side effects.

Multiple Sclerosis For over a hundred years published reports have described the anti-spasmodic effects of cannabis. Several surveys have evaluated the prevalence of medicinal cannabis use among patients seeking treatment for multiple sclerosis (MS). In the year 2000 it was determined that 16% of Alberta's MS patients had used cannabis medicinally. A 2002 study of MS patients in Nova Scotia revealed that 14% had used cannabis for medical purposes. People with MS reported using cannabis to manage symptoms including spasticity, chronic pain, anxiety, and depression. Patients also reported improvements in sleep. The role of cannabis in the management of MS has received considerable attention in recent years and is beyond the scope of this chapter. For a comprehensive review of current clinical and basic science research in this field we recommend reading the Health Canada document *Information for Health Care Professionals: Cannabis (Marihuana, Marijuana) and the Cannabinoids.*[29]

Amyotrophic Lateral Sclerosis The endocannabinoid system has been theorized to play a role in the pathogenesis of amyotrophic lateral sclerosis (ALS). In animal models of ALS cannabinoids have been reported to delay disease progression. However, there have been very few related clinical trials and the results are mixed. Anecdotal reports suggest decreased muscle cramps and fasciculation's in ALS patients who smoke herbal cannabis or drink cannabis tea. Up to 10% of ALS patients use cannabis for symptom control.

Epilepsy

Current evidence has led researchers to theorize a role for the endocannabinoid system in the modulation of neuronal tone and excitability. Both human and animal studies suggest epileptic activity is associated with changes in the levels and distribution of CB_1 receptors in the hippocampus, and reduced levels of the endocannabinoid anandamide have been detected in the cerebrospinal fluid of patients with untreated newly diagnosed temporal lobe epilepsy. Collectively these studies have suggested that dysregulation of the endocannabinoid system may play a role in epileptogenesis and therefore could provide future targets for antiepileptic therapies. However, a recent systematic review performed to assess the efficacy and safety of cannabinoid treatment for patients with epilepsy concluded that the current evidence is not sufficient to be able to draw reliable conclusions regarding the efficacy of cannabinoids as a treatment for epilepsy. The Marihuana for Medical Purposes Regulations currently allow the use of dried marijuana in the context of epilepsy in patients who experience seizures and who have either not benefited from, or would not be considered to benefit from, conventional treatments.

Pain

There is now strong evidence that the endocannabinoid system plays an important role in the modulation of pain and that elements of the endocannabinoid system can be found at supraspinal, spinal, and peripheral levels of pain pathways. Furthermore, the distribution of cannabinoid receptors provides an anatomical basis to explain many of the analgesic effects of cannabinoids. Although the mechanism of action underlying these analgesic effects requires further determination, a number of pre-clinical studies support a clinical role for cannabis in suppressing pain in certain diseases.

Pain from Cancer Few properly controlled clinical trials of smoked marijuana for the treatment of cancer pain have been conducted. Two randomized, double-blind, placebo-controlled studies suggested oral THC (dronabinol, Marinol) provided an analgesic effect in people with moderate to severe continuous pain caused by advanced cancer. In Canada, Sativex is approved as an adjunctive treatment for pain in adults with advanced cancer who experience moderate to severe pain even with the highest tolerated dose of strong opioid therapy. The Marihuana for Medical Purposes Regulations currently allow the use of dried marijuana in cancer patients experiencing severe pain and who have either not benefited from, or would not be considered to benefit from, conventional treatments.

Pain from Causes Other Than Cancer Chronic pain not caused by cancer is a complex syndrome that involves physical, psychological, and psychosocial factors. The analgesic effects of smoked cannabis on the pain associated with neuropathology, rheumatoid arthritis, osteoarthritis, headache, and fibromyalgia have been inconclusive, in large part due to poor study design and conflicting results.

Psychiatric Disorders

There are anecdotal and historical claims regarding the beneficial effects of cannabis in the treatment of anxiety, depression, and sleep disorders, as well as for the treatment of alcohol and opiate withdrawal symptoms. However, insufficient clinical evidence exists at this time to recommend the use of cannabinoids in the treatment of such disorders. Clinical trials of marijuana or oral THC to treat anxiety or depression show either a lack of improvement or worsening of the condition.

Other Diseases and Symptoms

In addition to the use of marijuana in the treatment of the medical conditions described above, there are many, many other reports (anecdotal and scientific) of its potential effects in other diseases and conditions.

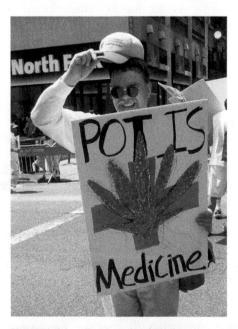

The potential medical benefits of marijuana are an issue with a long and controversial history.

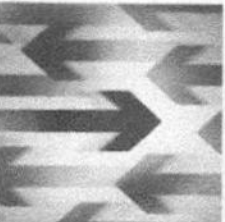

TAKING SIDES

The Legal Sanctions Related to Cannabis Possession/Use Position Statement

The Centre for Addiction and Mental Health (CAMH) does not encourage or promote cannabis use. CAMH emphasizes that the most effective way to avoid cannabis-related harms is by not using cannabis and encourages people to seek treatment when its use has become a problem.

Cannabis is not a benign drug. Cannabis use, and in particular frequent and long-term cannabis use, has been associated with negative health and behavioural consequences, including respiratory damage, problems with physical coordination, difficulties with memory and cognition, prenatal and postnatal development problems, psychiatric effects, hormone, immune, and cardiovascular system defects, as well as poor work and school performance. The consequences of use by youth and those with a mental disorder are of particular concern. However, most cannabis use is sporadic or experimental and hence not likely to be associated with serious negative consequences.

CAMH thus holds the position that the criminal justice system in general, and the Controlled Drugs and Substances Act (CDSA) specifically, under which cannabis possession is a criminal offence, has become an inappropriate control mechanism. This conclusion is based on the available scientific knowledge on the effects of cannabis use, the individual consequences of a criminal conviction, the costs of enforcement, and the limited effectiveness of the criminal control of cannabis use.

CAMH thus concurs with similar recent calls from many other expert stakeholders who believe that the control of cannabis possession for personal use should be removed from the realm of the CDSA and the criminal law/criminal justice system. While harmful health consequences exist with extensive cannabis use, CAMH believes that the decriminalization of cannabis possession will not lead to its increased use, based on supporting evidence from other jurisdictions that have introduced similar controls.

CAMH recommends that a more appropriate legal control framework for cannabis use be put into place that will result in a more effective and efficient control system, produce fewer negative social and individual consequences, and maintain public health and safety. CAMH recommends serious consideration of conversion of cannabis possession to a civil violation under the federal Contraventions Act.

CAMH further recommends that such an alternative framework be explored on a temporary and rigorously evaluated trial basis, and that an appropriate level of funding be provided/maintained for prevention and treatment programs to minimize the prevalence of cannabis use and its associated harms.

Do you think the federal government needs to change the laws as they relate to cannabis possession? Why or why not?

Source: Adapted from the Centre for Addiction and Mental Health. *The Legal Sanctions Related to Cannabis Possession/Use Position Statement.* 2009. Retrieved February 24, 2011, from http://www.camh.net/Public_policy/Public_policy_papers/cannabis.html.

A comprehensive review of all claims is beyond the scope of this chapter; however, below we consider two better known cases, glaucoma and asthma.

Glaucoma Glaucoma is a multifactorial disease characterized by the progressive degeneration of the optic nerve and the death of retinal ganglion cells. If left untreated the condition can lead to irreversible blindness. Marijuana has long been purported to provide relief from the symptoms of this disease and current evidence suggests that the ocular (as well as systemic) administration of cannabinoids can lower IOP by up to 30%. However, cannabinoid-based therapy appears to be limited by the short duration of cannabinoid action and unwanted physical and psychotropic effects. At this time neither the Canadian Ophthalmological Society nor the American Glaucoma Society recommend the use of cannabinoids for the treatment of glaucoma because of the availability of other effective therapeutic options.

Asthma The benefits of smoking marijuana for asthmatics are likely to be minimal. Although smoking marijuana has been shown to decrease bronchospasm, increase bronchodilation, and modestly improve respiratory function in some persons with asthma, its effects are short-term. More importantly, marijuana smoke contains noxious gases and particulates known to damage respiratory systems; hence, it is not a viable long-term therapy for asthma. Ongoing animal studies with classical and synthetic cannabinoids suggest a promising role for cannabis-based medicines in the treatment of asthma. More questions need to be answered if cannabinoids are to become indicated for the treatment of this condition.

Contraindications

The contraindications that apply to those considering using Sativex or Marinol also apply to the use of marijuana. Marijuana is contraindicated in any person under the age of 18 and anyone who has a history of hypersensitivity to any cannabinoid or to smoking. Marijuana should not be used by people with liver, kidney, or cardiopulmonary disease, or a history of psychiatric disorders, particularly schizophrenia. It is also contraindicated in women of childbearing age not on a reliable contraceptive, as well as those planning pregnancy, those who are pregnant, or women who are breastfeeding. Men intending to start a family are also discouraged from using marijuana. Marijuana may also exacerbate the CNS depressant effects of sedatives, including alcohol. Concomitant use of marijuana with other drugs may increase the incidence of adverse effects.

LO8 Causes for Concern

The euphoric effect produced by cannabis is not as intense as that produced by other psychoactive drugs, such as cocaine or heroin. However, it does possess a dependency syndrome and withdrawal symptoms with cessation of frequent or high-potency use.

Abuse and Dependence

Can regular marijuana use produce a withdrawal syndrome? According to the DSM-5 (the standard diagnostic instrument), the answer is no. The DSM-5 does not recognize a diagnosis of cannabis withdrawal. Data from a variety of human laboratory and clinical studies, however, demonstrate that an abstinence syndrome can be observed following abrupt cessation of several days of smoked marijuana administration or oral delta-9-THC administration. Cannabinoid withdrawal is not life threatening, but symptoms can be unpleasant. Marijuana withdrawal syndrome in humans may include negative mood states (e.g., anxiety, restlessness, depression, and irritability), disrupted sleep, decreased food intake, and in some cases, aggressive behaviour. These symptoms have been reported to begin 1 day after cannabinoid cessation and persist from 4 to 12 days, depending on an individual's level of marijuana dependence. Clearly, the majority of marijuana users do not experience withdrawal symptoms and do not meet DSM-5 criteria for cannabis-use disorders. But these findings indicate that regular marijuana use may not be as innocuous as previously perceived.[30]

The evidence now suggests that if high levels of marijuana are used regularly over a sustained period, tolerance can develop to many marijuana-related effects, including the cognitive-impairing, physiological, and subjective effects. However, tolerance may not develop uniformly across each of these variables. For example, it has been demonstrated that heavy marijuana smokers exhibit minimal cognitive impairment following acute marijuana smoking while showing dramatic heart rate increases and reporting significant levels of euphoria. These findings suggest that tolerance may develop more readily to marijuana-related cognitive effects than to heart rate responses and subjective effects.[15]

Relative to other drugs of abuse, many people perceive marijuana to be an innocuous drug with limited abuse potential. Other people have made comparisons between marijuana abuse and abuse of other drugs, such as crack cocaine. However, the social consequences associated with marijuana use and those associated with crack cocaine use are dissimilar, making one-to-one comparisons imperfect. Research showing that THC and marijuana produce robust self-administration in laboratory animals and in human research participants clearly demonstrates that the drug has some abuse potential. In addition, of the 7 million Americans classified with dependence on or abuse of illicit drugs in 2006, 4.2 million were dependent on or abused marijuana.[31] Although this number represents a relatively small fraction of current marijuana users (less than 30%), it shows that a significant number of marijuana smokers do suffer ill effects from using the drug.

Toxicity Potential

Frequent and long-term cannabis use is associated with negative health and behavioural consequences.

Acute Physiological Effects The acute physiological effects of marijuana, primarily an increase in heart rate, have not been thought to be a threat to health. However, as the marijuana-using population ages, there is concern that individuals with high blood pressure,

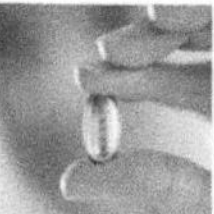

DRUGS IN DEPTH

Canadian Bar Association, British Columbia Branch: Possession of Marijuana

Is possession of marijuana a criminal offense?

Yes. Possession of marijuana is a criminal offense under the *Controlled Drugs and Substances Act* (available at laws.justice.gc.ca—click on "English", then on "Consolidated Acts", then on letter "C", and then scroll down to the Act). You don't have to own the marijuana—you just have to have, or possess, it. There are medical exceptions. If you are charged with possession of marijuana, you should speak to a lawyer.

What must the prosecutor prove to convict you? What can you do?

In court, the prosecutor, also called the crown counsel (Crown), must prove—beyond a reasonable doubt—that you had control of the marijuana—for example, the police found it on you or in an area you controlled, such as a car, suitcase, or bedroom, and knew the marijuana was there.

If the Crown proves both these things, the judge will convict you. To prove these things, the Crown will have witnesses—normally the police officer who arrested you—tell the court (or testify) about the situation when they found the marijuana on you. Witnesses testify under oath, meaning they promise to tell the truth. You can question, or cross-examine, each witness the Crown uses.

After the Crown finishes, you—and your witnesses, if you have any—can tell the court what happened. To do this, you have to take an oath promising to tell the truth, and then give evidence as a witness. If you have any witnesses who saw what happened and who can support your story, you can call them to testify, or give evidence. They also have to promise to tell the truth. You then question them about what they know. When you and your witnesses finish giving evidence, the Crown can question, or cross-examine, you and them.

Lastly, you and the Crown summarize your positions by making "submissions" to the court. For more information, check script 211, called "Defending Yourself Against a Criminal Charge" (www.cbabc.org/For-the-Public/Dial-A-Law/Scripts/Criminal-Law/211) and script 212, called "Pleading Guilty to a Criminal Charge" (www.cbabc.org/For-the-Public/Dial-A-Law/Scripts/Criminal-Law/212).

Is the amount of marijuana important?

Yes—a small amount is less serious. The more you have, the greater the chance that you may be charged with possession for the purpose of trafficking, a more serious offense with more serious penalties. The way the marijuana is packaged is also important.

What are the penalties?

For a first conviction, if you had less than 30 grams of marijuana, the maximum penalties are a fine of $1000 or 6 months in jail, or both. But the penalty for a first offense is usually much less.

You may also get a criminal record. That can prevent you from traveling to other countries, getting certain jobs, being bonded (which some jobs require), and applying for citizenship. Check script 205, called "Criminal Records and Applying for a Record Suspension" (www.cbabc.org/For-the-Public/Dial-A-Law/Scripts/Criminal-Law/205), for more information.

If it is your first offence, ask the judge for a discharge or ask the Crown for diversion (or alternative measures). If you meet the conditions of the discharge or if you complete the alternative measures, you will not get a criminal record. For more on discharges, check script 203, called "Conditional Sentences, Probation and Discharges" (www.cbabc.org/For-the-Public/Dial-A-Law/Scripts/Criminal-Law/203). For more on diversion, check script 212, called "Pleading Guilty to a Criminal Charge" (www.cbabc.org/For-the-Public/Dial-A-Law/Scripts/Criminal-Law/212).

The legal issues for this crime can be complex and a conviction can seriously harm you. If you are charged with this crime, you should talk to a lawyer.

Source: Used with permission of the Canadian Bar Association.

heart disease, or hardening of the arteries might be harmed by smoking marijuana.[32] The lethal dose of THC has not been extensively studied in animals, and no human deaths have been reported from "overdoses" of cannabis.

Driving Ability The 2004 *Canadian Addiction Survey* (CAS) indicated that 4.8% of Canadians drove a motor vehicle within two hours of using cannabis at least once in the past year.[33] This and other studies have also revealed that the prevalence of driving after using cannabis is considerably higher among young people. For example, the 2004 CAS also revealed that 20.6% of drivers aged 16 to 18 years drove a motor vehicle after using cannabis. Similar rates were determined in the 2001 *Ontario Student Drug Use Survey*, where 19.3% of students in grades 10 through 12 reported driving after using cannabis.[34] Finally, data from the 2002/2003 *Student Drug Use Survey for the Atlantic Provinces* revealed that 15.1% of senior students drove after using cannabis.[35] In each of these surveys more young people reported driving after using cannabis than driving after consuming alcohol.

A roadside survey was conducted in British Columbia to determine the extent of driving under the influence of alcohol and cannabis. Examination of oral fluid and breath samples collected from a random sample of nighttime drivers identified 4.6% of drivers testing positive for cannabis. Of these, 20% also tested positive for alcohol.[36] Male drivers and persons between the ages of 25 and 34 were most likely to test positive for cannabis.

There is growing demand for greater understanding of the association between cannabis use and motor vehicle collisions. In an early study of seriously injured drivers admitted to a regional trauma unit in Toronto it was determined that 13.9% tested positive for cannabis.[37] Subsequent investigations in Quebec revealed that 19.7% of drivers killed in road crashes had tested positive for cannabis.[38] Finally, a national study of fatally injured drivers in Canada between 2000 and 2006 revealed that 14.9% of those tested were positive for cannabis.[39]

A large number of studies have also investigated the effects of marijuana on driving performance, but the findings have been inconsistent. Some studies have reported marijuana-related driving impairments, while others have not. Traditionally, two types of studies have been conducted: (1) Epidemiological studies determine whether marijuana use is overrepresented among drivers involved in automobile accidents; and (2) Laboratory studies determine the direct effects of marijuana on skills related to driving performance. Findings from the majority of the epidemiological studies show little evidence that drivers who use marijuana alone are more likely to be involved in an accident than drivers who haven't used drugs. But data from laboratory studies of computer-controlled driving simulators indicate that marijuana produces significant impairments.[40] Most of the laboratory studies have employed relatively infrequent marijuana users as participants, a group that would be expected to show marked impairments. Because tolerance can develop to many of the cognitive-impairing effects of marijuana, further laboratory studies should include heavy marijuana smokers.

It has been suggested that experienced users may be aware that they are high and endeavour to compensate by slowing down and increasing headway when operating a motor vehicle.[41] Future investigation is necessary to determine whether or not these techniques are sufficient to compensate for the impairing effects of cannabis—especially higher-order cognitive functions such as divided attention tasks and decision making.[42]

Panic Reactions The other major behavioural problem associated with acute marijuana intoxication is the panic reaction. Much like many of the bad trips with hallucinogens, the reaction is usually fear of loss of control and fear that things will not return to normal. This reaction is more common among less-experienced marijuana users. Even Baudelaire understood this and advised his readers to surround themselves with friends and a pleasant environment before using hashish. Although many people do seek emergency medical treatment for marijuana-induced panic and are sometimes given sedatives or tranquillizers, the best treatment is probably "talking down," or reminding the person of who and where the person is, that the reaction is temporary, and that everything will be all right.

Chronic Lung Exposure There has been a great deal of concern about the possible long-term effects of chronic marijuana use. A couple of physiological concerns merit attention. One is the effect on lung function and the concern about lung cancer. Experiments have shown that chronic, daily smoking of marijuana impairs air flow in and out of the lungs.[43] It is hard to tell yet whether years of such an effect results in permanent, major obstructive lung disease in the same way that smoking tobacco cigarettes does. A recent study investigated the association between lung function and marijuana smoking in about 1000 adults aged 40 years and older. Marijuana was not associated with an increased risk of respiratory symptoms or lung disease.[44] Also, no direct evidence links marijuana smoking to lung cancer in humans. Remember that it took many years of cigarette smoking by millions of people before the links between tobacco and lung cancer and other lung diseases were shown.

Marijuana smoke has been compared with tobacco smoke.[45] Some of the constituents differ (there is no nicotine in marijuana smoke and no THC in tobacco), but many of the dangerous components are found in both. Total tar levels, carbon monoxide, hydrogen

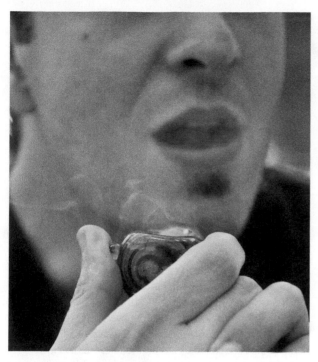

Inhaling marijuana smoke.

cyanide, and nitrosamines are found in similar amounts (except for tobacco-specific nitrosamines, which are carcinogens). Another potent carcinogen, *benzopyrene*, is found in greater amounts in marijuana than in tobacco. Everyone suspects that marijuana smoking will eventually be shown to cause cancer, but how much of a problem this will be compared with tobacco is hard to say. On the one hand, few marijuana smokers smoke 20 marijuana cigarettes every day, whereas tobacco smokers regularly smoke this much. On the other hand, the marijuana cigarette is not filtered and the user generally gets as much concentrated smoke as possible as far down in the lungs as possible and holds it there. So, while some wait to see when the data will come out, others are participating in the experiment.

Reproductive Effects Another area of concern is reproductive effects in both men and women. Heavy marijuana smoking can decrease testosterone levels in men, although the levels are still within the normal range and the significance of those decreases is not known. Diminished sperm counts and abnormal sperm structure in heavy marijuana users has been reported, perhaps because anandamide plays a role in normal sperm function.[46] A number of studies have reported either lower birthweight or shorter length at birth for infants whose mothers smoked marijuana during pregnancy, but because so many of the women also smoked tobacco or drank alcohol, it is not possible to determine the exact contribution of marijuana to these effects. It is, of course, wise to avoid the use of all drugs during pregnancy.

Immune System Effects There have also been reports that marijuana smoking impairs some measures of the functioning of the immune system.[47] Animal studies have found that THC injections can reduce immunity to infection, but at doses well above those obtainable by smoking marijuana. Some human studies of marijuana smokers have suggested reduced immunity, but most have not. If the effect were real, it could result in marijuana smokers being more susceptible to infections, cancer, and other diseases, such as genital herpes. We might suspect that such problems would eventually be reflected in the overall death rate of marijuana users. However, a report examining ten years of mortality data for more than 65 000 people found no relationship between marijuana use and overall death rates.[48]

Amotivational Syndrome Since 1971, when some psychiatric case reports were published identifying an *amotivational* syndrome in marijuana smokers, concern has been expressed about the effect of regular marijuana use on behaviour and motivation. A number of experiments and correlational studies have been aimed at answering this question. There does seem to be evidence for this diminished motivation, impaired ability to learn, and school and family problems in some adolescents who are chronic, heavy marijuana smokers. If they stop smoking and remain in counselling, the condition improves.[49] This probably implies a constant state of intoxication rather than a long-lasting change in brain function or personality.

Brain Damage For decades it has been speculated that amotivational or prolonged psychotic reactions could reflect an underlying damage to brain tissue produced by marijuana. For example, a 1972 report from England indicated that two individuals who demonstrated cerebral atrophy had a history of smoking marijuana. They also had a history of using many other illicit drugs, and had other medical problems, but it was suggested that the brain damage might have been caused by the marijuana. Several experiments have since been done, and all have failed to find a relationship between marijuana smoking and cerebral atrophy.

Ironically, some of the non-psychoactive ingredients in marijuana, such as cannabidiol, have been

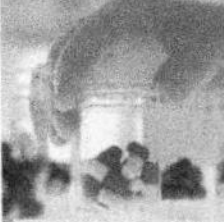

DRUGS IN THE MEDIA

Justin Trudeau Says Canada Should "Draw on Best Practices" from Marijuana Legalization in Colorado, Washington

Federal Liberal Leader Justin Trudeau thinks there are lessons to be learned from the legalization of marijuana in some U.S. states. Sales of marijuana to adults over 21 began January 1 in Colorado as the state legalized pot for recreational purposes. Washington's stores are expected to open in late spring. Last summer, Trudeau admitted to smoking pot after becoming an MP and has maintained that legalization in Canada is a good idea. He said Canada would benefit from keeping a close eye on the experiences in Colorado and Washington State.

He said there are all sorts of questions to be asked about how it actually works in practice.

"It's just how they balance the need to protect people and control a substance and respect people's freedoms," Trudeau told reporters after a 90 minute meet-and-greet with 200 supporters in Okotoks, south of Calgary. "I'm very interested in drawing on best practices and not repeating mistakes that other people might make."

What matters now, Trudeau said, is ending a marijuana prohibition policy that he says costs law enforcement $500-million a year and has left 475,000 people with criminal records since the Conservatives took office in 2006. "It is not protecting our kids from the negative impacts of marijuana on the developing brain. . .we are funneling millions upon millions of dollars each year into organized crime and criminal gangs."

"The fact of the matter is our current approach on marijuana—the prohibition that Stephen Harper continues to defend—is failing in two primary ways. The first one is it is not protecting our kids from the negative impacts of marijuana on the developing brain," said Trudeau. "Secondly, we are funneling millions upon millions of dollars each year into organized crime and criminal gangs. We do not need to be funding those organizations."

Trudeau said he has smoked pot five or six times in his life and never really liked it much. The local RCMP were called to the community centre over reports that two men were smoking pot outside the venue where Trudeau was speaking but the individuals produced licences proving it was medicinal and no arrests were made.

Source: The National Post. Canadian Politics. "Justin Trudeau Says Canada Should 'Draw on Best Practices' from Marijuana Legalization in Colorado, Washington." Canadian Press, 2014.

shown to have powerful antioxidant properties that protect brain cells from the toxic effects of other chemicals.[50] This effect was strong enough that the U.S. National Institute of Mental Health filed a patent in 1988 entitled "Cannabinoids as Antioxidants and Neuroprotectants."

Emotion has played an obvious and influential role on the research on brain damage and marijuana. Scientists on both sides have become crusaders for their cause. Some individuals seem to think it is their professional duty to seek out and publicize every potential evil associated with marijuana, even if no strong scientific evidence supports their views. Others seem to automatically question the negative reports and look for ways to discredit them. We can predict that the emotion, the premature announcements of new scary findings, the repeating of long discredited stories, and the conflicting reports will continue.

Although marijuana is known to cause memory deficits in humans and laboratory animals, the mechanisms responsible for this action remain unclear. Because administration of marijuana and cannabinoids to rodents causes a reduction in neuron density in the hippocampus, it has been hypothesized that memory deficits might be attributable to neurotoxicity. Treatment of rats and other laboratory animals with THC elicits several responses, including decreases in memory. The hippocampus is pivotal for memory, and damage to this area of the brain in humans or rodents decreases the ability to acquire new information or recover previously learned knowledge. The hippocampus is also rich in CB_1 receptors.

Research has demonstrated that binding of THC to cannabinoid CB_1 receptors in cultured neurons or hippocampus slices leads to neuronal cell death.[51] For example, THC is neurotoxic at concentrations as low as 0.5–1.0 micromole. This concentration is comparable to THC levels measured in human plasma after smoking marijuana. These findings have led scientists to theorize that memory loss associated with marijuana exposure, in rodents, may be attributable to THC neurotoxicity. Whether these findings will translate to the human case is yet to be seen.

Cannabis and Psychosis

Psychosis describes a mental state characterized by delusions, which involve having beliefs that are not true; hallucinations, which involve sensing things that are not there, such as hearing voices; and gross disorganization of speech or behaviour such that the person's speech and actions do not make sense. Although psychosis is typically associated with schizophrenia, it is important to realize that psychosis is present in many other mental health disorders.[52]

The 1936 cult classic film *Reefer Madness* depicted how smoking marijuana could turn nice middle-class youth into psychotic killers. Today, this cautionary tale is mocked and spoofed for its outrageous assertions. At the same time, however, some researchers are collecting data that they claim show that marijuana indeed causes psychosis. Were the statements made in 1930s about the dangers of marijuana accurate? The connection between marijuana use and psychosis was one of the main arguments for outlawing the drug. It seems that the marijuana-psychosis link is similar to other emotionally arousing drug issues in the past–they return in slightly different forms periodically. Given this situation, we feel that it might be useful to discuss this topic in some detail.

In our attempt to understand the relationship between marijuana use and psychosis, we must first know something about how studies investigating this issue are conducted. Typically, a few thousand adults are separated into groups based on their reported use of marijuana: marijuana users in one group and nonusers in the other. Then, researchers see if the groups differ on the outcome measure of interest–psychosis. An important question that you should ask is: How do they define psychosis in these studies? Remember from Chapter 8 that psychosis is a mental disorder involving a loss of contact with reality and is characterized by hallucinations, irrational beliefs, and disorganization of speech and behaviours. We typically think of psychosis in association with schizophrenia, but it can also be present in other disorders. In order for a person to be given a diagnosis of psychosis, they must be evaluated by a psychiatrist or psychologist. This can be a rather involved and time-consuming evaluation. As such, participants in the overwhelming majority of these studies are not assessed for a psychosis disorder. Instead, they are asked to complete a questionnaire, containing about 20 items, that probes psychotic symptoms.

Some studies have found a correlation between marijuana use and psychotic symptoms. That is, participants in the marijuana group were more likely to admit to having experienced at least one psychotic symptom. This type of finding has fuelled sensational media headlines such as "Even infrequent use of marijuana increases risk of psychosis." Here, we'd like to make two important points that will better help you evaluate the veracity of these claims and of research in this area in general. First, you should know that someone could endorse psychotic symptoms without meeting criteria for a disorder. Indeed, in some of these studies marijuana users reported an average of fewer than five symptoms; the specific symptoms endorsed are usually not made clear by researchers. This makes it impossible to determine whether the marijuana users reported symptoms that were clinically meaningful (e.g., I hear voices that others do not) or those that were not (e.g., I sometimes feel uncomfortable in public). In addition, many of the symptoms contained on these questionnaires can be experienced only for a brief period and are not necessarily an indication of a permanent disorder.

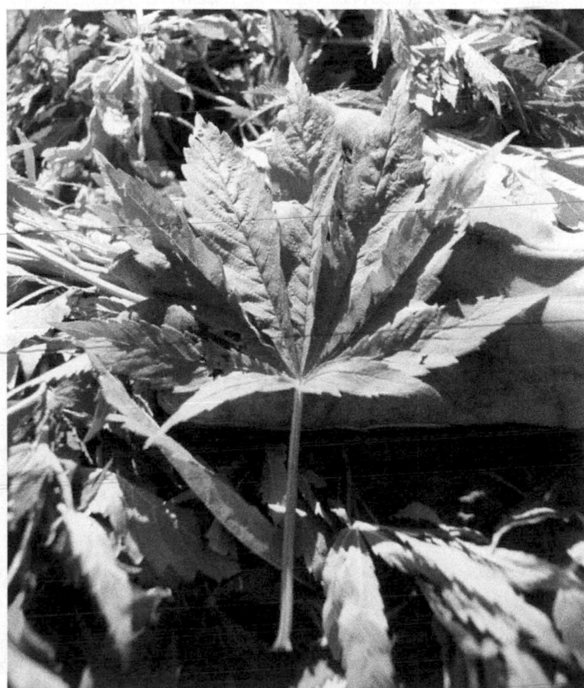

Federal laws and penalties related to marijuana possession tend to reflect other social trends, becoming more severe in periods of social and political conservatism.

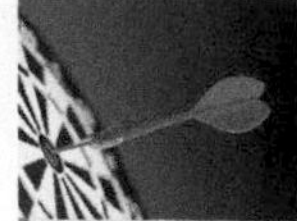

TARGETING PREVENTION

Synthetic Cannabis: The Devil You Know or the One You Don't

Over the past several decades, our knowledge about marijuana's effects on human behaviour has increased dramatically. Such knowledge affords us the ability to maximize beneficial effects while minimizing deleterious ones. Recently, a new generation of synthetic cannabinoid agonists has been reported to be used recreationally, especially by teens and young adults. The products are marketed as natural herbal incense or potpourri under various brand names such as "Spice" or "K2," and have been sold legally in "head shops," convenience stores, and through the Internet to those seeking the "marijuana-like high." The poorly labelled contents have been found to include a mixture of psychoactive herbs and aromatic extracts sprayed with synthetic cannabinoid compounds. The ingredient that has generated the most interest is JWH-018, a synthetic cannabinoid developed by chemist John W. Huffman (JWH). Anecdotal reports indicate that when one of these products is inhaled, it produces psychoactive effects similar to those produced by marijuana. While the truthfulness of such claims is difficult to confirm because there are no published studies investigating this product in humans, the fact that many young people around the country readily pay about $40 per gram to obtain such products suggest that they do something. There is real concern, however, that synthetic cannabinoids may cause negative effects on human health. Relative to delta-9-THC, the synthetic compounds are more potent and efficacious agonists, which could lead to greater toxicity. Marijuana, the most frequently used cannabis agent, contains over 60 identified cannabinoids that may modulate delta-9-THC-related effects, including negative ones. Anecdotal case reports and increasing calls to poison control centres suggest potential adverse effects of synthetic cannabinoid exposure such as anxiety, rapid heart rates, and psychosis, coupled with the abuse potential of the substances, recently led to Drug Enforcement Agency (DEA) control of several synthetic cannabinoids under the Controlled Substances Act. In addition, lawmakers in several states, alarmed by growing concerns about synthetic cannabinoids, have banned these products. At present, the long-term effects of inhaling synthetic cannabinoids on brain functioning and behaviour is unknown. Thus, it seems less than wise to consume these products when so little is known about their potential harmful effects.

Our second point deals with the question of how we determine causation in science. In general, the conclusion drawn from these studies is that marijuana causes psychosis. Is this necessarily the case? It could be that psychosis causes people to smoke marijuana. It is difficult to determine what came first, because research participants' psychotic symptoms are not usually assessed before the initiation of marijuana use. So, it is possible that psychotic individuals may have exhibited symptoms prior to using marijuana. Finally, because marijuana users typically use other psychoactive drugs at higher rates than non-marijuana users, it is extremely difficult to disentangle the influence of other drug use on psychotic symptoms. Together, these issues lead us to conclude that the evidence supporting a causal role for marijuana use in psychosis of otherwise healthy individuals is weak and difficult to interpret. There is, however, better evidence showing that marijuana can increase the likelihood of psychotic episodes in individuals with a history of psychiatric problems.

Cannabidiol

There is growing evidence that the average content of THC in cannabis may be increasing.[53] This is potentially important because the psychoactive effects of cannabis vary according to its THC content. Cannabidiol, another constituent in cannabis, is interesting because rather than producing psychoactive effects it produces anxiolytic and antipsychotic effects. As such it may have the potential to offset some of the adverse effects of THC.[54] Just as there is variability in the THC content of cannabis, there can also be variability in the cannabidiol content. Thus, if the negative effects of cannabis use are related to THC content and if cannabidiol offsets some of the negative effects of THC, then exposure to cannabis with a higher THC content or low cannabidiol content might be associated with greater negative consequences. Some experimental evidence supports this theory.[55]

Summary

- Marijuana, hashish, and hash oil are all obtained from the cannabis plant. Marijuana is a preparation of leafy material from the cannabis plant and is primarily smoked.
- Three species of cannabis exist. *Cannabis sativa* originated in Asia but now grows worldwide. *Cannabis indica* is grown for its psychoactive resins and is cultivated worldwide. *Cannabis ruderalis* grows primarily in Russia and not at all in North America.
- Manually scraping exuded resin off the plant to make hashish is a tedious process, and more efficient methods for separating the resin exist. Products of these processes are referred to as "red oil of cannabis" or *hash oil*. These products vary widely in their potency but can contain more than 50% THC.
- The primary psychoactive agent, delta-9-tetrahydrocannabinol (THC), is concentrated in the resin of the *Cannabis* plant; most of the resin is in the flowering tops, less is in the leaves, and little is in the fibrous stalks. The psychoactive potency of a cannabis preparation depends on the amount of resin present and therefore varies depending on the part of the plant used.
- Marijuana is cultivated in both indoor and outdoor grow operations in Canada, although indoor production is now more common. Increasingly sophisticated indoor cultivation methods, including improved growing techniques and equipment have contributed to increasing production and potency.
- While illicit marijuana production takes place in all provinces and territories, it predominantly occurs in British Columbia, Ontario, and Quebec. The amount of marijuana produced in Canada exceeds domestic demand and organized crime produce it for foreign markets, such as the United States.
- Hash and hash oil smuggled into Canada originates mainly from South Asia, the Middle East, Africa, and the Caribbean. Morocco and Pakistan are primary sources for hash destined for Canada. Jamaica has been the primary supplier of hash products, especially hash oil, to Canada.
- A survey conducted by the Canadian Centre on Substance Abuse of youth across Canada revealed the complexities surrounding the use of cannabis. Canadian youth appear puzzled with what they perceive as the diverse messaging pertaining to cannabis.
- Cannabis is the most widely consumed illicit drug in the world.
- Compassion clubs, cannabis clubs, or buyers' clubs are clubs in which individuals can purchase an assortment of strains of cannabis and cannabis products. Health Canada does not license compassion clubs to possess, produce, or distribute marijuana for medicinal purposes. In fact, purchasing marijuana from compassion clubs falls outside the requirements of the Controlled Drugs and Substances Act. This means that individuals who purchase marijuana through these clubs can be subject to law enforcement measures.
- There are more than 400 chemicals in marijuana, but only 66 of them are unique to the *Cannabis* plant—these are called cannabinoids. One of them, delta-9-tetrahydrocannabinol (THC), was isolated and synthesized in 1964 and is clearly the most pharmacologically active.
- THC and other cannabinoids bind to two receptors, designated CB_1 and CB_2. The CB_1 receptors are found primarily in the brain. The locations of CB_1 receptors in the brain may provide some clues about their functions. For example, the highest density of CB_1 receptors has been found in cells of the basal ganglia, which is involved in coordinating body movements. CB_2 receptors are found mainly outside the brain in immune cells, suggesting that cannabinoids may play a role in the modulation of the immune response.
- Marinol® (dronabinol) is indicated for the treatment of severe nausea and vomiting associated with cancer chemotherapy and for AIDS-related anorexia in Canada. Sativex® is marketed in Canada as an adjunctive treatment for the symptomatic relief of neuropathic pain in adults with multiple sclerosis and as an adjunctive analgesic in adults with advanced cancer. Cesamet® (nabilone) is a synthetic cannabinoid with antiemetic properties that has been found to be of value in the management of nausea and vomiting associated with cancer chemotherapy.
- While there are many anecdotal reports of the therapeutic value of smoked marijuana, scientific studies supporting the safety and efficacy of marijuana for many therapeutic claims are currently inconclusive.
- Research has demonstrated that THC and marijuana produce robust self-administration in laboratory animals and in human research participants, demonstrating its abuse potential. Data from a

variety of human laboratory and clinical studies demonstrate that an abstinence syndrome can be observed following abrupt cessation of several days of smoked marijuana administration or oral delta-9-THC administration. Cannabinoid withdrawal is not life threatening, with symptoms that include negative mood states, disrupted sleep, decreased food intake, and, in some cases, aggressive behaviour.

- The acute physiological effects of marijuana, primarily an increase in heart rate, have not been thought to be a threat to health. However, as the marijuana-using population ages, there is concern that individuals with high blood pressure, heart disease, or hardening of the arteries might be harmed by smoking marijuana. The lethal dose of THC has not been extensively studied in animals, and no human deaths have been reported from "overdoses" of cannabis
- A 1972 report indicated that two individuals who demonstrated cerebral atrophy had a history of smoking marijuana. The report suggested that the brain damage might have been caused by the marijuana. However, no other studies since then have been able to demonstrate the same finding. Although marijuana is known to cause memory deficits in humans and laboratory animals, the mechanisms responsible remain unclear. Because administration of marijuana and cannabinoids to rodents causes a reduction in neuron density in the hippocampus, it has been hypothesized that memory deficits might be attributable to neurotoxic effects of marijuana.
- Currently, little doubt exists of a relationship between substance use and psychotic illness. National mental health surveys have repeatedly found more substance use (especially cannabis) among people with such a diagnosis. Over the past years, the publication of studies assessing the relationship between cannabis and psychosis has attracted considerable attention in the research literature, popular media, and community generally. Existing reviews have concluded that cannabis has a causal relationship to psychosis or that the possibility of such a relationship cannot be excluded. Further research is necessary to determine whether or not cannabis and other substances can trigger psychosis by direct neurotoxic effects.
- Several reports suggest that the average THC content of cannabis may be increasing. Cannabidiol, another constituent in cannabis, has been shown to have anxiolytic and antipsychotic effects. This has led to the suggestion that cannabidiol may offset some of the adverse effects of THC. Just as there is variability in the THC content of cannabis, so too is there variability in the cannabidiol content of cannabis.

Review Questions

1. What are the major differences between *C. sativa* and *C. indica*?
2. How is hashish produced?
3. When and where was the earliest recorded medical use of cannabis?
4. What have brain imaging studies told us about the effects of cannabis on cognition?
5. What is a *cannabinoid*, and about how many are there in cannabis? What is the cannabinoid found in brain tissue?
6. How is the action of THC in the brain terminated after about 30 minutes, when the half-life of metabolism is much longer than that?
7. What are the two most consistent physiological effects of smoking marijuana?
8. What is cannabidiol? What is its role in anxiety and psychosis?
9. What is Sativex, and for which conditions is it indicated as an adjunctive?

CHAPTER 16

PERFORMANCE-ENHANCING DRUGS

OBJECTIVES

When you have finished this chapter, you should be able to

- **LO1** Relate historical uses of performance-enhancing drugs by athletes.
- **LO2** Describe the history of the use of stimulants to enhance performance.
- **LO3** Describe the development and current state of drug testing in sports.
- **LO4** Describe the performance-enhancing effects and primary dangers of stimulant drugs.
- **LO5** Distinguish between androgenic and anabolic effects of testosterone and other related steroid hormones.
- **LO6** Describe the desired effects and undesirable side effects of steroids in men, women, and adolescents.
- **LO7** Explain the rationale behind athletes' use of human growth hormone and its associated dangers.
- **LO8** Explain the performance-enhancing effects of blood doping and its associated risks.

Why is there so much concern over drug use by athletes? Why not focus on drug use by clarinet players or muffler repair people? There are several answers to this question, and together they demonstrate the special reasons to be concerned about drug use in sports. First, well-known athletes are seen as role models for young people, portraying youth, strength, and health. When a famous athlete is reported to be using steroids or some other illicit substance, there is concern that impressionable young people will see drug use in a more positive light. Corporate sponsors pay these athletes to endorse their products, from shoes to breakfast cereal, based on this presumed influence over young consumers.

Second, some of the drugs used by athletes are intended to give the user an advantage over the competition, an advantage that is clearly viewed as being unfair. This is inconsistent with our tradition of fair play in sports, and widespread cheating of any kind tends to diminish a sport and public interest in it. Professional wrestling, which is widely viewed as being rigged or staged, is enjoyed more as a form of comic entertainment than as an athletic contest. Most professional and amateur athletes guard their honour carefully, and the use of performance-enhancing drugs is seen as a threat to that honour.

Third, there is a concern that both the famous and the not-so-famous athletes who use drugs are endangering their health and perhaps their lives for the sake of a temporary burst of power or speed. Athletes should be aware of the risks associated with the use of these drugs. Because these drugs are often obtained illicitly, we can assume that the providers of the drugs do not present a balanced cost–benefit analysis to the potential user but, instead, probably maximize any possible benefit and minimize the dangers.

LO1, LO2, LO3

Historical Use of Drugs in Athletics

Although we tend to think of drug use by athletes as a recent phenomenon, the use of chemicals to enhance performance might be as old as sport itself. As with many early drugs, some of these concoctions seemed to make sense at the time but probably had only placebo value. We no longer think that the powdered hooves of an ass will make our feet fly as fast as that animal's, but perhaps it was a belief in that powder that helped the ancient Egyptian competitor's self-confidence. Also, if all the others are using it, why take chances?

Ancient Times

The early Greek Olympians used various herbs and mushrooms that might have had some pharmacological actions as stimulants, and Aztec athletes used a cactus-based stimulant resembling strychnine. Athletic competitions probably developed in tribal societies as a means of training and preparing for war or for hunting, and various psychoactive plants were used by tribal peoples during battles and hunts, so it is not surprising that the drugs were also used in athletic contests from the beginning.

Early Use of Stimulants

During the 1800s and early 1900s, three types of stimulants were reported to be in use by athletes. *Strychnine*, which became famous as a rat poison, can at low doses act as a central nervous system stimulant. However, if the dose is too high, seizure activity will be produced in the brain. The resulting convulsions can paralyze respiration, leading to death. At least some boxers were reported to have used strychnine tablets. This might have made them more aggressive and kept them from tiring very quickly, but it was a dangerous way to do it. We'll never know how many of them were killed in this way, but there must have been a few. Thomas Hicks won the marathon in the 1904 St. Louis Olympics, then collapsed and had to be revived. His race was partly fuelled by a mixture of

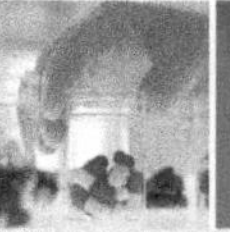

DRUGS IN THE MEDIA

Banned Substances and How to Avoid Them

Television and other media from the past several Olympic games reported multiple instances of athletes being disqualified for using banned substances. In some cases, the disqualification was not contested, but in others the athletes thought they had been disqualified unfairly because they had taken something prescribed for them or something that they were not aware had been banned. The following list, from an article in *Technique* magazine by Jack Swarbick, lawyer for USA Gymnastics, includes tips for athletes on how to avoid the problem. Even if you aren't an Olympic competitor, these tips should give you an idea of how complex and difficult this problem can be.

1. Be familiar with the banned substances list of the governing body, the International Olympic Committee. This means knowing not only what drugs are on the list but also the types of medications or even foods in which those drugs are often found.
2. Make certain that others who ought to know, such as your parents, physician, and school nurse, are also familiar with the banned substances list.
3. Know what medications you are using. Athletes should consult with the governing body regarding the potential for any medications to contain elements of banned substances and should be careful to list all medications when completing the screening form as part of the drug-testing program.
4. At competitions, drink only out of containers that were sealed when you got them, and once you have begun drinking out of a container do not leave it unattended. Several sports have implemented fairly rigorous security measures for the handling of coolers and water bottles.
5. When you are required to produce a urine sample as part of the drug-testing procedures, never surrender possession of the sample or leave it unattended until after you have sealed it inside the shipping canister provided by the officials.
6. If there are any irregularities in the process by which you give a urine sample and place that sample in the sealed container (e.g., a cracked beaker, a spilled sample, or unauthorized individuals on-site), immediately bring those irregularities to the attention of the drug-control administrator on-site.
7. If you are informed that you have tested positive for a banned substance (and you dispute that result), you will be invited to witness the testing of the second half (i.e., the "B sample") of your urine sample. Attend the test of the B sample, take with you an individual qualified to evaluate the process, and consider videotaping the test.

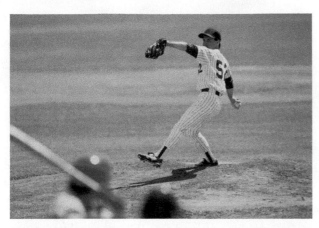

One of the major concerns with the use of performance-enhancing drugs is that they violate the tradition of fair play in sports.

brandy and strychnine.[1] Although the availability of amphetamines later made highly dangerous drugs, such as strychnine, less attractive, some evidence indicates the occasional use of strychnine continued at the level of world competition into the 1960s.

Cocaine was also available in the 1800s, at first in the form of Mariani's Coca Wine (used by the French cycling team), which was referred to in some advertisements as "wine for athletes."[2] When pure cocaine became available, athletes quickly adopted this more potent form. Many athletes used coffee as a mild stimulant, and some added pure *caffeine* to their coffee or took caffeine tablets. There were numerous reports of the suspected doping of swimmers, cyclists, boxers, runners, and other athletes during this period. Then, as now, some of the suspicions were raised by the losers, who might or might not have had any evidence of doping. Our use of the word *dope* for illicit drugs is derived from a Dutch word used in South Africa to refer to a cheap brandy, which was sometimes given to racing dogs or horses to slow them down. From this came the term for doping horses and then people, more often in an effort to improve rather than impair performance. Dogs and horses received all the substances used by humans, including coca wine and cocaine, before the days of testing for drugs.

Amphetamines

It isn't clear when athletes first started using amphetamines for their stimulant effects, but it was probably not long after the drugs were introduced in the 1930s. Amphetamines were widely used throughout the world during World War II, and in the 1940s and 1950s there were reports of the use of these pep pills by professional soccer players in England and Italy. Boxers and cyclists also relied on this new synthetic energy source. More potent than caffeine, longer lasting than cocaine, and safer than strychnine, it seemed for a while to be the ideal **ergogenic** (energy-producing) drug for both training and competition.

In 1952, the presence of syringes and broken ampules in the speed-skating locker room at the Oslo Winter Olympics was an indication of amphetamines' presence in international competition. There were other reports from the 1952 summer games in Helsinki and the 1956 Melbourne Olympics. Several deaths during this period were attributed to overdoses of amphetamines or other drugs. By the time of the 1960 Rome games, amphetamine use had spread around the world and to most sports. On opening day a Danish cyclist died during time trials. An autopsy revealed that his death from sunstroke was aided by the presence of amphetamines, which reduce blood flow to the skin, making it more difficult for the body to cool itself. Three other cyclists collapsed that day, and two were hospitalized.[1] This and other examples of amphetamine abuse led to investigations and to antidoping laws in France and Belgium. Other nations, including Canada and the United States, seemed less concerned.

International Drug Testing

Some sports, especially cycling, began to test competitors for drugs on a sporadic basis. Throughout the 1960s, some athletes refused to submit to tests or failed tests and were disqualified. These early testing efforts were not enough to prevent the death of cyclist Tommy Simpson, an ex-world champion, who died during the 1967 Tour de France. His death was seen on television, and weeks later it was reported that his body contained two types of amphetamines and that drugs had been found in his luggage. This caused the International Olympic Committee in 1968 to establish rules requiring the disqualification of any competitor who refuses to take a drug test or who is found guilty of using banned drugs. Beginning with fewer than 700 urine tests at the 1968 Mexico City

ergogenic: producing work or energy; a general term for performance enhancement.

Olympics, each subsequent international competition has had more testing, more disqualifications, and more controversy.

North American Football

Most people did not seem to be very concerned about drug use by athletes until reports surfaced in the late 1960s and early 1970s that professional football players were using amphetamines during games. Before that, people might not have been very concerned about it even if they had known. Remember from Chapter 6 that the amphetamines underwent a major status change in 1973. For years an increasing number of Canadians had used amphetamines to keep them awake, to provide extra energy, or to lose weight. They were seen by most people as legal, harmless pep pills. It was in that context that the physicians for professional football teams ordered large quantities of the drugs as a routine part of their supplies, and trainers dispensed them liberally.

At the end of the 1960s, amphetamines were widely considered to be drugs of abuse, dangerous drugs that could lead to violent behaviour. In this context, revelations that many professionals were playing high made for sensational headlines. Of particular note was a June 1957 article published on the front page of the *New York Times* reporting that amphetamines were being used by athletes in the United States, Canada, and Australia. The article quoted the team physician of the Ottawa Rough Riders of the Canadian Football League (CFL) as stating that players on all the major Canadian football teams were using pep pills.[3] Subsequently several National Football League (NFL) players sued their teams for injuries received while playing under the influence of drugs, and the NFL officially banned the distribution of amphetamines by team physicians and trainers in 1971. Although the drugs were no longer condoned by the league, the NFL did little at that time to enforce the ban, except to request copies of each team's orders for medical supplies. Athletes who wanted amphetamines still obtained and used them, often through a legal prescription from their own physicians. The attitude seemed to be that if the players wanted to use pep pills and obtained them on their own, that was their business, but team physicians and trainers shouldn't be using medications to push the athletes beyond their normal endurance. The current CFL and NFL policies, of course, restrict all use of amphetamines, as well as many other drugs, no matter where they are obtained.

anabolic: promoting constructive metabolism; building tissue.

Steroids

During and after World War II, it was found that malnourished people could gain weight and build themselves up more rapidly if they were given the male hormone testosterone. The Soviets were the first to put this hormone to use on a wide scale to build up their athletes. An American team physician at the 1956 Olympics reported that the Soviet athletes were using straight testosterone, sometimes in excessive doses and with unfortunate side effects. Testosterone helps both men and women become more muscular, but its masculinizing effects on women and enlargement of the prostate gland in men are definite drawbacks. The American physician at the 1956 Olympics returned to the United States and helped develop and test **anabolic** steroids, which were quickly adopted by American weight lifters and bodybuilders.[4]

American and British athletes in such events as discus and shotput were the first to acknowledge publicly that they had used steroids, and there was evidence that steroid use was widespread during the 1960s in most track and field events. These drugs were not officially banned, nor were they tested for in international competition until the early 1970s, mainly because a sensitive urine test was not available until then. Of the 2000 urine samples taken during the 1976 Olympics, fewer than 300 were tested for the presence of steroids, and 8 of those were positive.[1] The first international athletes to be found guilty of taking steroids were a Bulgarian discus thrower, a Romanian shotputter, a Polish discus thrower, and weight lifters from several countries. By that time, individual Western athletes might have chosen to use steroids, but some of the eastern European countries seemed to have adopted their use almost as a matter of official policy. When the East German swimming coach was asked during the 1976 Olympics why so many of their women swimmers had deep voices, the answer was, "We have come here to swim, not sing."[5]

Perhaps the best-known Canadian athlete to run afoul of the steroid prohibition was sprinter Ben Johnson. Johnson, who set consecutive 100-metre world records at the 1987 World Championships in Athletics and the 1988 Summer Olympics, had his world records and Olympic gold rescinded after testing positive for use of the anabolic steroid stanozolol.

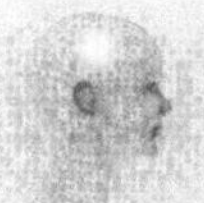

MIND/BODY CONNECTION

Baseball: Seeking Alternatives to Amphetamines

Psychologically, amphetamine increases feelings of alertness and well-being and improves attention, focus, reaction time, and vigilance. The drug also reverses psychological decrements caused by fatigue and sleep deprivation. Physically, it increases motor and cardiovascular activity. Undoubtedly, these features have contributed to the use of this drug in Major League Baseball for at least half a century. It is important to note that amphetamine use in baseball has continued, despite the fact that it has been available only by prescription in Canada since the late 1950s and the United States since 1970. According to investigations of drug use in baseball, this legal technicality did not seem to interfere with the widespread use of amphetamine. However, under baseball's new drug policy, which took effect at the start of the 2006 season, amphetamine was banned. While penalties associated with amphetamine infractions are not as severe as steroid violations, players consistently testing positive for the substance run the risk of being banned from the game.

The Major League Baseball season is a gruelling endurance test, comprising seven weeks of spring training followed by 162 games in six months. There are also double-headers (two games in one day), rain delays, cross-country flights, and the expectation that players perform at their peak each game. Given this situation, it is not difficult to see why amphetamine use was common.

One frequently asked question is what impact the ban will have on the players and the game. Some observers have speculated that ultimately it will be a positive development, prompting players to seek healthier and natural alternatives. For example, some players might adapt strategies to improve their physical conditioning. Others may seek out sport psychologists to learn mental skills necessary to perform consistently in training and competition. Some may alter their lifestyles such that they decrease their alcohol intake and attend more carefully to their diet and sleep habits.

Another view is that players will continue to use pharmacological tools to aid them through marathon seasons. It has been suggested that high-caffeine-containing energy drink consumption will increase, as will the use of over-the-counter stimulants. Although it is difficult to track this type of stimulant use, information is available regarding the number of players granted therapeutic-use exemptions for attention-deficit/hyperactivity disorder (ADHD). As discussed in Chapter 6, stimulants, including amphetamine, are used to treat this disorder, and its diagnosis provides a legal avenue through which a player can obtain amphetamine. In 2006, for example, of the 1354 Major League Baseball players, 28 were granted therapeutic-use exemptions for ADHD. In 2007, this number dramatically increased to 103.[6] It is worth noting that the North American adult prevalence rate for ADHD is substantially lower than baseball's 2007 exemption rate.

It is too early to know for certain the impact of baseball's ban on amphetamine. But judging from these early indications, a significant number of individuals will employ strategies, both pharmacological and nonpharmacological, to circumvent the ban.

The Johnson Olympic scandal led the Government of Canada to establish a Commission of Inquiry into the Use of Drugs and Banned Practices Intended to Increase Athletic Performance. The inquiry, held in 1989, was headed by Ontario Appeal Court Chief Justice Charles Dubin. During the inquiry hundreds of testimonies were presented, attesting to the widespread use of performance-enhancing drugs by athletes. In his testimony Ben Johnson's coach, Charlie Francis, told the inquiry that Johnson had been using steroids since 1981. He then went on to charge that Johnson was only one of many steroid users and that he just happened to get caught. It is important to note that no Canadian athlete has been caught using performance-enhancing drugs at a winter or summer Olympic games since 1988.

The BALCO Scandal

For years, rumours had circulated around professional baseball that certain players were using steroids, but Major League Baseball (MLB) did not test for them. When Barry Bonds came into the 2001 season looking bigger and stronger–and went on to hit a record 79 home runs–some speculated that he might have used steroids, but the rumours were always denied. In 2002,

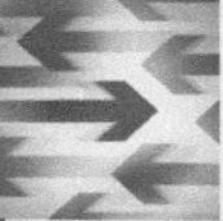

TAKING SIDES

Should We Be Concerned about Steroid Use by Entertainers?

In recent years much attention has been focused on Major League Baseball players' alleged use of performance-enhancing drugs. However, some are warning that steroids and human growth hormone are being illegally prescribed throughout the country at an alarming rate under the belief they will aid healing, enhance physical attractiveness, and slow aging. The list of people accused of using these drugs is extensive and ranges from ordinary citizens to prominent entertainers. For example, in March 2007, Sylvester Stallone was required to pay a fine of nearly $3000 to Australian officials after they discovered in his luggage several vials of human growth hormone. The use of anti-aging, anti-obesity, and anti-fatigue agents in the entertainment industry has been known and accepted for decades. But recent claims that some members of the industry are using steroids and related compounds raise similar questions to those mentioned regarding the use of these drugs by athletes. Entertainers are role models for young people. Will their steroid use suggest to impressionable youngsters that this type of drug use is acceptable? Performance-enhancing drugs are usually taken to create an advantage over the competition. For example, professional models may take amphetamines in an effort to decrease body weight and enhance their chances of landing the "supermodel" contract. This is clearly viewed as being unfair to models not taking anti-obesity drugs. And of course, these drugs carry health-related risks, especially when taken illicitly. As a result of these issues, should we increase our monitoring of performance-enhancing drug use by members of the entertainment industry? Should governments conduct investigations of drug use in the entertainment industry? Or should governments refrain from such drug-use investigations altogether?

former player Ken Caminiti admitted to using steroids and claimed that "half" the MLB players were doing so. MLB did institute a limited testing program that was generally considered to be too weak to have much effect.

In June 2003, an unidentified track coach delivered to the U.S. Anti-Doping Agency a syringe containing an "undetectable" steroid, naming the source as Victor Conte, founder of BALCO Laboratories. Analysis determined that the syringe contained tetrahydrogestrinone (THG), a steroid previously unknown to the agency and that did not show up in agency tests. The BALCO investigation led to a raid on the laboratory and the discovery of other steroids and human growth hormone.[7] Conte testified before a grand jury in San Francisco after being given immunity from prosecution and named a long list of Olympic and professional athletes who had been his clients, including Barry Bonds and many other professional baseball players.

As a result of this and other developments, at the start of the 2006 season the MLB instituted more frequent testing and toughened penalties for drug policy violations. In addition, testing for amphetamines was included as part of the new policy for the first time (see the Mind/Body Connection box). Under the current policy, each player is tested at least twice: once during the preseason and once during the regular season. All players are also subjected to additional random tests throughout the season. Table 16.1 summarizes the penalties associated with violations.

The Battle over Testing

During the 1980s, public revelations of drug use by athletes became common and cocaine was often mentioned. Professional basketball, baseball, and football

Table 16.1 Penalties for Violating Major League Baseball Drug Policy

Substance	Penalty
Steroid	
first positive test	50-game suspension
second positive test	100-game suspension
third positive test	lifetime suspension—may seek reinstatement after two years
Amphetamine	
first positive test	mandatory follow-up testing
second positive test	25-game suspension
third positive test	80-game suspension
fourth positive test	commissioner's discretion

players in the United States were being sent into treatment centres for cocaine dependence, and several either dropped out or were kicked out of professional sports. Most amateur and professional sports organizations have adopted longer and more complicated lists of banned substances and rules providing for more and more participants to be tested. The Canadian Centre for Ethics in Sport publishes an annual *Substance Classification Booklet*, a quick reference of the status in sport of Canadian brand-name medications and ingredients.[8] This status is based on the World Anti-Doping Agency's *Prohibited List*, an international standard that defines the substances and methods that are prohibited both in and out of competition.[9] In many events around the world, all contestants must now be subjected to urine tests as a matter of routine.

Because of both the expense and the inconvenience, some have questioned the wisdom of trying to test every athlete for everything. Despite the enormous expense to which sports organizations have gone, the use of steroids, stimulants, and other performance-enhancing substances seems to be as great as ever. Both the extent of testing and the ingenuity of athletes trying to beat the tests continue to escalate. The BALCO scandal demonstrates that chemists will keep coming up with new ways to help the athletes avoid detection.

LO4 Stimulants as Performance Enhancers

The first question to be answered about the use of a drug to increase energy or otherwise enhance athletic performance is, Does it work? We might not worry so much about unfair competition if we didn't feel that the use of a drug would really help the person using it. Also, if we could prove that these drugs were ineffective, then we could presumably convince young people not to take the risk of using drugs because there would be no gain to be had. But experiments can never prove that a drug has no effect–you might have done a hundred experiments and not used the right dose or the right test (peak output? endurance? accuracy?). The possibility always exists that someone will come along later with the right combination to demonstrate a beneficial effect. Therefore, be wary when someone tries to use scientific evidence to argue that a drug doesn't work, has no effect, is not toxic, or is otherwise inactive.

We've had a pretty good idea of the effectiveness of the amphetamines since 1959, when Smith and Beecher published the results of a double-blind study comparing amphetamines and placebos in runners, swimmers, and weight throwers.[10] They concluded that most of the athletes performed better under amphetamines, but the improvement was small (a few percentage points' improvement). Several studies have reported no differences or very small differences in performance, and some medical experts in the 1960s wanted to argue that amphetamines were essentially ineffective and there was no reason for people to use them. An excellent 1981 review of the existing literature put it all into perspective. Pointing out that it had been taking athletes an average of about seven years to attain each 1% improvement in the world record speed for the mile run (1.6 kilometres), if amphetamines produced even a 1% improvement, they could make an important difference at that level of competition. The study concluded that there is an amphetamine margin. It is usually small, amounting to a few percent under most circumstances. But even when that tiny, the advantage can spell the difference between a gold medal and sixth place.[11]

Whether amphetamines or other stimulants increase physical ability (provide pep or energy) or produce their actions only through effects on the brain is an interesting question, which might not be answerable. Surely a person who feels more confident will train harder, compete with a winning attitude, try harder, and keep trying longer. With amphetamines, improvements have been seen both in events requiring brief, explosive power (shotput) and in events requiring endurance, such as distance running. In laboratory studies, increases have been found in isometric strength and in work output during endurance testing on a stationary bicycle (the subjects rode longer under amphetamine conditions). This endurance improvement could be due to the masking of fatigue effects, allowing a person to compete to utter exhaustion.

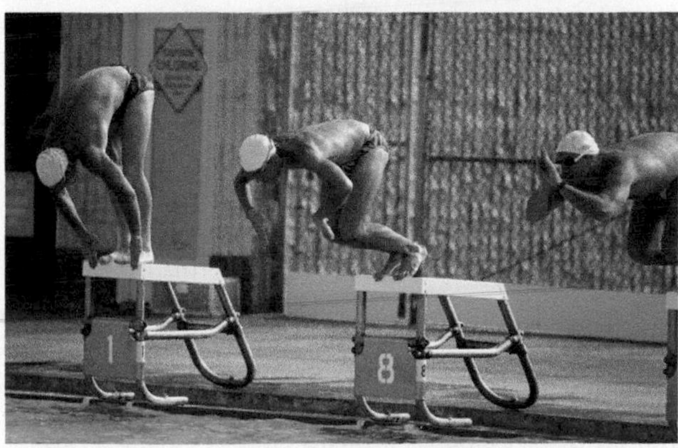

Stimulants have been shown to improve endurance.

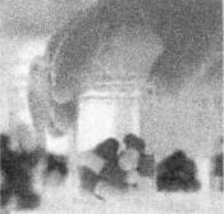

DRUGS IN THE MEDIA

When Taking Over-the-Counter Medication, Read the Label

Perhaps the best-known Canadian athlete to run afoul of stimulant prohibition was former women's rowing World Champion and Olympic medal winner Silken Laumann. Following a gold medal win in the 1995 Pan American quadruple rowing event, Laumann and her teammates were stripped of their gold medals when Laumann's antidoping tests showed illegal levels of the banned stimulant pseudoephedrine. Laumann lashed out at the action, saying that she had unintentionally used the prohibited substance.

Her troubles began when, just before the Pan American Games, she began to experience cold symptoms. She consulted the rowing team physician who recommended she purchase Benadryl, an over-the counter (OTC) antihistamine that did not contain banned substances. Inadvertently Laumann purchased the wrong type of Benadryl, buying a form that contained pseudoephedrine. Once again, immediately before her event, Laumann asked another team physician if it was okay to take Benadryl. The physician said yes without checking the type Laumann had purchased. Laumann explained that she did not read the OTC's label, which clearly indicated that it contained the banned substance.

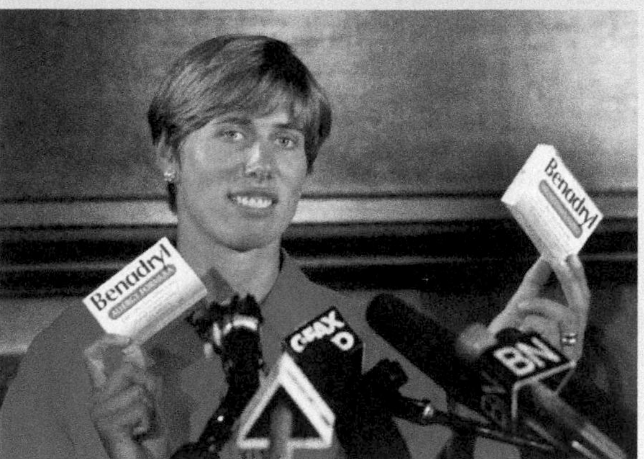

Canadian athlete Silken Laumann.

While assuming partial responsibility for the incident, Laumann also laid heavy blame on the team physicians, accusing them of providing flippant advice. The International Olympic Commission's medal committee concurred, calling for sanctions against the Canadian team's physicians. So what's the moral of this story? *When taking an OTC medication, always read the label.*

Source: Chidley, J., and J. Deacon. "Laumann Fails Drug Test." *Maclean's Magazine* April 3 (1995).

Caffeine has also been shown to improve endurance performance under laboratory conditions. In one experiment, 330 milligrams of caffeine (approximately equivalent to three cups of brewed coffee) increased the length of a stationary bicycle ride by almost 20%. In another experiment, when subjects rode for two hours, their total energy output was 7% higher after 500 milligrams of caffeine than in the control condition.[12] The effectiveness of caffeine might depend on other factors: For example, one study reported no benefit from caffeine when athletes ran long distances (19 kilometres/12 miles) in hot, humid conditions.[13] Small amounts of caffeine are acceptable in most sports, but a urine level of more than 12 micrograms/millilitre will lead to disqualification in many competitions. The doses needed to produce large performance increases produce much higher levels than that, but there could still be a slight improvement even at legal levels.

Apparently no controlled laboratory or field experiments have tested the performance-enhancing capabilities of cocaine, but especially during the 1980s many athletes believed in its power. Cocaine's stimulant properties are generally similar to those of the amphetamines, so we can assume that cocaine would be effective under some circumstances. Given cocaine's shorter duration of action, it would not be expected to improve endurance over a several-hour period as well as either amphetamines or caffeine.

For years, athletes had another readily available stimulant in the form of ephedrine, either as a drug or as an ephedra extract. Ephedra (*ma huang*) is mentioned in Chapter 12 as the herbal source of ephedrine, and it was the ephedrine molecule that was modified in the 1920s to produce amphetamine. When Olympic officials developed lists of banned substances, ephedrine was soon included (except for people whose physicians said they had asthma–ephedrine relaxes bronchial passages and is an ingredient in asthma medications). Professional sports organizations were at first less concerned about ephedrine, but eventually the CFL and NFL also banned it. MLB did not, and baseball players used it to provide extra energy, or in some cases to reduce weight, since ephedra was also found in many weight-control dietary supplements. In 2003, Baltimore Orioles pitcher Steve Bechler collapsed during practice and died later in hospital. Before he died, his temperature rose to 42°C, which was attributed to heatstroke caused by the ingestion of "significant amounts" of ephedrine from a dietary supplement.[14] This widely publicized death finally gave the U.S. Food and Drug Administration enough political backing to go along with the years of evidence it had been accumulating, leading to the 2004 ban on ephedra and ephedrine in dietary supplements. In Canada ephedrine (low dose, 8 milligrams per tablet) remains available as a natural health product (NHP) and is present in some OTC cold medicines (see Chapter 12 for a detailed discussion).

With all these and several other CNS stimulants banned by most sports associations, some athletes have continued to use them during training, to allow them to run, ride, or swim harder. They then do not use the drug for several days before the competition or during the competition, hoping that traces of the substance will not appear in the urine test. This might make sense, but no one knows whether training under one drug condition has an effect on competition under another condition. Also, overexertion under the influence of a fatigue-masking drug might be most dangerous during training, leading to muscle injury, a fall or another accident, or heat exhaustion.

Athletes and others who use amphetamines or cocaine regularly run the risk of developing a dependence on the drug, developing paranoid or violent behaviour patterns, and suffering from the loss of energy and the psychological depression that occur as the drugs wear off (see Chapter 6).

LO5, LO6 Steroids

The male sex hormone testosterone has two major types of effects on a developing boy. **Androgenic** effects are masculinizing actions: Initial growth of the penis and other male sex glands, deepening of the voice, and increased facial hair are examples. This steroid hormone also has anabolic effects. These include increased muscle mass, increases in the size of various internal organs, control of the distribution of body fat, increased protein synthesis, and increased calcium in the bones. In the 1950s, drug companies began to synthesize various steroids that have fewer of the androgenic effects and more of the anabolic effects than testosterone. These are referred to as *anabolic steroids,* although none of them is entirely free of some androgenic (masculinizing) effect.

Whether these drugs are effective in improving athletic performance has been controversial: For many years the medical position was that they were not, whereas the lore around the locker room was that they would make anyone bigger, stronger, and more masculine looking. A lot of people must have had more faith in the locker-room lore than in the official word. The 1989 *Physician's Desk Reference* contained the following statement in boldface type: "Anabolic steroids have not been shown to enhance athletic ability." Try telling that to any MLB player, sportswriter, or fan.

There is no doubt that testosterone has a tremendous effect on muscle mass and strength during puberty, and experiments on castrated animals clearly show the muscle-developing ability of the synthetic anabolics.[15] What is not as clear is the effect of adding additional anabolic stimulation to adolescent or adult males who already have normal circulating levels of testosterone.

Laboratory research on healthy men who are engaged in weight training and are maintained on a proper diet has often found that anabolic steroids produce small increases in lean muscle mass and sometimes small increases in muscular strength. There is no evidence in those studies for an overall increase in aerobic capacity or endurance. However, it might never be possible to conduct experiments demonstrating the effectiveness of the high doses used by some athletes. Many athletes report that they take ten or more times the dose of a steroid that has been tested and recommended for treatment of a deficiency disorder.[16] It is also common for athletes to take more than one steroid at a time (both an oral and an injectable form, for example). This practice is known as "stacking." To expose research subjects to such massive doses would clearly be unethical.

Another impediment to doing careful research on this topic is that these steroids produce detectable psychological effects. When double-blind experiments have been attempted, almost always the subjects have known when they were on steroids, thus destroying the blind control.[17] This is important because steroid users report that they feel they can lift more or work harder when they are on the steroids. This may be due to CNS effects of the steroids leading to a stimulant-like feeling of energy and loss of fatigue or to increased aggressiveness expressed as more aggressive training. There is a further possibility of what is known as an *active placebo effect,* with a belief in the power of steroids, enhanced

androgenic: masculinizing.

by the clear sensation that the drug is doing something because the user can "feel" it. Until recently, many of the scientists studying steroid hormones believed that their main effects were psychological, combined with a "bloating" effect on the muscle, in which the muscle retains more fluids, is larger, weighs more, but has no more physical strength.[1]

Mechanism of Action

Anabolic steroids, technically known as anabolic-androgenic steroids, are drugs that mimic the effects of the endogenous hormones testosterone and dihydrotestosterone. Anabolic steroids are fat-soluble hormones and as such are capable of penetrating plasma cell membranes. As illustrated in Figure 16.1, the pharmacological action of steroids begins when the steroid penetrates the plasma membrane of a target cell and binds to its receptor located in the cell's cytoplasm. Once bound, the steroid-receptor complex moves into the cell's nucleus, where it binds to a regulatory site on the DNA. This interaction leads to gene transcription, which directs the production of proteins.

How do anabolic steroids affect skeletal muscle size? They do so through two actions: (1) They promote gene transcription in muscle cells leading to the

Figure 16.1 Steroid Mechanism of Action

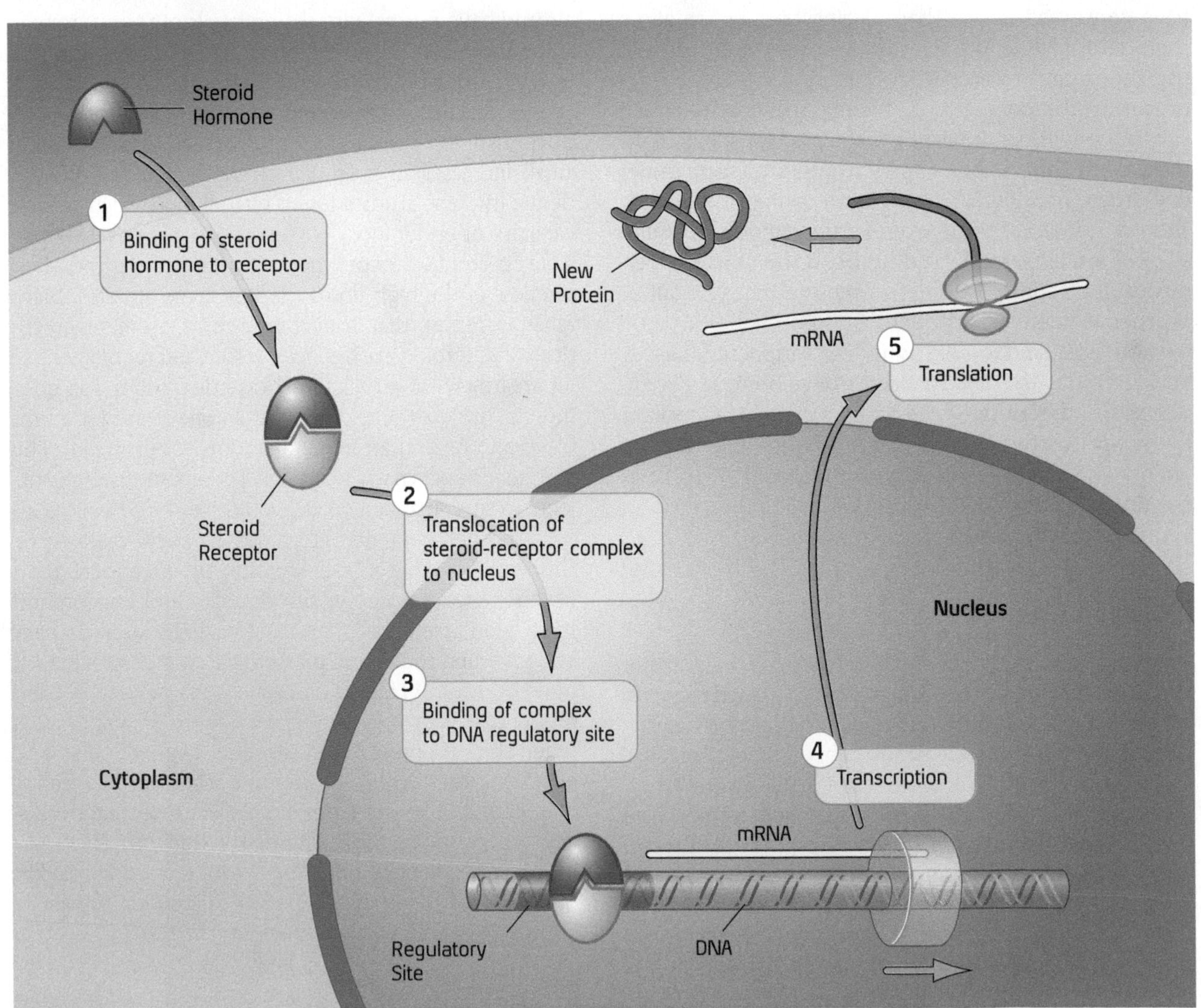

Source: The Pharmacology Education Partnership, "Steroids and Athletes: Genes Work Overtime" (Module 6). Courtesy of Rochelle D. Schwartz-Bloom, Duke University Medical Center. Retrieved from: http://www.thepepproject.net.

synthesis of muscle proteins. More muscle protein means bigger muscle cells. (2) They bind to glucocorticoid receptors, preventing endogenous glucocorticoids from performing their normal function: the breakdown of muscle (also known as catabolism). Collectively, these actions lead to increased muscle size.[18]

Prevalence of Illicit Steroid Use in Canada

Steroid use is surprisingly high among Canada's youth. Since 1989 the *Ontario Student Drug Use Health Survey* has asked students (in grades 7-12) if they have ever used steroids to enhance their athletic performance or to change their physical appearance. Data in Figure 16.2 show the percentage of reported steroid use in lifetime by students (grades 9-12). In 2013 an estimated 2.0% of students reported having used steroids. This was a significant decrease from 1999 estimates of 4.3%. Reports indicate that males are more likely than females to use steroids. In 2013 the Canadian Association of College and University Student Services published results of the *ACHA National College Health Assessment* survey, which reported selected drug use trends among 34 039 students from 32 postsecondary Canadian institutions. The 2013 *ACHA National College Health Assessment* data provided a snapshot of current anabolic steroid use among postsecondary students. In 2013, 98% of students self-reported as lifetime abstainers. Of those who self-reported lifetime use of anabolic steroids, all were males; only 1% reported use in the past 30 days.[19] For the general population, the 2004 *Canadian Addiction Survey* revealed that approximately 0.6% of Canadians 15 years of age and older have used illicit steroids at some point in their lives.[20] General population data on the use of illicit steroids has not been collected since 2004.

Figure 16.2 Lifetime Steroid Use in the Total Population and by Sex, OSDUHS, 1999–2013 (Grades 9–12)

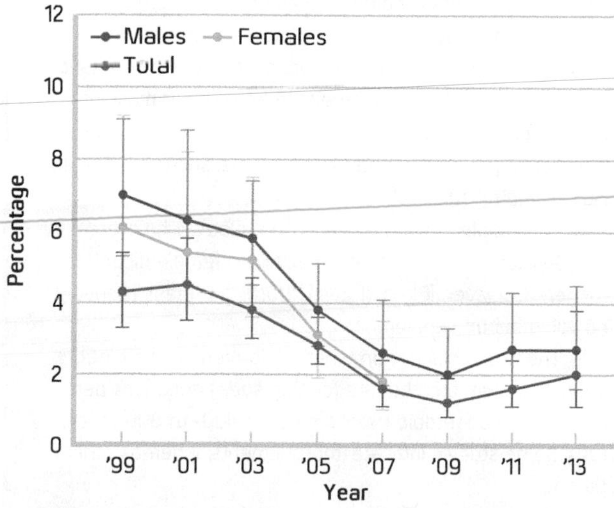

Note: Confidence intervals are shown.

Source: Boak, A., and others. (2013) *Drug Use among Ontario Students, 1977–2013: Detailed OSDUHS Findings* (CAMH Research Document Series No. 36). Toronto: ON, Centre for Addiction and Mental Health. Retrieved December 12, 2013, from http://www.camh.ca/en/research/news_and_publications/ontario-student-drug-use-and-health-survey/Documents/2013%20OSDUHS%20Docs/2013OSDUHS_Detailed_DrugUseReport.pdf.

Psychological Effects of Steroids

The reported psychological effects of steroids, including a stimulant-like high and increased aggressiveness, might be beneficial for increasing the amount of work done during training and for increasing the intensity of effort during competition. However, preclinical, clinical, and anecdotal reports suggest that steroid use, especially at high doses, may lead to the development of psychiatric dysfunctions.

Research has shown that abuse of anabolic steroids may lead to extreme aggression, mood swings, paranoid jealousy, delusions, extreme irritability, and violence.[21] There has been a great deal of discussion about "roid rage," a kind of manic rage that has been reported by some steroid users.[22] We should be careful about attributing instances of violence to a drug on the basis of uncontrolled retrospective reports, especially when the perpetrator of a violent crime might be looking for an excuse.[23] However, there are a sufficient number of reports of violent feelings and actions among steroid users for us to be concerned and to await further research. Says Dr. William Taylor, a leading authority on anabolic steroids, "I've seen total personality changes. A passive, low-key guy goes on steroids for muscle enhancement, and the next thing you know, he's being arrested for assault or disorderly conduct."[24]

It is not entirely clear whether steroid use can lead to dependency in the way that cocaine, heroin, or nicotine do. However, certain findings suggest that substance dependency may occur:

- Steroid users frequently report experiencing withdrawal symptoms when they stop taking their drug. Symptoms include fatigue, restlessness, insomnia, loss of appetite, depression, and steroid craving.[25]
- Animal studies have shown that anabolic steroids are reinforcing. This is based on findings that, as is seen for other addictive substances, mice and hamsters will self-administer anabolic steroids when given the opportunity.[26,27]

- Many steroid users continue their drug taking even in the face of steroid-induced physical, psychological, and social problems.[28]
- Steroid users typically spend considerable time and money obtaining the drug.

In Chapter 2 we were introduced to a tool, the DSM-5, used in the diagnosis of substance dependency. Based on these criteria, what is your opinion about the addictive potential of steroids?

Adverse Effects on the Body

There are many concerns about the effects of steroid use on the body. In young users who have not attained their full height, steroids can cause premature closing

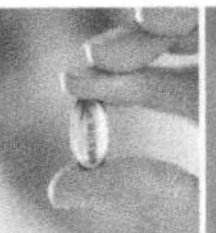

DRUGS IN DEPTH

Nutritional Ergogenic Aids

If athletes can't get or refuse to use pharmacological aids in athletic competition, most believe that certain foods or natural health products (NHPs) are a "natural" way to enhance their performance. Following is a very abbreviated description of a more complete review of this topic.[29]

Amino acids are the natural building blocks of the protein required to build muscle, and people certainly require a basic minimum intake. There is some evidence that very active people can benefit from a somewhat increased intake of dietary protein, slightly above the recommended daily allowances, but there is no demonstrated need to purchase expensive amino acid supplements to achieve this. Marketers of these "muscle-building" NHPs walk an ambiguous line, describing intended uses as "helps to assist in muscle cell repair after exercise" or "a nonessential amino acid that is involved in protein synthesis." Usually nearby posters or pamphlets link amino acids to the idea of muscle growth. These NHPs are probably of little or no value to an athlete who is receiving proper nutrition.

Carbohydrates are burned as fuels, especially during prolonged aerobic exercise. Carbohydrates taken two to four hours before an endurance performance lasting for more than an hour may enhance the performance by maintaining blood glucose levels and preventing the depletion of muscle stores of glycogen. Carbohydrate loading before marathon runs consists of resting for the last day or two while ingesting extra carbohydrates, increasing both muscle and liver stores of carbohydrates. In either case, there is not much evidence to support the value of carbohydrate supplements for athletic performances lasting less than an hour.

Fats, in experiments with fat supplements, have not been found to be a useful ergogenic aid.

Vitamins, especially the water-soluble B vitamins, are necessary for normal utilization of food energy. Deficiencies in these vitamins, such as might result when a wrestler is dieting to meet a weight limit, can clearly impair physical performance. However, once the necessary minimum amount is available for metabolic purposes, further supplements are of no value. Many experiments have been done with supplements of C, E, and B-complex vitamins or with multivitamin supplements, the so-called vitamin B15, and with bee pollen, and there is no evidence for enhanced performance or faster recovery after workouts. Again, these supplements are probably of no value to an athlete who is receiving proper nutrition.

Minerals, in the form of various mineral supplements, are widely used by athletes. Once again, most are probably not needed or useful, but there may be some exceptions. Electrolyte drinks are designed to replace both fluids and electrolytes, such as sodium and chloride, that are lost in sweat. Actually, sweat contains a lower concentration of these electrolytes than does blood, so it is more important to replace the fluids than the electrolytes under most circumstances. Sodium supplementation may be useful for those engaged in ultra-endurance events, such as 100-mile (161-kilometre) runs.

Iron supplements are helpful in athletes who are iron-deficient, as may occur especially in female distance runners. However, if iron status is normal, there is probably no value in iron supplements.

The jury is still out on whether "buffering" the blood pH with sodium bicarbonate (baking soda) enhances performance in anaerobic events, such as 400- to 800-metre runs. Some studies indicate improvements, whereas others do not.

Water is needed by endurance athletes to keep their body temperatures down, especially in a warm environment. Drinking water both before and during prolonged exercise can deter dehydration and improve performance.

of the growth plates of the long bones, thus limiting their adult height. For all users the risks of peliosis hepatitis (bloody cysts in the liver) and the changes in blood lipids, such as increases in LDL (bad cholesterol) and decreases in HDL (good cholesterol), possibly leading to atherosclerosis, high blood pressure, and heart disease, are potentially serious concerns. Acne and baldness are reported, as are atrophy of the testes and breast enlargement (gynecomastia) in men using anabolic steroids.

There are also considerations for women who use anabolic steroids. Because women usually have only trace amounts of testosterone produced by the adrenals, the addition of even relatively small doses of anabolic steroids can have dramatic effects, in terms of both muscle growth and masculinization (e.g., facial hair growth, male pattern baldness, changes in the menstrual cycle). Some of the side effects, such as mild acne, decreased breast size, and fluid retention, are reversible. The enlargement of the clitoris might be reversible if steroid use is stopped soon after it is noticed. Other effects, such as increased facial hair and deepening of the voice, might be irreversible.[17]

Finally, persons who inject illicit steroids are at increased risk of contracting or transmitting HIV or hepatitis.

Regulation

As we found in Chapter 2, when a drug produces dependence, violent behaviour, and toxic side effects, society may feel justified in trying to restrict the drug's availability. Such is the case for the anabolic steroids, which, along with their derivatives, are controlled substances in Canada listed under Schedule IV of the Controlled Drugs and Substances Act. As such they cannot be sold in Canada as either drugs or natural health products. Unfortunately, these products can be purchased illegally over the Internet. The penalty for buying or selling anabolic steroids in Canada is imprisonment for up to 18 months. Import and export carry similar penalties.[30]

LO7 Other Hormonal Manipulations

Whereas the anabolic steroids have been in wide use, other treatments have been experimented with on a more limited basis. Female sex hormones have been used to feminize men so that they could compete in women's events. The women's gold medal sprinter in the 1964 Olympics was shown by chromosome testing to have been a man, and he had to return the medal. Hormone receptor–blocking drugs have probably been used to delay puberty in female gymnasts. In women, puberty shifts the centre of gravity lower in the body and changes body proportions in ways that adversely affect performance in some gymnastic events. Smaller women appear to be more graceful, spin faster on the uneven bars, and generally have the advantage, which is why top female gymnasts are usually in their teens. However, the Soviets were suspected of tampering with nature: Their top three international gymnasts in 1978 were all 17 or 18 years old, but the following were their heights and weights: 135 centimetres, 29 kilograms; 154 centimetres, 40 kilograms; and 145 centimetres, 36 kilograms.

We have certainly not seen the end of growth-promoting hormonal treatments. **Human growth hormone**, which is released from the pituitary gland, can potentially increase the height and weight of an individual to gigantic proportions, especially if administered during childhood and adolescence. In rare instances, the excessive production of this hormone creates giants more than two metres tall. These giants usually die at an early age because their internal organs continue to grow. However, administration of a few doses of this hormone at the right time might produce a more controlled increase in body size. Likewise, the growth-hormone-releasing hormone, and some of the cellular intermediary hormones by which growth hormone exerts its effects, might work to enhance growth. It is difficult to test for the presence of these substances. Despite the possible dangers, the lure of an otherwise capable basketball player growing a couple of centimetres taller or of a football player being 15 kilograms heavier has no doubt caused many young athletes to experiment with these substances. Studies have shown that growth hormone increases lean body mass but may not improve strength.[31] Unlike anabolic steroids, which are scheduled in Canada's Controlled Drugs and Substances Act, human growth hormone is not and is available through prescription. In 2013 13 Major League Baseball players were accused of obtaining performance-enhancing drugs, specifically human growth hormone, from the now-defunct clinic

human growth hormone: a pituitary hormone responsible for some types of gigantism.

Biogenesis of America. The 13 players involved in the "Biogenesis baseball scandal" received suspensions of 50 or more games.

Beta-2 Agonists

At the beginning of the 1992 Olympics, the leader of the British team was disqualified because of the detection of a new drug. Clenbuterol was developed as a treatment for asthma and is a relative of several other bronchodilators that are found in prescription inhalers. These drugs have sympathomimetic effects on the bronchi of the lungs but are designed to be more specific than older sympathomimetics, such as ephedrine or the amphetamines (see Chapter 6). Their specificity comes from a selective stimulation of the beta-2 subtype of adrenergic receptors. Research with cows had revealed an increase in muscle mass, and speculation was beginning that this might represent a new type of nonsteroidal anabolic agent. Apparently someone in Great Britain was keeping an eye on the animal research literature and decided to try the anabolic actions on at least one Olympic athlete. Presumably it was hoped that such a new drug would not be tested for, but the Olympic officials were also well informed and ready, at least for clenbuterol. Human studies have shown some increases in strength of selected muscle types with clenbuterol or a similar drug, but there is no evidence that beta-2 agonists improve athletic performance.[32]

LO8 Blood Doping

Blood doping in sports is not a new practice, having been used for over 40 years. It is defined as the misuse of substances or certain techniques to increase the number of red blood cells in the bloodstream. Because red blood cells carry oxygen from the respiratory system to the skeletal muscles, higher concentrations in the blood improve aerobic capacity and therefore endurance. Its widespread use among athletes stems from its proven efficacy in improving performance in sports activities. Blood doping can be achieved through a variety of mechanisms including blood transfusion, administration of erythropoiesis-stimulating agents (which increase production of red blood cells) or blood substitutes (synthetic oxygen carriers), and gene manipulations.[33,34,35]

Blood doping is extremely dangerous and is suspected of having caused the death of many athletes since its inception. In 1984 the enhancement of oxygen transfer through blood transfusions was declared a prohibited method by the International Olympic Committee. The following references provide excellent description of the history of blood doping in sport, its associated risks, and regulation by the World Anti-Doping Agency.[35,36,37]

Creatine

One widely used substance among bodybuilders has been creatine, a natural substance found in meat and fish. In Canada this compound can be purchased as a licensed NHP for the intended use to "increase muscle mass when used in conjunction with a resistance training regimen. Improves performance in repetitive bouts of brief, highly intense physical activity." There is clear evidence that creatine helps regenerate ATP, which provides the energy for muscle contractions. Users of creatine tend to gain weight, some of which is water weight. There is considerable evidence that the use of creatine can improve strength and short-term speed in sprinting. However, studies of longer-distance running, cycling, and swimming often find no effect, and in one case a significant slowing was reported, probably because of weight gain.[5]

Getting "Cut"

If getting "cut," "ripped," and "shredded" sounds like something you'd want to avoid, then you're probably not into bodybuilding. These terms refer to the appearance of someone who is both muscular and lean. Because amateur wrestlers compete in weight classes and they need to be strong, they have always had the problem of eating well to build strength and train hard, but then needing to "cut" weight before the weigh-ins for matches. Jockeys have had a similar problem. Over the years, some of these athletes have engaged in fairly extreme methods to achieve short-term weight reduction, such as purging, taking diuretic drugs to lose water weight, and exercising in a heated environment or wearing nonporous clothing to maximize sweating. The entire list of weight-control drugs mentioned in Chapters 6 and 12 have been used as well, ranging from amphetamine to ephedrine to caffeine.

Increasingly, bodybuilders are seeking the look of someone who is both strong and lean, with lots of muscle definition. That appearance is referred to as looking "cut," probably derived from the idea of cutting weight or cutting fat, but perhaps also carrying the connotation of "sculpted." A more extreme version of looking

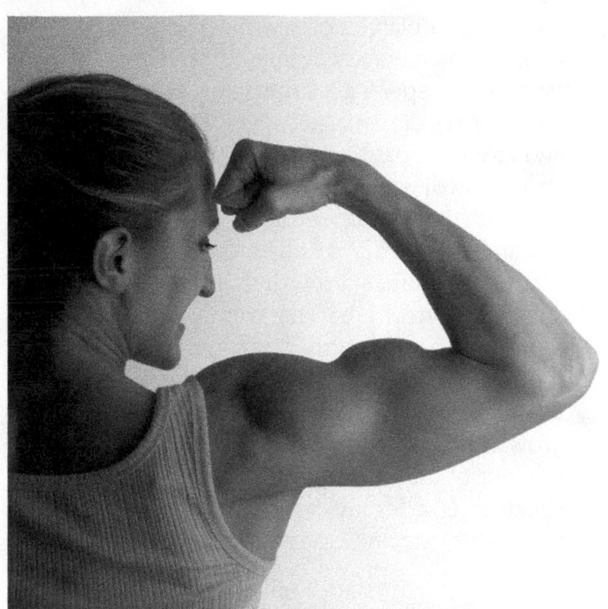

Bodybuilders and other athletes have used steroids or other supplements to develop a lean, strong, muscular body—to become "cut" or "ripped."

cut is looking "ripped," or sometimes "shredded." These are the men and women whose every muscle fibre and vein can be seen through the skin, perhaps with a body fat percentage down to an unhealthy 6%–9% (14%–20% is considered ideal for a healthy male). They also are using drugs and NHPs to help achieve this appearance. Steroids increase muscle mass, but they don't produce this kind of lean definition. A brisk market has developed in products containing the word *ripped* in their name, such as Ripped Fuel and Ripped Fast. For many years these products relied mainly on ephedra, a natural source of the alkaloids ephedrine and pseudoephedrine, as the main active ingredient. In 2002 the Canadian government restricted the amount of ephedra allowed in OTC products and NHPs, significantly reducing the ability of *ripped* products to promote weight loss. However, these profitable products did not go away; their manufacturers simply changed their formulas and kept making the same claims about being "fat burners" and promising incredible results. They contain a bewildering variety of plant extracts, many of which contain caffeine in unknown amounts (e.g., guarana extract, green tea extract, and coffee bean extract).

Remember that these substances are listed as non-medicinal ingredients and do not have to be demonstrated to be effective. If an included ingredient should turn out to be dangerous, it might take a long time for this to come to the attention of Health Canada, and it would then take a long time for the agency to build a case to remove the ingredient from the market. No such product has ever been shown to actually be a "fat burner," so it's unlikely that these are either. If you buy them, the closest you'll get to being "ripped" as a result is probably feeling "ripped off" when the magic pill doesn't deliver what you hoped.

Summary

- Performance-enhancing drugs have been used by athletes throughout history. The early Greek Olympians used various herbs and mushrooms as stimulants. Aztec athletes used a cactus-based stimulant resembling strychnine.
- During the 1800s and early 1900s, strychnine, cocaine, and caffeine were used as stimulants by athletes, including swimmers, cyclists, boxers, runners, and other athletes. Some evidence indicates the occasional use of strychnine continued at the level of world competition into the 1960s.
- Amphetamines began to be used as stimulants in the 1930s. In the 1940s and 1950s, there were reports of the use of these pep pills by professional soccer players, boxers, and cyclists. Use later spread to professional football.
- Use of stimulants by athletes continued and reached those at the Olympic level in the 1950s. By the time of the 1960 Rome games, amphetamine use had spread around the world and to most sports, amateur and professional.
- Testosterone and other steroids began to be used, particularly by bodybuilders and weightlifters.
- Some sports, especially cycling, began to test competitors for drugs on a sporadic basis. Throughout the 1960s, some athletes refused to submit to tests or failed tests and were disqualified.
- The International Olympic Committee in 1968 established rules requiring the disqualification of any competitor who refuses to take a drug test or who is found guilty of using banned drugs. Beginning with fewer than 700 urine tests at the 1968 Mexico City Olympics, each subsequent international competition has had more testing, more disqualifications, and more controversy.

- Steroids were not officially banned or tested for in international competition until the early 1970s, mainly because a sensitive urine test was not available until then.
- Today, recognition of the dangers associated with the use of many such substances has led to the creation of strict regulations prohibiting their use in sports.
- Drug testing of athletes in professional sports developed, in part, because of public revelations of widespread drug use (e.g., cocaine) by athletes.
- Because of both the expense and the inconvenience, some have questioned the wisdom of trying to test every athlete for everything.
- Amphetamines and caffeine have both been shown to increase work output and to mask the effects of fatigue.
- Some athletes continue to use stimulants for training, despite the dangers of injury and overexertion. Anabolic steroids are capable of increasing muscle mass and probably strength, although it has been difficult to separate the psychological stimulant-like effect of these drugs from the physical effects on the muscles themselves.
- The steroid hormone testosterone produces both androgenic and anabolic actions on the human body. Androgenic actions promote the development of masculine characteristics, while anabolic actions lead to such changes as increased muscle mass and internal organ size.
- The popularity of anabolic steroids lies in their ability to increase body weight and muscle mass. Unfortunately use of anabolic steroids can also lead to the development of dangerous and sometimes irreversible side effects, such as heart disease, atherosclerosis, and balding.
- Research has shown that abuse of anabolic steroids may lead to extreme aggression, mood swings, paranoid jealousy, delusions, extreme irritability, and violence.
- Steroid use in young people may permanently stunt their growth. Men risk atrophy of the testes and breast enlargement, while women face masculinization, decreased breast size, increased facial hair, and deepening of the voice. All users are at risk of peliosis hepatitis, changes in blood lipids, and HIV or hepatitis if the drugs are injected using shared needles.
- It is difficult to do ethical and well-controlled research on the effects of steroids.
- Misuse of human growth hormone and related substances might be the next problem to arise. While human growth hormone can potentially increase the height and weight of an individual, its use in people with normal blood levels of human growth hormone may lead to the abnormal development of internal organs.
- Creatine is a legally available nutritional supplement that can increase strength but might slow distance runners because of resultant weight gain.

Review Questions

1. What was the first type of stimulant drug reported to be used by boxers and other athletes in the 1800s?
2. What was the first type of drug known to be widely used in international competition and that led to the first Olympic urine-testing programs?
3. When and in what country were the selective anabolic steroids first developed?
4. Do amphetamines and caffeine actually enhance athletic performance? If so, how much?
5. How was ephedrine used by athletes, and what happened to it?
6. What muscle effect do we know for certain that anabolic steroids can produce in healthy men?
7. What is meant by "roid rage," and what double-blind studies have been done on this phenomenon?
8. What specific effect of anabolic steroids might be of concern to young users? to females?
9. Why do "pituitary giants" often die at an early age?
10. How does creatine increase strength?

SECTION

7

CHAPTER 17

Preventing Substance Abuse

What kinds of prevention programs have been tested in schools, and which ones seem to be effective? What can families and communities do?

CHAPTER 18

Treating Substance Abuse and Dependence

What are the differences among the various approaches to treating alcohol, opioid, cocaine dependence, and others? How well do these programs work?

PREVENTION AND TREATMENT

This final section on prevention and treatment comes at the end of the book for a reason. Now that you're more familiar with the wide spectrum of substances that people can abuse, and also with the wide variety of forms of substance abuse and dependence, we are better able to talk about what we're trying to prevent and what we're trying to treat. Because many of the medication-based treatments depend on specific interactions with the targeted substances of abuse, you now should understand how those medications have been developed and used.

CHAPTER 17

PREVENTING SUBSTANCE ABUSE

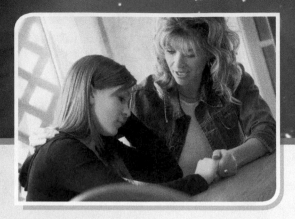

OBJECTIVES

When you have finished this chapter, you should be able to

- **LO1** Distinguish between education and propaganda programs based on their goals and approaches.
- **LO2** Describe two systems for classifying prevention programs: one based on stages of involvement, the other based on target populations defined by risk for drug use.
- **LO3** Explain why focusing prevention efforts on youth is essential to reducing substance abuse in later life.
- **LO4** Describe the historical shifts in substance abuse prevention programs from the knowledge-attitudes-behaviour model to affective education to antidrug norms.
- **LO5** Describe how Canada's current National Anti-Drug Strategy is failing to promote prevention-focused initiative.
- **LO6** Explain how the social influence model for smoking prevention led to the development of DARE and similar programs.
- **LO7** Give some examples of peer, family, and community approaches to prevention.

Why can't we *do* something to keep people from ruining their lives with drugs? As our society seeks to prevent drug abuse by limiting the availability of such drugs as heroin and cocaine, we are forced to recognize several other facts. First, as long as there is a sizable market for these substances, there will be people to supply them. Thus, only if we can teach people not to want the drugs can we attack the source of the problem. Second, these substances will never disappear, so we should try to teach people to live in a world that includes them. Third, our society has accepted the continued existence of tobacco and alcohol, yet some people are harmed by them. Can we help people to coexist with both legal and illegal substances and to live in such a way that their lives and health are not impaired by them?

According to the Canadian Centre on Substance Abuse, investment in evidence-based substance abuse prevention initiatives not only reduces the harm associated with substance abuse to individuals, families, and communities but also greatly reduces the cost of substance abuse and dependency to our society. Cost-benefit analysis across a variety of prevention programs has shown savings of $15 to $18 on every dollar spent on drug abuse prevention.[1,2] One youth substance abuse prevention program alone showed a cost-benefit ratio of 37:1.[3]

Despite a growing recognition of the social and economic benefits associated with evidence-based substance abuse prevention, Canada's investment continues to be limited. This is best exemplified in a recent informal audit of Canada's National Anti-Drug Strategy that determined funding for prevention-focused initiatives accounted for only 4% of strategy spending.[4]

LO1 Defining Goals and Evaluating Outcomes

Think about the process you are engaged in while reading and studying this book. The text is aimed at teaching its readers about drugs: their effects, how they are used, and how they relate to society. The goal of the authors is *education*. A person who understands all this information about all these drugs will perhaps be better prepared to make decisions about personal drug use, more able to understand drug use by others, and better prepared to participate in social decisions about drug use and abuse. We hope that a person who knows all this would be in a position to act more rationally, neither glorifying a drug and expecting miraculous changes from using it nor condemning it as the essence of evil. But our ultimate goal is not to change readers' behaviour in a particular direction. For example, the chapter on alcohol, although pointing out the dangers of its use and the problems it can cause, does not attempt to influence readers to avoid all alcohol use. The success of this book is measured by how much a person knows about alcohol, hallucinogens, marijuana, opioids, stimulants, and tobacco, not whether he or she is convinced never to use any of these substances.

Conversely, a tradition exists, going back to the "demon rum" programs of the late 1800s, of presenting negative information about alcohol and other drugs in the public schools with the clear goal of *prevention* of use. Some of these early programs presented information that was so clearly one-sided that they could have been classified as propaganda rather than education. We would not measure the success of such a program by how much objective information the students gained about the pharmacology of cocaine, for example. A more appropriate index might be how many of the students did subsequently experiment with the drugs against which the program was aimed. Until the early 1970s, it was simply assumed that these programs would have the desired effect, and few attempts were made to evaluate them.

LO2 Types of Prevention

The goals and methods of a prevention program also depend on the drug-using status of those served by the program. The programs designed to prevent young people from starting to smoke might be different from those used to try to prevent relapse in smokers who have quit, for example. Until recently, drug-abuse prevention programs have been classified according to a public health model:

- *Primary prevention* programs are those aimed mainly at young people who have not yet tried the substances in question or who may have tried tobacco or alcohol a few times. As discussed in the section "Defining Goals and Evaluating Outcomes,"

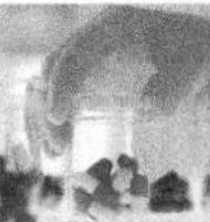

DRUGS IN THE MEDIA

To Be a Patsy or Not

A few years ago, prevention program advocates began running an advertisement campaign called "Don't be a Patsy." During these spots, Patsy, a mother of teenage children, confidently advises viewers on how to determine if their children are using drugs. In one advertisement, she clumsily demonstrates the "Patsy pat-down." As her daughter descends the stairs before leaving the house, Patsy asks for a hug with the supposedly hidden purpose of conducting a frisk search. Of course, the daughter looks bewildered by her mother's strange demonstration of affection. Nonetheless, Patsy looks into the camera and claims that this is an effective way to check your kids for drugs without their knowledge. Then, toward the end of the commercial, a voice-over announces, "Don't be a Patsy. Learn a better way at drugfree.org."

The Patsy spots were intended to get viewers' attention through humour and not to exaggerate the harms associated with drug use. This is quite a departure from previous prevention campaigns. Some may recall public service announcements in the late 1980s, "This is your brain on drugs." During the original spot, a man holds up an egg and says, "This is your brain." Then, he picks up a frying pan and says, "This is drugs." Then, he cracks open the egg, fries the contents, and says, "This is your brain on drugs." Finally, he asks, "Any questions?" While this is perhaps the most memorable anti-drug-use advertisement, it is frequently ridiculed because it overstates the potential harmful effects of drugs used by its target audience, namely young people. Indeed, a major concern of drug educators is that these types of embellishments decrease their credibility and may lead some young people to reject all drug-related information from so-called informed sources.

Perhaps the Patsy advertisements signal that the prevention advocates have learned to frame their drug use prevention message in more realistic terms. In this way, they decrease the likelihood of alienating their target audience. What do you think? Should drug prevention efforts exaggerate drug effects to discourage their use? Or should such efforts be more realistic, even if the positive effects of a drug outweigh the negative ones?

such programs might encourage abstinence from specific drugs or might have the broader goal of teaching people how to view drugs and the potential influences of drugs on their lives, emotions, and social relationships. Because those programs are presented to people who have little personal experience with drugs, they might be expected to be especially effective. But, there is the danger of introducing large numbers of children to information about drugs that they might otherwise never have heard of, thus arousing their curiosity.

- *Secondary prevention* programs can be thought of as designed for people who have tried the drug in question or a variety of other substances. The goals of such programs are usually the prevention of the use of other, more dangerous substances and the prevention of the development of more dangerous forms of use of the substances they are already experimenting with. We might describe the clientele here as more "sophisticated" substance users who have not suffered seriously from their drug experiences and who are not obvious candidates for treatment. Many postsecondary students fall into this category, and programs aimed at encouraging responsible use of alcohol among postsecondary students are good examples of this stage of prevention.
- *Tertiary prevention*, in our scheme, is relapse prevention, or follow-up programs. For alcohol- or heroin-dependent individuals, treatment programs are the first priority. However, once a person has been treated or has stopped the substance use without assistance, we enter another stage of prevention.

The Institute of Medicine has proposed a new classification of the continuum of care, which includes prevention, treatment, and maintenance.[5] Prevention efforts are categorized according to the intended target population, but the targets are not defined only by prior drug use:

- *Universal prevention* programs are designed for delivery to an entire population–for example, all schoolchildren or an entire community.
- *Selective prevention* strategies are designed for groups within the general population that are deemed to be at high risk–for example, students who are not doing well academically or the poorest neighbourhoods in a community.
- *Indicated prevention* strategies are targeted at individuals who show signs of developing problems, such as a child who began smoking cigarettes at a young age or an adult arrested for a first offence of driving under the influence of alcohol.

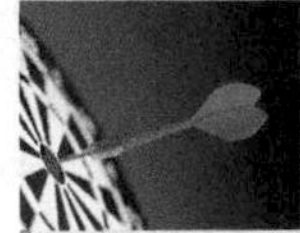

TARGETING PREVENTION

Preventing Inhalant Abuse

The abuse by children of spray paints and other products containing solvents appears to have increased somewhat in recent years (see Chapter 7). Several characteristics of this type of abuse make it an interesting problem for prevention workers. First, the variety of products and their ready availability in stores, the home, and even in schools make preventing access to the inhalants impossible. Second, most of the kids who use these substances probably know it's unhealthy and dangerous to do so, and further information of that sort may not add much in the way of preventing their use. Third, this use is very "faddish"—a group of students in grade 8 in one school might start inhaling cleaning fluid; a group of students in grade 6 in another neighbourhood might be into gold paint (in distinct preference to black, yellow, or white).

Given these characteristics, where does a school-based prevention education program begin to attack the problem? Does it focus on a particular product and try to talk kids out of using gold paint? Does it talk about a whole variety of products and thereby perhaps introduce the kids to new things they hadn't thought of? One videotape (*Inhalants: Kids in Danger, Adults in the Dark*) took the approach of attempting to inform parents and teachers of the varieties of paints, perfumes, solvents, and other spray products used by abusers and to inform them of some of the subterfuge used by some of the kids (carrying a small cologne vial to school, spraying paint into empty soft drink cans, etc.). However, this video is not meant to be shown to children, because it describes exactly what to do and how to do it. Probably the best idea in prevention classes is to reinforce to children in general terms the dangers of inhalants without describing a particular substance or method of use.

LO3, LO4, LO5, LO6

Prevention Programs in Schools

Why Invest in Young People?

Substantial changes occur during youth and early adulthood, including significant brain growth and development. As we recall from earlier chapters, while parts of the brain associated with impulsivity and motivation mature early, areas of the brain that moderate risk and reward typically mature later.[6,7,8,9] This delay means that young people can be more prone to risk-taking behaviour. Consider the fact that young people are also disproportionately more likely to use substances and to engage in risky patterns of use, and it should come as no surprise that reports of harm from use are very high.[10] In fact, the prevalence of reported harm due to their own drug use is four times higher among youth aged 15 to 24 years (5.5%) than adults aged 25 years and older (1.4%).[11]

As we have seen in previous chapters, in Canada:

- 57% of young people ages 15–24 have used drugs sometime in their life[12]
- The average age at which students grades 7–12 consumed their first alcoholic beverage was 13 years[13]
- The average age at which students grades 7–12 first used cannabis was 13.7 years[13]
- 49% of students grades 10–12 reported binge drinking in the past 12 months[13]
- 36% of university/college students reported binge drinking in the past two weeks[14]
- 32.6% of university students reported that, in the past 12 months, while drinking alcohol they did something they later regretted[14]
- 16.4% of university students reported that in the past 12 months while drinking alcohol they physically injured themselves[14]

Rates of recovery from substance dependency in adults are low, and for many afflicted by this disease harm reduction is the only option. This may reflect the fact that most substance dependent individuals developed brain pathways that caused their disease during their youth, when brain pathways were capable of change. In fact, the median age for developing substance dependence is 18 years. As adults, however, the ability to easily modify brain pathways is substantially diminished and therefore recovery from dependency is extremely difficult. Such hypotheses may be supported by recent neuroimaging studies which suggest that the development of healthy neuronal pathways may be circumvented by exposure to addictive substances,[6,7] leading to development of pathways that make substance dependency.[8,9] In Chapter 18 you will learn something about current approaches for the treatment of substance dependence; however, as alluded to above, for most adults dependency will remain a lifelong struggle. As such, the need for development, implementation, and evaluation of effective prevention programs, services, and policies is paramount. Despite this recognized need, funding toward prevention-focused initiatives accounted for only 4% of spending under Canada's National Anti-Drug Strategy.[4]

There are many approaches to prevention. In this chapter we concentrate on individual programs used in the primary prevention of substance abuse and dependency in youth, placing particular emphasis on school and family programs. However, our choice of focus should not detract from the importance of broader philosophies and approaches, including those of health promotion and population health.[15]

The Knowledge-Attitudes-Behaviour Model

After the increase in the use of illegal drugs by young middle-class people in the 1960s there was a general sense that society was not doing an adequate job of drug education, and most school systems increased their efforts. However, there was confusion over the methods to be used. Traditional antidrug programs had relied heavily on representatives of the local police, who went into schools and told a few horror stories, describing the legal trouble due anyone who got caught with illegal drugs. Sometimes the officers showed what the drugs looked like or demonstrated the smell of burning marijuana, so that the kids would know what to avoid. Sometimes, especially in larger cities, a former user described how easy it was to get "hooked," the horrible life of the junkie, and the horror of withdrawal symptoms. The 1960s saw more of that, plus the production of a large number of scary antidrug films.

Teachers and counsellors knew little about illegal drugs, and many teachers attended courses taught by experts. Some of the experts were enforcement-oriented and presented the traditional scare-tactics information, whereas others were pharmacologists who presented the "dry facts" about the classification and effects of various drugs. The teachers then brought many of these facts into their classrooms. It was later pointed out that the programs of this era were based on an assumed model: that providing information about drugs would increase the students' *knowledge* of drugs and their effects, that this increased knowledge would lead to changes in *attitudes* about drug use, and that these changed attitudes would be reflected in decreased drug-using *behaviour*.[16]

In the early 1970s, this model began to be questioned. A 1971 study indicated that students who had more knowledge about drugs tended to have a more positive attitude toward drug use.[17] Of course, it may have been that pro-drug students were more interested in learning about drugs, so this was not an actual assessment of the value of drug education programs. A 1973 report by the same group indicated that four different types of drug education programs were equally effective in producing increased knowledge about drugs and equally ineffective in altering attitudes or behaviour.[18] Nationwide, drug use had increased even with the greater emphasis on drug education. Concern arose about the possibility that drug education may even have contributed to increased drug use. Before the 1960s, the use of marijuana and LSD was rare among school-age youngsters. Most of them didn't know much about these things, had given them little thought, and had probably never considered using them. Telling them over and over not to use drugs was a bit like telling a young boy not to put beans in his nose. He probably hadn't thought of it before, and your warning gives him the idea. These concerns led many governments to stop supporting the production of drug-abuse films and educational materials until it could determine what kinds of approaches would be effective.

The question of effectiveness depended greatly on the goals of the program. Did we want all students *never to experiment* with cigarettes, alcohol, marijuana, or other drugs? Or did we want students to be prepared *to make rational decisions* about drugs? For example, a 1976 report indicated that students in drug education programs did increase their use of drugs over the two years after the program, but they were less likely to show drastic escalation of the amount or type of drug use over that period when compared with a control group.[19] Perhaps by giving the students information about drugs, we make them more likely to try them, but we also make them more aware of the dangers of excessive use. For a time in the 1970s, it seemed as though teaching students to make rational decisions about their own drug use with the goal of reducing the overall harm produced by misuse and abuse could be a possible goal of prevention programs.

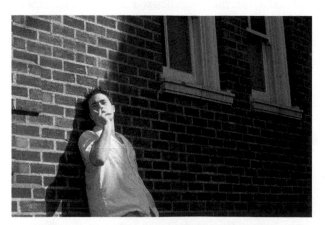

Helping young people learn to deal with emotions in healthy ways and giving them successful experiences may reduce their rates of smoking, drinking, and drug use.

Affective Education

Educators have been talking for several years about education as including both a "cognitive domain" and an "affective domain," the domain of emotions and attitudes. One reason that young people might use psychoactive drugs is to produce certain feelings: of excitement, of relaxation, of power, of being in control. Or perhaps a child might not really want to take drugs but does so after being influenced by others. Helping children know their own feelings and express them, helping them achieve altered emotional states without drugs, and teaching them to feel valued, accepted, and wanted are all presumed to be ways of reducing drug use.

Values Clarification The values clarification approach makes the assumption that what is lacking in drug-using adolescents is not factual information about drugs but, rather, the ability to make appropriate decisions based on that information.[20] Perhaps drug use should not be "flagged" for the students by having special curricula designed just for drugs but, instead, emphasis should be placed on teaching generic decision-making skills. Teaching students to analyze and clarify their own values in life is accomplished by having them discuss their reactions to various situations that pose moral and ethical dilemmas. Groups of parents or other citizens who are concerned about drug abuse sometimes have great difficulty understanding and accepting these approaches because they do not take a direct antidrug approach. In the 1970s, when these programs were developed, it seemed important that the schools not try to impose a particular set of values but, rather, allow for differences in religion, family background, and so on. For this reason, the programs were often said to be *value free*.

To many parents, the purpose of **values clarification** training is not immediately clear, and teaching young children to decide moral issues for themselves may run contrary to the particular set of values the parents want their children to learn. The Canadian Home and School Federation supports the application of formal values clarification programs in all Canadian schools. It has recommended that such programs be developed, in consultation with parents, and as teachers become available who are qualified in values clarification techniques.[21]

Alternatives to Drugs Along with values clarification, another aspect of affective education involves the teaching of **alternatives** to drug use. Under the assumption that students might take drugs for the experience, for the altered states of consciousness that a drug might produce, students are taught about so-called natural highs, or altered states, that can be produced through relaxation exercises, meditation, vigorous exercise, or an exciting sport. Students are encouraged to try these things and to focus on the psychological changes that occur. These alternatives should be discussed with some degree of sensitivity to the audience; for example, it would make little sense to suggest to many inner-city 13-year-olds that expensive activities such as scuba diving and downhill skiing would be good alternatives to drugs.

Personal and Social Skills Several studies indicate that adolescents who smoke, drink, or use marijuana also get lower grades and are less involved in organized sports or school clubs. One view of this is that students might take up substance use in response to personal or social failure. Therefore, teaching students how to communicate with others and giving them success experiences is another component of affective education approaches. For example, one exercise that has been used is having the students operate a school store. This is done as a group effort with frequent group meetings. The involved students are expected to develop a sense of social and personal competence without using drugs. Another approach is to have older students tutor younger students, which is designed to give the older students a sense of competence. An

values clarification: teaching students to recognize and express their own feelings and beliefs.

alternatives: alternative nondrug activities, such as relaxation exercises or dancing.

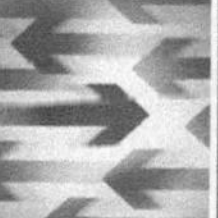

TAKING SIDES

Are "Alternatives to Drugs" Really Alternatives?

As one part of many drug education programs, students are taught that they can produce natural highs—that is, altered states of consciousness similar to those produced by drugs, but without using drugs.

One such alternative that has been mentioned in these programs is skydiving. Obviously an activity of that sort has all the glamour, danger, and excitement most of us would want. Maybe if the kids could do this whenever they wanted, they wouldn't want to try cocaine or marijuana. But let's examine this as an alternative for a bunch of junior high school kids. First, there's the matter of cost and availability. How realistic is it to think that most of these kids would have access to skydiving? Second, there's the issue of convenience. Even if you were a rich kid, with your own airplane, parachute, and pilot, it's unlikely that you'd be able to go skydiving every afternoon after school. Drugs and alcohol may not provide the best highs in the world, but often they are easy to get and use, compared with such activities as skydiving.

Maybe skydiving isn't a *practical* alternative to drugs for many people. Still, it seems more wholesome and desirable. Let's become social philosophers and ask ourselves why the image of a person skydiving is more positive than the image of a person snorting cocaine. After all, skydiving doesn't make any obvious contributions to society. Let's play devil's advocate and propose that skydiving is not preferable to taking cocaine. Either way, the person is engaged in dangerous, expensive, self-indulgent activity. Contrast skydiving with cocaine, and see if you can answer for yourself why skydiving has a more positive image than cocaine use. You may have to talk about this with several people before you get a consistent feeling for why our society respects one of these activities so much more than the other. What about skiing? bungee jumping?

experiment carried out in Napa, California, combined these approaches with a drug education course, small-group discussions led by teachers, and classroom management techniques designed to teach discipline and communication skills and to enhance the students' self-concepts.[22] Although a small effect on alcohol, marijuana, and cigarette use was found among the girls, the effects were gone by the one-year follow-up.

Antidrug Norms

A 1984 review of prevention studies concluded the following:

> (1) Most substance abuse prevention programs have not contained adequate evaluation components; (2) increased knowledge has virtually no impact on substance abuse or on intentions to smoke, drink, or use drugs; (3) affective education approaches appear to be experiential in their orientation and to place too little emphasis on the acquisition of skills necessary to increase personal and social competence, particularly those skills needed to enable students to resist the various interpersonal pressures to begin using drugs; and (4) few studies have demonstrated any degree of success in terms of actual substance abuse prevention.[23]

This last point is not entirely a criticism of the programs themselves but reflects the difficulty of demonstrating statistically significant changes in behaviour over time after the programs.

Refusal Skills In response to the third point, that affective education approaches were too general and experiential, the next efforts at preventing drug use focused on teaching students to recognize peer pressure to use drugs and on teaching specific ways to respond to such pressures without using drugs. This is sometimes referred to as psychological inoculation. In addition to the focus on substance use, "refusal skills" and "pressure resistance" strategies are taught in a broader context of self-assertion and social skills training. The first successful application of this technique was a film in which young actors acted out situations in which one person was being pressured to smoke cigarettes. The film then demonstrated effective ways of responding to the pressure gracefully without smoking. After the film, students discuss alternative strategies and practise the coping techniques presented in the film. This approach has been demonstrated to be successful in reducing cigarette smoking in adolescent populations. It has been adapted for use with groups of various ages and for a wider variety of drugs and other behaviours.

National Anti-Drug Strategy Canada's approach to prevention is directed through the National Anti-Drug Strategy, which was launched October 2007. The Strategy is a collaborative effort among Health Canada, the Department of Justice, and Public Safety Canada. It includes three action plans: preventing illegal drug use, treating those with illegal drug dependencies, and combating the production and distribution of illegal drugs.[24] As part of the prevention plan, Health Canada has developed a campaign, called DrugsNot4Me, aimed at equipping young people (ages 15–24) with coping and refusal skills to support their decision not to experiment with illegal drugs. In addition to an interactive and informative Web site, not4me.ca, the campaign includes television and movie theatre commercials; advertisements in buses, trains, subways, and shopping malls across Canada; and Internet banners on Web sites popular with teens. The DrugsNot4Me commercials entitled "Fast Forward" and "Mirror" aim to make youth consider the stark reality of experimenting with drugs and to recognize that addiction can happen to anyone—even them. The commercials lead viewers to the DrugsNot4Me Web site, where they are given an opportunity to learn more about the effects of drugs and how to say no. The effectiveness of this program in achieving its prescribed outcomes is yet to be evaluated.

Drug-Free Schools In the 1980s the U.S. federal government created a program to support "drug-free schools and communities." Among other things, the government provided millions of dollars' worth of direct aid to local school districts to implement or enhance drug-prevention activities. Along with this, the Department of Education produced a small book called *What Works: Schools Without Drugs*,[25] which made specific recommendations for schools to follow. This book did not recommend a specific curriculum; its most significant feature was the emphasis on factors other than curriculum, such as school policies on drug and alcohol use. It suggested policies regarding locker searches, suspension, and expulsion of students. The purpose was not so much to take a punitive approach to alcohol or drug use as to point out through example and official policy that the school and community were opposed to drug and alcohol use by minors. Following this general drug-free lead, schools adopted "tobacco-free" policies, stating that not only the students but also teachers and other staff people were not to use tobacco products at school or on school-sponsored trips or activities.

According to this approach, the curriculum should include teaching about the laws against drugs and about school policies. In other words, as opposed to the

1970s values clarification approach of teaching students how to make responsible decisions for themselves, this approach wants to make it clear to the students that the society at large, the community in which they live, and the school in which they study have already made the decision not to condone drug use or underage alcohol use. This seems to be part of a more general educational trend away from "value-free" schools toward teaching values that are generally accepted in our society. For schools to be eligible for federal U.S. Drug-Free Schools funding, they must certify that their program teaches that "illicit drug use is wrong and harmful."

Development of the Social Influence Model

Some of the most sophisticated prevention research in recent years has been focused directly on cigarette smoking in adolescents. This problem has two major advantages over other types of drug use, as far as prevention research is concerned. First, a large enough fraction of adolescents do smoke cigarettes so that measurable behaviour change is possible in a group of reasonable size. In contrast, we would have to perform an intervention with tens of thousands of people before significant alterations in the proportion of heroin users would be statistically evident. Second, the health consequences of smoking are so clear with respect to cancer and heart disease that there is a fairly good consensus over goals: We'd like to prevent adolescents from becoming smokers. One research advantage is the relatively simple verification available for self-reported use of tobacco: Saliva samples can be measured for cotinine, a nicotine metabolite.

Virtually all the various approaches to drug-abuse prevention have been tried with smoking behaviour; in fact, Evans's 1976 smoking prevention paper introduced the use of the psychological inoculation approach based on the **social influence model**.[26] Out of all this research, certain consistencies appear. The most important of these is that it *is* possible to design smoking prevention programs that are effective in reducing the number of adolescents who begin smoking. Some practical lessons about the components of those programs have also emerged.[27] For example, presenting information about the delayed consequences of smoking (possible lung cancer many years later) is relatively ineffective. Information about the immediate physiological effects (increased heart rate, shortness of breath) is included instead. Some of the most important key elements that were shown to be effective were the following:

- *Training refusal skills* (for example, eight ways to say no). This was originally based on films demonstrating the kinds of social pressures that peers might use to encourage smoking and modelling a variety of appropriate responses. Then the students engage in role-playing exercises in which they practise these refusal skills. By using such techniques as changing the subject or having a good excuse handy, students learn to refuse to "cooperate" without being negative. When all else fails, however, they are taught to be assertive and insist on their right to refuse.
- *Public commitment*. Researchers found that having each child stand before his or her peers and promise not to start smoking and sign a pledge not to smoke are effective prevention techniques.
- *Countering advertising*. Students are shown examples of cigarette advertising, and then the "hidden messages" are discussed (young, attractive, healthy, active models are typically used; cigarette smoking might be associated with dating or with sports). Then the logical inconsistencies between these hidden messages and the actual effects of cigarette smoking (e.g., bad breath, yellow teeth, shortness of breath) are pointed out. The purpose of this is to "inoculate" the children against cigarette advertising by teaching them to question its messages.
- *Normative education*. Adolescents tend to overestimate the proportion of their peers who smoke. Presenting factual information about the smoking practices of adolescents provides students with a more realistic picture of the true social norms regarding smoking and reduces the "everybody is doing it" attitude. When possible, statistics on smoking from the specific school or community should be used in presenting this information.
- *Use of teen leaders*. Presenting dry facts about the actual proportion of smokers should ideally be reinforced by example. If you're presenting the program to junior high students, it's one thing to *say* that fewer than one-fifth of the high school students in that community smoke, but it's another to bring a few high school students into the room and have them discuss the fact that neither they nor their friends smoke, their attitudes about smokers, and ways they have dealt with others' attempts to get them to smoke.

social influence model: a prevention model adopted from successful smoking programs.

Possible improvements to those approaches are offered by the *cognitive developmental* approach to smoking behaviour. McCarthy criticized the social influence or social skills training model for assuming that all students should be taught social skills or refusal skills without regard to whether they need such training.[28] The model "is that of a defenceless teenager who, for lack of general social skills or refusal skills, passively accedes to social pressures to smoke." Alternative models have been proposed in which the individual makes active, conscious decisions in preparation for trying cigarettes or trying smoking and becoming an occasional or regular user. The decision-making processes, and thus the appropriate prevention strategy, might be different at each of these "stages of cognitive development" as a smoker. Furthermore, smokers who begin smoking very young behave differently from smokers who begin as older adolescents (e.g., those who start young show more unanimity in selecting the most popular brand). Unfortunately, adolescents continue to initiate smoking, and the risk and protective factors reviewed in Chapter 1 have more influence on smoking behaviour (and on alcohol and other drug use) than any information or education programs yet devised.[29]

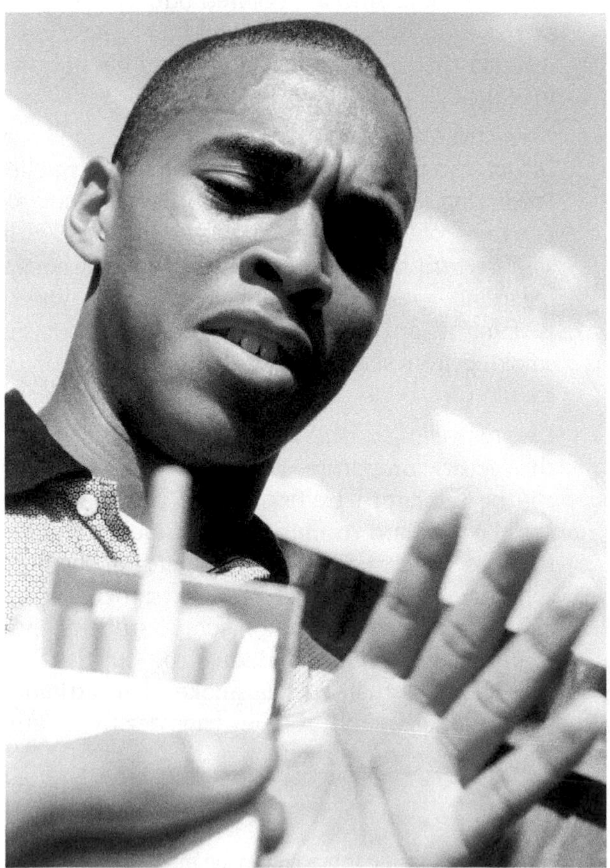

Training in refusal skills, including role-playing exercises, is a key component of the social influence model.

Prevention Programs That Work

Current research indicates that prevention strategies that employ multifaceted approaches are the most effective (i.e., strategies in which media messages are delivered in tandem with prevention programs in schools, communities, and families, sustained over time).[30] In 2010 the Canadian Centre on Substance Abuse released the *Portfolio of Canadian Standards for Youth Substance Abuse Prevention*. This document was constructed to guide schools, communities, and families in the prevention and reduction of illegal drug use by Canadian youth ages 10–24.[30] The *Portfolio* comprises standards for prevention in schools (Building on Our Strengths) and communities (Stronger Together), along with guidelines for families (Strengthening Our Skills). This resource addresses everyday environments and provides teams with step-by-step guidance, based on the best available evidence, for the planning, implementation, and evaluation of their prevention efforts. The portfolio is funded through Canada's National Anti-Drug Strategy.

Today many evidence-based approaches to drug prevention have been developed. These programs can, if contextualized and delivered judiciously, significantly impact youth substance abuse and dependency and contribute to the improved overall health and well-being of young people.[30] In the sections that follow we will consider a few of the programs currently employed by some Canadian schools, families, and communities. As you read the following stories we encourage you to reflect on the programs you have participated in. Did you find them effective? Were they based on evidence?

School-Based Prevention Programs

Most programs for the prevention of illegal drug use are school-based. Schools are considered an appropriate setting for drug use prevention programs. Reasons for this include the following:

- As we have seen repeatedly throughout this text, illicit drug use is highly prevalent before adulthood.[31] Therefore, prevention programs for substance use must focus on school-age children and adolescents, before their beliefs and expectations about substance use are established.

- School systems theoretically provide a systematic and efficient way for reaching the majority of young persons, every year.
- Schools are generally well equipped for adopting and enforcing a broad spectrum of educational programs.[32]

Many school-based drug-use prevention programs have been modelled after the successful social influence model. Some of these programs have been evaluated for their effectiveness in reducing the incidence of first-time use, the frequency and amount of illegal drug use, and the prevalence of use among youth. Others have been evaluated for their ability to deliver knowledge or promote change in attitudes and behaviours. Some studies have demonstrated beneficial effects of these programs; others have not.[32,33,34,35,36] It should be noted that the vast majority of peer-reviewed programs used in Canada were developed in Europe and the United States and are therefore influenced by social context and drug policies of those jurisdictions. Recent systematic reviews are demonstrating that school-based prevention programs that are evidence-based, targeted, interactive, youth-focused, and engaging can have success in reducing drug abuse.

Project ALERT

Project ALERT was first tested in 30 junior high schools in California and Oregon.[37] The program targeted cigarette smoking, alcohol use, and marijuana use. Before the program, each student was surveyed and classified as a nonuser, an experimenter, or a user for each of the three substances. The curriculum was taught either by health educators or by educators with the assistance of trained teen leaders. Control schools simply continued whatever health or drug curriculum they had been using. The program was delivered in grade 7, and follow-up surveys were done 3, 12, and 15 months later. Three "booster" lessons were given in grade 8.

The program surprisingly had no measurable effect on initiation of smoking by nonusers. However, those who were cigarette experimenters before the program began were more likely to quit or to maintain low rates of smoking than the control group. The group with teen leader support showed the largest reduction: 50% fewer students were weekly smokers at the 15 month follow-up.

The experimental groups drank less alcohol soon after the program was presented, for previous alcohol nonusers, experimenters, and users. However, this

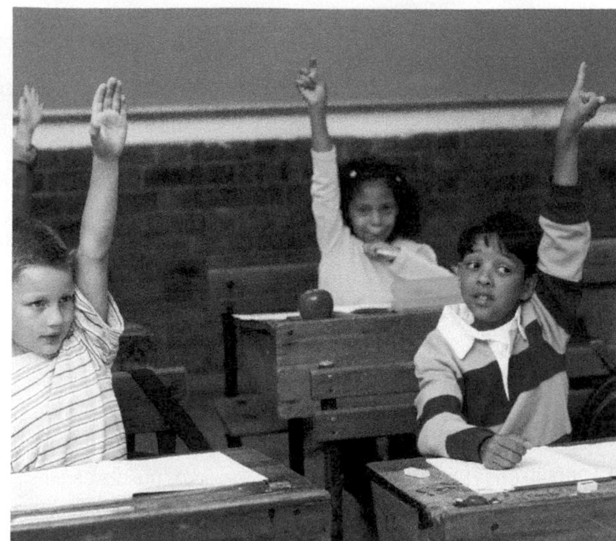

Some school-based drug-use prevention programs have been shown to reduce initiation and levels of drug use; others have not.

effect diminished over time and disappeared by the end of the study.

The most consistent results were in reducing initiation of marijuana smoking and reducing levels of marijuana smoking. For example, among those who were not marijuana users at the beginning, about 12% of the control-group students had begun using marijuana by the 15 month follow-up. In the treatment groups, only 8% began using during that time, representing a one-third decrease in initiation to marijuana use.

Drug Abuse Resistance Education (DARE)

Perhaps the most substantive educational phenomenon in a long time had fairly modest beginnings in 1983 as a joint project of the Los Angeles police department and school district. Those who are familiar with the Drug Abuse Resistance Education (**DARE**) program will have recognized its components described under the social influence model of smoking cessation. The difference here is that the educational program with DARE is delivered by police officers, originally in grade 5 and grade 6 classrooms. By basing the curriculum on sound educational research, by maintaining strict training standards for the officers who present the curriculum, and by encouraging the classroom teacher

DARE: Drug Abuse Resistance Education, the most popular prevention program in schools.

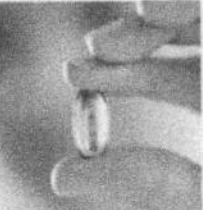

DRUGS IN DEPTH

Effective Prevention Programs

Canada does not have a program for the routine evaluation and publication of exemplary prevention programs for youth. The most recent comprehensive review of Canadian and international programs, *Preventing Substance Use Problems Among Young People: A Compendium of Best Practices,* was published in 2001.[38] However, the Center for Substance Abuse Prevention, a branch of the Substance Abuse and Mental Health Services Administration (SAMHSA) in the U.S. Department of Health and Human Services, maintains an ongoing program for the evaluation of research on effective prevention programs. It has developed a National Registry of Evidence-Based Programs and Practices (NREPP). Some of the programs on this partial list are described within this chapter, and more information on the others can be obtained from the SAMHSA Web site. As new programs are approved, they are added to the registry, so for the most current list, check on the Web.[39]

Model Programs

- Across Ages
- Athletes Training and Learning to Avoid Steroids (ATLAS)
- Communities Mobilizing for Change on Alcohol
- Creating Lasting Family Connections
- Dare to Be You
- Families and Schools Together
- Keep a Clear Mind
- Life Skills Training
- Project ALERT
- Project Northland
- Project Towards No Tobacco Use
- Reconnecting Youth
- Residential Student Assistance Program
- Safe Dates
- SMART Team
- Strengthening Families Program
- Too Good for Drugs
- Brief Intervention for College Students (BASICS)
- Good Behavior Game
- Unplugged

to participate, some of the old barriers to having nonteachers responsible for curriculum were overcome. The officers are in uniform, and they use interactive techniques as described for the social influence model. Most of the components are there: refusal skills, teen leaders, and a public commitment not to use illegal drugs. In addition, some of the affective education components are included: self-esteem building, alternatives to drug use, and decision making. The component on consequences of drug abuse is, no doubt, enhanced by the presence of a uniformed officer who can serve as an information source and symbol for concerns over gang activity and violence and can discuss arrest and incarceration. The 17-week program is capped by a commencement assembly at which certificates are awarded.

This program happened to be in place at just the right time, both financially and politically. With the assistance of drug-free schools money and with nationwide enthusiasm for new drug-prevention activities in the 1980s, the program spread rapidly across the United States. By the early 1990s DARE programs were found in every state and all Canadian provinces, except Quebec. Currently, there are approximately 75 000 students being taught the DARE program in 1600 Canadian schools by 855 active DARE Officers.[40]

This program was accepted quickly by many schools, and endorsed enthusiastically by educators, students, parents, and police participants, even though its effectiveness in preventing drug use was not evaluated extensively until 1994.

In 1994, two important, large-scale studies of the effects of DARE were reported. One was based on a longitudinal study in rural, suburban, and urban schools in Illinois, comparing students exposed to DARE with students who were not.[41] Although the program had some effects on reported self-esteem, there was no evidence for long-term reductions in self-reported use of drugs. The other report was based on a review of eight smaller outcome evaluations of DARE, selected from 18 evaluations based on whether the reports had a control group, a pretest-posttest design, and reliable outcome measures.[42] The overall impact of these eight programs was to increase drug

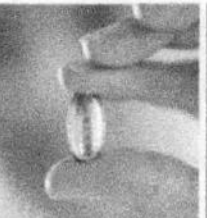

DRUGS IN DEPTH

How Much Do You Know about DARE?

1. Many Canadians have heard of DARE. What do the letters stand for?
2. One component of DARE is practising how to refuse using drugs. Do you know the origin of DARE's eight ways to say no?
3. DARE has been implemented in more schools than any other substance-abuse prevention program. Does research on its effectiveness show that it's one of the best at preventing drug abuse?
4. Besides school-based programs, what other kinds of substance-abuse prevention programs have been developed?
5. The Institute of Medicine has a relatively new way of categorizing prevention programs into various types. Do you know what factor is used to differentiate among the types?

Answers

1. Drug Abuse Resistance Education
2. This and most components of DARE were adopted from smoking prevention programs developed in the 1970s.
3. Research on the effectiveness of DARE has not demonstrated a strong impact on preventing drug use. Other programs described in this chapter appear to be more effective.
4. Parent, family, and community programs and public media campaigns have also been developed to prevent drug abuse.
5. The target population (the entire population, at-risk populations and individuals with early signs of problems) is the factor used.

knowledge and knowledge about social skills, but the effects on drug use were marginal at best. There was a very small but statistically significant reduction of tobacco use and no reliable effect on alcohol or marijuana use.

A more recent review of 20 studies on DARE published in peer-reviewed journals found an average effect size that was small and not statistically significant.[43] The repeated failures to demonstrate a significant impact of the DARE program on drug use remain a dilemma in light of its widespread popularity. Communities have not abandoned the program. Instead, the DARE organization has developed additional programs, including DARE 1 PLUS (Play and Learn Under Supervision) as an extension to the elementary program, and curriculum for middle school and high school DARE programs designed to follow up with these older adolescents. We cannot yet evaluate the effectiveness of these additional programs.

Project Life Skills Training

Another program, the Life Skills Training program, has been subjected to several tests and has shown long-term positive results.[44] This three-year program is based on the social influence model and teaches resistance skills, normative education, and media influences. Self-management skills and general social skills are also included. One study of this program found significantly lower use of marijuana, alcohol, and tobacco after six years. A subsequent application of this program among ethnic minority youth (Latino and African American) in New York City found reduced use on a two-year follow-up.[45]

LO7 Programs That Target Peers, Parents, and the Community

Our country's schools are clearly the most convenient conduit for attempts to achieve widespread social changes among young people, and that is why most efforts at drug-abuse prevention have been carried out there. However, peers, parents, and the community at large also exert powerful social influences on young people. Because these groups are less accessible than the schools, fewer prevention programs have been based on using parent and community influences. Nevertheless, important efforts have been made in all these areas.[46,47,48,49,50]

Peer Programs

Most peer programs have occurred in the school setting, but some have used youth-oriented community service programs (such as YMCA, YWCA, and recreation centres) or have focused on street youth by using them in group community service projects.

- *Peer influence* approaches start with the assumption that the opinions of an adolescent's peers are significant influences on the adolescent's behaviour. Often using an adult group facilitator or coordinator, the program's emphasis is on open discussion among a group of children or adolescents. These discussions might focus on drugs, with the peer group discussing dangers and alternatives, or they might simply have the more general goal of building positive group cohesiveness, a sense of belonging, and communication skills.
- *Peer participation* programs often focus on groups of youth in high-risk areas. The idea here is that young people participate in making important decisions and in doing significant work, either as "peers" with cooperating adults or in programs managed almost entirely by the youth themselves. Sometimes participants are paid for community service work, in other cases they engage in money-making businesses, and sometimes they provide youth-oriented information services. These groups almost never focus on drug use in any significant way; rather, the idea is to help people become participating members of society.

The benefits of these "extracurricular" peer approaches are measurable in terms of acquired skills, improved academic success, higher self-esteem, and a more positive attitude toward peers and school. As to whether they alter drug use significantly, the data either are not available or are inconclusive for the most part.

Parent and Family Programs

The various programs that have worked with parents have taken at least one of four approaches.[51] Most of the programs include more than one of these approaches.

- *Informational* programs provide parents with basic information about alcohol and drugs, as well as information about their use and effects. Although the parents often want to know simply what to look for, how to tell if their child is using drugs, and what the consequences of drug abuse are, the best programs provide additional information. One important piece of information is the actual extent of the use of various types of drugs among young people. Another goal might be to make parents aware of their own alcohol and drug use to gain a broader perspective of the issue. A basic rationale is that well-informed parents will be able to teach appropriate attitudes about drugs, beginning when their child is young, and will be better able to recognize potential problems relating to drug or alcohol use.
- *Parenting skills* might be taught through practical training programs. Communication with children, decision-making skills, how to set goals and limits, and when and how to say no to your child can be learned in the abstract and then practised in role-playing exercises. One risk factor for adolescent drug and alcohol use is poor family relationships, and improving family interaction and strengthening communication can help prevent alcohol and drug abuse.
- *Parent support groups* can be important adjuncts to skills training or in planning community efforts. Groups of parents meet regularly to discuss problem solving, parenting skills, their perceptions of the problem, actions to be taken, and so on.
- *Family interaction* approaches call for families to work as a unit to examine, discuss, and confront issues relating to alcohol and drug use. Other exercises might include more general problem solving or response to emergencies. Not only do these programs attempt to improve family communication, but they also place parents in the roles of teacher of drug facts and coordinator of family action, thus strengthening their knowledge and skills.

Strengthening Families for the Future

One selective prevention program, called Strengthening Families for the Future (SFF), targets elementary school children (between the ages of 7 and 11) and their parents who may be at risk for substance abuse, depression, violence, delinquency, and school failure. The children's risks of these problems may be due in part to their parents' substance use or mental health problems.[52] This program has been successfully implemented several times within diverse populations. It has three major goals: improving parenting skills, increasing children's skills (such as communication skills, refusal

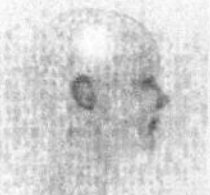

MIND/BODY CONNECTION

Integrating Treatment and Prevention with Pregnancy Services

Does your community provide needed services and compassionate support for pregnant women who use alcohol and drugs? An emerging consensus views alcohol, tobacco, and other drug use during pregnancy as a community problem. During this period when women anticipate major life change, prevention initiatives can enhance their motivation to have a healthy baby. And for women with substance-abuse problems, pregnancy provides a similarly strong motivation to seek help.

Fear of blame, legal intervention, and loss of child custody prevent many women from getting help. To counteract these barriers to services, prevention initiatives should promote services that are safe and confidential. Services should be not only physically accessible but also culturally accessible. Efforts that recognize the importance of relationships to women can call on the support of family members and others for alcohol-free and other drug-free pregnancies. Prevention strategies that combine information with options for change have shown promising results in reducing drug use during pregnancy.

Find out if women in your area have access to an integrated system of alcohol, tobacco, and other drug treatment and maternal and child health care.

skills, awareness of feelings, and emotion expression skills), and improving family relationships (decreasing conflict, improving communication, increasing parent-child time together, and increasing the planning and organizational skills of the family). Children and parents attend evening sessions weekly for 14 weeks to learn and practise these skills. Evaluations of this program indicate that it reduces tobacco and alcohol use in the children and reduces substance abuse and other problems in the parents.[51,53] SFF can also serve as a primary prevention for families.

Community Programs

Two basic reasons exist for organizing prevention programs at the community level. The first is that a coordinated approach using schools, parent and peer groups, civic organizations, police, newspapers, radio, and television can have a much greater impact than an isolated program that occurs only in the school, for example. Another reason is that drug-abuse prevention and drug education are controversial and emotional topics. Parents might question the need for or the methods used in drug education programs in the schools. Jealousy and mistrust about approaches can separate schools, police, church, and parent groups. A program that starts by involving all these groups in the planning stages is more likely to receive widespread community support. Clearly, the spread of the DARE program in the schools is based partly on the fact that it demonstrates and encourages cooperation between the police and the schools, and encourages parental involvement.

Community-based programs can bring other resources to bear. For example, the city council and local businesses can be involved in sponsoring alcohol-free parties, developing recreational facilities, and arranging field trips so that when the school-based program talks about alternatives, the alternatives are available. The media can be enlisted not only to publicize public meetings and programs but also to present drug- and alcohol-related information that reinforces what is learned in the other programs.

Communities Mobilizing for Change on Alcohol is a prevention program developed at the University of Minnesota and included in the SAMHSA NREPP. The program works for change in alcohol ordinances in the community and alcohol policies of schools, universities, and civic organizations. It encourages parents, faith organizations, the police, city government, and all businesses and organizations within the community to promote the idea of limiting alcohol availability for 13- to 18-year-olds. The program was studied in 15 communities over a five-year period and resulted in decreased alcohol sales to minors, decreases in friends providing alcohol to minors, and decreases in self-reported drinking in the targeted age group.

Prevention in the Workplace

As a part of its efforts to reduce the demand for drugs, the federal government has encouraged private

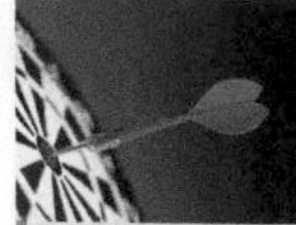

TARGETING PREVENTION

Prevention in First Nations and Inuit Communities

Approximately 1 million people in Canada (3%) identify themselves as Aboriginal. For generations Canada's Aboriginal peoples have faced a variety of significant health issues, and although recent years have seen improvements in many areas of Aboriginal health, specific challenges remain. Of these challenges substance abuse appears paramount.

Obtaining a truly representative view of substance use problems across Canada's Aboriginal peoples has proven difficult, and data that currently exist have their limitations. The challenge in collecting truly representative data is fuelled in part by the broad diversity of ancestry, history, residence, and culture of Canada's Aboriginal population. For example, there are 630 First Nation bands, comprising 52 nations and 50 languages. Furthermore, 70% of Aboriginal peoples live off reserve, making them difficult to follow. Despite the lack of clear national statistics, regional and population-specific data do exist. Surveys in Nunavik, conducted by the Nunavik Inuit Health Society, have shown that Inuit communities have been seriously affected by illicit drugs, namely cannabis, cocaine, and solvents. The 2004 *Inuit Health Survey* estimated that 60% of people had used cannabis in the past year, a use four times the Canadian national average.[54,55] Higher than national use was also reported for cocaine (7.5%), solvents (5.9%), hallucinogens (2.7%), and injection drugs (2%). The survey data also revealed that the use of cannabis, cocaine, and solvents increased considerably between 1992 and 2004, going from 38% to 60% for cannabis, from 5.1% to 7.5% for cocaine, and from 3.0% to 5.9% for solvents. In a recent study, researchers compared the use of tobacco (nontraditional), alcohol, and other drugs among 2620 Aboriginal youth living off reserve against 26 223 non-Aboriginal youth (grades 9–12). This work demonstrated that the prevalence of current smoking among the Aboriginal youth was more than double that among non-Aboriginal youth (24.9% versus 10.4%). Furthermore, Aboriginal youth were more likely than non-Aboriginal youth to have tried marijuana and other illicit drugs, and to have engaged in binge drinking.[56]

Numerous risk factors have been identified as contributors to the level of substance abuse in Aboriginal populations. Issues of poverty, low education, unemployment, unstable family structure, physical abuse, lack of social support networks, barriers to health care, the effects of residential schools, and discrimination have created significant challenges for Canada's Aboriginal peoples. To put the level of risk into perspective, consider the following Canadian facts:

- One in four Aboriginal children lives in poverty compared with the non-Aboriginal rate of one in six.
- 23% of Aboriginal people live in houses in need of major repairs, compared with 7% for the non-Aboriginal population.
- More than half of Aboriginal people are not employed, and the unemployment rate for Aboriginal people was 13.9% in 2009, compared with 8.1% for non-Aboriginal people.
- High school graduation rates for Aboriginal youth are half the Canadian rate.
- 12% of Aboriginal people ages 15 years and older reported an incident involving sexual assault, robbery, or physical assault committed by someone other than a spouse or common-law partner. This proportion is more than double that reported by non-Aboriginal people (5%).[57,58]

Substance use often becomes a coping mechanism for dealing with these challenges. Logically, any drug-use prevention strategy must begin by eradicating risk factors that contribute to a population's substance abuse.

Since the 1970s the Government of Canada has supported the National Native Alcohol and Drug Abuse Program.[59] This program, now largely controlled by First Nations communities, has worked to assist communities to create and operate treatment and prevention programs for reducing high levels of alcohol, drug, and solvent abuse. Today the program supports more than 550 prevention programs whose activities include public awareness campaigns, public speaking, developing school prevention programs, news media work, and cultural and spiritual events. These programs, which have received considerable monies, time, and efforts, have seen little formal evaluation of their abilities to achieve their objective: preventing illicit drug use.

In 2008 the Government of Canada, as part of its National Anti-Drug Strategy, committed $141.5 million, delivered over five years, to improve the effectiveness of, and access to, addiction prevention and treatment services for First Nations and Inuit. What impact do you think enhanced treatment and prevention services will have, given the multitude and degree of risk factors faced by Aboriginal peoples? What approach might you recommend?

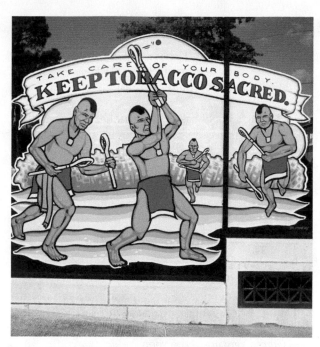

Community-based programs work best when they have widespread community support. This anti-tobacco mural is tied to the values of a local community and focuses on the traditional sacred origins of tobacco use among many First Nations peoples.

employers, especially those who do business with the government, to adopt policies to prevent drug use by their employees. One area of debate is the possibility of legislation for compulsory employee drug testing, as a means of ensuring workplaces are drug and alcohol free, especially in safety-sensitive sectors.[60] Whether Canada takes the path of the United States, where the most consistent feature of these programs is random urine screens, remains to be seen. At a minimum, the Government of Canada expects employers to state clearly that drug use on the job is unacceptable and to notify employees of the consequences of violating company policy regarding drug use. The ultimate goal is not to catch drug users and fire them but to prevent drug use by making it clear that it is not condoned.

What Should We Be Doing?

By now you have picked up some ideas for things to do to reduce drug use, as well as some things to avoid doing. But the answer as to what needs to be done in a particular situation depends on the motivations for doing it. All provinces and territories support drug- and alcohol-abuse prevention education as part of a health curriculum, for example. If that is the primary motive for doing something, and if there doesn't seem to be a particular problem with substance abuse in the schools, then the best thing would be to adopt one of the modern school-based programs that have been developed for this purpose, to make sure the teachers and other participants are properly trained in it, and to go ahead. In selecting from among the curricula, a sensible, balanced approach that combines some factual information with social skills training, perhaps integrated into the more general themes of health, personal values, and decision making, would be appropriate. The ones mentioned in the section "Prevention Programs That Work" fit this general description, and each deserves a careful look. Above all, avoid sensational scare stories, preachy approaches from the teacher to the student, and untrained personnel developing their own curricula. Another good thing to avoid is the inadvertent demonstration of how to do things you don't want students to do.

If, however, there is a public outcry about the "epidemic" of drugs and alcohol abuse in the community, speakers have inflamed passions, and there is a widespread fervour to do something about it, this presents both a danger and an opportunity. The danger is that this passionate group might attack and undermine the efforts already being made in the schools, substituting scary, preachy, negative approaches, which can have negative consequences. The opportunity lies in the possibility that this energy can be organized into a community planning effort, out of which could develop cooperation, increased parent understanding, a focus on family communication, interest in the lives of the community's young people, and increased recreational and creative opportunities.

The key to making this happen is convincing the aroused citizenry of the possibly negative consequences of doing what seems obvious and selling them on the idea of studying what needs to be done. A good place to start is by visiting the Web site of the Canadian Centre on Substance Abuse or the U.S. Substance Abuse and Mental Health Services Administration. These agencies produce updated materials for groups interested in developing drug- and alcohol-abuse prevention programs and provide technical assistance and training to communities interested in developing programs.

Summary

- We can distinguish between education and propaganda approaches to prevention. Traditionally, prevention programs took the form of propaganda in that they focused solely on the presentation of negative information about alcohol and other drugs. Education programs strive to teach individuals about drugs: the good and bad effects, how they are used, and how they relate to society. The goal of education is to prepare people to make appropriate decisions about personal drug use and abuse.
- Most of the research over the past 30 years has failed to demonstrate that prevention programs can produce clear, meaningful, long-lasting effects on drug-using behaviour.
- The affective education programs of the 1970s have been criticized for being too value free.
- Two systems are used for classifying prevention programs. One is based on stages of involvement and includes primary prevention programs aimed mainly at young people who have not yet tried the substances in question; secondary prevention programs designed for people who have tried the drug in question or a variety of other substances; and tertiary prevention programs or relapse prevention and follow-up programs. The second includes prevention efforts categorized according to the intended target population, but the targets are not defined only by prior drug use. They include universal prevention programs designed for delivery to an entire population, selective prevention strategies designed for groups within the general population that are deemed to be at high risk, and indicated prevention strategies targeted at individuals who show signs of developing problems.
- Early drug prevention programs were based primarily on a knowledge-attitudes-behaviour model. By the 1970s studies began to show the effectiveness of such programs in altering attitudes and behaviour about drugs. This led to the development of interest and research in affective education.
- Based on the success of the social influence model in reducing cigarette smoking, a variety of school-based prevention programs have used the same techniques with illegal drugs.
- The DARE program has been adopted rapidly and widely, despite research showing limited impact on drug-using behaviour. In response to the lack of evidence in support of their program, DARE proponents have developed extensions to the program, including DARE 1 PLUS. The effectiveness of these extensions has yet to be demonstrated.
- Current school-based approaches teach refusal skills, counter advertising, require public commitments, and use teen leaders. Several of these programs have been demonstrated to be effective.
- Other nonschool programs are peer-based, after-school groups or activities (e.g., YMCA/YWCA programs), parent-based family training (e.g., Strengthening Families for the Future), or community-based programs (e.g., Communities Mobilizing for Change on Alcohol).
- In the United States one of the most consistent features of workplace prevention programs is urine drug testing. Whether Canada will take this path, legislating workplace drug testing in security-sensitive sectors, remains to be seen.

Review Questions

1. What is the distinction between secondary and tertiary prevention?
2. What is the knowledge-attitudes-behaviour model, and what information first called it into question?
3. Describe what is meant by "value-free" values clarification programs and explain why they fell out of favour in the 1980s.
4. When the Drug-Free Schools programs began in 1986, the emphasis shifted away from curriculum to what?
5. What were the five successful components of the social influence model for smoking prevention?
6. In Project ALERT, what was the impact of using teen leaders to assist the instructors?
7. What distinguishes DARE from other similar programs based on the social influence model?
8. What do ALERT and Life Skills Training have in common, besides their effectiveness?
9. What are some of the parenting skills that might be taught and practised in a prevention program?
10. What is the most common component of drug-free workplace plans?

CHAPTER 18

TREATING SUBSTANCE ABUSE AND DEPENDENCE

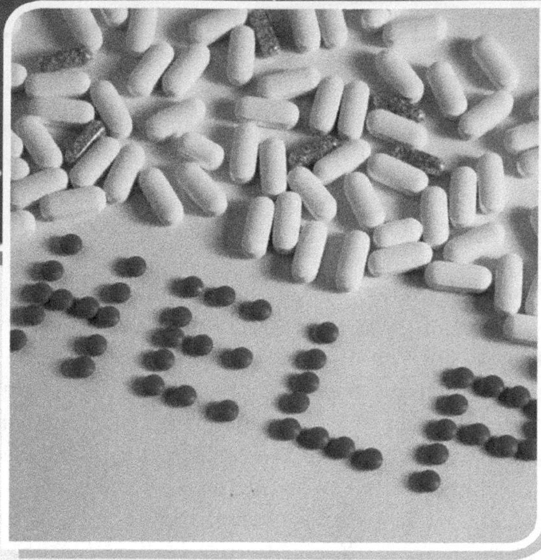

OBJECTIVES

After you have studied this chapter, you should be able to:

- **LO1** Discuss the social and economic costs of alcohol and other drugs in Canada.
- **LO2** Describe selected pharmacological approaches used to help substance abusers deal with withdrawal symptoms and maintain abstinence from alcohol, nicotine, the opioids, cocaine, and cannabis.
- **LO3** Discuss some of the behavioural and psychosocial treatment approaches used to help individuals deal with their substance abuse problems.
- **LO4** Discuss concurrent disorders in Canada.
- **LO5** Explain how substance abuse treatment is organized and funded in Canada.
- **LO6** Explain the systems approach to substance use in Canada.

Every year, hundreds of thousands of Canadians undergo treatment for substance-related disorders, substance abuse, and addictions. In 2009–2010 in Nova Scotia alone, 12 384 clients received specialized addiction treatment services and supports in the province. This accounts for 1.3% of all Nova Scotians and approximately 1.6% of Nova Scotians ages 15 and older.[1] The word *treatment* conjures up images of hospitals, nurses, and physicians, but traditional medical approaches form only a small part of the overall treatment picture. As we will see, the variety of treatment approaches reflects the variety of substance-related disorders, as well as the variety of theories about such disorders. There are also many who question whether drug treatment is effective. It certainly is for some, but multiple treatment attempts may be required. Nonetheless, you should be wary of "experts" who claim to have a complete understanding of what works for everyone. You should also be suspicious of those who have simple, definitive answers. Addiction is a complex problem that requires individualized treatment and, in some cases, various treatment approaches may need to be combined for the optimal outcome. The sections that follow provide a snapshot of approaches currently used in the treatment of selected substance-related disorders in Canada and elsewhere.

LO1 The Social and Economic Costs of Alcohol and Other Drugs in Canada

We have learned throughout this text how alcohol and other drug abuse is of serious concern to all Canadians. We have seen that approximately 2 million Canadians may meet the diagnostic criteria for being dependent on or having abused alcohol and other drugs and that the burden of alcohol and other drug abuse, at $40 billion per year, creates a substantial drain (both direct and indirect) on Canada's economy. To put the significance of this burden into further perspective, consider the impact of substance abuse on a small province like Nova Scotia—where, with a population of less than one million people, the associated financial burden estimated in terms of death, illness, and economic costs caused in whole or in part by the use of tobacco, alcohol, and illegal drugs totalled $1.244 billion.[2] Of these costs, $625.5 million (50.3%) were attributed to tobacco use, $418.9 million (33.7%) to alcohol abuse, and $200.2 million (16.1%) to abuse of illegal drugs.

LO2 Pharmacotherapies (Medication Treatments)

Substance abuse and dependence are increasingly being viewed as "brain diseases," much like, for example, Parkinson's disease. But the overwhelming majority of individuals who use substances do not become dependent, whereas virtually all the individuals who lose greater than 80% of nigrostriatal dopamine neurons will exhibit symptoms of Parkinson's disease. Nevertheless, an intense amount of research effort has focused on developing medications to treat substance abuse and dependence. The rationale is that as we increase our understanding of the brain mechanisms mediating substance abuse, we should be better able to use medications to target these mechanisms, thereby blocking the reinforcing effects of drugs of abuse (i.e., the "magic bullet approach"). Despite the enthusiasm accompanying medication development efforts, most experts do not believe that pharmacotherapies alone will cure a chronic, relapsing disorder such as substance abuse, in part because the problem of substance abuse is expressed behaviourally. Thus, a major hope is that pharmacotherapies will provide a window of opportunity by relieving withdrawal symptoms, for example, so that behavioural or psychosocial treatments can be used. Below we describe some medications that have been used to help substance abusers deal with withdrawal symptoms and maintain abstinence. The focus of our discussion will be limited to alcohol, nicotine, the opioids, cocaine, and cannabis. These substances were selected for their public health importance and because a large amount of research has been conducted regarding their use. Table 18.1 summarizes selected medications used to treat substance-related disorders in Canada.

Detoxification (Withdrawal Management) and Maintenance Phase

Pharmacological interventions are typically initiated at two different phases of the dependence cycle: detoxification and maintenance. Detoxification can be viewed as an *initial and immediate goal* during which medications are administered to alleviate unpleasant withdrawal symptoms that may appear following abrupt cessation of drug use (e.g., the nicotine patch and nicotine gum have been used to treat individuals experiencing cigarette smoking abstinence symptoms). Medications used in the detoxification phase are also sometimes used in the maintenance phase (e.g., nicotine replacement medications). Thus, the distinction between a detoxification medication and a maintenance medication is sometimes less clear.

Maintenance on pharmacological agents can be viewed as a *longer-term strategy* used to help the dependent individual avoid relapsing to the abused drug. Three major maintenance strategies are used. First, *agonist or substitution therapy* is used to induce cross-tolerance to the abused drug. Methadone, a long-acting μ-opioid agonist, for opioid dependence and nicotine replacement medications for tobacco dependence

Table 18.1 Medications Used to Treat Substance-Related Disorders in Canada

Substance	Treatment Medication	Proposed Mechanism of Action
Alcohol	benzodiazepines diazepam (Valium) lorazepam (Ativan)	Increase the activity of GABA
	barbiturates phenobarbital	Increase the activity of GABA
	naltrexone (Revia)	Opioid receptor antagonist
	acamprosate (Campral)	Normalizes basal GABA concentrations; blocks alcohol-withdrawal-induced glutamate increases
Nicotine	nicotine replacements	Full agonists at nicotine receptors
	bupropion (Zyban)	Inhibits the reuptake of dopamine and norepinephrine; acetylcholine receptors antagonist
	varenicline (Champix)	Partial nicotine-receptor agonist
Opioids	methadone	Full agonist at opioid receptors
	buprenorphine	Partial agonist at opioid receptors
	buprenorphine/naloxone (Suboxone)	Partial agonist at opioid receptors

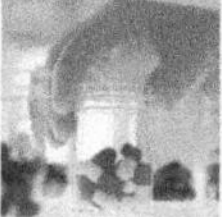

DRUGS IN THE MEDIA

Celebrity Rehab

It seems that every few weeks another well-known celebrity or politician is caught in some kind of public misbehaviour, followed by the explanation that the famous person is suffering from a substance-related disorder and will be entering a treatment program. Rob Ford, Mel Gibson, Russell Brand, Britney Spears, Lindsay Lohan, and others have made public confessions of their substance abuse and have gone to expensive residential treatment programs. This has become such a part of our culture that the cable channel VH1 began a reality TV series in 2008 called *Celebrity Rehab with Dr. Drew.* Eight somewhat less well-known celebrities checked in for treatment with Dr. Drew Pinsky and his staff and were followed for 10 episodes until they "graduated." Whether or not these individuals will be successful in abstaining from future substance use, the series itself was apparently successful enough that six seasons were completed.

In May 2013, Dr. Drew stated that he would not return for another season because of intense pressure from public criticism. To date, at least five of Dr. Drew's "Celebrity Rehab" patients have died and some blame him for being less than competent. Do you think that Dr. Drew deserves blame for the death of his patients? Do you think that drug addiction is a life-threatening disease and the focus on Dr. Drew is misplaced?

have been used as agonist maintenance treatments to prevent relapse and cravings in individuals attempting to maintain abstinence. Agonist maintenance agents typically have safer routes of administration and diminished psychoactive effects. Second, *antagonist therapy* is used to produce extinction by preventing the user from experiencing the reinforcing effects of the abused drug (e.g., the opioid antagonist naltrexone, which selectively blocks opioid effects). Finally, *aversion therapy* is used to produce an aversive reaction following ingestion of the abused drug. Disulfiram (Antabuse) for the treatment of alcohol dependence is an example of aversion therapy. Disulfiram inhibits aldehyde dehydrogenase, a major enzyme involved in alcohol metabolism, which, in the presence of alcohol, can produce unpleasant symptoms, including headache, vomiting, and breathing difficulties. In Canada, disulfiram (Antabuse) was discontinued in 2001 by the manufacturer. However, disulfiram is available as a bulk powder and most pharmacies will compound it for customers.

Alcohol

Pharmacotherapies have become increasingly important in the treatment of alcohol dependence, in part because of the serious nature of the acute alcohol withdrawal syndrome. This syndrome is typically characterized by tremors, tachycardia (rapid heartbeat), and hypertension, profuse sweating, insomnia, hallucinations, and seizures. Medical risks associated with the alcohol withdrawal process often require an inpatient medical setting. Symptoms usually present themselves within 6 to 24 hours after cessation of alcohol intake and peak by about 72 hours.[3,4,5] During detoxification, two of the central tasks for the clinician are to prevent the development of seizures and reduce autonomic hyperactivity. For several reasons, administration of a benzodiazepine during alcohol detoxification is the standard treatment approach. There is a high degree of cross-tolerance between alcohol and the benzodiazepines. Because benzodiazepines can serve as substitutes for alcohol and generally have longer half-lives than alcohol, the withdrawal process can be safely completed. Benzodiazepines, by potentiating the inhibitory actions of GABA on the central nervous system, significantly decrease the risk of seizures during detoxification. In addition, the increased autonomic arousal that occurs during alcohol withdrawal is similar to the initiation of the "stress response" (i.e., increased heart rate, blood pressure, respiration, and anxiety). This suggests the mechanisms that mediate the stress response may also play a role in alcohol withdrawal symptoms. Because it is well documented that increased GABA-ergic transmission markedly diminishes the stress response,[6] it is not surprising that benzodiazepines are also effective in attenuating the autonomic hyperactivity that accompanies alcohol withdrawal symptoms.

While benzodiazepines are effective and safe in managing withdrawal in a variety of clinical settings, they have limitations and liabilities in the addiction treatment setting.[7] The high doses of benzodiazepines typically required to manage alcohol withdrawal symptoms may cloud the sensorium, potentially affecting multiple areas of cognition; most notably, interfering with the formation and consolidation of memories of new material and may induce complete anterograde amnesia.[7] This can create a challenge to the development of effective therapeutic relationships between patients and clinical staff. Furthermore, when administered at doses outside the therapeutic range, common in the management of alcohol withdrawal symptoms, benzodiazepines are liable to abuse and dependency.[8,9,10,11] Unfortunately, there is no other equally effective anxiety management agent better suited to this population.

Three medications have received approval by Health Canada for the treatment of alcohol abuse and dependence: disulfiram (Antabuse), naltrexone (Revia), and acamprosate (Campral). All these medications are used during the maintenance phase. Typically, these medications are used for weeks or months; indefinite maintenance for years is unusual with these approaches. Nearly a half century ago it was discovered that ingestion of disulfiram in the presence of alcohol resulted in an unpleasant reaction, including facial flushing, accelerated pulse, throbbing headache, nausea, and vomiting.[12] These symptoms occur as a result of the increased amount of acetaldehyde in the body following inhibition of aldehyde dehydrogenase by disulfiram. Since this initial observation, several studies have assessed disulfiram as a pharmacotherapeutic option in treating alcohol-use disorders. In general, disulfiram has not been shown to be effective in achieving abstinence or delaying relapse; most individuals simply do not take the medication.

Naltrexone was developed as an opioid antagonist and has been used in the treatment of opioid dependence. In the early 1990s, data from two large studies of naltrexone for the treatment of alcohol dependence showed that the medication substantially reduced days of alcohol drinking per week, the rate of relapse among those who drank, and alcohol craving.[13] The precise mechanism of action for naltrexone-related reductions in alcohol drinking is not fully understood, but it has been suggested that the medication blocks opioid receptors, thereby preventing the release of alcohol-induced dopamine, which in turn blocks the reinforcing effects of alcohol.[14] Although great fanfare accompanied the approval of naltrexone and many alcohol-dependent individuals were treated with this medication, it has not had a big impact on overall treatment success.

The latest medication to receive approval for the treatment of alcohol-use disorders is acamprosate, a compound that bears a structural resemblance to GABA. Acamprosate exerts at least two actions that have been proposed to be important for its clinical utility in treating alcohol dependence: normalizing basal GABA concentrations, which are proposed to be disrupted in alcohol-dependent individuals, and blocking the glutamate increases observed during alcohol withdrawal.[15] In several studies, acamprosate has been shown to be effective in decreasing alcohol relapse. But because the medication only recently received Health Canada approval, its efficacy in treating alcohol-use disorder in broader clinical populations has yet to be determined.

Nicotine

More than 98% of tobacco users are cigarette smokers. Despite the declining social acceptability and rates of cigarette smoking, a substantial proportion of individuals remain dependent. Tobacco smoke contains as many as 4000 chemical constituents, but nicotine is thought to be the primary component responsible for the maintenance of continued use. When most smokers attempt to quit, they experience withdrawal symptoms such as anxiety, depression, dysphoria, irritability, decreased concentration, insomnia, increased food intake, and cigarette craving. Pharmacotherapies have been used primarily to attenuate these symptoms. Currently, five nicotine-replacement therapies have received approval from Health Canada for treating nicotine dependence: transdermal nicotine patch, nicotine gum, nicotine vapour inhaler, nicotine spray, and nicotine lozenge. Before initiating nicotine-replacement treatments, smokers are advised to discontinue the use of other nicotine-containing products because of concerns about nicotine toxicity that might result from concurrent use of nicotine-containing products (e.g., cigarettes in combination with the nicotine patch). All these treatments have been demonstrated to increase quit rates in controlled clinical studies.[16] These studies have been conducted under fairly strict conditions, with a prescribed quitting period, several visits to the clinic to assess progress, and the usual trappings of a clinical research study, often including the collection of saliva (the validation of self-reported smoking status can be verified by measuring cotinine, the primary metabolite of nicotine in saliva) or other samples to detect tobacco use. That's a far cry from buying nicotine gum at the corner store, with no plan for quitting, no follow-up interviews, and no monitoring. Thus, it is not surprising that the average person might have great difficulties quitting even with the aid of nicotine-replacement medications.

In March 2009, Health Canada issued a statement advising Canadians not to purchase or use electronic smoking products. Their stated concern included that these products may pose health risks and have not been fully evaluated for safety, quality, and efficacy by Health Canada.[17] Electronic smoking products can be purchased in a variety of forms, including but not limited to electronic cigarettes, cigars, cigarillos, and pipes. Despite repeated calls for closer scrutiny of electronic smoking products from sources ranging from provincial governments to the Canadian Cancer Society, Health Canada has yet to take decisive action.

Health Canada approved the use of bupropion (Zyban), the first non-nicotine pharmacotherapy for smoking cessation, in 1998. Bupropion is also used in the treatment of depression, where it is referred to as Wellbutrin. While the mechanism of action specific to bupropion's smoking cessation has not been definitively proven, it is believed to be inhibition of dopamine and norepinephrine reuptake and, to a lesser extent, blockade of acetylcholine receptors.[18] Unlike nicotine-replacement therapies, there is no absolute requirement for the smoker to abstain from the use of nicotine-containing products. Bupropion has been shown to gradually decrease cigarette craving and use in some clinical trials. Because nicotine-replacement medications and bupropion have been demonstrated to decrease cigarette smoking when administered alone, it has been suggested that greater treatment success might be achieved if the two strategies were combined. Recently, a study evaluated the relative efficacies of five smoking cessation pharmacotherapy interventions (nicotine lozenge, nicotine patch, sustained-release bupropion, nicotine patch plus nicotine lozenge, and bupropion plus nicotine lozenge) using placebo-controlled, head-to-head comparisons. Additionally, all research participants received individual counselling sessions along with the pharmacotherapy interventions. Results from the study indicated that the nicotine patch plus lozenge produced the greatest benefit relative to placebo for smoking cessation. The nicotine lozenge, bupropion, and bupropion plus nicotine lozenge groups produced results similar to what has been previously reported.[19]

Health Canada approved the smoking cessation product varenicline (Champix) for sale in Canada in 2007. Varenicline is a partial nicotinic-receptor agonist, meaning that, even at large doses, it does not produce the full response of nicotine. As a result of its properties, it should be able to reduce symptoms of

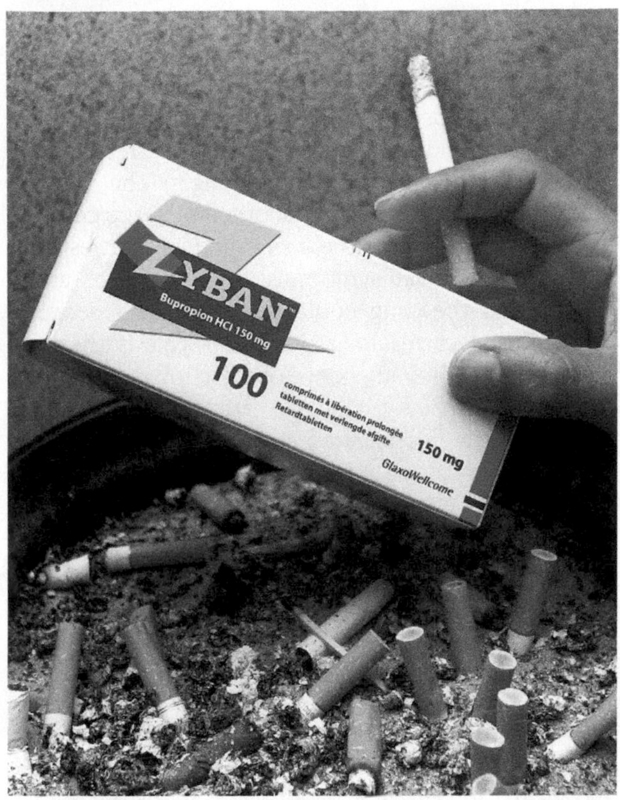

Zyban (bupropion) was the first non-nicotine pharmacotherapy for smoking cessation. The drug, also used to treat depression, appears to gradually reduce cravings for cigarettes.

withdrawal and craving, while blocking the effects of nicotine should the smoker relapse (see Chapter 10 for a fuller description of how varenicline works). Varenicline was found to be more effective than placebo or bupropion and is a viable option for smoking cessation therapy.[20] People choosing Champix as a smoking cessation medication pick a date to start the medication one week after they have stopped smoking. Typical dosage schedules for the medication suggest 0.5 milligram once a day for the first week of treatment. From the second week of treatment onward, individuals can choose between 0.5 milligram twice daily and 1.0 milligram twice daily. Currently, there is no evidence to suggest one dosage form is superior to the other. In June 2011, Health Canada announced that it was undertaking a review of Champix because of the possibility of an increased risk of heart-related side effects in patients who have cardiovascular disease. The U.S. Food and Drug Administration (FDA) had recently reported results from its review of a clinical trial involving 700 smokers with cardiovascular disease. It announced that the risk for patients with cardiovascular disease taking Champix was 2%, compared with 1% for those taking no drug. Health Canada announced it would update Canadians with any new safety recommendations regarding Champix use after the review process had been completed.[21]

Interest in immunotherapy for the treatment of substance use disorders is emerging.[22] The majority of currently available pharmacotherapies act centrally in the brain to block the rewarding properties of or reduce withdrawal symptoms from drugs of abuse. Yet what if the drug could be neutralized peripherally before ever reaching the brain? This is the basic premise on which the development of nicotine vaccines lies. Currently, all vaccinations for nicotine in the pipeline are conjugates, meaning nicotine is linked to a carrier protein capable of mounting an immune response. To date, three companies have begun clinical trials of their anti-nicotine vaccines. Two studies have demonstrated efficacy as long as a sufficient antibody level is achieved.[23,24]

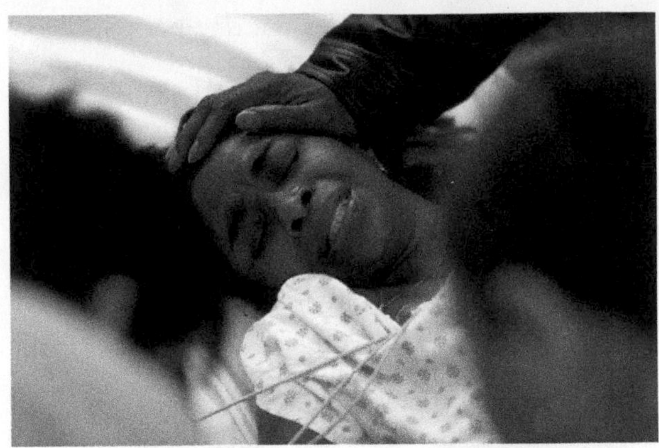

Drug withdrawal can have unpleasant and potentially dangerous symptoms. Drugs may be administered to reduce withdrawal symptoms.

Opioids

Although opioid withdrawal is not life threatening, such symptoms as nausea, vomiting, diarrhea, aches, and pain can be unpleasant. Medications are administered to minimize discomfort. Historically, anticholinergic drugs, like belladonna, were used in the treatment of opioid dependence.[25] The idea was that anticholinergics would produce a state of delirium for several days, after which the dependent person would emerge cured of dependence without remembering the dreadful experience of the withdrawal process. A more recent version of this approach is "rapid opioid detoxification." Opioid-dependent individuals are anaesthetized and, while unconscious, are given an opioid antagonist, so that withdrawal will occur while they are unconscious. After 24 hours the patient is released and enters a period of counselling, combined with continued opioid antagonist treatment. This procedure has been vehemently criticized because it increases the risk of problems during the withdrawal process and because aftercare (behavioural or psychosocial treatment) is often de-emphasized.

Methadone (Metadol), an opioid analgesic developed in Germany during World War II, is commonly used in this capacity. It has a long duration of action, which means that it needs to be taken less frequently to prevent withdrawal symptoms. Another medication that has been shown to decrease opioid withdrawal symptoms is buprenorphine, a partial opioid agonist. Buprenorphine has a relatively large margin of safety and a low overdose potential. In addition, it has a long duration of action and blocks the effects of other opioid agonists, such as heroin. As a result of these features, both methadone and buprenorphine are approved by Health Canada as opioid-dependence treatment medications. These medications are used not only during detoxification but during maintenance as well. Methadone maintenance, the most common form of treatment for opioid dependence, may continue for months or years or even indefinitely, as long as the person benefits from being on the medication. The duration of buprenorphine maintenance might be similar, but because the medication has only recently received approval, this is not yet known.

One major concern in the treatment of opioid dependence is opioid-induced overdose, which could lead to a coma and eventual death via respiratory depression. Because the short-acting opioid antagonist naloxone has a greater affinity for brain opioid receptors than do most opioid agonists, including heroin, it is often used for treating opioid overdose. Following its administration, naloxone displaces the opioid agonist from the receptors and thereby rapidly reverses the overdose. This observation led to speculations about the use of opioid antagonists in treating opioid dependence. That is, if a user takes heroin, for example, while being maintained on an opioid antagonist, the effects of heroin would not be felt. This rationale provided the basis for the approval of the long-acting opioid antagonist naltrexone for treating opioid dependence. Although naltrexone therapy has been shown to be effective in the treatment of opioid dependence, this therapy appears to be appropriate for only highly motivated individuals because most opioid abusers enrolled in naltrexone therapy prematurely discontinue treatment. To circumvent compliance problems, a new depot formulation of naltrexone, which requires one administration per month, is being studied as a potential opioid-dependence treatment medication. Initial findings are encouraging, as depot naltrexone has been demonstrated to block heroin-related effects for up to six weeks.[26] An interesting problem arises if a patient on naltrexone is involved in an accident and requires some pain relief. Current practice is to give high doses of hydromorphone (Dilaudid) to overcome the antagonism. This should be done only in a hospital and with extreme caution.

Methadone Methadone is a synthetic opioid. It was developed in 1937 by German scientists searching for an internal source of opioids. An analogue of heroin and morphine, methadone acts on the same opioid receptors as these drugs. Shortly after World War II, the American researchers Vincent Dole, Marie Nyswander, and Mary Jeanne Kreek at Rockefeller University discovered that methadone could be used to treat heroin withdrawal symptoms and serve as a maintenance treatment. However, it was a Canadian researcher, Dr. Robert Halliday, who would in 1963 set up perhaps the world's first methadone maintenance treatment program in British Columbia.[27]

Canadian guidelines for methadone maintenance were introduced in 1972. As awareness and concern about opioid dependence and its related health risks grew, notably the high risk of infection with HIV and HCV, the number of people with opioid dependence and who are receiving methadone, or buprenorphine, maintenance treatment increased (see Table 18.2).

In Canada, as in many other countries, there is a national-level regulatory framework for prescribing methadone. In recent years the Office of Controlled Substances, Health Canada, in conjunction with provincial and territorial governments and medical licensing bodies, has increased efforts to improve access to methadone maintenance treatment. To date, several provinces have developed guidelines and training for practitioners interested in providing methadone maintenance treatment. Currently methadone maintenance therapy can be prescribed only by physicians who have received an exemption to do so under the Controlled Drugs and Substances Act.

In recent years much has been written about the various types of methadone maintenance programs in Canada. A 2010 national survey of substance use treatment programs collected information from 870 programs, representing approximately 70% of Canadian programs. Of these programs 38 reported that they provide methadone maintenance treatment. The prevalence of, and perceived need for, such treatment varies across the country.

How Does Methadone Maintenance Treatment Work? Methadone works through a variety of mechanisms. It supports the withdrawal from opioids by alleviating symptoms including severe insomnia, nausea, vomiting, diarrhea, violent yawning, weakness, chills, fever, muscle spasms, flushing, and abdominal pain. As maintenance therapy methadone decreases the client's chronic craving for opioids, and due to its oral activity and long half-life, once-a-day oral dosing can prevent the onset of opioid withdrawal for 24–36 hours. Of equal importance is the fact that methadone reduces the euphoric effects of other opioids, through the development of cross-tolerance. Because of cross-tolerance, injection of other opioids while on methadone will not lead to euphoria. This decreases client use of other opioids while on methadone maintenance treatment. This reduction in other opioid use significantly reduces the health risks associated with injection drug use. Finally, tolerance to the beneficial effects associated with methadone maintenance develops very slowly. As a result, many individuals can be maintained on the same dose of methadone for many years.

What Is Methadone Maintenance Treatment? Canadians have yet to agree on a formal definition for methadone maintenance treatment. What is clear however is that methadone substitution, in and of itself, **does not** constitute effective treatment for opioid dependency and that methadone must be used in combination with other supports and services. Current guidelines, albeit broadly defined and in need of greater specificity, suggest the following as essential components to an effective methadone maintenance treatment program:

- Medical care
- Methadone
- Medical treatment for other substance-related disorders
- Counselling (for mental health and substance-related disorders)
- Health promotion, disease prevention, and education
- Community-based supports and services
- Outreach and advocacy

Consensus on how or in which settings to deliver methadone maintenance treatment has yet to be

Table 18.2 Methadone Maintenance Treatment Comparison across Canada (2010)

Province, Territory, or Population	Number of Patients	Number of Doctors with Exemption	Provincial Guidelines?	Service Models	On Drug Formulary?
Nova Scotia	Approx. 1000	29	Only for using methadone for treating chronic pain	Four provincially funded clinics (Halifax [2], Sydney and Truro), family practice, private clinics, and prison	Methadone: yes Buprenorphine: no
New Brunswick	1423 in 4 provincially funded clinics; 300–500 elsewhere	42	Yes (physicians and pharmacists)	4 provincially funded MMT programs (Moncton, Miramichi, Fredericton, Saint John); family practice, CHC, prison, and private clinic	Methadone: yes Buprenorphine: no
Newfoundland and Labrador	Approx. 700	4	Yes (physicians and pharmacists)	One provincially funded MMT clinic and two family physicians prescribe in St. John's; one physician in Grand Falls/Windsor; and prison	Methadone: yes Buprenorphine: no
PEI	160 patients at Addiction Services clinic; number in family practice is N/A	Over 10	Only for using MMT for treatment of chronic pain	One provincially funded MMT clinic (Addiction Services), three physicians in family practice, and prison.	Methadone: yes Buprenorphine: no
Quebec	2533 (2008)	Approximately 230	Yes for MMT and buprenorphine	MMT provided in addiction treatment centres, hospitals, regional health authorities, and family practice	Methadone: yes Buprenorphine: no
Ontario	29 743 (Oct 18, 2010)	309	Yes for MMT (physicians, pharmacists, nurses, and case management), buprenorphine guidelines in development	Private clinics, provincially funded clinics (in addiction treatment centres, CHC, needle exchange program, CAMH), family practice, prison setting; Ontario Addiction Treatment Centre, a for-profit network of clinics serving more than 7500 patients with just fewer than 40 affiliated physicians	Methadone: yes Buprenorphine: no
Manitoba	Estimated at 820; AFM has 380, private clinics, approx. 420	15	Yes for MMT (for prescribing and management of MMT-related care)	Two provincially funded clinics, two private clinics, family practice, and prison setting	Methadone: yes Buprenorphine: no
Saskatchewan	Approx. 2200	34	Yes for MMT (physicians, pharmacists, and counsellors)	Family practice, prison, and 3 provincially funded clinics; also have 2nd-level prescriber, which is a physician whose exemption allows him or her only to maintain the dose for stable patients in primary care	Methadone: yes Buprenorphine: yes

continued

Table 18.2 *Continued*

Province, Territory, or Population	Number of Patients	Number of Doctors with Exemption	Provincial Guidelines?	Service Models	On Drug Formulary?
Alberta	Approx. 2000 patients in 2009	80 physicians with exemptions, only 20 with general exemption who can initiate treatment	Yes for MMT (physicians and pharmacists)	Two provincially funded clinics (Edmonton and Calgary); six private clinics (Calgary, Medicine Hat, Lethbridge, Red Deer and two in Edmonton); family practice and prison. Also have 2nd-level prescriber, which is a physician whose exemption allows him or her only to maintain the dose for stable patients in primary care	Methadone: yes Buprenorphine: yes
British Columbia	11 033 as of December 31, 2009	390 have exemptions, 218 active caseloads	Yes for MMT (physicians and pharmacists)	Family practice; multidisciplinary models (including community health clinics and population specific clinics), private clinics and prison	Methadone: yes Buprenorphine: no
Nunavut	No MMT		N/A		
NWT	No MMT		N/A		
Yukon	Approx. 32	2		Family practices	
First Nations	N/A	N/A		National Native Alcohol and Drug Abuse Program does not offer MMT; some reserve communities have arrangements with provincial health departments for MMT; some private practices establish program just outside of reserve	Methadone: yes Buprenorphine: no
Federal Corrections	August 2010, 759 on methadone; 4 on Suboxone	Unknown. All are contractors with CSC.	Yes for MMT and buprenorphine	Federal prisons offer MMT to inmates who are already on methadone or who want to initiate treatment in jail	Methadone: yes Buprenorphine: yes

Note: Formulary coverage may not extend to all residents of a province. MMT = methadone maintenance therapy

Sources: *A Cross-Canada Scan of Methadone Maintenance Treatment Policy Developments: A Report Prepared for the Canadian Executive Council on Addictions.* Prepared by Janine Luce, MA, Centre for Addiction and Mental Health; and Carol Strike, PhD, University of Toronto. April 2011.

Disclaimer: The data presented above reflect information available in 2010 and may have changed since that time reached. In Canada methadone maintenance treatment programs are currently delivered within a variety of services and settings including:

- Substance-use treatment services and clinics (outpatient and inpatient)
- Community and hospital-based health centres
- Private substance-use treatment clinics
- Physicians' offices (linked with community-based pharmacies)
- HIV/AIDS services and clinics
- Mental health treatment services and clinics
- Correctional facilities

Finally, there appears to be significant variation both within Canadian jurisdictions and internationally with regard to program philosophies, type and level of services provided, patient groups served, level of patient involvement, program policies, and program settings.[27] Obviously, we have much work to do.

Buprenorphine In 2007, Canadians who were dependent on opioids such as heroin and opioid-based medications gained access to a second effective and safe substitution treatment option for opioid dependence. Suboxone (a combination of buprenorphine and naloxone) was approved by Health Canada as a tool for suppressing the symptoms of opioid withdrawal and reducing the cravings for opioid drugs. Buprenorphine is an opioid agonist/antagonist or partial agonist with high affinity for mu receptors. It has 25 to 50 times the potency of morphine. Buprenorphine also acts as an antagonist of kappa receptor. Through this action it can displace a full opioid agonist, such as heroin or methadone, from the mu receptor. Buprenorphine helps to manage the cravings associated with opioid withdrawal, while the naloxone component reduces the potential for misuse by causing unpleasant withdrawal symptoms if the product is misused by intravenous injection.[28] Suboxone is a tablet that dissolves under the tongue.

To help ensure appropriate use of Suboxone its manufacturer, Schering-Plough Canada, developed an online education program, accredited by the College of Family Physicians of Canada. This program provides health care professionals with guidance for product use and for creating dialogue with patients regarding the risk and benefits of therapy. Perhaps most important is that this educational material encourages an approach to care that includes the careful monitoring of patients within a framework of medical, social, and psychological support, essential components to any comprehensive opioid dependence treatment program. The Suboxone Education Program can be viewed at SuboxoneCME.ca.

anhedonia: a lack of emotional response; especially an inability to experience joy or pleasure.

off-label: use of a prescription drug to treat a condition for which the drug has not received approval from Health Canada.

Cocaine

Although a cocaine withdrawal syndrome does not appear to be a major feature of cocaine dependence,[29] some investigators have documented symptoms of depression, nervousness, dysphoria, **anhedonia**, fatigue, irritability, sleep and activity disturbances, and craving for cocaine.[30] Behavioural and mood changes that accompany cocaine withdrawal might be related to a decrease in the activity of monoamine neurotransmitters, which play an important role in movement and mood regulation. Accordingly, medications that increase monoaminergic activity may be useful in treating withdrawal symptoms and thereby prevent relapse. A plethora of medications, ranging from selective agonists of monoamine neurotransmitters to agents that simultaneously enhance the activity of multiple neurotransmitters, have been evaluated according to this theory. Unfortunately, to date the vast majority of medications assessed have not been effective at treating cocaine withdrawal symptoms or dependence.[31] The outlook is not completely bleak, however, as recent data from investigations of modafinil (Chapter 6) suggest that the medication is useful in treating cocaine dependence.[32,33] In these studies, cocaine use and cocaine-related subjective effects (e.g., euphoria and craving) were markedly reduced when cocaine abusers were taking modafinil compared with placebo. While the mechanisms underlying modafinil's therapeutic actions are unknown, the drug appears to increase the activity of several neurotransmitters (e.g., dopamine, norepinephrine, and glutamate) and decrease the release of GABA.[34,35,36] Although modafinil is not approved by Health Canada for the treatment of cocaine abuse or dependence, some physicians may use the medication for this purpose (**off-label**). No medications are currently approved to treat cocaine abuse or dependence in Canada or the United States.

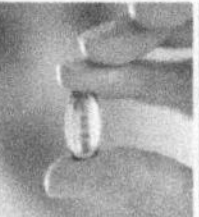

DRUGS IN DEPTH

Crack Pipe Vending Machines Draw Ire of Tory Minister Who Wants to Limit "Access to Drug Paraphernalia"

A pair of vending machines stocked with crack pipes for drug users in Vancouver's Downtown Eastside elicited blunt words from the Harper government over the weekend, with Public Safety Minister Steven Blaney reaffirming the government's quest to end drug use and limit "young people's access to drug paraphernalia." The project, run by a non-profit resource centre, has seen the two machines dispense sterile pipes for 25 cents in an attempt to prevent users from cutting their lips on broken pipes and potentially transmitting such diseases as HIV and hepatitis C.

It had gone unnoticed by the public for eight months, selling more than 22,000 pipes until this weekend when CTV News questioned the minister's office about the initiative. "While the NDP and Liberals would prefer that doctors hand out heroin and needles to those suffering from addiction, this government supports treatment that ends drug use," read the minister's statement — an apparent reference to the two parties' opposition of a bill currently in the House of Commons that would make it harder to open safe injection sites, like Vancouver's high-profile InSite centre. The centre was the subject of a controversial standoff between a provincial health authority and the federal government in 2011, when the Supreme Court ruled against the government's long-standing attempt to shutter it.

Outreach workers responsible for the crack pipe vending machines said they weren't surprised by the Minister's reaction, claiming Vancouver's resources for drug users have become "a convenient whipping boy" for the Conservative party. "Criticizing [the vending machines] is easy marketing because it does seem strange if you don't know all the details," said Mark Townsend, a manager at the Portland Hotel Society, which operates the machines.

"But it's much more complicated," he said, adding that the machines are an "access point" to introduce users to resources. "We're just trying to take action to make sure that people live for another day to get to detox and treatment."

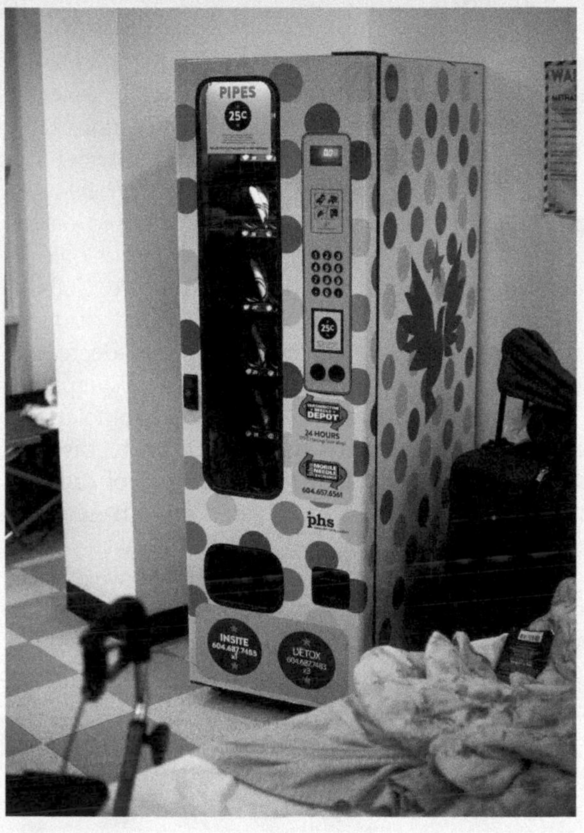

A drug resource centre in Vancouver is operating two "crack pipe vending machines" at its facilities, offering sterile crack pipes for $0.25 each in an attempt to prevent transmission of HIV and hepatitis C.

The initiative began as a pilot project in 2011 when the Vancouver Coastal Health Authority, which runs the InSite centre, circulated 60,000 clean crack pipes across the city. After extensive studies, the project was deemed a success and continues to operate, the authority said Sunday. When the pilot project was announced three years ago, then-Health Minister Leona Aglukkaq issued a statement saying "this is an area of provincial jurisdiction, so that's their call."

Cannabis

Most users of cannabis consume the drug infrequently and without apparent negative consequences. A small proportion, however, experience problems related to frequent cannabis use. An estimated 1 in 11 cannabis users will become dependent.[37] Rates of cannabis dependence in several countries have increased substantially over the past decade as has the number of individuals seeking treatment. Many individuals seeking treatment for cannabis dependence report experiencing withdrawal symptoms and that these symptoms made it more difficult to maintain abstinence. As a result, efforts to develop medication for cannabis dependence have primarily focused on relieving withdrawal symptoms. Cannabis withdrawal is characterized by symptoms of irritability, anxiety, sleep disruptions, and aches.[38] A growing number of medications have been tested for efficacy in relieving these symptoms, but only one has been demonstrated to be effective–oral delta-9-THC (dronabinol).

The primary reason for evaluating the effects of dronabinol on cannabis withdrawal was based on the idea of substituting a longer-acting pharmacologically equivalent drug for the abused substance, stabilizing the individual on that drug, and then gradually withdrawing the substituted drug, thus decreasing the likelihood of precipitating abstinence symptoms. It was recently demonstrated that dronabinol markedly reduced symptoms associated with cannabis abstinence, including self-reported ratings of cannabis craving, anxiety, misery, and sleep disturbance. The medication also reversed the withdrawal-associated psychomotor performance decrements, as well as the anorexia and weight loss, associated with cannabis withdrawal. These results indicate that moderate doses of oral dronabinol might be beneficial in the treatment of cannabis dependence.[39] To date, no medications are approved for the treatment of cannabis dependence, although dronabinol is sometimes used off-label for this purpose in Canada and the United States.

Management of Problematic Substance Use in Pregnancy

The Society of Obstetricians and Gynecologists of Canada has developed clinical practice guidelines for the care of pregnant women with substance-related disorders.[40] These guides are intended to inform and direct health care providers in their decision making, improving women's access to evidence-based practices that decrease maternal and neonatal morbidity and mortality (see Table 18.3).

There are two phases to the management of substance use disorders. The first addresses treatment of withdrawal syndromes. Pregnant women who are dependent on alcohol, opioids, or high-dose benzodiazepines ($\geq$50 mg daily diazepam equivalent) may require medical detoxification under the supervision of a physician. Women who are in withdrawal from other substances, such as cocaine or marijuana, may also

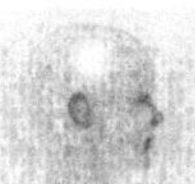

MIND/BODY CONNECTION

The Nature of Dependence

Is drug dependence strictly a matter of neurotransmitters and neural adaptation, as seems increasingly to be the accepted viewpoint, or will it ultimately be impossible to understand such a complex set of behaviours by reducing the problem to its biochemical correlates? This has been a huge and ongoing debate among proponents of the various views of drug dependence, but currently the research funding and most of the information seen in the popular media favour biological approaches to understanding these problems. This chapter's focus on drug treatments for substance dependence seems to be based on an implied acceptance that some biochemical imbalance is at the heart of people who are seemingly unable to exert control over their own drug-using behaviour.

However, many, including proponents of the Alcoholics Anonymous philosophy, believe that substance dependence is a "spiritual" disorder—essentially that an individual human is not recognizing the need to draw on either God or some other source of spiritual strength to help win the struggle with the bottle or needle or pill. For these people, drug treatments, especially of the substitution or maintenance type, are often seen as a crutch that does not address the individual's basic problem and cannot therefore be of much long-term benefit.

To others, substance abuse and dependence can be approached through behavioural techniques, such as contingency management, or through a variety of psychosocial approaches, such as group therapy. For them, medication might be seen as a temporary aid in assisting the person to "reprogram" his or her thinking, routines, and social interactions, but it is ultimately these changes in relationships, attitudes, and activities that are the key to longer-term success.

How do you feel about the evidence showing that former heroin users can often be maintained for years on methadone, a legal substitute, while they attend school, work, and otherwise enjoy more productive and less dangerous lives than if they had continued to use heroin?

Table 18.3 Council of the Society of Obstetricians and Gynecologists of Canada Guideline for the Use of Screening Tools, General Approach to Care, and Recommendations for Clinical Management of Problematic Substance Use in Pregnancy

Screening and assessment

1. All pregnant women and women of childbearing age should be screened periodically for alcohol, tobacco, and prescription and illicit drug use.
2. When testing for substance use is clinically indicated, urine drug screening is the preferred method. Informed consent should be obtained from the woman before maternal drug toxicology testing is ordered.
3. Policies and legal requirements with respect to drug testing of newborns may vary by jurisdiction, and caregivers should be familiar with the regulations in their region.

Components of office management

4. Health care providers should employ a flexible approach to the care of women who have substance use problems, and they should encourage the use of all available community resources.
5. Women should be counselled about the risks of periconception, antepartum, and postpartum drug use.

Nicotine dependence

6. Smoking cessation counselling should be considered as a first-line intervention for pregnant smokers. Nicotine replacement therapy and/or pharmacotherapy can be considered if counselling is not successful.

Opioid dependence

7. Methadone maintenance treatment should be standard of care for opioid-dependent women during pregnancy. Other slow release opioid preparations may be considered if methadone is not available.
8. Opioid detoxification should be reserved for selected women because of the high risk of relapse to opioids.
9. Opiate-dependent women should be informed that neonates exposed to heroin, prescription opioids, methadone, or buprenorphine during pregnancy are monitored closely for symptoms and signs of neonatal withdrawal (neonatal abstinence syndrome). (II-2B) Hospitals providing obstetric care should develop a protocol for assessment and management of neonates exposed to opiates during pregnancy.

Peripartum pain management

10. Antenatal planning for intrapartum and postpartum analgesia may be offered for all women in consultation with appropriate health care providers.

Breastfeeding

11. The risks and benefits of breastfeeding should be weighed on an individual basis because methadone maintenance therapy is not a contraindication to breastfeeding.

Source: Used with the permission of the Council of the Society of Obstetricians and Gynecologists of Canada, 2014.

benefit from a supportive admission to a non-medical withdrawal management centre, if available. The second phase focuses on relapse prevention by encouraging substance abuse treatment and development of a supportive network.

Pharmacotherapies for Adolescents with Substance-Related Disorders

High-level evidence in support of pharmacotherapy for adolescents with substance-related disorders is sparse.[41] As a consequence, we currently lack comprehensive evidence-based guidance to inform decisions on when to initiate treatment or about which pharmacotherapy confers the greatest benefit and least risk profile for a given psychoactive substance of abuse. An extrapolation from the adult literature may guide future directions in research, but the generalizability to adolescents is cautioned. For strictly short-term detoxification from various substances, such as alcohol, benzodiazepines, barbiturates, and opioids, it may be reasonable to assume that the same closely followed protocols in adults would also be applicable to adolescents, as long as consent for such treatment is obtained.[42] Despite the current paucity of evidence, recently published case reports and uncontrolled studies support the call for controlled investigations that would evaluate pharmacotherapy efficacy safety and tolerability, potential for abuse, possible interactions with other medications, and factors related to patient compliance.[43,44,45]

LO3 Behavioural and Psychosocial Treatments

Many early theories of substance dependence were based primarily on studying alcohol-dependent individuals, so it should come as no surprise that the history of behavioural and psychosocial treatment approaches also began with the treatment of alcohol dependence. However, most behavioural and psychosocial treatment programs today are not designed for a particular substance but treat a variety of types of substance dependence. Here, we present some behavioural and psychosocial treatment approaches often used in helping individuals deal with their substance abuse problems.

Defining Treatment Goals

The particular theoretical view a person has of substance abuse influences not only the treatment approaches that person is likely to take but also the goals of treatment. For example, if someone accepts the increasingly predominant view of alcohol dependence as a biological disease, which someone either has or does not have and which has an inevitable progression to more and more drinking, then the only acceptable treatment goal is total **abstinence**. Other experts view alcohol dependence as representing one end of a continuum of drinking, with no clear dividing line. For some of these theorists, a possible beneficial outcome of treatment is **controlled use**. Likewise, if someone views opioid dependence as inherently evil, undermining the physical and mental health of its victims (a common view until fairly recently), then abstinence from opioids is the only acceptable goal. North Americans seem to have accepted dependence on the legal opioid methadone as preferable to heroin dependence, so the goal has changed from eliminating opioid use to eliminating heroin use. The case with cigarette smoking is similar; some programs have focused on cutting down on smoking, whereas most programs aim for complete abstinence.

When we look for indicators of a treatment program's success, if we find that some people are still using, but using less, should we claim any benefit? Or should we assume, as some do, that any decreases will be temporary and that, unless the person quits entirely, there has been no real improvement? Although the answer depends on your goals, the DSM-5 (see Chapter 1) can provide a useful guide for answering this question. Researchers have begun to estimate the cost savings resulting from increased employment and decreased crime after treatment, and to compare these savings with the cost of treatment itself, to develop a cost-benefit analysis of the effectiveness of treatment.

abstinence: no alcohol or drug use at all.

controlled use: the idea that substance abusers may be able to use the substance under control.

stages of change: a model for decision making consisting of precontemplation, contemplation, preparation, action, maintenance, and relapse.

Motivational Enhancement Therapy

For many years, the predominant theories on why people seek treatment for substance abuse were based on the anecdotal experiences of alcohol-dependent individuals. According to the conventional wisdom, most substance abusers use the defence mechanism of *denial* and are obstinately unwilling to admit either that their substance use is unusual or that it has serious consequences for them or others. In this context, only when the abuser "hits bottom"—that is, suffers sufficient consequences that the reality of the problem finally sinks in—will he or she be ready to seek help. The obvious problem with this perspective is that grave consequences (e.g., death) may occur before the abuser's perception of "hitting bottom."

One relatively new treatment approach, motivational enhancement therapy, attempts to shift the focus away from denial and toward motivation to change.[46] The idea is that targeting the abuser's degree of motivation to quit substance use could enhance the effectiveness of treatment. Hence, ambivalent or less ready substance abusers should first receive *motivational interviewing*. During this nonconfrontational process, an assessment of the substance-using behaviour and its consequences is completed to determine the abuser's current **stage of change** because, according to this view, to help someone move from one stage to another through motivational interviewing, you need to know where he or she is in the decision-making process. In the *precontemplation* stage, the individual does not recognize that a problem exists. In the *contemplation* stage, the individual believes that a problem might exist and gives some consideration to the possibility of changing her or his behaviour. In the *preparation* stage, the individual decides to change and makes plans to do so. In the *action* stage, the individual takes active steps toward change, such as entering treatment. The *maintenance* stage involves activities intended to maintain the change. The motivational interviewer attempts to help the client focus on the concerns and problem behaviour but does not directly tell the client what to do. Ideally, if the therapist knows which stage of change the client is in, the discussion can be guided appropriately to help move the client to the next stage. Although this approach has been demonstrated to decrease substance use,[47] it is probably best conceptualized as a preparation for other therapies rather than as a stand-alone treatment. Finally, *relapse* is an expected part of the process; individuals can cycle and recycle through the stages. These stages are discussed in more detail below.

Contingency Management

A behavioural approach to treating substance abuse that has received substantial attention in recent years is *contingency management*. This approach has produced consistent reductions in substance-using behaviours among diverse substance-abusing populations.[48] In this approach, individuals receive immediate rewards (e.g., vouchers redeemable for goods or services) for providing drug-free urine samples, and the value of the rewards is increased with consecutive drug-free urine samples. However, rewards are withheld if the client's urine sample is positive for an illicit drug. In addition to receiving rewards, clients participate in counselling sessions weekly, where they learn a variety of skills to help them minimize substance use. A weakness of contingency management is the cost of the rewards, which could preclude the use of this procedure by small, less well-funded treatment programs. Another criticism of this approach is that some people think it is unfair to those who "do the right thing" by not taking drugs to see drug users being paid to abstain from drug use.

Ken Silverman and his colleagues at Johns Hopkins University conducted a series of innovative studies to address these issues.[49] These researchers developed a "therapeutic workplace" in which contingency management was used to train drug users for jobs in data entry. Study participants attended the therapeutic workplace for three hours a day during the workweek. Each day, when participants came to work, they were required to submit a urine sample. If it was negative, they were allowed to work that day. After their shift, they received a $7 voucher on the first day, and this amount was increased by $0.50 for each consecutive drug-free day, to a maximum of $27 per day. If a participant submitted a drug positive urine sample or failed to attend the workplace on a scheduled workday, voucher values were reset back to $7.

Participants were also paid as they were taught basic jobs skills, being paid for punctuality, professional demeanour, successful learning, and productivity. Importantly, Silverman and his colleagues used repeated quizzes to ensure that participants clearly understood the procedures, thereby increasing the probability that the vouchers would have their intended effects. In total, over the course of six months, participants could earn a maximum of $4030 in vouchers (or about $168 per week). The data showed that 40% of the participants in the contingency management group had drug-free results on 75% or more of testing occasions; in contrast, only 10% of the control group did so. While there are multiple benefits to this line of research, one of the most important is that participants' drug-taking behaviours are being replaced with employable skills. In this way, these programs ultimately pay for themselves as many who were formerly unemployable become taxpaying workers.

Relapse Prevention

Another behavioural strategy is called relapse prevention, an approach that uses cognitive-therapy techniques with behavioural-skills training. Individuals learn to identify and change behaviours that may lead to continued drug use, such as going out to bars or associating with users. Relapse prevention has been shown to be more effective at decreasing substance use than most standard psychotherapies, and the beneficial effects persist for as long as a year following treatment.[50] This approach is criticized for placing greater demands on the patients compared with other substance abuse treatments, and it may be particularly challenging for individuals who have cognitive limitations.[51] However, findings from a recent critical review of cognitive functioning of methamphetamine abusers suggest that this assumption should be reevaluated.[52] For example, the dominant view had been that cognitive impairments seen in this group compromised their ability to engage in, and benefit from, cognitive-behavioural therapy. The results from the review made a convincing case that such concerns are not warranted. Perhaps this is why cognitive-behavioural therapy remains one of the most effective and widely used substance-abuse treatment strategies.

Transtheoretical Model (Stages of Change) and Substance Abuse Treatment

In recent years there has been growing interest in processes purported to support intentional behaviour change. Numerous studies have attempted to outline the behaviour change processes, and perhaps the best known, and debated, theory was proposed by Prochaska and DiClemente. These researchers, in 1983, proposed the transtheoretical model (TTM) of behaviour change, which is the stages-of-change model described above. The TTM became widely viewed as a guide for clinical interventions across a range of health problems, including substance-related disorders.[53] The stages of change, defined below, include precontemplation, contemplation, preparation, action, maintenance, and relapse. The model attempts to outline behavioural change by defining the tasks, steps, experiences, contexts, and main processes through which change occurs. It also attempts to define success: In each phase of the change, success is associated with task accomplishment, which promotes engagement with the targets in the subsequent phase.

Inherent to the TTM is the premise that intentional change does not occur at a specific moment. The model recognizes that each person will have different experiences prior to and during their change processes and that these experiences will affect the time it takes to move through the defined stages. Another premise is that behavioural change can be dissected into four components: stage, processes, context, and signs of change, and that the signs of change have objective and subjective aspects. Movements through stages are cyclical, with persons moving into and out of earlier or later stages until achieving behavioural consistency and stability (see Figure 18.1). One caution with the TTM noted by Prochaska and

Figure 18.1 Stages of Change in Addiction

In this circular representation of the stages of change, the preparation stage is referred to as the decision stage.

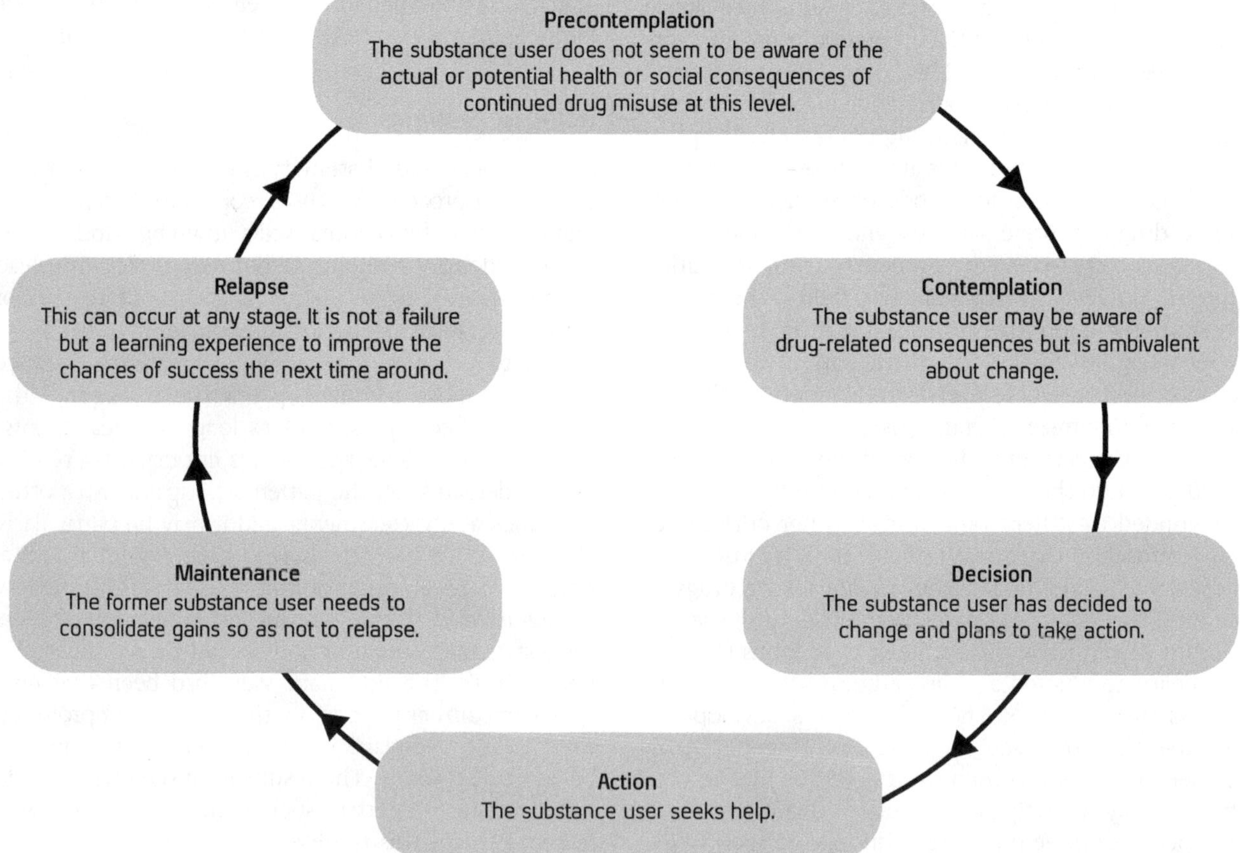

Source: InnovAiT by Royal College of General Practitioners Reproduced with permission of OXFORD UNIVERSITY PRESS in the format republish in a book/journal via Copyright Clearance Center.

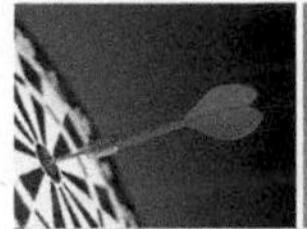

TARGETING PREVENTION

Avoiding Relapse

One important type of substance abuse prevention involves those who have been in treatment and are trying to avoid relapsing, or going back to their previously abusive behaviour. Think about the messages these people receive each day from public media (such as television, movies, newspapers, and the Web) and from other individuals. Which of these messages support relapse prevention and which tend to encourage relapse? Have a conversation with a friend, relative, or classmate who has been in treatment for substance abuse and has had to deal with the problem of relapse prevention. Ask what was helpful for him or her and what made it more difficult to avoid substance abuse.

DiClemente is that their description of the process of behaviour change is derived from their own clinical cases, observations, and practices and therefore may not be not generalizable.[54]

- *Precontemplation:* In this stage there is no intention to change the behaviour. Individuals may still not realize that their behaviour is a problem, or they have minimized it thereby avoiding the reality of their situation and their need for change. As such, during the *precontemplation* stage the main goal is for the person to come to the realization that a problem exists and that a habitual pattern of behaviour needs to be changed.
- *Contemplation:* In this stage change comes under consideration, albeit without a commitment to action. For many individuals ambivalence will be an important impediment. Before a person can begin to contemplate change they must first come to realize that the benefits resulting from the considered changes might exceed the benefits of the problem behaviour. In other words, they must justify, to themselves, why change is beneficial. Once this has occurred the person may be ready for transition to the next stage, *preparation.* Clinically, to support people in transitioning to the next stage, a therapist might focus on motivating them to act on their decision and to envision the benefits that might occur. Assisting persons in the development of self-evaluation and self-efficacy is also considered important at this stage.
- *Preparation:* During the *preparation* stage a commitment to action is made. Tasks to be accomplished include strengthening the commitment to change and establishing a realistic action plan for making change happen. Clinically, support generally involves assisting the person in the identification of an approach to change that is best suited (contextualized) to them.
- *Action:* In the *action* stage the first steps toward modification of previous behavioural patterns are taken. During this stage it is important that the individual becomes engaged and adopts a new attitude. Over a period of time, new behavioural patterns should be developed, in accordance with the action plan.
- *Maintenance:* The *maintenance* stage focuses on sustaining and integrating new habits. Goals of this stage include avoiding relapses and consolidation of gains made in the *action* stage. For a behaviour to be considered established it must be executable without the need for excessive energy or effort to maintain it. *Maintenance* is a continual process.
- *Relapse:* Relapse is an inherent part of the change process and therefore it is not considered unusual if a person goes back and forth among stages. During relapses the persons should be supported in returning to the previous plan. Recognition of their self-efficacy and regaining confidence are important in this stage.

Description of transformation are often depicted in a circle (Figure 18.1) as this is believed to more accurately represents the reality of change, accounting for evolution through the stages as well as for the possibility of relapse.

Harm Reduction

In its broadest sense, harm reduction is a set of practical ideas and strategies aimed at reducing negative consequences associated with drug use.[55] It is guided by a number of principles that collectively support the development of pragmatic responses to dealing with drug use through interventions that place primary emphasis on reducing the health-related harms of continued drug use.[56,57] In Canada harm reduction is often defined as encompassing a range of interventions, policies, and programs that seek to reduce the health, social, and economic harms of drug use to individuals, communities, and societies. In practice, harm reduction is a *combination intervention,* comprising multiple selected interventions, tailored to local settings and needs, and aimed at reducing the harms of drug use. It is important to note that harm reduction approaches neither exclude nor presume a treatment goal of abstinence. Abstinence-oriented interventions can, and often do, fall within the hierarchy of harm reduction goals. In relation to reducing the harms of injecting drug use, for example, a combination of interventions might include needle and syringe programs, opioid substitution treatment, counselling services, the provision of drug consumption rooms, peer education and outreach, and the promotion of public policies conducive to protecting the health of populations at risk.[58] Selected examples of harm reduction programs and policies include:

- Syringe (needle) exchanges
- Methadone maintenance treatment programs
- Other pharmacological treatments for reducing illicit and/or harmful drug use (i.e., stimulants)
- Education and outreach programs
- "Tolerance areas" including safe injection sites and safe dealing areas
- Marijuana policies (e.g., promoting the de facto decriminalization of possession of small amounts of cannabis)

In the words of one expert:

> Harm reduction, in the final analysis, is concerned with ensuring the quality and integrity of human life, in all its wonderful, awful complexity. Harm reduction does not portray issues as polarities, but sees them as they really are, somewhere in between; it is an approach that takes into account the continuum of drug use and the diversity of drugs as well as of human needs. As such, there are no clear-cut answers or quick solutions. Harm reduction, then, is based on pragmatism, tolerance and diversity: in short, it is both a product and a measure of our humanity. Harm reduction is as much about human rights as it is about the right to be human.[55]

As we discovered above, one of the earliest harm reduction programs was methadone maintenance treatment, which began in the 1960s. Today methadone maintenance treatment programs are ascribed to the reduction of many harms. Some harm reduction programs were designed with the specific intent to reduce criminal activity associated with acquiring heroin or prescription opioids and to eventually help drug users to re-enter society and the workforce. One such program, often cited as providing the earliest evidence of effectiveness in decreasing crime rates, was developed by the Merseyside police force in the United Kingdom.[59] The success of that program is believed to lie in the fact that in the Mersey Region, services follow a philosophy that you can still care for drug users even if you cannot "cure" them. Dispensed through local pharmacists, drug users receive oral methadone, injectable methadone, injectable heroin, amphetamines, cocaine, or other drugs. By leading in the development of cooperative harm reduction strategies the Merseyside police have improved the prevention and treatment of drug problems in their jurisdiction.

Switzerland was the first country to prescribe heroin for harm reduction purposes. Between 1994 and 1996 a number of Swiss heroin users were treated in this manner. The initiative resulted in a decrease in cocaine and heroin use, a decrease in crime, and an improvement in users' physical and mental health.[60] This initiative began with 700 dependent drug users across eight cities, but was later expanded to include 1146 people in seven cities. The cost of operation was US$13 per day.[61] The initiative provided participants with medical access to injectable, oral, and in some cases smokeable heroin, morphine, and methadone, and under some conditions cocaine.[62] In addition to opioids, participants were also offered clean syringes, lodging, assistance in finding employment, medical treatment, and counselling. Program administrators did not place strict limits on dosages but did provide information on what constituted typical doses of cocaine in dependent users. Evaluation of the study suggested the following benefits to participants:

- Their housing situation rapidly improved and stabilized (in particular, there were no longer any homeless).
- Fitness for work improved substantially: Permanent employment rates more than doubled (from 14% to 32%), and the number of unemployed fell by more than half (from 44% to 20%).

- Income from illegal and semi-legal activities declined from 59% to 10%.
- Both the number of offenders and the number of criminal offences decreased 60% within the first six months of treatment (based on information obtained directly from the patients and from police records).[63]

Heroin assisted treatment was implemented in Switzerland in response to finding that many drug users were not responding to traditional abstinence-based treatments. Based upon British practices clients who were chronically dependent, who suffered from health and social problems as a consequence of their dependence, and who were unsuccessful in at least two alternative treatment programs were accepted for participation in the heroin assisted treatment program.[64]

Drug policy in the Netherlands has focused on reducing the risks that drug use poses for the drug users themselves, their immediate environment, and society as a whole. One misconception is that soft drugs are legal in the Netherlands. They are not. However, contrary to most countries Dutch police do not seek to detect possession of drugs for personal use or for selling or possessing up to 5 grams of cannabis products. Furthermore, in many of Dutch cities there is undisturbed sale of marijuana in coffee shops, where the use of alcohol and hard drugs is not allowed. Dutch authorities do however monitor coffee shops and youth centres where marijuana trade occurs to ensure that there is no sale of large quantities, no sale of other drugs, no advertisements, no encouragement to use, and no sale to minors.[59] Other programs have been developed in the Netherlands to address the public nuisance caused by hard drug users. These programs, developed in the 1990s, were in response to findings that 20% of the hard drug users were involved in petty crime and disorderly conduct. Among other things, the program included the development of better shelter facilities for problem addicts. Municipalities and addiction organizations assumed primary responsibility for implementing the program.[65]

In summary, European cities in which harm reduction measures have been implemented have proven such policies and programs capable of reducing overall harms to society from drug use. Amsterdam officials have estimated that they are saving US$40 per person with harm reduction measures.

Described in Chapter 13, the supervised injection facility (SIF) Insite, located in the Downtown Eastside of Vancouver, was the first SIF in North America. SIFs gained recognition in the 1980s in response to growing incidents of public injecting, drug overdoses, and sharing of syringes and injection equipment (which account for a large portion of people affected by hepatitis C, HIV, or AIDS).[66] Opened in 2003, Insite represents one of Canada's most innovative and controversial harm reduction programs. An exemption to Health Canada's Controlled Drugs and Substances Act permits Insite's operation despite the fact that users inject pre-obtained illicit drugs at the facility. Injection drug users are supported by nurse educators who provide guidance on issues related to injection health and safety (e.g., showing drug users how to find a vein and tie off properly; showing them how to heat the solution to dissolve solid constituents and filter properly; showing them how to inject safely; and giving them information about safer injecting).[67] The Health Canada exemption was based upon the expectation that research would be done to evaluate Insite's effectiveness. Included within the research infrastructure for Insite is an onsite database for tracking activities and health-related events at the facility. Insite users are registered anonymously and provide basic demographic information. Also collected are data pertaining to all overdoses and interventions that occur at Insite.[68] For example, between March 1, 2004, and August 30, 2005, there were 336 overdose events, revealing an average rate of 1.33 overdoses per 1000 injections.[69] Further analysis revealed that 285 unique participants accounted for these overdoses. Data pertaining to drugs involved in the overdoses were available for 318 (95%) cases and included:

- Heroin (71% of overdoses, or 201 of 318 cases)
- Cocaine (13% of overdoses)
- Speedballs (10% of overdose cases)
- Morphine (2% of overdose cases)
- Dilaudid (1.7% of overdose cases)
- Crack (1.4% of overdose cases)
- Methadone (0.7% of overdose)

It is important to note none of the above described overdoses resulted in a fatality.

The effects of Insite on new HIV infection and deaths has also been evaluated. Using mathematical models and secondary data analysis researchers compared the cost of illness and death prevented against

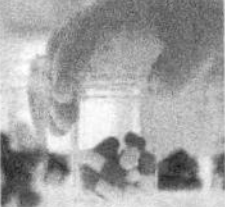

DRUGS IN THE MEDIA

Insite Survives 10 Years On: Supervised Injection Site Opened as Three-Year Experiment Sept. 21, 2003

The procedure is hard to watch: A 52-year-old woman takes a syringe filled with heroin and carefully inserts it into a vein in the side of her neck. As she pulls out the syringe, she checks herself in the mirror and notices a trickle of blood coming from the tiny wound. She wipes it with a sterile pad and she's done.

Gail Hunt is high.

She will complete the same procedure at least twice more on this day. And she will do it in the Insite supervised injection site, where she's been a client for nine years. "It's safe and if anything happens to me, there's trained professionals here who can help," she said, sitting in an injection booth last Thursday at the facility on East Hastings. "I've watched people go down in front of me—overdose—and the staff are there right away. We haven't lost one person in here."

Hunt, who began using heroin to mask the pain from breast cancer, is a regular at Insite, which marks its 10th anniversary of operation this month. The facility's longevity is a remarkable feat considering it originally opened Sept. 21, 2003 as a three-year scientific experiment. Ten years later, and after more than two million injections without an overdose death, Insite continues to be the only legal site of its kind in North America.

But keeping the facility's doors open has been a battle.

Prime Minister Stephen Harper and his government want Insite closed and fought unsuccessfully in the courts to shut down the service. Despite a Supreme Court of Canada ruling in 2011 to allow Insite to operate indefinitely, the Harper government tabled a bill in June aimed at making it difficult for Insite to renew its licence in 2014. The bill, called the Respect for Communities Act and supported by the Canadian Police Association, sets out a long list of criteria that critics say also dissuades other cities from applying for an exemption under the country's drug laws to open an injection site. The

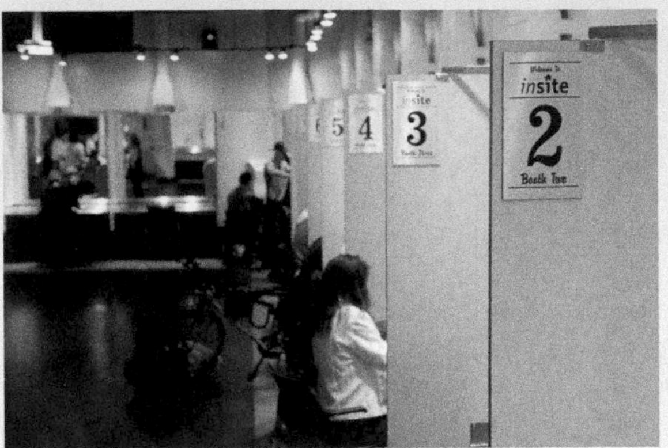

Insite opened as three-year experiment on Sept. 21, 2003.
Used with permission of the Vancouver Courier. Photo courtesy of Dan Toulgoet

federal government's campaign against Insite and advocates of injection sites comes despite a series of peer-reviewed studies showing the facility is doing some good for people.

Studies published in various medical journals including *The Lancet* and *The New England Journal of Medicine* concluded Insite saves lives and health care dollars, reduces disease transmission and does not increase crime or perpetuate active drug use. Additionally, a recent Vancouver Coastal Health report revealed Downtown Eastside residents, a portion of whom are addicts, are living longer—from a life expectancy of 69.4 years in 1996 to 79.9 in 2012.

For 62-year-old drug user Larry Love, who also visited Insite last Thursday to inject himself with heroin, the alternative to a supervised injection site is not something he wants to think about. He remembers the mid-1990s when upwards of 200 people per year died of drug overdoses in Vancouver. If Insite closed, he said, the city would "look like hell again."

"I just couldn't imagine if this place wasn't open, I just couldn't imagine it," said Love, overlooking the facility's injection booths busy with people getting their next fix.

Source: Used with permission of the Vancouver Courier.

the cost to run the SIF. Considered within the cost-benefit analysis were such factors as Insite's operational cost ($1.5 million), costs associated with individual HIV infection treatment ($150 000), and the loss to society for each new HIV infection ($500 000) and fatal overdose ($660 000). By combining HIV and fatal overdoses, the number of potential deaths prevented by Insite was 2.87, as well as 35 prevented new HIV infections each year.[70]

Collectively, such data suggest that SIF may serve an effective role in managing overdoses among injection drug users and highlight the need for further investigation of their impact of injection related infections and deaths.

LO4 Substance Abuse in Canada: Concurrent Disorders

The term *concurrent disorder* is used to describe conditions in which a person has both a mental health and a substance-related disorder. Concurrent disorders are a major health issue worldwide. Individuals with concurrent disorders are among the most complex and difficult to treat, often experiencing frequent relapses and recurring crises. It is not surprising, therefore, that persons with concurrent disorders consume significant health care resources–and account for a large proportion of the costs of care. The complex challenges of this highly vulnerable population cannot be overlooked. Because of their oftentimes limited capacity to cope with everyday challenges and the stigma attached to their conditions–many may have HIV or hepatitis C–persons with concurrent disorders experience higher unemployment, relationship difficulties and social anxiety. At the extreme many become homeless, socially marginalized, or criminally involved.

The first national assessment of the prevalence of concurrent mental health and substance-related disorders in Canada was drawn, via secondary analysis, from the 2002 *Canadian Community Health Survey: Mental Health and Well-Being*. These data have shown that 50% of persons who *seek help* for a substance-related disorder also have a mental health disorder, and 15%–20% of those *seeking help* from mental health services are also living with a substance-related disorder.[71,72] It is important to note, however, that the 12-month population prevalence of concurrent disorders is 1.7%. Although the researchers argued that cross-study comparisons are hampered by methodological differences, these Canadian data are at the lower end of the range reported internationally. This might have resulted from the exclusion of several disorders known to be highly comorbid with SUDs. Worldwide population health surveys of concurrent disorders have demonstrated similar prevalences and collectively support the need for integrated planning and delivery of services.

Canada's mental health and addiction systems are currently independent and compartmentalized. As a result, the focus of treatment for people with concurrent disorders tends to be on one component of their concurrent disorder, but not the other. Seeking a more effective treatment approach to improve overall client outcomes will require a focus on the following areas[71]:

- *Treatment and care:* A unified national approach for the treatment and care of those with concurrent disorders is urgently needed and should include integrated clinical practice guidelines.
- *Education and training:* A common educational platform with new specialized training programs–shared by health professionals from different sectors–needs to be created.
- *Research:* The addictions and mental health communities must come together to effectively seize the resources and momentum necessary to address gaps in research and research funding for concurrent disorders.
- *The system:* Currently, separate national treatment strategies exist in the addictions and mental health fields that highlight system needs and priorities. Integrating these national treatment strategies will go a long way toward developing a unified and coordinated system for addressing concurrent disorders.
- *Developmental considerations:* Because of the developmentally sensitive nature of many concurrent disorders and the fact that onset of substance use is common during adolescence, a focus on youth and early detection is needed.
- *Early detection:* There is a need to ensure that we have practices in place to identify individual and group risk factors early, and to intervene with integrated care programs aimed at preventing concurrent disorders or reducing the severity and progression of the symptoms and harms.

LO5 Treatment and Rehabilitation: The Big Picture in Canada

The delivery of prevention and treatment services for substance-related disorders is primarily the responsibility of Canada's provinces and territories. Canada is a vast nation with diverse social, economic, and political conditions. These differences contribute to a variety of patterns of substance use and variation in approaches to treatment across the country.[73]

In the 1990s, Canada's health care system underwent a dramatic transformation. At that time, most government addiction treatment services were integrated into community health and social services delivery systems. This integration was supported by adoption of a population health model by the provinces, territories, and federal government. This new approach changed the way in which health care services determined the health of populations, giving greater priority to broad socioeconomic factors. These changes were supported by an increased awareness of the need for better integration of substance abuse services into the general health and social support systems and social welfare policy.

The majority of funds for the treatment of substance-related disorders are provided by the provinces and territories. These funds are obtained from local taxes, provincial/territorial health insurance programs, and federal transfers under the Canada Health Act and other federal program opportunities. The Canada Health Act stipulates the criteria for the funding and administration of provincial/territorial health care services. Provinces and territories receive transfer payments to provide insured health services under each jurisdiction's health care insurance plan.[73] The federal government also provides direct funding for treatment and rehabilitation of members of the following groups:

- On-reserve First Nations Peoples and Inuit
- Members of the Royal Canadian Mounted Police (RCMP)
- Members of the Canadian Armed Forces
- Persons serving a term in a federal penitentiary
- Persons who have not lived in a province or territory long enough to receive insured health services

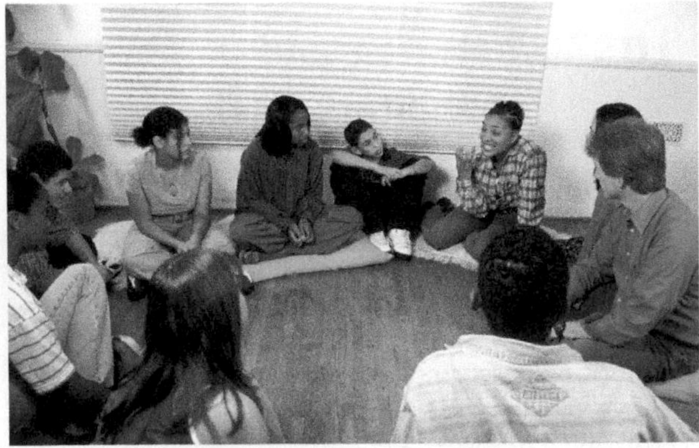

Drug treatment doesn't work for every person every time, but overall, treatment does reduce drug use, reduce associated criminal activity, and increase employment. By continuing to participate in outpatient drug rehabilitation meetings, these teens increase the likelihood that their substance-abuse treatment will be a success over the long term.

Is Treatment Effective?

There is common belief that treatments for substance-related disorders are ineffective. We've all heard about celebrities who have been in treatment programs and are later found to be using illegal drugs. We might also know an alcohol abuser who went into treatment but later began drinking again. Treatment doesn't work for every client every time, especially if our expectation is that a single course of treatment can eliminate the use of the substance for the rest of the person's life. The reality is that substance-related disorders are chronic illnesses and share the characteristics of other chronic illnesses, such as diabetes, hypertension, and asthma. There are no reliable "cures," and all these conditions may require continuing care throughout the client's life.

Do substance-abuse treatment programs have any beneficial effect–and, if they do, are their effects worth the cost? The answer is yes. In general, people who go into treatment fare better than those who do not. We know that people who participate in treatment have lower incidence of involvement in crime, better employment, and better health. One report by the California Department of Alcohol and Drug Programs concluded that, on average, seven dollars are saved for every dollar invested in the treatment of alcohol and other drug abuse.[74] Alcohol and other drug use was reduced by about two-fifths after treatment; treatment for crack cocaine, powder cocaine, and methamphetamine use was equally effective as for alcohol; and criminal activity declined by about two-thirds after treatment.

One report reviewed 53 studies of the effectiveness of substance abuse treatments for adolescents. Overall, most of the treated adolescents had significant reductions in substance use and problems in other life areas in the year following treatment, and an average of 32% remained abstinent at the end of a year. Successful program completion, involvement in outpatient therapy, and the inclusion of the family therapy as one treatment component all appeared to predict success.[75]

Overall, substance abuse treatment can work. It can save lives, save money, and is, therefore, a worthwhile investment.

Alcoholics Anonymous

The formation of Alcoholics Anonymous (AA) in 1935 can now be seen as an important milestone in

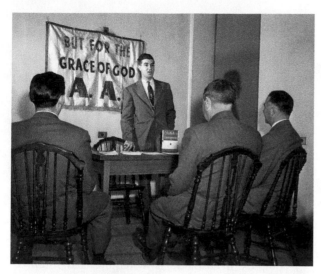

The major approach of Alcoholics Anonymous, founded in 1935, is group support and a buddy system.

treatment. This group, which has total abstinence as a goal, has given support to the disease model of alcohol dependence. One of the basic tenets of this group is that the "alcoholic" is biologically different from others and therefore can never safely drink any alcohol. Central to this disease model is the idea that the disease takes away the person's control of his or her own drinking behaviour and therefore removes the blame for the problem. AA members are quick to point out that removing blame for the disease does not remove responsibility for dealing with it. By analogy, we would not blame people with diabetes for having the disease, but we do expect people with diabetes to control their diets, take their medication, and so on. Thus, the alcohol-dependent person is seen as having the responsibility for managing the disease on a day-by-day basis but need not feel guilty about being different. The major approach used by AA has been group support and a buddy system. The members of AA help each other through difficult periods and encourage each other in their sobriety. Currently AA estimates membership in Canada and the United States to be over 1.3 million members and welcomes anyone interested in AA's program of recovery to attend open meetings in their community.

Although AA has been described as a loose affiliation of local groups, each with its own character, they have in common adherence to a method. Nevertheless, formal evaluations of the success of AA have been few and have not been very positive. For example, studies of court-ordered referrals to AA or to other types of interventions have not shown AA to be more effective. However, AA was developed by and for people

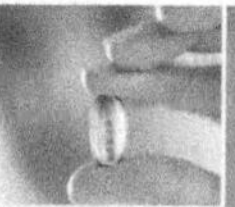

DRUGS IN DEPTH

The 12 Steps of Alcoholics Anonymous

1. We admitted we were powerless over alcohol—that our lives had become unmanageable.
2. Came to believe that a Power greater than ourselves could restore us to sanity.
3. Made a decision to turn our will and our lives over to the care of God *as we understand Him.*
4. Made a searching and fearless moral inventory of ourselves.
5. Admitted to God, to ourselves, and to another human being the exact nature of our wrongs.
6. Were entirely ready to have God remove all these defects of character.
7. Humbly asked Him to remove our shortcomings.
8. Made a list of all persons we had harmed and became willing to make amends to them all.
9. Made direct amends to such people wherever possible, except when to do so would injure them or others.
10. Continued to take moral inventory and when we were wrong promptly admitted it.
11. Sought through prayer and meditation to improve our conscious contact with God *as we understand Him* praying only for knowledge of His will for us and the power to carry that out.
12. Having had a spiritual awakening as the result of these steps, we tried to carry this message to alcoholics, and to practice these principles in all our affairs.

Source: The Twelve Steps are reprinted with permission of Alcoholics Anonymous World Services, Inc. Permission to reprint the Twelve Steps does not mean that AA has reviewed or approved the contents of this publication, nor that AA agrees with the views expressed herein. AA is a program of recovery from alcoholism *only*—use of the Twelve Steps in connection with programs and activities which are patterned after AA, but which address other problems, or in any other non-AA context, does not imply otherwise.

who have made a personal decision to stop drinking and who want to affiliate with others who have made that decision, and it might not be the most appropriate approach for individuals who are coerced into attending meetings as an alternative to jail. More appropriate (and more difficult and expensive) evaluations of AA should be done to determine which types of drinkers are most likely to benefit from this organization's program.

This point is particularly important because many treatment programs, such as the Betty Ford Center, Hazelden, and Phoenix House, rely mostly on the 12-step model of AA (see the Drugs in Depth box). Moreover, a wide variety of other self-help groups, including Cocaine Anonymous (CA), Narcotics Anonymous (NA), and Gamblers Anonymous (GA), have modelled the AA treatment approach.

LO6 A Systems Approach to Substance Use in Canada

In 2008 the National Treatment Strategy Working Group released a document entitled *A Systems Approach to Substance Use in Canada: Recommendations for a National Treatment Strategy*. This document was intended to provide recommendations for improving the quality, accessibility, and range of services and supports that address risks and harms associated with substance-related disorders and addiction. The strategy proposes the adoption of a "tiered" model for organizing services and supports and comprises five tiers. Each tier represents a cluster of services and supports that offer similar levels of eligibility, address problems of similar severity, and that are of similar intensity and specialization.

Services and supports associated with the lower tiers (Tiers 1 and 2) would have open eligibility criteria and be intended to meet the needs of a greater number of people than those in the more specialized upper tiers. Lower-tier services and supports are not focused exclusively on substance use, are integrated into communities, and are of relatively low intensity and cost. The intention is that such services would be available in most communities. People typically seeking services and supports in these lower tiers might include:

- Those at risk for developing substance-related disorders and addictions
- Those currently experiencing substance use problems but of low severity (i.e., low acuity, low chronicity, and low complexity)
- Those who have higher level needs but who, by choice, seek help from services in a lower tier (e.g., their physician, Tier 2) rather than specialized treatment program associated with upper tiers (Tier 4 or Tier 5)
- Those who have in the past required services and supports associated with the upper tiers, for more complex needs, but now require less intensive supports to maintain their well-being

Services and supports associated with the upper tiers (Tiers 4 and 5) are designed to meet the needs of smaller numbers of people, are highly specialized and intensive, and address the needs of people with more severe substance-related disorders (i.e., high acuity, high chronicity, or high complexity). Consequently, such services and supports are more costly than those in the lower tiers.

Eligibility to use services in the upper tiers is oftentimes based on more structured admission criteria and may require a referral. Because of lower demand, higher cost, and the need for specialized training, such services and supports are frequently harder to provide than services and supports associated with the lower tiers (i.e., they are provided in fewer communities). These challenges oftentimes leave those in need of higher level care at a disadvantage.

A premise of the tiered model is that no two individuals' needs and wants are alike and that no person's needs or wants stays the same over time. As a result, individuals do not reside within a given tier but instead, at different points in one's life, may seek services and supports from different tiers, sequentially or simultaneously. The pathway a client takes within the proposed system is inherently client-centred.[76]

Summary

- The rapid-onset benzodiazepine diazepam is the pharmacological treatment of choice to effectively manage alcohol withdrawal symptoms.
- Alcohol withdrawal symptoms include anxiety, nausea and vomiting, tremors, paroxysmal sweat, agitation, tactile, auditory and visual disturbances, headaches, orientation, and clouding of sensorium and are potentially life-threatening.
- Five nicotine-replacement therapies have been approved by Health Canada to treat nicotine dependence: the transdermal nicotine patch, nicotine gum, the nicotine vapour inhaler, nicotine spray, and nicotine lozenges. These therapies have been demonstrated to increase quit rates in controlled clinical studies conducted under fairly strict clinical research conditions. Therefore, the average person might have difficulties quitting even with the aid of nicotine-replacement medications.
- In 1998 bupropion (Zyban) became the first non-nicotine pharmacotherapy for smoking cessation approved by Health Canada. Although bupropion's mechanism is not currently understood in treating nicotine dependence, the action most commonly attributed is its ability to inhibit dopamine and norepinephrine reuptake. Bupropion has been shown to gradually decrease cigarette craving and use in some clinical trials.
- Methadone alleviates the symptoms of opioid withdrawal and decreases the chronic craving for opioids. The advantage of using methadone for maintenance purposes is that it is orally active and has a long half-life. Once-a-day dosing prevents the onset of opioid withdrawal for 24-36 hours.
- Tolerance to the effects of methadone for maintenance purposes develops very gradually. As a result, many individuals can be maintained on the same dose of methadone for many years.
- Buprenorphine is an opioid agonist/antagonist or partial agonist at the mu receptor. Suboxone (a combination of buprenorphine and naloxone) was approved by Health Canada in 2007 and is available for substitution treatment in opioid drug dependence in adults.
- Suboxone is a tablet that dissolves under the tongue, suppressing the symptoms of opioid withdrawal and reducing the cravings for opioid drugs.
- Buprenorphine helps to manage the cravings associated with opioid withdrawal while the naloxone component reduces the potential for misuse by causing unpleasant withdrawal symptoms if the product is misused by intravenous injection.
- The Society of Obstetricians and Gynecologists of Canada developed clinical practice guidelines for substance use in pregnancy. The guidelines are intended to increase the knowledge and comfort level of health care providers caring for pregnant women who have substance use disorders.
- There are two phases to the management of substance use disorders during pregnancy. Pregnant women dependent on alcohol, opioids, or high-dose benzodiazepines may require medical detoxification under the supervision of a physician. The second phase focuses on relapse prevention by encouraging substance abuse treatment and development of a supportive network.
- The transtheoretical model (TTM) defines intentional change as a process that does not occur at a specific moment but is sensitive to the dynamic changes that an individual presents over time in terms of a motivational stage.
- The six stages of TTM are precontemplation (no intention to change the behaviour in the upcoming six months), contemplation (change under consideration but without a commitment to action), preparation (commitment to action), action (the first step toward modification of previous patterns), maintenance (sustaining and integrating new habits), and relapse (cycling back through the stages).
- Dividing the process of behaviour change into stages results in some arbitrariness since the limits of each phase were derived from the researchers' background in terms of clinical observation and practice.
- Harm reduction encompasses interventions, programs, and policies that seek to reduce the health, social, and economic harms of drug use to individuals, communities, and societies.
- A core principle of harm reduction is the development of pragmatic responses to dealing with drug use through a hierarchy of intervention goals that place primary emphasis on reducing the health-related harms of continued drug use. Harm reduction approaches neither exclude nor presume a treatment goal of abstinence, and this means that abstinence-oriented interventions can also fall within the hierarchy of harm reduction goals.
- Examples of harm reduction programs and policies include, but are not limited to, syringe exchange programs, methadone maintenance

treatment programs, tolerance areas (such as safe injection facilities), and marijuana policies, such as de facto decriminalization of small amounts of cannabis.

- The term *concurrent disorder* refers to individuals who have both a mental health and a substance use problem, and it is a major health issue in Canada. Individuals experiencing mental health and substance use problems concurrently are some of the most complex and difficult people to treat, with frequent relapses and recurring crises tending to be the norm.
- The 12-month prevalence of alcohol use problems among people with other mental disorders was about twice that of people with no other mental disorders, while the rate of illicit drug problems was three times higher based upon data from the 2002 *Canadian Community Health Survey: Mental Health and Well-Being*.
- The 12-month prevalence of other mental disorders among those with substance problems was two to three times greater than among those without substance problems. When illicit drugs are considered separately, the prevalence of co-occurring mental disorders was three to four times higher relative to those without drug problems based upon data from the 2002 *Canadian Community Health Survey: Mental Health and Well-Being*.
- Across all disorders, women were more likely than men to have a co-occurring mental disorder. Most notably, one-third of women with illicit drug use problems met criteria for a mood or anxiety disorder based upon data from the 2002 *Canadian Community Health Survey: Mental Health and Well-Being*.
- Canada's mental health and addiction systems are currently independent and compartmentalized. As a result, the focus of treatment for people with concurrent disorders tends to be on only one component of their concurrent disorder. Seeking a more effective treatment approach to improve overall client outcomes requires a focus on treatment and care, education and training, research, the system, developmental considerations, and early detection.
- The formation of Alcoholics Anonymous (AA) in 1935 can now be seen as an important milestone in treatment. This group, which has total abstinence as a goal, has given support to the disease model of alcohol dependence. One of the basic tenets of this group is that an alcoholic is biologically different from others and therefore can never safely drink any alcohol.
- Central to this disease model is the idea that the disease takes away the person's control of his or her own drinking behaviour and therefore removes the blame for the problem. AA members are quick to point out that removing blame for the disease does not remove responsibility for dealing with it.
- Although AA has been described as a loose affiliation of local groups, each with its own character, they have in common adherence to a method. Nevertheless, formal evaluations of the success of AA have been few and have not been very positive. However, AA was developed by and for people who have made a personal decision to stop drinking and who want to affiliate with others who have made that decision; it might not be the most appropriate approach for individuals who are coerced into attending meetings as an alternative to jail.
- *A Systems Approach to Substance Use in Canada: Recommendations for a National Treatment Strategy* is a comprehensive, collaborative report that provides direction and recommendations for improving the quality, accessibility, and range of services and supports to address risks and harms associated with substance use in Canada.
- The strategy proposes the adoption of a tiered model for organizing services and supports to address substance use problems. The model comprises five tiers, representing groupings of services and supports. Each tier is not an entity point per se, but rather a cluster of services and supports that offer similar levels of access or eligibility, that address problems of similar severity and that are of similar intensity and specialization.
- A key premise of the tiered model is that no two people—or their needs and wants—are alike, and indeed that no one person—or his or her needs or wants—stays the same over time. Rather, at given points in life, a person may seek services and supports from one or more tiers, sequentially or simultaneously. Pathways through the tiered system are thus individualized and inherently client-centred.

Review Questions

1. Give one example of a medication used for each therapeutic approach: agonist/substitution therapy, antagonist therapy, and punishment therapy.

2. What drugs are typically used to reduce and manage withdrawal symptoms during alcohol detoxification?
3. Compare and contrast the use of disulfiram with either naltrexone or acamprosate for alcohol dependence.
4. How are methadone and buprenorphine-naloxone similar to each other and different from naltrexone as treatments for opioid dependence?
5. List five types of approved nicotine-replacement therapies in Canada
6. Describe the kinds of contingencies used in contingency management: What happens if the client has several clean urine samples in a row? What happens if the client fails one of the urine sample tests?
7. Name and describe the six stages of the transtheoretical model (stages of change).
8. What is harm reduction? List some examples of harm reduction programs or policies.
9. What is the 12-month prevalence of alcohol use problems among people with other mental disorders? What is the prevalence of illicit drug problems?
10. List the 12 steps of Alcoholics Anonymous.
11. What are the five tiers of the systems approach to substance use in Canada? Describe their feature(s).

GLOSSARY

A

abstinence: no alcohol or drug use at all.

abuse: the use of a substance in a manner, amounts, or situations such that the drug use causes problems or greatly increases the chances of problems occurring. The problems may be social (including legal), occupational, psychological, or physical.

acetaminophen: an Aspirin-like analgesic and antipyretic.

acetylcholine: neurotransmitter found in the parasympathetic branch in the cerebral cortex.

acetylsalicylic acid: the chemical known as Aspirin.

action potential: the electrical signal transmitted along the axon when a neuron fires.

active metabolite: a metabolite that has drug actions of its own.

acute: referring to drugs, the short-term effects of a single dose.

addiction: a chronic relapsing condition characterized by compulsive drug seeking and abuse and by long-lasting chemical changes in the brain.

adenosine: an inhibitory neurotransmitter through which caffeine acts.

ADHD: attention-deficit/hyperactivity disorder.

agonist: a substance that facilitates or mimics the effects of a neurotransmitter on the postsynaptic cell.

AIDS: acquired immune deficiency syndrome.

Alcoholics Anonymous (AA): a worldwide organization of self-help groups based on alcoholics helping one another achieve and maintain sobriety.

alternatives: alternative nondrug activities, such as relaxation exercises or dancing.

amphetamine: a synthetic CNS stimulant and sympathomimetic.

anabolic: promoting constructive metabolism; building tissue.

anandamide: a chemical isolated from brain tissue that has marijuana-like properties.

androgenic: masculinizing.

angel dust: the street name for PCP sprinkled on plant material.

anhedonia: a lack of emotional response; especially an inability to experience joy or pleasure.

animism: the belief that objects attain certain characteristics because of spirits.

antagonist: a substance that prevents the effects of a neurotransmitter on the postsynaptic cell.

antecedent: a variable that occurs before some event, such as the initiation of drug use.

antihistamine: the active ingredient in OTC sleep aids and cough and cold products.

anti-inflammatory: reducing swelling and inflammation.

antipsychotics: a group of drugs used to treat psychosis; same as neuroleptics.

antipyretic: fever reducing.

antitussive: a medication used to suppress or relieve coughing.

anxiety disorders: mental disorders characterized by excessive worry, fears, or avoidance.

anxiolytics: drugs, such as Valium, used in the treatment of anxiety disorders; literally, "anxiety-dissolving."

ataxia: uncoordinated walking.

autonomic: the part of the nervous system that controls "involuntary" functions, such as heart rate.

B

barbiturates: a chemical group of sedative-hypnotics.

basal ganglia: subcortical brain structures controlling muscle tone.

behavioural tolerance: tolerance caused by learned adaptation to the drug.

behavioural toxicity: toxicity resulting from behavioural effects of a drug.

benzodiazepines: a chemical grouping of sedative-hypnotics.

biopsychosocial: a theory or perspective that relies on the interaction of biological, individual psychological, and social variables.

bipolar disorder: a type of mood disorder also known as manic-depressive disorder.

blood alcohol concentration (blood alcohol level): a measure of the concentration of alcohol in blood, expressed in grams per 100 mL (percentage).

blood-brain barrier: structure that prevents many drugs from entering the brain.

brand name: specifies a particular formulation and manufacturer of a drug.

bronchitis: inflammation of the main air passages to the lungs.

C

caffeinism: a condition caused by an excessive intake of caffeine; characteristics include insomnia, restlessness, excitement, tachycardia (fast heart rate), tremors, and diuresis (increased urination).

***Cannabis*:** the genus of plant known as marijuana.

catheters: plastic or other tubing implanted into the body.

central nervous system (CNS): the neurons and pathways of the brain and spinal cord.

chemical name: specifies the complete chemical description of a drug.

chlorpheniramine maleate: a common antihistamine in cold products.

chronic: referring to drugs, the long-term effects from repeated use.

chronic obstructive pulmonary disease (COPD): a chronic lung disease in which airways swell and are partly blocked by mucus; includes chronic bronchitis and emphysema.

cirrhosis: an irreversible, frequently deadly liver disorder associated with heavy alcohol use.

coca: a bush that grows in the Andes and produces cocaine.

coca paste: a crude extract containing cocaine in a smokeable form.

cocaethylene: a chemical formed when ethanol and cocaine are co-administered.

cocaine hydrochloride: the most common form of pure cocaine, it is stable and water soluble.

cocaine: the active chemical in the coca plant.

codeine: the secondary active agent in opium.

comatose: unconscious and unable to be aroused.

congeners: other alcohols and oils contained in alcoholic beverages.

controlled release: a dosage form for drugs that are released or are activated over time.

controlled use: the idea that substance abusers may be able to use the substance under control.

correlate: a variable that is statistically related to some other variable, such as drug use.

crack: a street name for a simple and stable preparation of cocaine base for smoking.

crank: a street name for illicitly manufactured methamphetamine.

cumulative effects: the effects of giving multiple doses of the same drug.

D

DARE: Drug Abuse Resistance Education, the most popular prevention program in schools.

DAWN: Drug Abuse Warning Network. System for collecting data on drug-related deaths or emergency room visits.

delirium tremens: an alcohol withdrawal syndrome that includes hallucinations and tremors.

dependence: a state in which the individual uses the drug so frequently and consistently that it appears it would be difficult for the person to get along *without* using the drug; stopping is very difficult and may cause severe physical and psychological withdrawal.

depolarized: when the membrane potential is less negative than resting potential.

depressants: drugs that slow activity in the CNS.

depression: a major type of mood disorder.

detoxification: an early treatment stage, in which the body eliminates the alcohol or other substance.

dextromethorphan: an OTC antitussive (cough control) ingredient.

distillation: the evaporation and condensing of alcohol vapours to produce beverages with higher alcohol content.

dopamine: neurotransmitter found in the basal ganglia and other regions.

dose-response curve: a graph comparing the size of response to the amount of drug.

double-blind procedure: an experiment in which neither the researcher nor the participant knows whether the drug or a placebo is being used.

dronabinol: the generic name for prescription THC in oil in a gelatin capsule.

drug: any substance, natural or artificial other than food, which by its chemical nature alters structure or function in the living organism.

drug absorption: the passage of a drug from the site of administration to the circulatory system.

drug disposition tolerance: tolerance caused by more rapid elimination of the drug.

drug distribution: the movement of drugs to and from the blood and various tissues of the body (for example, fat, muscle, and brain tissue).

drug excretion: the removal of drugs from the body.

drug metabolism: the process by which the body breaks down drugs.

drug misuse: refers to the use of prescribed drugs in greater amounts than, or for purposes other than, those prescribed by a physician or dentist. For nonprescription drugs or chemicals, such as paints, glues, or solvents, misuse might mean any use other than the use intended by the manufacturer.

duration of action: the length of time a drug is effective; how long a drug's effects last.

E

ED_{50}: in animal drug trials, the effective dose for half of the animals tested.

efficacy: a drug's ability to produce a desired behavioural effect.

electroconvulsive therapy (ECT): a medical procedure in which a cerebral seizure is induced by a brief electrical stimulus under controlled conditions; purpose is to treat major mental disorders.

emphysema: a chronic lung disease characterized by difficulty breathing and shortness of breath.

endorphin: opiate-like chemical that occurs naturally in the brain of humans and other animals.

enkephalins: morphine-like neurotransmitters found in the brain and adrenals.

enzyme: large molecule that assists in either the synthesis or metabolism of another molecule.

ephedrine: a sympathomimetic drug used in treating asthma.

epilepsies: disorders characterized by uncontrolled movements (seizures).

ergogenic: producing work or energy; a general term for performance enhancement.

ergot: from the French word *argo* meaning "cock's spur," because of the resemblance of *Claviceps purpurea*, the ergotism-inducing fungus, to the spurs on roosters' legs.

F

fermentation: the production of alcohol from sugars through the action of yeasts.

fetal alcohol effect: individual developmental abnormalities associated with the mother's alcohol use during pregnancy.

fetal alcohol syndrome: facial and developmental abnormalities associated with the mother's alcohol use during pregnancy.

freebase: a method of preparing cocaine as a chemical base so that it can be smoked.

G

GABA: inhibitory neurotransmitter found in most regions of the brain.

gateway: one of the first drugs (e.g., alcohol or tobacco) used by a typical drug user.

generic name: specifies a particular chemical but not a particular brand.

GHB: gamma-hydroxybutyrate; chemically related to GABA and used recreationally as a depressant.

glutamate: excitatory neurotransmitter found in most regions of the brain.

H

half-life: the time it takes for half of the drug to lose its pharmacological or physiological effects and to be eliminated from the body.

harm reduction: an initiative of Canada's Drug Strategy to use public education programs to significantly reduce the damage associated with alcohol and other drugs.

hashish: concentrated resin from the *Cannabis* plant.

heroin: diacetylmorphine, a potent derivative of morphine.

HIV: human immunodeficiency virus.

homeostasis: maintenance of an environment of body functions within a certain range (e.g., temperature, blood pressure).

human growth hormone: a pituitary hormone responsible for some types of gigantism.

hyperpolarization: occurs when the membrane potential is pushed below the resting potential.

hypnotics: drugs used to induce sleep.

I

ibuprofen: an Aspirin-like analgesic and anti-inflammatory.

ice, crystal meth: street names for crystals of methamphetamine hydrochloride.

illicit drug: a drug that is unlawful to possess or use; many drugs are available by prescription, but when they are manufactured or sold illegally, they are illicit.

indole: a particular chemical structure found in serotonin and LSD.

inhalants: volatile solvents inhaled for intoxicating purposes.

intramuscular: injection into a muscle.

intravenous (IV): injection directly into a vein.

L

laissez-faire: a hands-off approach to government interference in the workings of the market.

LD_{50}: in animal drug trials, the lethal dose for half of the animals tested.

leukoplakia: a whitening and thickening of the mucous tissue in the mouth, considered to be a precancerous tissue change.

lipid solubility: the tendency of a chemical to dissolve in fat, as opposed to in water.

lipophilic: the extent to which chemicals can be dissolved in oils and fats.

lithium: a drug used in treating mania and bipolar disorder.

longitudinal study: a study done over time (months or years).

M

marijuana: also spelled "marihuana." Dried leaves of the *Cannabis* plant.

Marinol: the brand name for dronabinol.

mescaline: the active chemical in the peyote cactus.

mesolimbic dopamine pathway: one of two major dopamine pathways; may be involved in psychotic reactions and in drug dependence.

metabolite: a product of enzyme action on a drug.

metabolize: to break down or inactivate a neurotransmitter (or a drug) through enzymatic action.

methadone: a long-lasting synthetic opioid.

methylphenidate (Ritalin): a stimulant used in treating ADHD.

moist snuff: finely chopped tobacco, held in the mouth rather than snuffed into the nose.

monoamine: a class of chemicals characterized by a single amine group; monoamine neurotransmitters include dopamine, norepinephrine, and serotonin.

monoamine oxidase (MAO) inhibitor: a type of antidepressant drug.

mood stabilizer: an agent that has efficacy in treating acute manic and depressive symptoms.

morphine: the primary active agent in opium.

N

naloxone: an opioid antagonist.

narcolepsy: a disease that causes people to fall asleep suddenly.

negative reinforcement: the reinforcing of a response by giving an aversive stimulus when the response is not made and omitting the aversive stimulus when the response is made.

neuroleptics: a general term for antipsychotic drugs.

neuromuscular junction: the synapse between a muscle and a neuron.

neurotransmitters: chemical messengers released from neurons and having brief, local effects.

nigrostriatal dopamine pathway: one of two major dopamine pathways; damaged in Parkinson's disease.

nitrosamine: a type of chemical that is carcinogenic; several are found in tobacco.

NSAIDs: nonsteroidal anti-inflammatory drugs, such as ibuprofen.

nucleus accumbens: a collection of neurons in the forebrain thought to play an important role in emotional reactions to events.

O

off-label: use of a prescription drug to treat a condition for which the drug has not received approval from Health Canada.

opioid: a drug derived from opium (e.g., morphine and codeine) or a synthetic drug with opium-like effects (e.g., oxycodone).

opioid antagonists: drugs that can block the actions of opioids.

opium: a raw plant substance containing morphine and codeine.

P

parasympathetic: the branch of the autonomic system that stimulates digestion, slows the heart, and has other effects associated with a relaxed physiological state.

Parkinson's disease: degenerative neurological disease involving damage to dopamine neurons in the basal ganglia.

passive smoking, second-hand smoke: the inhalation of tobacco smoke by individuals other than the smoker.

PCP: phencyclidine; originally developed as an anaesthetic; has hallucinogenic properties.

peripheral nervous system: a division of the nervous system containing all the nerves that lie outside the brain and spinal cord.

peyote: a type of hallucinogenic cactus.

phantastica: drugs that create a world of fantasy.

pharmacodynamic tolerance: tolerance caused by altered nervous system sensitivity.

phenothiazines: a group of drugs used to treat psychosis.

phenylpropanolamine (PPA): until 2002, an active ingredient in OTC weight-control products in Canada and the United States.

physical dependence: drug dependence defined by the presence of a withdrawal syndrome, implying that the body has become adapted to the drug's presence.

placebo: an inactive chemical or substance.

polarized: when the membrane potential is more negative.

positive reinforcement: the offering of desirable effects or consequences for a behaviour with the intention of increasing the chance of that behaviour being repeated in the future.

potency: measured by the amount of drug (dose) required to produce an effect.

precursors: chemicals that are acted on by enzymes to form neurotransmitters.

prodrugs: drugs that are inactive until acted on by enzymes in the body.

Prohibition: laws prohibiting all sales of alcoholic beverages from 1920 to 1933.

proof: a measure of a beverage's alcohol content; twice the alcohol percentage.

psilocybin: the active chemical in *Psilocybe* mushrooms.

psychedelic: "mind-viewing."

psychoactive: having effects on thoughts, emotions, or behaviour.

psychological dependence: behavioural dependence; indicated by a high rate of drug use, craving for the drug, and a tendency to relapse after stopping use.

psychosis: a serious mental disorder involving loss of contact with reality.

psychotherapeutic drugs: drugs that are prescribed for their effects in relieving symptoms of anxiety, depression, or other mental disorders.

psychotomimetic: mimicking psychosis.

R

receptors: recognition proteins that respond to specific chemical signals.

reinforcement: a procedure in which a behavioural event is followed by a consequent event, such that the behaviour is then more likely to be repeated. The behaviour of taking a drug may be reinforced by the effect of the drug.

rock: another name for crack.

Rohypnol: a benzodiazepine; the "date-rape drug."

S

safety margin: the dosage difference between an acceptable level of effectiveness and the lowest toxic dose.

schizophrenia: a mental disorder characterized by chronic psychosis.

sedatives: drugs used to relax, calm, or tranquillize.

selective serotonin reuptake inhibitor (SSRI): a type of antidepressant drug.

semipermeable: allowing some, but not all, chemicals to pass.

serotonin: neurotransmitter found in the raphe nuclei; may be important for impulsivity, mood, and cognition, and plays a role in depression.

side effects: the unintended effects that accompany therapeutic effects.

sinsemilla: "without seeds"; high-grade or more potent marijuana.

smokeless tobacco: a term used for chewing tobacco.

social influence model: a prevention model adopted from successful smoking programs.

somatic system: nerve cells that interact with the external environment to carry sensory information into the central nervous system and carry motor (movement) information back out.

speed: a street name for cocaine, and then later amphetamine.

speedball: the combination of heroin and cocaine injected together.

stages of change: a model for decision making consisting of precontemplation, contemplation, preparation, action, maintenance, and relapse.

subcutaneous: injection under the skin.

sympathetic: the branch of the autonomic system involved in flight or fight reactions.

sympathomimetic: a drug that stimulates the sympathetic branch of the autonomic nervous system.

synapse: the space between neurons.

synesthesia: a sensation that normally occurs in one sense modality occurs when another modality is stimulated (e.g., hearing colours or seeing sounds).

synthesis: the forming of a neurotransmitter by the action of enzymes on precursors.

T

temperance: the idea that people should drink beer or wine in moderation but drink no hard liquor.

THC: delta-9-tetrahydrocannabinol, the most psychoactive chemical in marijuana, hashish, and hash oil.

theobromine: a xanthine found in chocolate.

theophylline: a xanthine found in tea.

therapeutic index (TI): the ratio of LD_{50} to ED_{50}.

time course: the timing of the onset, duration, and termination of a drug's effect.

tolerance: condition that may follow repeated ingestion of a drug; occurs when a person's reaction to a psychopharmaceutical drug (such as a painkiller or an intoxicant) decreases so that larger doses are required to achieve the same effect.

topical administration: application of a drug directly to the area where it is needed.

toxic: poisonous, dangerous.

transporter: mechanism in the nerve terminal membrane responsible for removing neurotransmitter molecules from the synapse by taking them back into the neuron.

tricyclic: a type of antidepressant drug.

U

uptake: energy-requiring mechanism by which selected molecules are taken into cells.

V

values clarification: teaching students to recognize and express their own feelings and beliefs.

W

Wernicke-Korsakoff syndrome: chronic mental impairments produced by heavy alcohol use over a long period of time.

withdrawal: abnormal physical or psychological effects that occur after stopping a drug; symptoms may include sweating, tremors, vomiting, anxiety, insomnia, and muscle aches and pains.

withdrawal syndrome: symptoms (e.g., muscle aches, anxiety attacks, sweating, nausea, convulsion, death) resulting from weaning of substance dependence.

X

xanthines: the class of chemicals to which caffeine belongs.

CREDITS

Chapter 1
p. 2 Monkeybusinessimages/Dreamstime.com/Getstock.com
p. 3 THE CANADIAN PRESS/Ted Ostowski
p. 4 (top left) Creativestock/Dreamstime.com
p. 4 (top right) Getty Images
p. 4 (bottom) Svanhorn4245/Dreamstime.com
p. 7 Brand X Pictures
p. 9 THE CANADIAN PRESS/Adrian Wyld
p. 15 © The McGraw-Hill Companies, Inc./Gary He, photographer
p. 20 © Brand X Pictures/PunchStock
p. 22 © BananaStock/PunchStock

Chapter 2
p. 25 Brand X Pictures
p. 28 Photodisc Collection/Getty Images
p. 32 (top) Ingram Publishing
p. 32 (bottom) © Annie Griffiths Belt/Corbis
p. 34 © The McGraw-Hill Companies, Inc./Gary He, photographer
p. 38 © Alison Derry
p. 40 The Toronto Star/GetStock.com

Chapter 3
p. 44 National Library of Medicine
p. 46 (left) Library of Congress Prints and Photographs Division (3C3376U)
p. 46 (right) Library of Congress Prints and Photographs Division (09335u)
p. 53 PhotoLink/Getty Images

Chapter 4
p. 64 © Jim Wehtje/Getty Images
p. 71 (left) Dwong19/Dreamstime.com
p. 71 (right) Used with the permission of Dr. Ali Rajput
p. 76 Fomaa/Dreamstime.com
p. 77 (top) © David Hoffman Photo Library/Alamy
p. 77 (bottom) Snapper99/Dreamstime.com
p. 85 Guy Croft SciTech/Alamy

Chapter 5
p. 87 Toronto Star/Getstock.com
p. 89 (left) Don Farrall/Getty Images
p. 89 (right) Photodisc Collection/Getty Images
p. 91 © Alison Derry
p. 94 © Alison Derry
p. 105 © Alison Derry
p. 106 (left) © Royalty-Free/Corbis
p. 106 (right) © The McGraw-Hill Companies, Inc./Gary He, photographer
p. 114 © 2001-2014 Rogers Media. All rights reserved.

Chapter 6
p. 120 © The McGraw-Hill Companies, Inc./Suzie Ross, photographer
p. 121 Mary Evans Picture Library/Alamy
p. 122 National Library of Medicine
p. 125 © The McGraw-Hill Companies, Inc./Gary He, photographer
p. 128 S. Meltzer/PhotoLink/Getty Images
p. 130 Spike Mafford/Getty Images
p. 132 (bottom left) © Mikael Karlsson
p. 132 (bottom right) Drug Enforcement Administration
p. 142 (top) Used with permission of Medicalopedia. Retrieved from http://www.medicalopedia.org/1908/ritalin-abuse-among-students-is-increasing-alarmingly/
p. 142 (bottom left) Mdilsiz/Dreamstime.com
p. 142 (bottom right) Creative Commons License. Wikimedia.
p. 146 (top) Andresr/Dreamstime.com

Chapter 7
p. 151 Pixtal
p. 153 Fancy Collection
p. 158 © Sam Edwards/age fotostock
p. 161 Andresr/Dreamstime.com
p. 167 Ryan J. Mitchell
p. 170 © Michael Newman/PhotoEdit

Chapter 8
p. 174 Dragonchild/Dreamstime.com
p. 180 (left) © Author's Image/PunchStock
p. 180 (right) Burlingham/Dreamstime.com
p. 181 Image Source/Getty Images
p. 182 © iStockphoto.com/Stockphoto4u
p. 194 Kumar Sriskandan/Alamy
p. 198 Mel Curtis/Getty Images
p. 205 (top) Gary Moore/realworldimage.com
p. 205 (bottom) Brand X Pictures

Chapter 9
p. 208 © Alison Derry
p. 210 Dimmu/Dreamstime.com
p. 211 Onoky/SuperStock
p. 212 Library and Archives Canada/PA-134862
p. 215 National Photo Company Collection; Library of Congress Prints and Photographs Division (LC-USZ62-96757)
p. 221 © Stockbyte/Getty Images
p. 224 © Alison Derry
p. 228 Coprid/Dreamstime.com
p. 232 © BananaStock/PunchStock
p. 234 (left) Normal Liver Fletcher, C.D.M. and McKee, P.H. *An Atlas of Gross Pathology.* © 1987 Mosby-Wolfe Europe Limited, London, UK.
p. 234 (right) Cirrhotic Liver: Fletcher, C.D.M. and McKee, P.H. *An Atlas of Gross Pathology.* © 1987 Mosby-Wolfe Europe Limited, London, UK.
p. 236 © David H. Wells/Corbis

Chapter 10
p. 244 Laurent Hamels/Photoalto/PictureQuest
p. 245 Flora Torrance/Life File/Getty Images
p. 246 The Canadian Press/Alan Diaz-AP
p. 247 Toronto Reference Library/Special Collections
p. 248 Library of Congress Prints and Photographs Division (3b04259)
p. 250 Reproduced with permission of Simcoe Muskoka District Health Unit on behalf of Ontario's Tobacco Control Area Networks
p. 251 Creative Commons License. Wikimedia.com
p. 252 Greg Wohlford/Erie Times-News/Associated Press
p. 253 © BananaStock/PunchStock
p. 256 © iStockphoto.com/Ju-Lee
p. 259 (top left) © Neil Collishaw/Physicians for a Smoke-Free Canada <www.smoke-free.ca>
p. 259 (top right) © pojoslaw–Fotolia.com
p. 259 (bottom left) Licensed under Health Canada copyright
p. 259 (bottom right) Licensed under Health Canada copyright
p. 260 Getty Images
p. 263 IMS Communications Ltd./Capstone Design/FlatEarth Images
p. 265 © moodboard/Corbis

Chapter 11
p. 269 © Ingram Publishing/Alamy
p. 270 The McGraw-Hill Companies, Inc./John Flournoy, photographer
p. 271 Reprinted with permission of Just Us! Coffee Roasters Co-op
p. 272 (left) Pixtal/AGE Fotostock
p. 272 (right) McGraw-Hill Companies/Lissa Harrison
p. 273 © david pearson/Alamy
p. 274 Library of Congress Prints and Photographs Division (3A25022U)
p. 276 (top) Vicspacewalker/Dreamstime.com
p. 276 (bottom) L.Hobbs/PhotoLink
p. 277 © Royalty-Free/Corbis
p. 278 Library of Congress Prints and Phtoographs Division (3G1222U)
p. 279 © iStockphoto.com/Brasil2
p. 280 © The McGraw-Hill Companies/Jill Braaten, photographer
p. 282 The Canadian Press/Paul Sakuma-AP
p. 286 © Ned Frisk/Blend Images LLC
p. 287 © Juice Images/Alamy
p. 288 © Digital Vision/Getty Images

Chapter 12
p. 292 © Brand X Pictures/Punchstock
p. 294 (top) © The McGraw-Hill Companies/Jill Braaten, photographer
p. 294 (bottom) Mitch Hrdlicka/Getty Images
p. 298 (left) McGraw-Hill Companies Inc./Ken Karp, photographer
p. 298 (right) © Royalty-Free/Corbis
p. 305 © Alison Derry

Chapter 13
p. 312 Pixtal/AGE Fotostock
p. 314 Steven L. Raymer/Getty Images
p. 316 Drug Enforcement Administration
p. 318 © Scott Camazine/Alamy
p. 319 Medioimages/PictureQuest
p. 326 Used with permission. BC Centre for Disease Control.
p. 331 © Getty Images/Steve Miller
p. 333 Nick Procaylo/PNG

Chapter 14
p. 339 Drug Enforcement Administration
p. 346 Americanspirit/Dreamstime.com
p. 347 © Alison Derry
p. 351 Alexkurgano/Dreamstime.com
p. 352 Courtesy of the authors/Hart, Carl L. and Ksir, Charles (2011). Drugs, Society & Human Behavior, 14th Ed. New York: McGraw-Hill.
p. 355 Maljalen/Dreamstime.com
p. 357 Nenovbrothers/Dreamstime.com
p. 358 United States Drug Enforcement Administration
p. 361 (left) Courtesy of Dr. Perry Kendall, Provincial Health Officer, British Columbia, Canada
p. 361 (right) ©iStockphoto.com/evemilla (Camilla Wisbauer)
p. 363 © Steven P. Lynch
p. 365 Tinke Hamming/Ingram Publishing
p. 367 Courtesy of Pie4all88/http://en.wikipedia.org/wiki/File:Salvia Divinorum25xExtract.jpg

Chapter 15
p. 369 (top) Drug Enforcement Administration
p. 369 (bottom) © travelib india/Alamy
p. 371 Eldadcarin/Dreamstime.com
p. 372 © (2010) HER MAJESTY THE QUEEN IN RIGHT OF CANADA as represented by the Royal Canadian Mounted Police (RCMP). Reproduced with the permission of the RCMP.
p. 381 © Matthew Trace
p. 384 © The McGraw-Hill Companies, Inc./Lars A. Niki, photographer
p. 389 © Matthew Trace
p. 391 © Getty Images

Chapter 16
p. 395 Urmoments/Dreamstime.com
p. 397 Getty Images
p. 401 © PhotoLink/Getty Images
p. 402 The Canadian Press/Chuck Stoody
p. 409 © The McGraw-Hill Companies, Inc./Jill Braaten, photographer

Chapter 17
p. 412 Design Pics/Don Hammond
p. 416 Donna Day/Imagestate
p. 420 © Royalty-Free/Corbis
p. 421 Stockbyte/PunchStock
p. 427 © The McGraw-Hill Companies, Inc./John Flournoy, photographer

Chapter 18
p. 429 Nancy R. Cohen/Getty Images
p. 433 © Robert Vanden Brugge/BELGA/epa/Corbis
p. 434 © Ed Kashi/Corbis
p. 439 © BEN NELMS/Reuters/Corbis
p. 448 Used with permission of the Vancouver Courier. Photo courtesy of Dan Toulgoet
p. 450 © Mikael Karlsson/Arresting Images
p. 451 © Bettmann/Corbis

REFERENCES

Chapter 1

1. Health Canada. *Canadian Addiction Survey: Public Opinion, Attitudes and Knowledge: A National Survey of Canadians' Use of Alcohol and Other Drugs.* 2006. Retrieved October 31, 2011, from http://www.hc-sc.gc.ca/hc-ps/pubs/adp-apd/cas_opinions-etc/index-eng.php.
2. Centre for Addiction and Mental Health. *2013 Ontario Student Drug Use and Health Survey.* 2013. Retrieved October 31, 2013, from http://www.camh.ca/en/research/news_and_publications/ontario-student-drug-use-and-health-survey/Documents/2013%20OSDUHS%20Docs/2013OSDUHS_Detailed_DrugUseReport.pdf.
3. Health Canada. *Canadian Alcohol and Drug Use Monitoring Survey. Detailed Tables for 2012.* Ottawa: Controlled Substances and Tobacco Directorate, 2013. To obtain a copy, please send an e-mail request to CADUMS-ESCCAD@hc-sc.gc.ca.
4. Centre for Addiction and Mental Health. *Ecstasy Use Down, Cigarettes and LSD Continue to Decline, But Heavy Drinking Remains a Problem.* 2003. Retrieved October 31, 2011, from http://www.camh.net/News_events/News_releases_and_media_advisories_and_backgrounders/osdus2003_newsrelease.html.
5. Centre for Addiction and Mental Health. *Ecstasy Use Down, Cigarettes and LSD Continue to Decline, But Heavy Drinking Remains a Problem.* 2003. Retrieved October 31, 2011, from http://www.camh.net/News_events/News_releases_and_media_advisories_and_backgrounders/osdus2003_newsrelease.html.
6. Canadian Centre on Substance Abuse. *CCENDU Bulletin, No Confirmed Reports of Desomorphine ("Krocodil"/"Crocodile") in Canada.* 2013. Retrieved December 30, 2013, from http://www.ccsa.ca/2013%20CCSA%20Documents/ccsa-CCENDU-Desomorphine-Bulletin-2013-en.pdf.
7. Canadian Public Health Association. *Parents Be Aware: Sniffing Kids.* 2005. Retrieved October 31, 2011, from http://www.cpha.ca/en/portals/substance/article06.aspx#5.
8. Health Canada and Kaweionnehta Human Resource Group. *First Nations and Inuit Community Youth Solvent Abuse Survey and Study.* Ottawa: Author, 1994.
9. Dell, C., C. Hopkins, and D. Dell. "Resiliency and Holistic Inhalant Abuse Treatment." *Journal of Aboriginal Health* 2 (2005), pp. 4–12.
10. Canadian Centre on Substance Abuse. *Harm Reduction Overview.* 2008. Retrieved October 31, 2011, from http://www.ccsa.ca/Eng/Topics/HarmReduction/Pages/HarmReductionOverview.aspx.
11. Health Canada. *Canadian Addiction Survey: Public Opinion, Attitudes and Knowledge: A National Survey of Canadians' Use of Alcohol and Other Drugs.* 2006. Retrieved October 31, 2011, from http://www.hc-sc.gc.ca/hc-ps/pubs/adp-apd/cas_opinions-etc/index-eng.php.
12. Adlaf, E.M., P. Begin, and E. Sawka, eds. *Canadian Addiction Survey (CAS): A National Survey of Canadians' Use of Alcohol and Other Drugs: Prevalence of Use and Related Harms: Detailed Report.* Ottawa: Canadian Centre on Substance Abuse, 2005.
13. Health Canada. *Canadian Alcohol and Drug Use Monitoring Survey 2011. Microdata User Guide.* Ottawa: October 2012. Retrieved December 12, 2013, from http://abacus.library.ubc.ca/jspui/bitstream/10573/42749/6/cadums-user-guide-2011-eng-nov-2012.pdf.
14. Adlaf, E.M., A. Demers, and L. Gliksman, eds. *Canadian Campus Survey 2004.* Toronto: Centre for Addiction and Mental Health, 2005.
15. American College Health Association. *National College Health Assessment II: Canadian Reference Group Data Report.* Spring 2013. Hanover, MD: Author. Retrieved December 12, 2013, from http://www.cacuss.ca/_Library/documents/NCHA-II_WEB_SPRING_2013_CANADIAN_REFERENCE_GROUP_DATA_REPORT.pdf.
16. Paglia-Boak, A., and others. *Drug Use among Ontario Students, 1977–2013: Detailed OSDUHS Findings* (CAMH Research Document Series No. 36). Toronto: Centre for Addiction and Mental Health. 2013. Retrieved December 12, 2013, from http://www.camh.ca/en/research/news_and_publications/ontario-student-drug-use-and-health-survey/Documents/2013%20OSDUHS%20Docs/2013OSDUHS_Detailed_DrugUseReport.pdf.
17. Paglia-Boak, A., and others. *Drug Use among Ontario Students, 1977–2009: Detailed OSDUHS Findings.* (CAMH Research Document Series No. 27). Toronto: Centre for Addiction and Mental Health. 2009. Retrieved September 12, 2011, from http://www.camh.net/Research/Areas_of_research/Population_Life_Course_Studies/OSDUS/~Detailed_DrugReport_2009OSDUHS_Final.pdf.
18. Adlaf, E.M., A. Demers, and L. Gliksman, eds. *Canadian Campus Survey 2004.* Toronto: Centre for Addiction and Mental Health, 2005. Also available at http://www.camh.net/research/population_life_course.html.
19. Johnston, L.D., and others. *Monitoring the Future: National Survey Results on Drug Use, 1975–2007: Volume I, Secondary School Students* (NIH Publication No. 08-6418A). Bethesda, MD: National Institute on Drug Abuse, 2008.
20. Wright, D., and M. Pemberton. *Risk and Protective Factors for Adolescent Drug Use: Findings from the 1999 National Household Survey on Drug Abuse* (DHHS Publication No. SMA 04-3874, Analytic Series A-19). Rockville, MD: Substance Abuse and Mental Health Services Administration, Office of Applied Studies, 2004.

21. Alamian, A., and G. Paradis. "Correlates of Multiple Chronic Disease Behavioural Risk Factors in Canadian Children and Adolescents." *American Journal of Epidemiology* 170 (2009), pp. 1279–89.
22. Bibby, R. *The Emerging Millennials: How Canada's Newest Generation Is Responding to Change & Choice.* Lethbridge, AB: Project Canada Books, 2008.
23. Galambos, N.L., and L.C. Tilton-Weaver. "Multiple-Risk Behaviour in Adolescents and Young Adults." *Health Reports* 10, no. 2 (1998), Statistics Canada, Catalogue 82-003.
24. Vangsness, L., B.H. Bry, and E.W. LaBouvie. "Impulsivity, Negative Expectancies, and Marijuana Use: A Test of the Acquired Preparedness Model." *Addictive Behaviors* 30 (2005), pp. 1071–76.
25. Kreek, M.J., and others. "Genetic Influences on Impulsivity, Risk Taking, Stress Responsivity and Vulnerability to Drug Abuse and Addiction." *Nature Neuroscience* 8 (2005), pp. 1450–57.
26. Poikolainen, K. "Antecedents of Substance Use in Adolescence." *Current Opinion in Psychiatry* 15 (2002), pp. 241–45.
27. Ensminger, M.E., H.S. Juon, and K.E. Fothergill. "Childhood and Adolescent Antecedents of Substance Use in Adulthood." *Addiction* 97 (2002), pp. 833–44.
28. Tremblay, R.E., and others. *Multi-Level Effects on Behaviour Outcomes in Canadian Children.* Hull, QC: Human Resources Development Canada, Applied Research Branch, 2001.
29. Tremblay, R.E., and others. "Physical Aggression during Early Childhood: Trajectories and Predictors." *Pediatrics* 114 (2004), pp. e43–e50.
30. Kandel, D., and R. Faust. "Sequence and Stages in Patterns of Adolescent Drug Use." *Archives of General Psychiatry* 32 (1975), pp. 923–32.
31. Ginzler, J.A., and others. "Sequential Progression of Substance Use among Homeless Youth: An Empirical Investigation of the Gateway Theory." *Substance Use and Misuse* 38 (2003), pp. 725–58.

Chapter 2

1. Substance Abuse and Mental Health Services Administration. *Drug Abuse Warning Network, 2011: National Estimates of Drug-Related Emergency Department Visits.* Rockville, MD: U.S. Department of Health and Human Services, 2013. Retrieved January 3, 2014, from http://www.samhsa.gov/data/2k13/DAWN2k11ED/DAWN2k11ED.htm#2.1
2. Substance Abuse and Mental Health Services Administration. *Drug Abuse Warning Network, 2007: Area Profiles of Drug-Related Mortality.* Rockville, MD: Author, 2011. Retrieved January 3, 2014, from http://www.samhsa.gov/data/2k11/dawn/2k9dawnme/html/dawn2k9me.htm.
3. World Health Organization. *International Classification of Disease and Related Health Problems,* 10th ed., 1999. Retrieved January 2, 2011, from http://www.who.int/classifications/apps/icd/icd10online/search.aspx.
4. Spurr, K.F., and others. "Analysis of Hospital Discharge Data to Characterize Obstructive Sleep Apnea and Its Management in Adult Patients Hospitalized in Canada: 2006 to 2007." *Canadian Respiratory Journal* 17 (2010), p. 1.
5. Substance Abuse and Mental Health Services Administration. *Results from the 2008 National Survey on Drug Use and Health: National Findings.* Rockville, MD: Author, 2009. Retrieved September 12, 2011, from http://oas.samhsa.gov/nsduh/2k8nsduh/2k8Results.cfm.
6. Office of Drug and Alcohol Research and Surveillance, Substance and Tobacco Directorate, Health Canada. *Canadian Alcohol and Drug Use Monitoring Survey: Summary Results for 2009.* Ottawa: Controlled Substances and Tobacco Directorate, 2009. Retrieved December 30, 2010, from www.hc.gc.ca/hc-ps/drugs-drogues/stat/_2009/summary-sommaire-eng.php.
7. Single, E. *A Social Demographic Profile of Drug Users in Canada.* Ottawa: Health Canada, 2000.
8. Fischer, B. "Comparing Heroin Users and Prescription Opioid Users in a Canadian Multisite Population of Illicit Opioid Users." *Drug and Alcohol Review* 27 (2008), pp. 625–632.
9. Surveillance and Risk Assessment Division, Centre for Infectious Disease Prevention and Control. *Summary: Estimates of HIV Prevalence and Incidence in Canada, 2008.* Public Health Agency of Canada, 2009. Retrieved December 10, 2010, from www.phac.aspc.gc.ca/aids-sida/publication/survreport/estimat08-eng.php.
10. Surveillance and Risk Assessment Division, Centre for Infectious Disease Prevention and Control. *HIV and AIDS in Canada, Surveillance Report to December 31, 2008.* Public Health Agency of Canada, 2009. Retrieved December 10, 2010, from www.phac.aspc.gc.ca/aids-sida/publication/survreport/2008/decindex-eng.php.
11. Zou, S., L. Forrester, and A. Giulivi. "Hepatitis C Update." *Canadian Journal of Public Health* 94 (2003), pp. 127–129.
12. Surveillance and Risk Assessment Division, Centre for Infectious Disease Prevention and Control. *I-Track: Enhanced Surveillance of Risk Behaviour among People who Inject Drugs: Phase 1 Report.* Public Health Agency of Canada, 2006. Retrieved December 28, 2010, from www.phac.aspc.gc.ca/i-track/sr-re-1/index-eng.php.
13. Strike, C., and others. *Ontario Needle Exchange Programs: Best Practice Recommendations.* Toronto: Needle Exchange Coordinating Committee, 2006.
14. Ksobiech, K. "A Meta-Analysis of Needle Sharing, Lending, and Borrowing Behaviours of Needle Exchange Program Attenders." *AIDS Education and Prevention* 15 (2003), pp. 257–68.
15. Bruneau, J., and others. "Trends in Human Immunodeficiency Virus Incidence and Risk Behavior among Injection Drug Users in Montreal, Canada: A 16-Year Longitudinal Study." *American Journal of Epidemiology* 171 (2011), pp. 1049–58.

16. Katz, J.L., and S.T. Higgins. "What Is Represented by Vertical Shifts in Self-Administration Dose-Effect Curves?" *Psychopharmacology* 17 (2004), pp. 360–61.
17. Gable, R.S. "Toward a Comparative Overview of Dependence Potential and Acute Toxicity of Psychoactive Substances Used Nonmedically." *American Journal of Drug and Alcohol Abuse* 19 (1993), pp. 263–81.
18. Kilts, C.D., and others. "The Neural Correlates of Cue-Induced Craving in Cocaine-Dependent Women." *American Journal of Psychiatry* 161 (2004), pp. 233–41.
19. Kelly, T.H., and others. "Individual Differences in Drug Abuse Vulnerability: d-Amphetamine and Sensation-Seeking Status." *Psychopharmacology* 189 (2006), pp. 17–25.
20. White, T.L., D. Lott, and H. de Wit. "Personality and the Subjective Effects of Acute Amphetamine in Healthy Volunteers." *Neuropsychopharmacology* 31 (2006), pp. 1064–74.
21. Peele, S. "What Addiction Is and Is Not: The Impact of Mistaken Notions of Addiction." *Addictive Behaviours* 8 (2000), pp. 599–607.
22. Dr. Nora Volkow, What Do We Know about Addictions? Available at http://vimeo.com/30015129.
23. Blum, K., and others. "The Addictive Brain: All Roads Lead to Dopamine." *Journal of Psychoactive Drugs* 44 (2012), pp. 134–143.
24. Ross, S., and E. Peselow. "The Neurobiology of Addictive Disorders." *Clinical Neuropharmacology* 32 (2009), pp. 269–76.
25. Mroziewicz, M., and R.F. Tyndale. "Pharmacogenetics: A Tool for Identifying Genetic Factors in Drug Dependence and Response to Treatment." *Addiction Science & Clinical Practice* 5 (2010), pp. 17–29.
26. Stone, A.L., and others. "Review of Risk and Protective Factors of Substance Use and Problem Use in Emerging Adulthood." *Addictive Behaviors* 37 (2012), pp. 747–775.
27. Arria, A.M., and A.T. McLellan. "Evolution of Concept, But Not Action, in Addiction Treatment." *Substance Use Misuse* 47 (2012), pp. 1041–8.
28. Cunningham, J.A., and J. McCambridge. "Is Alcohol Dependence Best Viewed as a Chronic Relapsing Disorder?" *Addiction* 107 (2011), pp. 6–12.
29. Simpson, M. "The Relationship between Drug Use and Crime: A Puzzle inside an Enigma." *International Journal of Drug Policy* 14 (2003), pp. 307–19.
30. Bureau of Justice Statistics. *Drugs and Crime Facts.* (Pub. No. NCJ 165148). Washington, DC: U.S. Department of Justice, 2004.
31. Rehm, J.D., and others. *The Cost of Substance Abuse in Canada, 2002.* Ottawa: Canadian Centre on Substance Abuse. Retrieved December 10, 2010, from www.ccsa.ca/2006CCSADocuments/ccsa-011332-2006.pdf.
32. National Institute on Alcohol Abuse and Alcoholism. *Tenth Special Report to the U.S. Congress on Alcohol and Health.* (Pub. No. 00-1583). Bethesda, MD: National Institutes of Health, 2000.
33. Pernanen, K., and others. *Proportions of Crimes Associated with Alcohol and Other Drugs in Canada.* Ottawa: Canadian Centre on Substance Abuse, 2002. Retrieved October 31, 2011, from www.ccsa.ca/2003.
34. National Opinion Research Center. *Drug and Alcohol Use and Related Matters among Arrestees, 2003.* Washington, DC: U.S. Department of Justice, 2004.
35. Dauvergne, M. *Trends in Police-Reported Drug Offences in Canada.* Ottawa: Statistics Canada, 2009. Retrieved December 15, 2010, from www.statscan.gc.ca/pub/85-002-x/2009002/article/10847-eng.htm.
36. Motiuk L., and B. Vuong. *Homicide, Sex, Robbery and Drug Offences in Federal Corrections: An End-of-2004 Review.* Research Branch: Correctional Services of Canada, 2005.

Chapter 3

1. Solomon, R., and M. Green. "The First Century: The History of Non-Medical Opiate Use and Control Policies in Canada, 1870–1970." In *Illicit Drugs in Canada: A Risky Business,* J. Blackwell and P. Erickson, eds. Scarborough, ON: Nelson Canada, 1988, pp. 88–104.
2. Alexander, B. *Peaceful Measures: Canada's Way Out of the War on Drugs.* Toronto: University of Toronto Press, 1990.
3. Blackwell, J. "An Overview of Canadian Illicit Drug Use Epidemiology." In *Illicit Drugs in Canada: A Risky Business,* J. Blackwell and P.G. Erickson, eds. Scarborough, ON: Nelson Canada, 1988, pp. 230–232.
4. McPhee, J. "Pain Clinics May Require Urine Tests. Mandate Would Aim to Curb Drug Abuse." *The Chronicle Herald* (2011). Retrieved from http://thechronicleherald.ca/Front/1221625.html.
5. Smith, P. "What's Up with These 'Pain Contracts'?" (2006). Retrieved from http://stopthedrugwar.org/speakeasy/2006/oct/05/whats_these_pain_contracts.
6. Collen, M. "Opioid Contracts and Random Drug Testing for People with Chronic Pain–Think Twice." *The Journal of Law, Medicine and Ethics* 37, no. 4 (2009), pp. 841–845.
7. Association for Medical Education and Research in Substance Abuse (AMERSA). *Guidelines for Proper Opioid Prescribing Practice,* 2010. Retrieved from http://www.amersa.org/2010_Reg_Brochure_91510.pdf.
8. Tellioglu, T. "The Use of Urine Drug Testing to Monitor Patients Receiving Chronic Opioid Therapy for Persistent Pain Conditions." *Medicine and Health, Rhode Island* 91, no. 9 (2008), pp. 279–282.
9. Tenore, P.L. "Advanced Urine Toxicology Testing." *Journal of Addictive Diseases* 29, no. 4 (2010), pp. 436–438.
10. Kahan, M., A. Srivastava, L. Wilson, D. Gourlay, & Midmer D. "Misuse of and Dependence on Opioids: Study of Chronic Pain Patients." *Canadian Family Physician* 52, no. 9 (2006), pp. 1081–1087.
11. Savage, S.R. "Management of Opioid Medications in Patients with Chronic Pain and Risk of Substance

Misuse." *Current Psychiatry Reports* 11, no. 5 (2009), pp. 377–384.

12. Tooley, J. "Demon Drugs and Holy Wars: Canadian Drug Policy as Symbolic Action." Unpublished master's thesis, University of New Brunswick, 1999.
13. Health Canada. *Brief History of Drug Regulation in Canada.* 2007. Retrieved September 20, 2011, from http://www.hc-sc.gc.ca/dhp-mps/homologation-licensing/info-renseign/hist-eng.php.
14. Erickson, P. "Recent Trends in Canadian Drug Policy: The Decline and Resurgence of Prohibition." *Daedalus* 121 (1992), pp. 239–67.
15. Erickson, P., and R. Smart. "The Le Dain Commission Recommendations." In *Illicit Drugs in Canada: A Risky Business,* J. Blackwell and P. Erickson, eds. Scarborough, ON: Nelson Canada, 1988, pp. 336–343.
16. Parliament of Canada. Legislative Summary of Bill C-10: 4 Amendments to the Controlled Drugs and Substances Act [Bill C-10, Part 2, Clauses 32-33, 39-48 and 50-51] (Former Bill S-10). 2012. Retrieved May 12, 2014, from http://www.parl.gc.ca/About/Parliament/LegislativeSummaries/bills_ls.asp?ls=c10-04&Parl=41&Ses=1&source=library_prb&Language=E#a5.
17. Health Canada. *What Are Canada's Drug Laws? Controlled Drugs and Therapeutic Act.* Retrieved December 27, 2010, from http://www.hc-sc.gc.ca/hc-ps/pubs/adp-apd/straight_facts-faits_mefaits/drug_laws-lois_de_drogues-eng.php.
18. Parliament of Canada. "Legislative Summary of Bill S-10: An Act to amend the Controlled Drugs and Substances Act and to make related and consequential amendments to other Acts," by Tanya Dupuis and Robin MacKay, Legal and Legislative Affairs Division, May 17, 2010 and revised March 31, 2011. Retrieved October 23, 2013 from http://www.parl.gc.ca/About/Parliament/LegislativeSummaries/bills_ls.asp?Language=E&ls=s10&Parl=40&Ses=3&source=library_prb.
19. Vandermeer, J. "Senate Quietly Passes Bill S-10 and Mandatory Minimums for Marijuana," *Cannabis Culture.* December 14, 2010. Retrieved October 25, 2013 from http://www.cannabisculture.com/content/2010/12/14/Senate-Quietly-Passes-Bill-S-10-and-Mandatory-Minimums-Marijuana.
20. McLemore, M. "Why Canadians Should Reject Bill S-10," *Human Rights Watch.* February 16, 2011. Retrieved October 22, 2013, from http://www.hrw.org/news/2011/02/16/why-canada-should-reject-bill-s-10.
21. Health Canada. *Access to Therapeutic Products: The Regulatory Process in Canada.* 2006. Retrieved January 1, 2011, from http://www.hc-sc.gc.ca/ahc asc/pubs/hpfb-dgpsa/access-therapeutic_acces-therapeutique-eng.php.
22. Government of Canada. *Patent Protection for Pharmaceutical Products in Canada: Chronology of Significant Events.* 2002. Retrieved June 22, 2011, from http://dsp-psd.pwgsc.gc.ca/Collection-/LoPBdP/BP/prb9946-e.htm.
23. Elliott, R. *Global Access to Medicines: Canada's Law on Compulsory Licensing for Export.* Canadian HIV/AIDS Legal Network. Retrieved June 22, 2011, from http://www.aidslaw.ca/publications/interfaces/downloadFile.php?ref=658.
24. Health Canada. *Clinical Trials Regulatory Review: Targeted Measures for a Strengthened Framework.* 2008. Retrieved January 2, 2011, from http://www.hc-sc.gc.ca/dhp-mps/prodpharma/activit/consultation/clini-rev-exam/ct_regrev_ce_exareg-eng.php.
25. Boisvert, J. "The Canadian Clinical Trial Regulation Overview and Update." *GOR* 5 no.2 (2003), pp. 35–39. Retrieved December 26, 2010, from http://www.touchbriefings.com/pdf/15/ACF6EE9.pdf.
26. Industry Canada. *Canadian Pharmaceutical Industry Profile.* 2010. Retrieved December 31, 2010, from http://www.ic.gc.ca/eic/site/lsg-pdsv.nsf/eng/h_hn00021.html.
27. Health Canada. *Marijuana Medical Access Regulations: Daily Amount Fact Sheet (Dosage).* 2008. Retrieved December 22, 2010, from http://www.hc-sc.gc.ca/dhp-mps/marihuana/how-comment/medpract/help-aide/daily-quotidienne-eng.php.
28. Government of Canada. "Marihuana for Medical Purposes Regulations." *Canada Gazette* 147 (2013). June 19, 2013. Retrieved October 26, 2013 from http://gazette.gc.ca/rp-pr/p2/2013/2013-06-19/html/sor-dors119-eng.php#archived.

Chapter 4

1. Brunton, L.L., J.S. Lazo, and K.L. Parker, eds. *Goodman & Gilman's The Pharmacological Basis of Therapeutics,* 11th ed. New York, NY: McGraw-Hill, 2006, p. 596.
2. Fields, R.D., and B. Stevens-Graham. "New Insights into Neuron-Glia Communication." *Science* 298 (2002), pp. 556–62.
3. Canadian Institute of Neurosciences, Mental Health and Addiction. *The Brain from Top to Bottom: Neurons.* (n.d.). Retrieved November 11, 2011, from http://thebrain.mcgill.ca/flash/a/a_01/a_01_cl/a_01_cl_ana/a_01_cl_ana.html.
4. Azevedo, F.A., L.R. Carvalho, L.T. Grinberg, J.M. Farfel, R.E. Ferretti, R.E. Leite, W. Jacob Filho, R. Lent, and S. Herculano-Houzel. "Equal Numbers of Neuronal and Nonneuronal Cells Make the Human Brain an Isometrically Scaled-Up Primate Brain." *Journal of Comparative Neurology* 513 (2009), pp. 532–541.
5. Eriksen, N., and B. Pakkenberg. "Total Neocortical Cell Number in the Mysticete Brain." *Anatomical Record* (Hoboken) 290, no. 1 (2007), pp. 83–95.
6. Herculano-Houzel, S., and R. Lent. "Isotropic Fractionator: A Simple, Rapid Method for the Quantification of Total Cell and Neuron Numbers in the Brain." *Journal of Neuroscience* 25, no. 10 (2005), pp. 2518–2521.
7. Hilgetag, C., and H. Barbas. "Are There Ten Times More Glia Than Neurons in the Brain?" *Brain Structure Function* 213 (2009), pp. 365–366.

8. Kandel, E.R., J.H. Schwartz, and T.M. Jessell. *Principles of Neural Science,* 4th ed. McGraw-Hill, New York, 2000.
9. Jabr, F. "Know Your Neurons: What Is the Ratio of Glia to Neurons in the Brain?" *Scientific American* (2012). Retrieved from http://blogs.scientificamerican.com/brainwaves/2012/06/13/know-your-neurons-what-is-the-ratio-of-glia-to-neurons-in-the-brain/.
10. Häusser, M. *Lab Summary.* 2008. Retrieved September 20, 2011, from http://www.ucl.ac.uk/wibr/research/neuro/mh/index.htm.
11. Takada, M., Z.K. Li, and T. Hattori. "Astroglial Ablation Prevents MPTP-Induced Nigrostriatal Neuronal Death." *Brain Research* 509, no. 1 (1990), pp. 55–61.
12. Pitchers, K.K., and others. "Neuroplasticity in the Mesolimbic System Induced by Natural Reward and Subsequent Reward Abstinence." *Biological Psychiatry* 67, no. 9 (2010), pp. 872–79.
13. Canadian Council on Animal Care. *CCAC Training Module on Ethics in Animal Experimentation.* (n.d.). Retrieved September 20, 2011, from http://www.ccac.ca/en_/education/niaut/stream/cs-ethics.
14. Koob, G.F., and M. LeMoal. "Drug Abuse: Hedonic Homeostatic Dysregulation." *Science* 278 (1997), pp. 52–58.
15. Sizemore, G.M., and others. "Time-Dependent Recovery from the Effects of 6-Hydroxydopamine Lesions of the Rat Nucleus Accumbens on Cocaine Self-Administration and the Levels of Dopamine in Microdialysates." *Psychopharmacology* 171 (2004), pp. 413–20.
16. Ryan, D.H. "Clinical Use of Sibutramine." *Drugs Today* 40 (2004), pp. 41–54.
17. Lin, P.Y., and G. Tsai. "Association between Serotonin Transporter Gene Promoter Polymorphism and Suicide: Results of a Meta-Analysis." *Biological Psychiatry* 55 (2004), pp. 1023–30.
18. Cheng, V.Y., and others. "Alpha5GABAA Receptors Mediate the Amnestic But Not Sedative-Hypnotic Effects of the General Anesthetic Etomidate." *Journal of Neuroscience* 26, no. 14 (2006), pp. 3713–20.
19. Kalivas, P.W. "Glutamate Systems in Cocaine Addiction." *Current Opinions in Pharmacology* 4 (2004), pp. 23–29.
20. Liu, X.Y., and others. "Modulation of D2R-NR2B Interactions in Response to Cocaine." *Neuron* 52 (2006), pp. 897–909. Also found at http://www.neuron.org.
21. Health Canada. *Health Concerns: Lysergic Acid Diethylamide (LSD).* 2009. Retrieved November 11, 2011, from http://www.hc-sc.gc.ca/hc-ps/drugs-drogues/learn-renseigne/lsd-eng.php.
22. Seeman, P., F. Ko, and T. Tallerico. "Dopamine Receptor Contribution to the Action of PCP, LSD and Ketamine Psychotomimetics." *Molecular Psychiatry* 10 (2005), pp. 877–83.
23. Lidstone, S.C., and others. "Effects of Expectation on Placebo-Induced Dopamine Release in Parkinson Disease." *Archives of General Psychiatry* 67, no. 8 (2010), pp. 857–65.
24. Poulter, M.O., and others. "Altered Organization of $GABA_A$ Receptor mRNA Expression in the Depressed Suicide Brain." *Frontiers in Molecular Neuroscience* 3 (2010), pp. 1–10. Also found at http://www.frontiersin.org.
25. Bailey, C.D., and others. "The Nicotinic Acetylcholine Receptor Alpha5 Subunit Plays a Key Role in Attention Circuitry and Accuracy." *Journal of Neuroscience* 30, no. 27 (2010), pp. 9241–52. To visualize Ach pathways in the brain visit McGill University's site, The Brain from Top to Bottom, at http://thebrain.mcgill.ca/flash/a/a_01/a_01_cr/a_01_cr_fon/a_01_cr_fon.html.
26. Stocker, S. "Compounds Show Strong Promise for Treating Cocaine Addiction." *NIDA Notes,* May/June, pp. 1–4. Health Canada, 1997. Retrieved November 2, 2011, from http://www.hc-sc.gc.ca/hc-ps/pubs/adp-apd/cocaine_use-usage_cocaine/treatment-traitement-eng.php.

Chapter 5

1. *Industry Profile 2009.* Washington, DC: Pharmaceutical Research and Manufacturing Association.
2. Harris, G. "U.S. Moves to Halt Import of Drugs from Canada." *New York Times.* September 10, 2003, p. C2.
3. Wagner, J.L., and E. McCarthy. "International Differences in Drug Prices." *Annual Review of Public Health* 25 (2004), pp. 475–95.
4. Business Wire. *Research and Markets: Essential and Comprehensive Canada Pharmaceutical Industry Report.* 2009. Retrieved November 3, 2011, from http://www.allbusiness.com/pharmaceuticals-biotechnology/pharmaceutical/13550076-1.html.
5. Scherer, F.M. "The Pharmaceutical Industry: Prices and Progress." *New England Journal of Medicine* 351 (2004), pp. 927–32. Retrieved November 3, 2011, from http://www.nejm.org/doi/full/10.1056/NEJMhpr040117.
6. Douglas, K., and C. Jutras. *Patent Protection for Pharmaceutical Products in Canada—Chronology of Significant Events.* 2008. Retrieved November 12, 2011, from http://www.parl.gc.ca/Content/LOP/researchpublications/prb9946-e.htm.
7. Health Central. *Lifestyle Changes: St. John's Wort and Other Herbal Remedies.* 2006. Retrieved November 3, 2011, from http://www.healthcentral.com/depression/treatment-000008_10-145.html.
8. Medicinal Herbs Info. *Foxglove.* 2010. Retrieved November 3, 2011, from http://www.medicinalherbinfo.org/herbs/Foxglove.html.
9. Simon Fraser University. "Student Abuse of Ritalin Raises Questions about Familiar Drug." Burnaby, BC: *The Peak* 98, no. 7 (1998).
10. Public Health Agency of Canada. *Canadian Street Youth and Substance Use: Findings from Enhanced Surveillance of Canadian Street Youth, 1999–2003.* Public Health Agency of Canada, 2007. Also found at http://www.phac-aspc.gc.ca/sti-its-surv-epi/report07/pdf/csy07_e.pdf.
11. See http://www.brainchildmag.com/2013/05/brain-doping/0.

12. See CTV News, "Canadian Students Abusing Adderall to Get Edge in Studying," February 4, 2013. http://www.ctvnews.ca/health/canadian-students-abusing-adderall-to-get-edge-in-studying-1.1143205.
13. See http://oncampus.macleans.ca/education/2013/02/08/concentration-for-5-a-pill/.
14. See http://www.ccsa.ca/2007%20CCSA%20Documents/ccsa-011519-2007.pdf.
15. SDUS Summary 2007. See http://www.health.gov.nl.ca/health/publications/sdus_summary_report_2007_11_15_final_r_.pdf.
16. OSDUHS 2011–CAMH. See http://www.camh.ca/en/research/news_and_publications/ontario-student-drug-use-and-health-survey/Documents/2011%20OSDUHS%20Docs/2011OSDUHS_Highlights_DrugUseReport.pdf.
17. NBSDUS 2007. See http://www.gnb.ca/0378/pdf/SDUS-2007-e.pdf.
18. See http://acposb.on.ca/LearnChall/ADHD.html.
19. Maskalyk, J. "Grapefruit Juice: Potential Drug Interactions." *Canadian Medical Association Journal* 167, no. 3 (2002), pp. 279–80.
20. Health Canada. *The Effects of Grapefruit and Its Juice on Certain Drugs.* 2006. Retrieved November 3, 2011, from http://www.hc-sc.gc.ca/hl-vs/iyh-vsv/food-aliment/grapefruit-pamplemousse-eng.php.
21. Turner, E.H., and others. "Selective Publication of Antidepressant Trials and Its Influence on Apparent Efficacy." *New England Journal of Medicine* 358, no. 3 (2008), pp. 252–60.
22. http://globalnews.ca/news/482456/drug-reactions-the-effectiveness-of-antidepressants/.
23. Gottlieb, S. "Placebo Response Not All in the Mind." *The Scientist* 3, no. 1 (2002). Retrieved November 12, 2011, from http://classic.the-scientist.com/news/20020111/03/.
24. Zhou, M. "Central Inhibition and Placebo Analgesia." *Molecular Pain* 1, no. 21 (2005). Retrieved November 12, 2011, from http://www.molecularpain.com/content/1/1/21.
25. Lidstone, S.C., R. de la Fuente, and A.J. Stoessl. "The Placebo Response as a Reward Mechanism." *Seminars in Pain Medicine* 3 (2005), pp. 37–42.
26. For more information, refer to www.mofed.org/Animal_Research.htm.
27. Campbell, J.A. "Time Release Preparations for Oral Medication." *Canadian Medical Association Journal* 80 (1959), p. 462. Also found at http://www.ncbi.nlm.nih.gov/pmc/articles/PMC1830696/pdf/canmedaj00801-0041b.pdf.
28. Hu, H., and M. Wu. "Mechanism of Anesthetic Action: Oxygen Pathway Perturbation Hypothesis." *Medical Hypotheses* 57 (2001), p. 619.
29. Health Canada. *Risk of Important Drug Interactions between St. John's Wort and Prescription Drugs.* 2000. Retrieved September 25, 2011, from http://www.hc-sc.gc.ca/dhp-mps/medeff/advisories-avis/prof/_2000/hypericum_perforatum_hpc-cps-eng.php.
30. Lin, K.-M., and R.E. Poland. "Ethnicity, Culture, and Psychopharmacology." *Neuropsychopharmacology: The Fifth Generation of Progress.* 2000. Retrieved November 3, 2011, from http://www.acnp.org/g4/GN401000184/CH180.html.
31. American Psychological Association. "Pavlovian Psychopharmacology." *Monitor* 35, no. 3 (2004), p. 18. Retrieved November 3, 2011, from http://www.science.mcmaster.ca/psychology/pdfs/mar-2004-monitor-siegel.pdf.

Chapter 6

1. Dillehay, T.D., and others. "The Nanchoc Tradition: The Beginnings of Andean Civilization." *American Scientist* 85 (1997), pp. 46–55.
2. Taylor, N. *Flight from Reality.* New York, NY: Duell, Sloan & Pearce, 1949.
3. Freud, S. "On the General Effect of Cocaine." Lecture before the Psychiatric Union, March 5, 1885. Reprinted in *Drug Dependence* 5 (1970), p. 17.
4. Doyle, A.C. "The Sign of the Four." In *The Complete Sherlock Holmes.* New York, NY: Garden City, 1938.
5. Musto, D.F. "Opium, Cocaine and Marijuana in American History." *Scientific American* (July 1991), p. 40.
6. Bourne, P.G. "The Great Cocaine Myth." *Drugs and Drug Abuse Education Newsletter* 5 (1974), p. 5.
7. Grinspoon, L., and J.B. Bakalar. "Drug Dependence." In *The Comprehensive Textbook of Psychiatry,* 3rd ed., H.I. Kaplan, A.M. Freedman, and B.J. Sadock, eds. Baltimore, MD: Williams & Wilkins, 1980, pp. 50–51.
8. Freud, S. "Über Coca." *St. Louis Medical and Surgical Journal* 47 (1884), pp. 502–50. Also published in S.A. Edminster, and others. *The Cocaine Papers.* Vienna: Dunquin, 1963.
9. United Nations Office on Drugs and Crime. *World Drug Report 2009.* 2009. Retrieved November 3, 2011, from http://www.unodc.org/unodc/en/data-and-analysis/WDR-2009.html.
10. Riley, K.J. *Snow Job?* New Brunswick, NJ: Transaction, 1996.
11. Royal Canadian Mounted Police. *Drug Utilization Report 2007.* Retrieved November 3, 2011, from http://www.rcmp-grc.gc.ca/drugs-drogues/index-eng.htm.
12. Feldman, R.S., J.S. Meyer, and L.F. Quenzer. *Principles of Neuropsychopharmacology.* Sunderland, MA: Sinauer, 1997.
13. Williams, S. "Cocaine's Harmful Effects." *Science* 248 (1990), p. 166.
14. Hart, C.L., and others. "Comparison of Intravenous Cocaethylene and Cocaine in Humans." *Psychopharmacology* 149 (2000), p. 153.
15. Faruque, S., and others. "Crack Cocaine Smoking and Oral Sores in Three Inner-City Neighborhoods." *Journal of Acquired Immune Deficiency Syndromes and Human Retrovirology* 13 (1996), pp. 87–92.
16. Brady, K.T., and others. "Cocaine-Induced Psychosis." *Journal of Clinical Psychiatry* 52 (1991), p. 509.

17. Bunn, W.H., and A.J. Giannini. "Cardiovascular Complications of Cocaine Abuse." *American Family Physician* 46 (1992), p. 769.
18. Substance Abuse and Mental Health Services Administration. *Treatment Episode Data Set (TEDS) Highlights: 2006 National Admissions to Substance Abuse Treatment Services.* OAS Series #S-40. DHHS Publication No. (SMA) 08-4313. Rockville, MD: Substance Abuse and Mental Health Services Administration, Office of Applied Studies, 2007.
19. Haney, M., and others. "Effects of Pergolide on Intravenous Cocaine Self-Administration in Men and Women." *Psychopharmacology* 137 (1998), p. 15.
20. Johanson, C.E., and others. "Self-Administration of Psychomotor Stimulant Drugs: The Effects of Unlimited Access." *Pharmacology Biochemistry and Behavior* 4 (1976), p. 45.
21. Frank, D.A., and others. "Growth, Development, and Behavior in Early Childhood Following Prenatal Cocaine Exposure: A Systematic Review." *Journal of the American Medical Association* 285 (2001), p. 1613.
22. Northwest Territories Health and Social Services. *Northwest Territories Addiction Survey 2006.* 2006. Retrieved November 11, 2011, from http://www.hlthss.gov.nt.ca/english/publications/pubresult.asp?ID=165.
23. Poulin, C., and D. Elliott. *Student Drug Use Survey in the Atlantic Provinces (SDUSAP) 2007: Atlantic Technical Report.* Dalhousie, NS: Dalhousie University and Communication Nova Scotia, 2007. Retrieved November 3, 2011, from http://www.gov.pe.ca/photos/original/doh_sds_tech.pdf.
24. Brecher, E.M. *Licit and Illicit Drugs.* Boston, MA: Little, Brown, 1972.
25. Office of the Air Surgeon. "Benzedrine Alert." *Air Surgeon's Bulletin* 1, no. 2 (1944), pp. 19–21.
26. Manhard, F.R. "A History of Speed." In *The Facts about Amphetamines.* Tarrytown, NY: Marshall Cavendish Benchmark, 2006.
27. Burgess, J.L. "Phosphine Exposure from a Methamphetamine Laboratory Investigation." *Journal of Toxicology and Clinical Toxicology* 39 (2001), p. 165.
28. Drug Abuse Warning Network. *The DAWN Report: Club Drugs.* 2002.
29. Community Epidemiology Work Group (CEWG). "Epidemiologic Trends in Drug Abuse, Volume I." *Proceedings of the Community Epidemiology Work Group.* NIH Pub. No. 04-5364. Washington, DC: U.S. Government Printing Office, 2004.
30. Royal Canadian Mounted Police, National Intelligence Analysis, Criminal Intelligence. *Drug Situation in Canada 2007.* Retrieved November 3, 2011, from http://www.rcmp-grc.gc.ca/drugs-drogues/drg-2007-eng.htm, Cat. No. PS61-14/2007E-PDF.
31. Guevara, R.E. *Facing the Methamphetamine Problem in America.* Statement of Rogelio E. Guevara, Chief of Operations, Drug Enforcement Administration Before the House Committee on Government Reform Subcommittee on Criminal Justice, Drug Policy and Human Resources, July 18, 2003. Washington, DC: Drug Enforcement Administration, 2003.
32. Royal Canadian Mounted Police, Criminal Intelligence Directorate. *Federal and International Operations: Coming into Force of the Precursor Control Regulations, Beginning January 9, 2003.* Ottawa: Royal Canadian Mounted Police, 2003.
33. Royal Canadian Mounted Police, Criminal Intelligence Directorate. *Drug Situation in Canada 2003.* Ottawa: Royal Canadian Mounted Police, 2004.
34. Sevick, J.R. *Precursor and Essential Chemicals in Illicit Drug Production: Approaches to Enforcement.* Washington, DC: National Institute of Justice, 1993.
35. Cunningham, J.K., L.M. Liu, and R. Callaghan. "Impact of US and Canadian Precursor Regulation on Methamphetamine Purity in the United States." *Addiction* 104, no. 3 (2009), pp. 441–53.
36. Partilla, J.S., and others. "Interaction of Amphetamines and Related Compounds at the Vesicular Monoamine Transporter." *Journal of Pharmacology and Experimental Therapeutics* 319 (2006), pp. 237–46.
37. Han, D.D., and H.H. Gu. "Comparison of the Monoamine Transporters from Human and Mouse in Their Sensitivities to Psychostimulant Drugs." *BMC Pharmacology* 6, no. 6 (2006). Retrieved November 2, 2011, from http://www.biomedcentral.com/content/pdf/1471-2210-6-6.pdf.
38. Rothman, R.B., and M.H. Baumann. "Monoamine Transporters and Psychostimulant Drugs." *European Journal of Pharmacology* 479 (2003), pp. 23–40.
39. Sulzer, D., and others. "Mechanisms of Neurotransmitter Release by Amphetamines: A Review." *Progress in Neurobiology* 75 (2005), pp. 406–33.
40. Brauer, L.H., and H. deWit. "High Dose Pimozide Does Not Block Amphetamine-Induced Euphoria in Normal Volunteers." *Pharmacology Biochemistry and Behavior* 56 (1997), p. 265.
41. Rothman, R.B., and others. "Amphetamine-Type Central Nervous System Stimulants Release Norepinephrine More Potently Than They Release Dopamine and Serotonin." *Synapse* 39 (2001), p. 32.
42. Antoniou, T., and Juurlink, D. "Five Things to Know about 'Bath Salts.'" *Canadian Medical Association Journal* 184, issue 15 (2012), p. 1713. http://www.ncbi.nlm.nih.gov/pubmed/?term=%22Five%20things%20to%20know%20about%20bath%20salts%22.
43. CBC News. "Bath Salts Drug Arrests in Pictou County, Nova Scotia." CBC/Radio Canada, October 31, 2012. Retrieved January 21, 2014, from http://www.cbc.ca/news/canada/nova-scotia/bath-salts-drug-arrests-in-pictou-county-1.1156648.
44. Government of Canada, Health Canada. "Bath Salts." August 14, 2013. Retrieved January 20, 2014, from http://www.healthycanadians.gc.ca/health-sante/addiction/bath_salts-sels_bain-eng.php.
45. Black, M. "What Are 'Bath Salts'? A Look at Canada's Newest Illegal Drug." CBC/Radio Canada, June 25, 2012.

Retrieved January 20, 2014, from http://www.cbc.ca/news/canada/what-are-bath-salts-a-look-at-canada-s-newest-illegal-drug-1.1143407.

46. CTV News. "Canadian Health Authorities Warn of 'Bath Salts' Drug." June 1, 2012. Retrieved January 20, 2014, from http://www.ctvnews.ca/canadian-health-authorities-warn-of-bath-salts-drug-1.834524.
47. Canadian Centre on Drug Abuse. Canadian Community Epidemiology Network on Drug Use Alerts and Bulletins: "CCENDU Drug Alert: 'Bath Salts.'" June 5, 2012. http://www.ccsa.ca/2012%20CCSA%20Documents/CCSA-CCENDU-Drug-Alert-Bath-Salts-2012-en.pdf.
48. CTV News. "Feds Seek to Ban 'Bath Salts' Drug after U.S. Incident." June 5, 2012. Retrieved January 19, 2014 from http://www.ctvnews.ca/feds-seek-to-ban-bath-salts-drug-after-u-s-incident-1.835568.
49. CBC News. "Hallucinogenic 'Bath Salts' Entering Canada." CBC/Radio Canada, December 29, 2011. Retrieved January 20, 2014, from http://www.cbc.ca/news/canada/hallucinogenic-bath-salts-entering-canada-1.1041023.
50. Metro News. "Bath Salts Drug Has Experts on High Alert." June 1, 2012. Retrieved January 21, 2014. http://metronews.ca/news/kitchener/246504/bath-salts-drug-has-experts-on-high-alert/.
51. Truro Daily News. "Nova Scotia Man Gets 17-Month Sentence for Trafficking Bath Salts." June 27, 2013. Retrieved January 18, 2014 from http://www.trurodaily.com/News/Local/2013-06-27/article-3294032/Nova-Scotia-man-gets-17-month-sentence-for-trafficking-bath-salts/1.
52. Pace, N., and N. Logan. "N.S. Bath Salts Seizure Possibly Largest in Canada: Police." Global News. January 25, 2013. Retrieved January 18, 2014, from http://globalnews.ca/news/384061/n-s-bath-salts-seizure-possibly-largest-in-canada-police/.
53. *The News* (New Glasgow). "Record Bath Salts Bust in Pictou County." January 25, 2013. Retrieved January 18, 2014, from http://www.ngnews.ca/News/Local/2013-01-25/article-3163573/Record-bath-salts-bust-in-Pictou-County/1.
54. Tjepkema, M. *Obesity in Canada: Measured Height and Weight.* Ottawa: Statistics Canada, 2008. Retrieved September 11, 2011, from http://www.statcan.gc.ca/pub/82-620-m/2005001/article/adults-adultes/8060-eng.htm.
55. *Physician's Desk Reference,* 61st ed. Oradell, NJ: Medical Economies, 2007.
56. Health Canada. *Meridia (Sibutramine) Capsules: Voluntary Withdrawal from the Canadian Market for Health Professionals.* Retrieved September 10, 2011, from http://www.hc-sc.gc.ca/dhp-mps/medeff/advisories-avis/prof/_2010/meridia_hpc-cps-eng.php.
57. Rush, C.R., and others. "Acute Behavioral and Physiological Effects of Modafinil in Drug Abusers." *Behavioral Pharmacology* 13 (2002), p. 1055.
58. U.S. Modafinil in Narcolepsy Multicenter Study Group. "Randomized Trial of Modafinil as a Treatment for the Excessive Daytime Somnolence of Narcolepsy." *Neurology* 54 (2002), p. 1166.
59. American Psychiatric Association. *Diagnostic and Statistical Manual of Mental Disorders,* 4th ed. Washington, DC: American Psychological Association, 2000.
60. Spencer, T.L., and others. "Overview and Neurobiology of Attention-Deficit/Hyperactivity Disorder." *Journal of Clinical Psychiatry* 63, suppl. 12 (2003).
61. Caballero, J., and M.C. Nahata. "Atomoxetine Hydrochloride for the Treatment of Attention-Deficit/Hyperactivity Disorder." *Clinical Therapeutics* 25 (2003), p. 3065.
62. Picard, A. (2013). "Spending on Drugs Slowing Down in Canada." *The Globe and Mail.* Retrieved from http://www.theglobeandmail.com/life/health-and-fitness/health/spending-on-drugs-slowing-down-in-canada/article11073846/.
63. *Prescription Monitoring Act* (2004, c. 32, s. 1). Retrieved from the Nova Scotia Legislature Website: http://nslegislature.ca/legc/statutes/prescmon.htm.
64. Richard, G., V. Ojala, A. Ojala, S. Bowles, and H.L. Bahn. "Monitoring Programs for Drugs with Potential for Abuse or Misuse in Canada." *Canadian Pharmacists Journal 145,* 4 (2012), pp. 168–171.
65. Vik, S., D. Ozegovic, and S. Samanani. *Literature Review to Support Conceptualization of a Prescription Drug Misuse Surveillance System in Alberta.* Edmonton: OKAKI Health Intelligence Inc., 2011.
66. The Nova Scotia Prescription Monitoring Program. (n.d.). "About Us: History." Retrieved from the Nova Scotia Prescription Monitoring Program Website: http://www.nspmp.ca/history.php.
67. The Nova Scotia Prescription Monitoring Program. (2007). "PMP Bulletin." Retrieved from http://www.pdbns.ca/Resources/Docs/patient%20info.pdf.
68. Report of the Auditor General. (2012). *Health and Wellness: Nova Scotia Prescription Monitoring Program.* Retrieved from http://oag ns.ca/index.php/publications?task=document.viewdoc&id=719.
69. National Advisory Committee on Prescription Drug Misuse. (2013). *First Do No Harm: Responding to Canada's Prescription Drug Crisis.* Ottawa: Canadian Centre on Substance Abuse.
70. Health Canada. *Non-Insured Health Benefits Prescription Monitoring Program (NIHB-PMP).* 2014. Retrieved from the Health Canada Website: http://www.hc-sc.gc.ca/fniah-spnia/pubs/nihb-ssna/_drug-med/pmp-psm/index-eng.php.
71. Health Canada. *Non-Insured Health Benefits Program Update.* 2014. Retrieved from the Health Canada Website: http://www.hc-sc.gc.ca/fniah-spnia/nihb-ssna/benefit-prestation/newsletter-bulletin-eng.php#mar2014_a12.
72. Downey, J., S. Outram, and F. Campbell. "*Caveat Emptor, Venditor, et Praescribor:* Legal Liability Associated with Methylphenidate Hydrochloride (MPH) Use by Post-secondary Students." *Health Law Journal* 18. Retrieved from http://www.hli.ualberta.ca/HealthLawJournals/~/

media/hli/Publications/HLJ/HLJ18-03_Downie-Outram-Campbell.pdf.

73. Canadian Centre on Substance Abuse. "Prescription Stimulants." 2013. Retrieved from the Canadian Centre on Substance Abuse Website: http://www.ccsa.ca/Resource%20Library/CCSA-Prescription-Stimulants-2013-en.pdf.
74. Canadian ADHD Resource Alliance. *CADDRA Guide to ADHD Pharmacological Treatments in Canada, 2014*. Retrieved from http://www.caddra.ca/pdfs/Medication_Chart_English_CANADA.pdf.
75. *The Controlled Drugs and Substances Act* (1996, c.19). Retrieved from http://laws-lois.justice.gc.ca/eng/acts/c-38.8/page-26.html#docCont.
76. Health Canada. *Buying Drugs over the Internet*. 2009. Retrieved from the Health Canada Website: http://www.hc-sc.gc.ca/hl-vs/iyh-vsv/med/internet-eng.php#th.
77. National Association of Pharmacy Regulatory Authorities. *Internet Pharmacy Standards*. 2001. Retrieved from the NAPRA Website: http://napra.ca/pages/Practice_Resources/internet_pharmacy_standards.aspx.
78. Bergeron-Oliver, A. *Regulatory Gap Leaves Canadians at Risk as Online Pharmacies Multiply*. 2014. Retrieved from http://www.ipolitics.ca/2014/04/23/regulatory-gap-leaves-canadian-at-risk-as-online-pharmacies-multiply/.
79. Fung, C.H., H.E. Woo, and S.M. Asch. "Controversies and Legal Issues of Prescribing and Dispensing Medications Using the Internet," *Mayo Clinic Proceedings* 79, vol. 2 (2004), pp. 188–194.
80. The U.S. Food and Drug Administration. *Know the Risks*. 2013. Retrieved from the FDA Website: http://www.fda.gov/Drugs/ResourcesForYou/Consumers/BuyingUsingMedicineSafely/BuyingMedicinesOvertheInternet/BeSafeRxKnowYourOnlinePharmacy/ucm294167.htm.
81. Dawe, S., and others. "Mechanisms Underlying Aggressive and Hostile Behavior in Amphetamine Users." *Current Opinion in Psychiatry* 22 (2009), pp. 269–73.
82. Marek, G.J., and others. "Dopamine Uptake Inhibitors Block Long-Term Neurotoxic Effects of Methamphetamine upon Dopaminergic Neurons." *Brain Research* 513 (1990), p. 274.
83. Moore, K.A., and others. "Alpha-Benzyl-N-methylphenethylamine (BNMPA), an Impurity of Illicit Methamphetamine Synthesis: Pharmacological Evaluation and Interaction with Methamphetamine." *Drug and Alcohol Dependence* 39 (1995), p. 83.
84. See DSM-5, pp. 561-570.
85. Griffiths, R.R., and others. "Predicting the Abuse Liability of Drugs with Animal Self-Administration Procedures: Psychomotor Stimulants and Hallucinogens." In *Advances in Behavioral Pharmacology*, Vol. 2, T. Thompson and P. Dews, eds. New York, NY: Academic Press, 1979.

Chapter 7

1. Richardson, B.W. "Chloral and Other Narcotics, I." *Popular Science* 15 (1879), p. 492.
2. e-CPS (Compendium of Pharmaceuticals and Specialties, online version). 2013. Retrieved from http://www.e-therapeutics.ca.
3. See http://www.cbc.ca/news/health/old-pain-drug-pulled-from-canadian-market-over-overdose-risk-1.1415188.
4. See http://www.drugs.com/librax.html.
5. Rosenblatt, S., and R. Dobson. *Beyond Valium*. New York: G.P. Putnam's Sons, 1981.
6. Neutel, C.I. "The Epidemiology of Long-Term Benzodiazepine Use." *International Review of Psychiatry* 17 (2005), pp. 189–197.
7. Hollister, L.E., B. Muller-Oerlinghausen, K. Rickels, and others. "Clinical Uses of Benzodiazepines." *Journal of Clinical Psychopharmacology* 13 (1993), pp. 1S–169S.
8. Uwe, R., and K. Frederic. "Beyond Classical Benzodiazepines: Novel Therapeutic Potential of GABA-A Receptor Subtypes." *Nature Reviews Drug Discovery* 10 (2011), pp. 685–97.
9. Hale, L., and others. "Does Mental Health History Explain Gender Disparities in Insomnia Symptoms among Young Adults?" *Sleep Medicine* 10 (2009), pp. 1118–23.
10. Kripke, D. "Greater Incidence of Depression with Hypnotic Use Than with Placebo," *BMC Psychiatry* 7 (2007), pp. 42–45.
11. Substance Abuse and Mental Health Services Administration, Center for Behavioral Health Statistics and Quality. *Emergency Department Visits for Adverse Reactions Involving the Insomnia Medication Zolpidem*. Rockville, MD: Author, 2013.
12. Griffiths, R.R., G. Bigelow, and I. Liebson. "Human Drug Self-Administration: Double-Blind Comparison of Pentobarbital, Diazepam, Chlorpromazine and Placebo." *Journal of Pharmacology and Experimental Therapeutics* 210 (1979), pp. 301–10.
13. Lader, M. "Benzodiazepines Revisited–Will We Ever Learn?" *Addiction* 106 (2011), pp. 2086–109.
14. Tripodianakis, J., and others. "Zolpidem-Related Epileptic Seizures: A Case Report." *European Psychiatry* 18 (2003), pp. 140–41.
15. Marin, M., and others. "New Agents for the Benzodiazepine Withdrawal Syndrome." *European Psychiatry* 25 (2010), p. 1286.
16. Health Canada, 2005. *Drug Utilization Review of Benzodiazepine Use in First Nations and Inuit Populations*. Minister of Public Works and Government Services Canada, 2011.
17. Hindmarch, I., M. ElSohly, J. Gambles, and S. Salamone. "Forensic Urinalysis of Drug Use in Cases of Alleged Sexual Assault." *Journal of Clinical Forensic Medicine* 8 (2001), pp. 197–205.
18. Slaughter, L. "Involvement of Drugs in Sexual Assault." *Journal of Reproductive Medicine* 45, vol. 5 (2000), pp. 425–30.
19. Jamieson, M.A. "Rohypnol, Gamma Hydroxybutyrate, and Drug Rape." *Journal of Obstetrics and Gynaecology Canada* 23, vol. 1 (2001), pp. 38–42.

20. Anglin, D., K.L. Spears, and H.R. Hutson. "Flunitrazepam and Its Involvement in Date or Acquaintance Rape." *Academy of Emergency Medicine* 4, no. 4 (1997), pp. 323–26.
21. Elsohly, M., and S. Salamone. "Prevalence of Drugs Used in Cases of Alleged Sexual Assault." *Journal of Analytical Toxicology* 23 (1999), pp. 141-6.
22. McGregor, M.J., J. Ericksen, L.A. Ronald, P.A. Janssen, A. Van Vliet, and M. Schulzer. "Rising Incidence of Hospital-Reported Drug-Facilitated Sexual Assault in a Large Urban Community in Canada: Retrospective Population-Based Study." *Canadian Journal of Public Health* 95, no. 6 (2004), pp. 441-5.
23. Burgess, A., P. Donovan, and S.E.H. Moore. "Understanding Heightened Risk Perception of Drink 'Spiking.'" *British Journal of Criminology* 49 (2009), pp. 848–62.
24. Spina, S.P., and M.H.H. Ensom. "Clinical Pharmacokinetic Monitoring of Midazolam in Critically Ill Patients." *Pharmacotherapy* 27, no. 3 (2007), pp. 389-398.
25. Hung, O.R., J.B. Dyck, J. Varvel, S.L. Shafer, and D.R. Stanski. "Comparative Absorption Kinetics of Intramuscular Midazolam and Diazepam." *Canadian Journal of Anaesthesia* 43, no. 5 (1996), pp. 450–455.
26. Fraser, A.D., W. Bryan, and A.F. Isner. "Urinary Screening for Midazolam and Its Major Metabolites with the Abbott ADx and TDx Analyzers and the EMIT d.a.u. Benzodiazepine Assay with Confirmation by GC/MS." *Journal of Analytical Toxicology* 15 (1991), pp. 8–12.
27. Stewart, S.H., S.E. Buffett-Jerrott, G.A. Finley, K.D. Wright, and T.V. Gomez. "Effects of Midazolam on Explicit vs Implicit Memory in a Pediatric Surgery Setting." *Psychopharmacology* 188 (2006), pp. 489-497.
28. See http://www.cbc.ca/news/canada/nova-scotia/drug-theft-from-halifax-hospital-a-suspected-inside-job-1.2743038.
29. Stewart, S.H., S.E. Buffett-Jerrott, G.A. Finley, K.D. Wright, and T.V. Gomez. "Effects of Midazolam on Explicit vs Implicit Memory in a Pediatric Surgery Setting." *Psychopharmacology* 188 (2006), pp. 489-497.
30. Schreiber, A., H. El Aribi, and J. Gibbons. "A Fast and Sensitive LC/MS/MS Method for the Quantitation and Confirmation of 30 Benzodiazepines and Nonbenzodiazepine Hypnotics in Forensic Urine Samples." *Application Note #114AP66-01, Cliquid Drug Screen & Quant Software [Applied Biosystems].* (2007). Retrieved from http://www3.appliedbiosystems.com/cms/groups/psm_marketing/documents/generaldocuments/cms_046758.pdf.
31. Walker, S.E., H.A. Grad, D.A. Haas, and A. Mayer. "Stability of Parental Midazolam in an Oral Formulation." *Anesthesia Progress* 44, no. 1 (1997), pp. 17–22. PMCID: PMC2148861.
32. First DataBank, Inc. *Midazolam–Oral Syrup.* 2010. Retrieved November 1, 2014, from https://myhealth.alberta.ca/health/medications/Pages/conditions.aspx?hwid=fdb1244.
33. Du Mont, J., S. Macdonald, N. Rotbard, D. Bainbridge, E. Asllani, N. Smith, and M.M. Cohen. "Drug-Facilitated Sexual Assault in Ontario, Canada: Toxicological and DNA Findings." *Journal of Forensic and Legal Medicine* 17, no. 6 (2010), pp. 333-8.
34. Brecher, E.M., *Licit and Illicit Drugs.* Boston: Little, Brown, 1972.
35. Johnston, L.D., P.M. O'Malley, J.G. Bachman, and J.E. Schulenberg. *Monitoring the Future National Survey Results on Drug Use, 1975–2012: Volume I, Secondary School Students.* Ann Arbor: Institute for Social Research, University of Michigan, 2013.
36. Beauvais, E., and others. "Inhalant Abuse among American Indian, Mexican American, and Non-Latino White Adolescents." *American Journal of Drug & Alcohol Abuse* 28 (2002), pp. 477–95.
37. Adlaf, E.M., P. Begin, and E. Sawka, eds. *Canadian Addiction Survey (CAS): A National Survey of Canadians' Use of Alcohol and Other Drugs: Prevalence of Use and Related Harms: Detailed Report.* Ottawa: Canadian Centre on Substance Abuse, 2005.
38. Goodman, D. *Youthlink Inner City. Hepatitis C Support Program. Final Report.* Toronto: Toronto CAS, in Research Group on Drug Use, 2004; Research Group on Drug Use. *Drug Use in Toronto.* Toronto: Toronto Public Health, 2005.
39. Manitoba Office of the Children's Advocate. *Pauingassi First Nation Report on Solvent Abuse.* 2003. In D. O'Brien, "Manitoba's Sniff Crisis Has Given Birth to a Tragic Trend . . . Babies That Smell Like Gas." *Winnipeg Free Press,* August 24, 2005, pp. A1-A2.
40. Kaweionnehta Human Resource Group. *First Nations and Inuit Community Youth Solvent Abuse Survey and Study.* Ottawa: National Native Alcohol and Drug Abuse Program/Addictions and Community-Funded Programs, 1993.
41. Canadian Centre on Substance Abuse. *Frequently Asked Questions Series: Youth Volatile Solvent Abuse.* 2006. Retrieved from http://www.ccsa.ca/2006%20CCSA%20Documents/ccsa-011326-2006.pdf.
42. Johnston, L.D., P.M. O'Malley, J.G. Bachman, and J.E. Schulenberg. *Monitoring the Future National Survey Results on Drug Use, 1975–2010: Volume I, Secondary School Students.* Ann Arbor: Institute for Social Research, University of Michigan, 2011.

Chapter 8

1. Institute of Health Economics. *How Much Should We Spend on Mental Health?* Edmonton: Institute of Health Economics, 2008.
2. http://wptheme.cameronhelps.ca/wp-content/uploads/2011/12/Mental-Health-Statistics.pdf
3. Centre for Addiction and Mental Health. *1999 Depressive Illness: A Guide for People with Depression and their Families.* Retrieved November 4, 2011, from http://www.camh.net/About_Addiction_Mental_Health/Mental_Health_Information/Depressive_Illness/depressive_illness_infoguide.pdf.
4. Canadian Centre on Substance Abuse. *Substance Abuse in Canada: Concurrent Disorders.* Ottawa: Canadian Centre on Substance Abuse, 2009.

5. Centre for Addiction and Mental Health. *About CAMH.* 2011. Retrieved November 11, 2011, from http://www.camh.net/About_CAMH/index.html.
6. Government of Canada. The Human Face of Mental Health and Mental Illness in Canada. 2006.
7. Brady, K.T., and S.C. Sonne. "The Relationship between Substance Abuse and Bipolar Disorder." *Journal of Clinical Psychiatry* 56, suppl. 3 (1995), pp. 19–24.
8. Regier, D.A., and others. "Comorbidity of Mental Disorders with Alcohol and Other Drug Abuse. Results from the Epidemiologic Catchment Area (ECA) Study." *Journal of the American Medical Association* 264, no. 19 (1990), pp. 2511–18.
9. Selzer, J.A., and J.A. Lieberman. "Schizophrenia and Substance Abuse." *Psychiatric Clinics of North America* 16 (1993), pp. 401–12.
10. George, T.P., and J.H. Krystal. "Comorbidity of Psychiatric and Substance Abuse Disorders." *Current Opinion in Psychiatry* 13, no. 3 (2000), pp. 327–62.
11. Ziedonis, D.M., and others. "Improving the Care of Individuals with Schizophrenia and Substance Use Disorders: Consensus Recommendations." *Journal of Psychiatric Practice* 11, no. 5 (2005), pp. 315–39.
12. Colp, R. "History of Psychiatry." In *Kaplan and Sadock's Comprehensive Textbook of Psychiatry,* 8th ed., B.J. Sadock and V.A. Sadock, eds. Baltimore, MD: Lippincott, Williams and Wilkins, 2004, pp. 4013–26.
13. Morrow, M., P. Dagg, and A. Manager. "Is Deinstitutionalization a 'Failed Experiment'? The Ethics of Re-institutionalization." *Journal of Ethics in Mental Health* 3, no. 2 (2008), pp. 1–7.
14. Centre for Addiction and Mental Health. *Mental Health and Addiction Statistics.* 2009. Retrieved November 4, 2011, from http://www.camh.net/News_events/Key_CAMH_facts_for_media/addictionmentalhealthstatistics.html.
15. Adlaf, E.M., A. Demers, and L. Gliksman, eds. *Canadian Campus Survey 2004.* Toronto: Centre for Addiction and Mental Health, 2005.
16. Schellinck, T., and others. *Seniors Survey: Prevalence of Substance Use and Gambling Among New Brunswick Adults Aged 55+.* New Brunswick Department of Health and Wellness, 2002. Retrieved November 4, 2011, from http://www.gnb.ca/0378/pdf/SeniorsFinalReport2002ENG.pdf.
17. American Psychiatric Association. *Diagnostic and Statistical Manual of Mental Disorders,* 5th ed. Washington, DC: American Psychiatric Association, 2013.
18. See http://pro.psychcentral.com/dsm-5-changes-anxiety-disorders-phobias/004266.html
19. Canadian Mental Health Association. *Understanding Mental Illness.* (n.d.). Retrieved November 4, 2011, from http://www.cmha.ca/bins/content_page.asp?cid=3.
20. Health Canada. *A Report on Mental Illnesses in Canada.* Ottawa: Health Canada, 2002.
21. Wedding, D., and M. Boyd. *Movies and Mental Illness.* New York, NY: McGraw-Hill, 1999.
22. See http://www.dsm5.org/Research/Documents/Craske_What%20is%20an%20Anxiety%20DO.pdf.
23. DSM-V, p. 161.
24. Hebb, A.L.O., and others. "The Myth of Panic Spontaneity: Consideration of Behavioural and Neurochemical Sensitization." *Open Psychiatry Journal* 1 (2007), pp. 1–25.
25. Dick, C.L., R.C. Bland, and S.C. Newman. "Epidemiology of Psychiatric Disorder in Edmonton: Panic Disorder." *Acta Psychiatrica Scandinavica* Suppl. 376 (1994), pp. 45–53.
26. Shugar, G., B.F. Hoffman, and J.D. Johnston. "Electroconvulsive Therapy for Schizophrenia in Ontario: A Report on Therapeutic Polymorphism." *Comprehensive Psychiatry* 25, no. 5 (1984), pp. 509–20.
27. Sibbald, B. "Quebec Tackles Electroconvulsive Therapy Issue." *Canadian Medical Association Journal* 168, no. 12 (2003), p. 1583.
28. Enns, M.W., J.P. Reiss, and P. Chan. "Electroconvulsive Therapy. Canadian Psychiatric Association: Position Paper." *The Canadian Journal of Psychiatry* 55, no. 6 (2010), pp. 1–12.
29. Tharyan, P., and C.E. Adams. "Electroconvulsive Therapy for Schizophrenia." *The Cochrane Database of Systematic Reviews* 2005, Issue 2.
30. Bolwig, T.G. "How Does Electroconvulsive Therapy Work? Theories on Its Mechanism. *Canadian Journal of Psychiatry* 56, no. 1 (2011), pp. 13–18.
31. Scissons, H. "Shock Therapy Sees Advances." *The StarPhoenix* (Saskatoon). 2010. Retrieved November 4, 2011, from http://www2.canada.com/saskatoonstarphoenix/news/story.html?id=84956de6-2609-4467-a61e-901f6216b554.
32. Saskatoon Health Region. *Dubé Centre for Mental Health to Open Soon.* 2010. Retrieved November 4, 2011, from http://regionreporter.wordpress.com/2010/01/08/dube-centre-for-mental-health-to-open-soon; Saskatoon Health Region. *Programs & Services–Mental Health and Addiction Services.* 2010. Retrieved November 4, 2011, from http://www.saskatoonhealthregion.ca/your_health/ps_mhas_acute_services.htm.
33. Freyhan, F.A. "The Immediate and Long-Range Effects of Chlorpromazine on the Mental Hospital." In Smith, Kline and French Laboratories, *Chlorpromazine and Mental Health.* Philadelphia, PA: Lea & Febiger, 1955.
34. Compendium of Pharmaceuticals and Specialties. *eCPS/Electronic Compendium of Pharmaceuticals and Specialties.* Canadian Pharmacists Association, 2010. Retrieved November 4, 2011, from http://www.pharmacists.ca/function/store/PublicationDetail.cfm?pPub=5.
35. Pfizer Canada Inc. *New Schizophrenia Treatment Now Available in Canada.* 2010. Retrieved November 4, 2011, from http://www.drugs.com/news/new-schizophrenia-now-available-canada-7717.html.
36. Health Canada. *Zeldox.* 2007. Retrieved November 4, 2011, from http://www.hc-sc.gc.ca/dhp-mps/prodpharma/sbd-smd/phase1-decision/drug-med/pm_mp_2007_zeldox_078188_partiii-eng.php.

37. McIntyre, R.S., and others. "Comparison of the Metabolic and Economic Consequences of Long-Term Treatment of Schizophrenia Using Ziprasidone, Olanzapine, Quetiapine and Risperidone in Canada: A Cost-Effectiveness Analysis." *Journal of Evaluation in Clinical Practice* 16, no. 4 (2010), pp. 744-55.
38. Alessi-Severini, S., and others. "Utilization and Costs of Antipsychotic Agents: A Canadian Population-Based Study, 1996-2006." *Psychiatric Services* 59, no. 5 (2008), pp. 547-53. Also found at http://www.ps.psychiatryonline.org.
39. Doey, T., and others. "Survey of Atypical Antipsychotic Prescribing by Canadian Child Psychiatrists and Developmental Pediatricians for Patients Aged Under 18 Years." *Canadian Journal of Psychiatry* 52 (2007), pp. 363-68.
40. Panagiotopoulos, C., and others. "First Do No Harm: Promoting an Evidence-Based Approach to Atypical Antipsychotic Use in Children and Adolescents." *Journal of the Canadian Academy of Child and Adolescent Psychiatry* 19, no. 2 (2010), pp. 124-37.
41. http://www.bmscanada.ca/en/products/release/health-canada-approves-abilify-as-first-atypical-antipsychotic-in-the-treatment-of-adolescents-with
42. Gardner, D.M., R.J. Baldessarini, and P. Waraich. "Modern Antipsychotic Drugs: A Critical Overview." *Canadian Medical Association Journal* 172, no. 13 (2005), pp. 1703-11.
43. Bollini, P., and others. "Antipsychotic Drugs: Is More Worse? A Meta-Analysis of the Published Randomized Control Trials." *Psychological Medicine* 24 (1994), p. 307.
44. Rochon, P.A., and others. "Antipsychotic Therapy and Short-Term Serious Events in Older Adults with Dementia." *Archives of Internal Medicine* 168, no. 10 (2008), p. 1090-96.
45. Schneeweiss, S., and others. "Risk of Death Associated with the Use of Conventional versus Atypical Antipsychotic Drugs among Elderly Patients." *Canadian Medical Association Journal* 176, no. 5 (2007), pp. 627-32.
46. Yan, J. "FDA Extends Black-Box Warning to All Antipsychotics." *Psychiatric News* 43, no. 14 (2008), p. 1.
47. Fick, D.M., and others. "Updating the Beers Criteria for Potentially Inappropriate Medication Use in Older Adults: Results of a US Consensus Panel of Experts." *Archives of Internal Medicine* 163, no. 22 (2003), pp. 2716-24.
48. CBC News. "Avoid Antipsychotic Drugs for Elderly, Experts Urge, After Death Risk Study." 2009. Retrieved November 4, 2011, from http://www.cbc.ca/news/health/story/2009/01/09/anti-psychotic-risks.html.
49. Avorn, J., and others. (1989). "Use of Psychoactive Medication and the Quality of Care in Rest Homes: Findings and Policy Implications of a Statewide Study." *New England Journal of Medicine* 320 (1989), pp. 227-32; Buck, J.A. "Psychotropic Drug Practice in Nursing Homes." *Journal of the American Geriatrics Society* 36 (1988), pp. 409-18; Ray, W.A., C.F. Federspiel, and W. Schaffner. "A Study of Antipsychotic Drug Use in Nursing Homes: Epidemiologic Evidence Suggesting Misuse." *American Journal of Public Health* 70 (1980), pp. 485-91.
50. Hagen, B., and others. "Antipsychotic Drug Use in Canadian Long-Term Care Facilities: Prevalence, and Patterns Following Resident Relocation." *International Psychogeriatrics* 17, no. 2 (2005), pp. 179-93.
51. Hughes, C., and others. "The Impact of Legislation on Psychotropic Drug Use in Nursing Homes: A Cross-National Perspective." *Journal of the American Geriatrics Society* 48 (2000), pp. 931-7; McGrath, A.M., and G.A. Jackson. "Survey of Neuroleptic Prescribing in Residents of Nursing Homes in Glasgow." *British Medical Journal* 312, no. 7031 (1996), pp. 611-13; Sorensen, L., and others. "Determinants for the Use of Psychotropics among Nursing Home Residents." *International Journal of Geriatric Psychiatry* 16 (2001), pp. 147-54.
52. Earthy, A., and others. "Ensuring the Appropriate Use of Neuroleptics." *Canadian Nursing Home* 11 (2000), pp. 5-10.
53. Lieberman, J.A., and others. "Effectiveness of Antipsychotic Drugs in Patients with Chronic Schizophrenia." *New England Journal of Medicine* 353 (2005), pp. 1209-23.
54. Lieberman, J.A. "Comparative Effectiveness of Antipsychotic Drugs." *Archives of General Psychiatry* 63 (2006), pp. 1069-72.
55. Compendium of Pharmaceuticals and Specialties. *eCPS/Electronic Compendium of Pharmaceuticals and Specialties,* 2010 online version. Canadian Pharmacists Association, 2010.
56. Kurdyak, P.A., D.N. Juurlink, and M.M. Mamdani. "The Effect of Antidepressant Warnings on Prescribing Trends in Ontario, Canada." *American Journal of Public Health* 97, no. 4 (2007), pp. 750-54.
57. Yan, J. "Canada Sees Troubling Trend in Antidepressant Prescribing." *Psychiatric News* 43, no. 10 (2008), p. 14. Also found at http://pn.psychiatryonline.org/content/43/10/14.1.full.
58. U.S. Food and Drug Administration. "FDA Launches a Multi-Pronged Strategy to Strengthen Safeguards for Children Treated with Antidepressant Medications." *FDA News*, 2004.
59. McManus, T. "Antidepressants: New Black Box Warnings Unlikely to Significantly Threaten Sales." *Pharmaceutical Business Review*. 2007. Online newsletter available at http://www.pharmaceutical-business-review.com.
60. Kinnon, D. *Improving Population Health, Health Promotion, Disease Prevention and Health Protection Services and Programs for Aboriginal People. 2002.* National Aboriginal Health Organization. Retrieved January 28, 2008, from http://www.naho.ca/english/pdf/research_pop_health.pdf.
61. Chambers, C.D., and others. "Birth Outcomes in Pregnant Women Taking Fluoxetine." *New England Journal of Medicine* 335 (1996), pp. 1010-15.
62. Currie, J. *The Marketization of Depression: The Prescribing of SSRI Antidepressants to Women.* 2005. Retrieved November 4, 2011, from http://www.whp-apsf.ca/pdf/SSRIs.pdf;

Health Canada. Health Canada Advises Canadians of Stronger Warnings for SSRIs and Other Newer Anti-Depressants. Ottawa: Health Canada, 2004. Available at http://www.hc-sc.gc.ca/ahc-asc/media/advisories-avis/2004/2004_31_e.html.

63. Ramos, É., M. St-André, and A. Bérard. "Association between Antidepressant Use during Pregnancy and Infants Born Small for Gestational Age." *Canadian Journal of Psychiatry* 55, no. 10 (2010), pp. 643–52.
64. Kirsch, I., and others. "Initial Severity and Antidepressant Benefits: A Meta-Analysis of Data Submitted to the Food and Drug Administration." *PLoS Medicine* 5, no. 2 (2008), p. e45 EP. Retrieved November 4, 2011, from http://www.plosmedicine.org/article/info:doi/10.1371/journal.pmed.0050045.
65. Turner, E.H., and others. "Selective Publication of Antidepressant Trials and Its Influence on Apparent Efficacy." *New England Journal of Medicine* 358, no. 3 (2008), pp. 252–60.
66. Kennedy, S.H., and S.J. Rizvi. "Emerging Drugs for Major Depressive Disorder." *Expert Opinion on Emerging Drugs* 14, no. 3 (2009), pp. 439–53.
67. Lavoie, K.L., and R.P. Fleet. "Should Psychologists Be Granted Prescription Privileges? A Review of the Prescription Privilege Debate for Psychiatrists." *Canadian Journal of Psychiatry* 47 (2002), pp. 443–49.
68. O'Connor, D.W., and others. "The Effectiveness of Continuation-Maintenance ECT in Reducing Depressed Older Patients' Hospital Re-admissions." *Journal of Affective Disorders* 120 (2010), pp. 62–66.
69. Shorter, E. "The History of Lithium Therapy." *Bipolar Disorders* 11, suppl. 2 (2009), pp. 4–9.
70. Kingston, E. "The Lithium Treatment of Hypomanic and Manic States." *Comprehensive Psychiatry* 1 (1960), pp. 317–20.
71. Parkinson, R. "Lithium Therapy in Canada before the 1970s" [Letter to the Editor]. *Canadian Medical Association Journal* 134, no. 1 (1986), p. 13. Retrieved November 1, 2011, from http://www.ncbi.nlm.nih.gov/pmc/articles/PMC1490598/pdf/cmaj00109-0015a.pdf.
72. Calabrese, J.R., and others. "International Consensus Group on Bipolar I Depression Treatment Guidelines." *Journal of Clinical Psychiatry* 65, no. 4 (2004), pp. 571–79.
73. Canadian Institute for Health Information. *Hospital Mental Health Services in Canada, 2003–2004*. Ottawa: Canadian Institute for Health Information, 2006; Madi, N., H. Zhao, and J.F. Li. "Hospital Readmissions for Patients with Mental Illness in Canada." *Healthcare Quarterly* 10, no. 2 (2007), pp. 30–32.
74. Brunette, M.F., and others. "Clozapine Use and Relapses of Substance Use Disorder among Patients with Co-occurring Schizophrenia and Substance Use Disorders." *Schizophrenia Bulletin* 32, no. 4 (2006), pp. 637–43; Coodin, S., and others. "Patient Factors Associated with Missed Appointments in People with Schizophrenia." *Canadian Journal of Psychiatry* 49, no. 2 (2004), pp. 145–48; Oehl, M., M. Hummer, and W.W. Fleischhacker, "Compliance with Antipsychotic Treatment." *Acta Psychiatrica Scandanavica,* suppl. 407 (2000), pp. 83–86.
75. Stahl, S.M. *Essential Psychopharmacology*. Cambridge, UK: Cambridge University Press, 2000.
76. Garnham, J., and others. "Prophylactic Treatment Response in Bipolar Disorder: Results of a Naturalistic Observation Study." *Journal of Affective Disorders* 104, nos. 1–3 (2007), pp. 185–90.
77. Isaac, R.J., and V.C. Armat. *Madness in the Streets: How Psychiatry and the Law Abandoned People with Mental Illnesses*. New York, NY: Free Press, 1990.
78. Holley, H.L., and J. Arboleda-Flórez. "Criminalization of People with Mental Illnesses: Part I. Police Perceptions." *Canadian Journal of Psychiatry* 33 (1988), pp. 81–86.
79. Morrissey, J.P., and H.H. Goldman. "The Enduring Asylum." *International Journal of Law and Psychiatry* 4 (1981), pp. 13–44.
80. Arboleda-Flórez, J. "Deinstitutionalization and Forensic Issues: Are We Flogging the Wrong Horse?" *Canadian Psychiatric Association Bulletin* 25, no. 6 (1993), pp. 29–31; Bland, R.C., and others. "Prevalence of Psychiatric Disorders and Suicide Attempts in a Prison Population." *Canadian Journal of Psychiatry* 35 (1990), pp. 407–13.
81. Davis, S. "Assessing the 'Criminalization' of People with Mental Illnesses in Canada." *Canadian Journal of Psychiatry* 37 (1992), pp. 532–38; Public Health Agency of Canada. *Mental Illness and Violence: Proof or Stereotype*. 2002. Retrieved November 4, 2001, from http://www.phac-aspc.gc.ca/mh-sm/pubs/mental_illness/critical-eng.php.
82. Mood Disorders Society of Canada. *Quick Facts: Mental Illness and Addiction in Canada*. 2009. Retrieved November 4, 2011, from http://www.mooddisorderscanada.ca/documents/Media%20Room/Quick%20Facts%203rd%20Edition%20Eng%20Nov%2012%2009.pdf.
83. Mental Health Commission of Canada. *The Homeless and Mental Illness: Solving the Challenge*. 2008. Retrieved November 4, 2011, from http://www.mentalhealthcommission.ca/SiteCollectionDocuments/Homelessness/Speech_kirbyVan_Apr2808_ENG.pdf.
84. CBC Canada. *Number of Prisoners with Mental Illness on Upswing: Report*. 2005. Retrieved November 4, 2011, from http://www.cbc.ca/canada/story/2005/11/04/MentalPrisoners_051104.html; Canwest News Service. *Mental Health Becoming Huge Challenge in Canada's Prisons*. 2007. Retrieved November 4, 2011, from http://www.canada.com/topics/news/national/story.html?id=c45d5f0b-4e84-4703-9285-5939b45fdec4&k=48813.

Chapter 9

1. Agriculture and Agri-food Canada. *The Canadian Brewing Industry*. 2007. Retrieved from http://www4.agr.gc.ca/AAFC-AAC/display-afficher.do?id=1171560813521#f1.

2. For more on this topic, see http://www.beercanada.com/statistics; http://www.agr.gc.ca/eng/industry-markets-and-trade/statistics-and-market-information/by-product-sector/processed-food-and-beverages/the-canadian-brewery-industry/?id=1171560813521#s3a; and http://www.ukessays.com/essays/economics/the-beer-industry-in-italy-and-canada-economics-essay.php.
3. Lender, M.E. *Drinking in America*. New York: The Free Press, 1987.
4. Levine, H.G. "The Alcohol Problem in America: From Temperance to Alcoholism." *British Addiction* 79 (1984), pp. 109–19.
5. CBC News. *A Timeline of Prohibition and Liquor Legislation in Canada*. 2005. Retrieved October 7, 2010, from http://www.cbc.ca/news/background/prohibition/.
6. Koren, J. *Economic Aspects of the Liquor Problem*. New York: Houghton Mifflin, 1899.
7. Clark, N.H. *The Dry Years: Prohibition and Social Change in Washington*. Seattle: University of Washington Press, 1965.
8. Canadian Centre on Substance Abuse. *Legal Drinking Age by Province in Canada*. 2008. Retrieved October 12, 2010, from http://www.ccsa.ca/eng/topics/legislation/legaldrinkingage/pages/default.aspx.
9. "Culture Shapes Young People's Drinking Habits." *Science Daily*, Sept. 23, 2008.
10. List of countries by beer consumption per capita. Retrieved from Wikipedia.com, January 23, 2013.
11. Kirin Holdings Company Limited. *Kirin Institute of Food and Lifestyle Report Vol. 29: Global Beer Consumption by Country 2009*. 2010. Retrieved September 24, 2011, from http://www.kirinholdings.co.jp/english/ir/news/2010/1222_01.html.
12. Statistics Canada. *Control and Sale of Alcoholic Beverages for the Year Ending March 31, 2013*. 2014. Retrieved from http://www.statcan.gc.ca/daily-quotidien/140410/dq140410a-eng.htm.
13. Centre for Addiction and Mental Health. *Canadian Campus Survey 2004*. 2005. Retrieved September 27, 2010, from http://www.camh.net/Research/Areas_of_research/Population_Life_Course_Studies/CCS_2004_report.pdf.
14. The Bottom Line. "Wet or Dry: Schools Ponder Variety of Strategies to Curb Alcohol Problems." *The Bottom Line* 18, no. 3 (1997), pp. 68–72.
15. Adlaf, E., P. Begin, and E. Sawka (eds.). *Canadian Addiction Survey (CAS): A National Survey of Canadians' Use of Alcohol and Other Drugs: Prevalence of Use and Related Harms: Detailed Report*. Ottawa: Canadian Centre on Substance Abuse, 2005. Retrieved December 2, 2013, from http://www.ccsa.ca/2005%20CCSA%20Documents/ccsa-004028-2005.pdf.
16. Adlaf, E., A. Demers, and L. Gliksman (eds.). *Canadian Campus Survey, 2004*. Toronto: Centre for Addiction and Mental Health, 2005. Retrieved December 2, 2013 from http://www.camh.ca/en/research/research_areas/community_and_population_health/Documents/CCS_2004_report.pdf.
17. Health Canada. *Canadian Alcohol and Drug Use Monitoring Survey (2012): Summary of Results*. 2014. Retrieved from http://www.hc-sc.gc.ca/hc-ps/drugs-drogues/stat/_2012/summary-sommaire-eng.php.
18. Frezza, M., and others. "High Blood Alcohol Levels in Women: The Role of Decreased Gastric Alcohol Dehydrogenase Activity and First-Pass Metabolism." *New England Journal of Medicine* 322 (1990), p. 95.
19. Azagba, S., D. Langille, and M. Asbridge. "The Consumption of Alcohol Mixed with Energy Drinks: Prevalence and Key Correlates among Canadian High School Students." *CMAJ Open*. 2013. doi: 10.9778/cmajo.20120017.
20. Brache, K., and T. Stockwell. "Drinking Patterns and Risk Behaviors Associated with Combined Alcohol and Energy Drink Consumption in College Drinkers." *Addictive Behaviors 36* (2011), pp. 1133–1140. doi: 10.1016/j.addbeh.2011.07.003.
21. Callaghan, R.C., M. Sanches, J.M. Gatley, and J.K. Cunningham. "Effects of the Minimum Legal Drinking Age on Alcohol-Related Health Service Use in Hospital Settings in Ontario: A Regression-Discontinuity Approach." *American Journal of Public Health* 103 (2013), pp. 2284–2291. doi: 10.2105/AJPH.2013.301320.
22. Graham, D. "Vodka Eyeballing: Is Seeing Believing?" *Toronto Star*. 2010. Retrieved November 20, 2014 from http://www.thestar.com/life/2010/06/08/vodka_eyeballing_is_seeing_believing.html.
23. Huffington Post Canada. "Vodka Tampons? Reported Alcohol Abuse Among Teens Also Includes 'Butt Chugging.'" 2011. Retrieved November 20, 2014 from http://www.huffingtonpost.ca/2011/11/14/vodka-tampon-teens_n_1092594.html.
24. McKinnon L.R., S.M. Hughes, S.C. De Rosa, J.A. Martinson, J. Plants, and others. "Optimizing Viable Leukocyte Sampling from the Female Genital Tract for Clinical Trials: An International Multi-Site Study." *PLOS ONE* 9, no. 1 (2014), p. e85675. doi:10.1371/journal.pone.0085675.
25. Romas, L.M., K. Hasselrot, L.G. Aboud, K.D. Birse, and T.B. Ball, and others. "A Comparative Proteomic Analysis of the Soluble Immune Factor Environment of Rectal and Oral Mucosa." *PLOS ONE* 9, no. 6 (2014), p. e100820. doi:10.1371/journal.pone.0100820.
26. Thombs, D.L., R.J. O'Mara, M. Tsukamoto, M.E. Rossheim, R.M. Weiler, M.L. Merves, and others. "Event-Level Analyses of Energy Drink Consumption and Alcohol Intoxication in Bar Patrons." *Addictive Behaviors* 35 (2010), pp. 325–330.
27. Dumas-Campagna, J., R. Tardif, G. Charest-Tardif, and S. Haddad. "Ethanol Toxicokinetics Resulting from Inhalational Exposure in Human Volunteers and Toxicokinetic Modeling." *Inhalational Toxicology* 26, no. 2 (2014), pp. 59–69.
28. Lange, R.T., J.R. Shewchuk, A. Rauscher, M. Jarrett, M.K.S. Heran, J.R. Brubacher, and G.L. Iverson. "A Prospective Study of the Influence of Acute Alcohol

Intoxication versus Chronic Alcohol Consumption on Outcome Following Traumatic Brain Injury." *Archives of Clinical Neuropsychology* 29, no. 5 (2014), pp. 478–495. doi:10.1093/arclin/acu027

29. Qureshi, S., S. Laganiere, G. Caille, D. Gossard, Y. Lacasse, and I. McGilveray. "Effect of Acute Dose of Alcohol on the Pharmacokinetics of Oral Nifedipine in Humans." *Pharmaceutical Research* 9, no. 5 (1992), pp. 683–686.
30. Ferguson, C.S., S. Miksys, R.M. Palmour, and R.F. Tyndale. "Differential Effects of Nicotine Treatment and Ethanol Self-Administration on CYP2A6, CYP2B6 and Nicotine Pharmacokinetics in African Green Monkeys." *Journal of Pharmacology and Experimental Therapeutics* 343, no. 3 (2012), pp. 628–637.
31. Kumar, S., and others. "The Role of GABA(A) Receptors in the Acute and Chronic Effects of Ethanol: A Decade of Progress." *Psychopharmacology (Berl)* 205 (2009), pp. 529–64.
32. Cruz, M., and others. "Shared Mechanisms of Alcohol and Other Drugs." *Alcohol Research and Health* 31 (2008), pp. 137–47.
33. Ron, D., and J. Wang. "The NMDA Receptor and Alcohol Addiction." In *Biology of the NMDA Receptor*, A.M. Van Dongen, ed. Boca Raton, FL: Florida CRC Press, 2009.
34. Steele, C.M., and R.A. Josephs. "Alcohol Myopia." *American Psychologist* 45 (1990), pp. 921–33.
35. Asbridge, M., and others. "The Criminalization of Impaired Driving in Canada: Assessing the Deterrent Impact of Canada's First Per Se Law." *Journal of Studies on Alcohol* 65 (2004), pp. 450–59.
36. Mann, R.E., and others. "Drinking-Driving Fatalities and Consumption of Beer, Wine and Spirits." *Drugs and Alcohol Review* 25 (2006), pp. 321–25.
37. Canada Safety Council. *Canada's Blood Alcohol Laws among the Strictest in the Western World*. 2009. Retrieved October 5, 2010, from http://www.safety-council.org/news/archives/canada-s-blood-alcohol-laws-among-the-strictest-2010.
38. George, W.H., and S.A. Stoner. "Understanding Acute Alcohol Effects on Sexual Behavior." *Annual Review of Sex Research* 11 (2000), pp. 1053–2528.
39. Crothers, T.D. "Alcoholic Trance." *Popular Science* 26 (1884), pp. 189, 191.
40. Pernanen, K. *Alcohol in Human Violence*. New York: Guilford Press, 1991.
41. Pernanen, K., and others. *Proportions of Crimes Associated with Alcohol and Other Drugs in Canada (R51)*. Correctional Services of Canada. 2002. Retrieved November 4, 2011, from http://www.csc-scc.gc.ca/text/rsrch/regional/smmry/summary0151-eng.shtml.
42. Mann, R., and others. "Alcoholics Anonymous Membership May Decrease Alcohol-Related Homicides." *Clinical and Experimental Research* 33 (2006), pp. 265–72.
43. Krebs, C.P., and others. "College Women's Experiences with Physically Forced, Alcohol- or Other Drug-Enabled, and Drug-Facilitated Sexual Assault Before and Since Entering College." *Journal of American College Health* 57 (2009), pp. 639–49.
44. Boenisch, S., and others. "The Role of Alcohol Use Disorder and Alcohol Consumption in Suicide Attempts–A Secondary Analysis of 1921 Suicide Attempts." *European Psychiatry* 25 (2010), pp. 414–20.
45. Centers for Disease Control and Prevention. "Alcohol-Attributable Deaths and Years of Potential Life Lost–United States, 2001." *Morbidity and Mortality Weekly Report* 53 (2004), pp. 866–70.
46. NIAAA. *Eighth Special Report to the US Congress on Alcohol and Health*. NIH Publication Number 94-3699. Washington, DC: U.S. Public Health Service, 1993.
47. Britton, A. "Alcohol and Heart Disease." *British Medical Journal* 341 (2010), pp. 1114–5.
48. Stockwell, T., J. Zhao, and G. Thomas. "Should Alcohol Policies Aim to Reduce Total Alcohol Consumption? New Analyses of Canadian Drinking Patterns." *Addiction Research and Theory* 17, no. 2 (2009, pp. 135–151.
49. Loxley, W., J. Toumbourou, T. Stockwell, B. Haines, K. Scott, C. Godfrey, and others. *The Prevention of Substance Use, Risk and Harm in Australia: A Review of the Evidence*. Canberra, Australia: National Drug Research Institute and the Centre for Adolescent Health, 2004.
50. Babor, T., R. Caetano, S. Casswell, G. Edwards, N. Giesbrecht, and others. "The Global Burden of Alcohol Consumption." In *Alcohol: No Ordinary Commodity: Research and Public Policy* (2nd ed.). Oxford University Press, 2010.
51. Floyd, R.J., and J.S. Sidhu. "Monitoring Prenatal Alcohol Exposure." *American Journal of Medical Genetics Part C (Seminars in Medical Genetics)* 127C (2004), pp. 3–9.
52. Mayo-Smith, M.E. "Pharmacological Management of Alcohol Withdrawal: A Meta-analysis and Evidence-based Practice Guideline." *Journal of the American Medical Association* 278 (1997), pp. 144–51.
53. American Psychiatric Association. *Diagnostic and Statistical Manual of Mental Disorders*, 5th ed., Washington, DC: American Psychiatric Association, 2013.
54. Kreusch, F., and others. "Assessing the Stimulant and Sedative Effects of Alcohol with Explicit and Implicit Measures in a Balanced Placebo Design." *Journal of Studies on Alcohol and Drugs* 74 (2013), pp. 923–30.

Chapter 10

1. Stewart, G.G. "A History of the Medicinal Use of Tobacco, 1492–1860." *Medical History* 11 (1967), pp. 228–68.
2. Sargent, J.D., and others. "Brand Appearances in Contemporary Cinema Films and Contribution to Global Marketing of Cigarettes." *The Lancet* 357 (2001), pp. 29–32.
3. Cole, L. *B.C. Group Calls for Restricted Ratings for Movies Featuring Smoking*. 2011. Retrieved November 5, 2011, from http://www.straight.com/article-375891/vancouver/bc-group-calls-restricted-ratings-movies-featuring-smoking.
4. Smoke Free Movies. *How Movies Sell Smoking*. (n.d.). Retrieved November 5, 2011, from http://smokefreemovies.ucsf.edu/problem/bigtobacco.html.

5. Vaughn, W. Quoted in Dunphy, E.B. "Alcohol and Tobacco Amblyopia: A Historical Survey." *American Journal of Ophthalmology* 68 (1969), p. 573.
6. International Development Research Centre. *Farmers on Tobacco Road.* 2004. Retrieved November 5, 2011, from http://ghri.gc.ca/waterdemand/ev-28833-201-1-DO_TOPIC.html.
7. Wyckman, R.G. "Smokeless Tobacco in Canada: Deterring Market Development." *Tobacco Control* 8 (1999), pp. 411–20.
8. The StarPhoenix (Saskatoon). "MLB Leaders Urged to Ban Chewing Tobacco." *The StarPhoenix* (Saskatoon). 2011. Retrieved October 12, 2011, from http://www2.canada.com/saskatoonstarphoenix/news/world/story.html?id=cb5c40c8-0275-465d-9d27-914b9958409d.
9. Brooks, J.E. *The Mighty Leaf.* Boston, MA: Little, Brown, 1952.
10. Canadian Centre on Substance Abuse. *The Costs of Substance Abuse in Canada.* 2002. Ottawa: Canadian Centre on Substance Abuse.
11. Canadian Centre on Substance Abuse. *Substance Abuse in Canada: Current Challenges and Choices.* 2005. Ottawa: Canadian Centre on Substance Abuse.
12. Clark, G., and A.M. Lavack. "Responding to the Global Tobacco Industry: Canada and the Framework Convention on Tobacco Control." *Canadian Public Administration* 50, no. 1 (2007), pp. 100–18.
13. Borio, G. *Tobacco Timeline.* 1998. Retrieved November 5, 2011, from http://academic.udayton.edu/health/syllabi/tobacco/history2.htm#Appendices.
14. Manfredi, C.P. "Expressive Freedom and Tobacco Advertising: A Canadian Perspective." *American Journal of Public Health* 92, no. 3 (2002), pp. 360–62.
15. Sherer, G. "Smoking Behaviour and Compensation: A Review of the Literature." *Psychopharmacology* 145 (1999), pp. 1–20.
16. Ferrence, R., P. Beck, and A. Mullins. *The Emerging Issue: Waterpipe/Hookah Usage* (2013), pp. 24–26. Retrieved from https://www.ptcccfc.on.ca/common/pages/UserFile.aspx?fileId=104483.
17. Alary, B., K. Toogood, B. Finegan, F. Hammal, and W. Kindzierski. "Herbal Shisha a Potential Health Hazard: Study." University of Alberta. November 8, 2013. Retrieved from http://news.ualberta.ca/newsarticles/2013/november/herbal-shisha-a-potential-health-hazard-study#sthash.C2RDHUMb.dpuf.
18. University of Saskatchewan Health Services. *Hookah: What You Need to Know.* May 13, 2014. Retrieved from http://students.usask.ca/current/life/health/stayhealthy/brochures/hookah.php.
19. Alberta Health Services. "Let's Talk About . . . Hookah." *Alberta Quits.* February 2014. Retrieved from http://www.albertaquits.ca/database/files/library/Hookah_final.pdf.
20. University of Saskatchewan Health Services. *Hookah: What You Need to Know.* May 13, 2014. Retrieved from http://students.usask.ca/current/life/health/stayhealthy/brochures/hookah.php.
21. University of Saskatchewan Health Services. *Hookah: What You Need to Know:* Figure 1.1. May 13, 2014. Retrieved from http://students.usask.ca/current/life/health/stayhealthy/brochures/hookah.php.
22. University of Saskatchewan Health Services. *Hookah: What You Need to Know.* May 13, 2014. Retrieved from http://students.usask.ca/current/life/health/stayhealthy/brochures/hookah.php.
23. *The Emerging Issue: Waterpipe/Hookah Usage.* Webinar. 2013. Retrieved from https://www.ptcc-cfc.on.ca/common/pages/UserFile.aspx?fileId=104483.
24. Adlaf, E.M., A. Demers, and L. Gliksman, eds. *Canadian Campus Survey 2004.* Toronto: Centre for Addiction and Mental Health, 2005.
25. Health Canada. *Canadian Tobacco Use Monitoring Survey, February–December 2006. Smoking and Education, Age 15 + Years, Canada 2006.* 2006. Retrieved November 5, 2011, from http://www.hc-sc.gc.ca/hc-ps/tobac-tabac/research-recherche/stat/_ctums-esutc_2006/ann-table8-eng.php.
26. Health Canada. *Canadian Tobacco Use Monitoring Survey.* 2010. Retrieved November 5, 2011, from http://www.hc-sc.gc.ca/hc-ps/tobac-tabac/research-recherche/stat/_ctums-esutc_2010/w-p-1_sum-som-eng.php.
27. Health Canada. *Summary of Results of the 2008–09 Youth Smoking Survey.* 2009. Retrieved November 5, 2011, from http://www.hc-sc.gc.ca/hc-ps/tobac-tabac/research-recherche/stat/_survey-sondage_2008-2009/result-eng.php.
28. Health Canada. *Tobacco.* 2006. Retrieved November 5, 2011, from www.hc-sc.gc.ca/fnih-spni/substan/tobac-tabac/index_e.html; Retnakaran, R., and others. "Cigarette Smoking and Cardiovascular Risk Factors among Aboriginal Canadian Youths." *Canadian Medical Association Journal* 173 (2005), pp. 885–89.
29. The Canadian Press. *Smoking Declines among Teens, Young Adults.* 2010. Retrieved November 5, 2011, from http://www.cbc.ca/health/story/2010/09/27/health-smoking-teens.html.
30. Poulin, C., and W. McDonald. *Nova Scotia Student Drug Use 2007.* 2007. Retrieved November 5, 2011, from http://www.gov.ns.ca/hpp/publications/NS_Highlights_2007.pdf.
31. CBC News. *Timeline of Canadian Tobacco Laws.* 2007. Retrieved November 5, 2011, from http://www.cbc.ca/news/background/smoking/timeline.html.
32. "Province to Outlaw Under-18 Smoking." *Calgary Herald.* 2003. Retrieved November 5, 2011, from http://www.saskdebate.com/media/3047/tobaccopossession.pdf.
33. Health Canada. *Toolkit for Responsible Tobacco Retailers–Atlantic Region.* 2009. Retrieved November 5, 2011, from http://www.hc-sc.gc.ca/hc-ps/pubs/tobac-tabac/rtr-dtr/part1-eng.php.

34. Gibson, B. "Tough Tobacco-Control Legislation Begins to Have an Impact in Ontario." *Canadian Medical Association Journal* 154 (1996), pp. 230–32.
35. Centre for Addiction and Mental Health. *About Tobacco.* 2009. Retrieved November 5, 2011, from http://www.camh.net/about_addiction_mental_health/drug_and_addiction_information/about_tobacco.html.
36. Canadian Cancer Society. *New Smoking Rates for Canada and Quebec.* 2009. Retrieved November 5, 2011, from http://www.cancer.ca/quebec/about%20us/media%20centre/qc-media%20releases/qc-quebec%20media%20releases/qc_taux_tabagisme.aspx.
37. Health Canada. *Canadian Tobacco Use Monitoring Survey.* 2003. Retrieved November 5, 2011, from http://www.hc-sc.gc.ca/hc-ps/tobac-tabac/research-recherche/stat/ctums-esutc_2008-eng.php.
38. First Nations Centre. *Differentiating Traditional Use of Tobacco from Its Recreational Use.* 2010. Retrieved November 5, 2011, from http://www.naho.ca/firstnations/english/public_tobacco.php.
39. CBC News. *Fewer Tax-Free Cigarettes for First Nations.* 2010. Retrieved November 5, 2011, from http://www.cbc.ca/news/canada/saskatchewan/story/2010/03/24/sk-first-nations-tobacco-1003.html.
40. Wardman, D., and others. "Tobacco Cessation Drug Therapy among Canada's Aboriginal People." *Nicotine & Tobacco Research* 9 (2006), pp. 607–11.
41. Health Canada. *Summary of Results of the 2004–05 Youth Smoking Survey.* 2006. Retrieved November 5, 2011, from http://www.hc-sc.gc.ca/hl-vs/tobac-tabac/research-recherche/stat/surveysondage/2004-2005/result e.html.
42. Baliunas, D., and others. "Smoking-Attributable Mortality and Expected Years of Life Lost in Canada 2002: Conclusions for Prevention and Policy." *Chronic Diseases in Canada* 27, no. 4 (2007), pp. 154–62.
43. Makomaski Illing, E.M., and M.G. Kaiserman. "Mortality Attributable to Tobacco Use in Canada and Its Regions, 1998." *Canadian Journal of Public Health* 95, no. 1 (2004), pp. 38–44.
44. Hirayama, T. "Non-Smoking Wives of Heavy Smokers Have a Higher Risk of Lung Cancer: A Study from Japan." *British Medical Journal* 282 (1981), pp. 183–85.
45. CBC News. *Truro Bans Smoking on Downtown Street.* 2009. Retrieved November 5, 2011, from http://www.cbc.ca/news/canada/nova-scotia/story/2009/01/13/truro-smoking-ban.html.
46. Behnke, M., and V.C. Smith. "Prenatal Substance Abuse: Short- and Long-Term Effects on the Exposed Fetus." *Pediatrics* 131, no. 3 (2013), pp. e1009–e1024.
47. Centers for Disease Control. "Annual Smoking-Attributable Mortality, Years of Potential Life Lost, and Economic Costs–United States, 1997–2001." *Morbidity and Mortality Weekly Report* 54 (2005), pp. 625–628.
48. Slotkin, T.A., and others. "Prenatal Nicotine Exposure Alters the Responses to Subsequent Nicotine Administration and Withdrawal in Adolescence: Serotonin Receptors and Cell Signaling." *Neuropsychopharmacology* 31 (2006), pp. 2462–75.
49. Hurt, R.D., and C.R. Robertson. "Prying Open the Door to the Tobacco Industry's Secrets about Nicotine: The Minnesota Tobacco Trial." *Journal of the American Medical Association* 280, no. 13 (1998), pp. 1173–81.
50. Spring, B., and others. "Altered Reward Value of Carbohydrate Snacks for Female Smokers Withdrawn from Nicotine." *Pharmacology, Biochemistry and Behaviour* 76 (2003), pp. 351–60.
51. Kalman, D. "The Subjective Effects of Nicotine: Methodological Issues, a Review of Experimental Studies, and Recommendations for Future Research." *Nicotine & Tobacco Research* 4 (2002), pp. 25–71.
52. U.S. Department of Health and Human Services. *The Health Consequences of Smoking: Nicotine Addiction, A Report of the Surgeon General.* DHHS Pub. No. (CDC) 88-8406. Washington, DC: U.S. Government Printing Office, 1988.
53. Kessler, D. *A Question of Intent.* New York, NY: Public Affairs, 2001, pp. 113–39.
54. Hart, C., and C. Ksir. "Nicotine Effects on Dopamine Clearance in Rat Nucleus Accumbens." *Journal of Neurochemistry* 66 (1996), pp. 216–21.
55. Fowler, J.S., and others. "Inhibition of Monoamine Oxidase B in the Brains of Smokers." *Nature* 379 (1996), p. 733.
56. Centre for Addiction and Mental Health. *Turning Smokers into Quitters: Nurses Prepare to Help Clients Butt Out: Cross-currents Winter 2002/03.* 2002. Retrieved November 5, 2011, from http://www.camh.net/Publications/Cross_Currents/Winter_2002-03/smokersquitters_crcuwinter 2002_0.html.
57. Gonzalez, D., and others. "Varenicline, an $\alpha 4\beta 2$ Nicotinic Acetylcholine Receptor Partial Agonist, vs. Sustained-Release Bupropion and Placebo for Smoking Cessation: A Randomized Controlled Trial." *Journal of the American Medical Association* 296 (2006), pp. 47–55.
58. Health Canada. "Health Canada Reviewing Stop-Smoking Drug Champix (Varenicline Tartrate) and Potential Risk of Heart Problems in Patients with Heart Disease." 2011. Retrieved October 17, 2011, from http://www.hc-sc.gc.ca/ahc-asc/media/advisories-avis/_2011/2011_84-eng.php.
59. Market Watch Canada. *Ontario May Be Next Canadian Province to Pay for Anti-Smoking Drugs.* 2011. Retrieved November 5, 2011, from http://blogs.marketwatch.com/canada/2011/02/14/ontario-may-be-next-canadian-province-to-pay-for-anti-smoking-drugs/.
60. The reader is referred to Alpert, H.R., G.N. Connolly, and L. Biener. *Tobacco Control* (2012). doi:10.1136/tobaccocontrol-2011-050129.
61. Shorter, D., and T.R. Kosten. "Antidrug Vaccines: Fact or Science Fiction?" *Psychiatric Times* 28, no. 4 (2011), pp. 28, 30–33. Retrieved November 5, 2001, from http://www.psychiatrictimes.com/display/article/10168/1846987.

62. Lamburg, L. "Patients Need More Help to Stop Smoking." *Journal of the American Medical Association* 292 (2004), p. 1286.

Chapter 11

1. Fredholm, B.B., and others. "Actions of Caffeine in the Brain with Special Reference to Factors That Contribute to Its Widespread Use." *Pharmacological Reviews* 51, no. 1 (1999), pp. 83–133.
2. Centre for Addiction and Mental Health. *Do You Know . . . Caffeine.* 2009. Retrieved November 5, 2011, from http://www.camh.net/about_addiction_mental_health/drug_and_addiction_information/caffeine_dyk.html;CBC News. "Our Growing Appetite for a Boost." 2010. Retrieved October 20, 2011, from http://www.cbc.ca/news/health/story/2010/07/26/f-caffeine-daily-intake.html.
3. Coffee Association of Canada. *Coffee in Canada. Highlights, 2003 Canadian Coffee Drinking Study.* 2004. Retrieved November 5, 2011, from http://www.coffeeassoc.com/coffeeincanada.htm.
4. Meyer, H. *Old English Coffee Houses.* Emmaus, PA: Rodale Press, 1954.
5. Moore, J. *Just Us! How Canada's First Fair Trade Coffee Was Born.* 2006. Retrieved March 17, 2011, from http://www.elements.nb.ca/theme/food06/jeff/jeff.htm.
6. CBC News. "Fair Trade: An Alternative Economic Model." 2007. Retrieved November 5, 2011, from http://www.cbc.ca/news/background/fair-trade/.
7. Spurgaitis, K. "Fair Trade Brew: Canadian Consumers Buy Alternative Commodities, Bolster Third World Economies." *Catholic New Times,* September 26, 2004, p. 5.
8. Agriculture and Agri-Food Canada. *The Canadian Coffee Industry.* 2010. Retrieved November 5, 2011, from http://www4.agr.gc.ca/AAFC-AAC/display-afficher.do?id=1172237152079&lang=eng.
9. U.S. Department of Commerce. *Statistical Abstract of the United States.* Washington, DC: U.S. Government Printing Office, 2010.
10. United States Department of Agriculture, Foreign Agricultural Service, Office of Global Analysis. *Coffee: World Markets and Trade.* 2009. Retrieved October 14, 2011, from http://www.fas.usda.gov/htp/coffee/2009/December_2009/2009_coffee_december.pdf.
11. Fineman, J., and D. Scanlan. "Tim Hortons Raises C$783 Million in Initial Offering." 2006. Retrieved November 5, 2011, from http://www.bloomberg.com/apps/news?pid=newsarchive&sid=aVbau_WUTixk&refer =news_index.
12. Tim Hortons. *Tim Hortons Brings a Taste of Home to Troops in Kandahar.* 2006. Retrieved October 21, 2011, from http://www.timhortons.com/ca/en/about/news_archive_2006h.html.
13. Canada Press. "Tim Hortons Aims for 600 New Canadian Stores, 300 in U.S. by 2013." *Ottawa Business Journal.* 2010. Retrieved November 5, 2011, from http://www.obj.ca/Canada---World/2010-03-05/article-885414/Tim-Hortons-aims-for-600-new-Canadian-stores%2C-300-in-U.S.-by-2013/1.
14. Tim Hortons. *The History of Tim Hortons.* 2011. Retrieved October 15, 2011, from http://www.timhortons.com/ca/en/about/media-history.html.
15. Stone, L. "Tim Hortons' Double-Double Comes to Dubai." *Toronto Star.* September 20, 2011. Retrieved October 14, 2011, from http://www.thestar.com/news/world/article/1056550–tim-hortons-double-double-comes-to-dubai?bn=1.
16. McGinley, S. "Canada's Tim Hortons Signs Deal for 120 Gulf Outlets." (Press release.) *Arabian Business.* February 6, 2011. Retrieved October 14, 2011, from http://www.arabianbusiness.com/canada-s-tim-hortons-signs-deal-for-120-gulf-outlets-378817.html.
17. First Research. *Coffee Shops Industry Profile.* Retrieved March 24, 2010, from http://www.firstresearch.com/industry-research/Coffee-Shops.html.
18. Statistics Canada. *Canada Food Stats: Analysis. Food Available for Consumption in Canada, 2008.* 2008. Retrieved November 5, 2011, from http://www.statcan.gc.ca/ads-annonces/23f0001x/hl-fs-eng.htm.
19. See http://www.tea.ca/tea-health/tea-for-your-health-january-2014/.
20. Health Canada. *It's Your Health–Caffeine.* 2010. Retrieved November 5, 2011, from http://www.hc-sc.gc.ca/hl-vs/iyh-vsv/food-aliment/caffeine-eng.php.
21. Knight, C.A., I. Knight, and D.C. Mitchell. "Beverage Caffeine Intakes in Young Children in Canada and the US." *Canadian Journal of Dietetic Practice and Research* 67, no. 2 (2006), pp. 96–99.
22. Huisking, C.L. *Herbs to Hormones.* Essex, CT: Pequot Press, 1968.
23. Health Canada. *Caffeine.* 2010. Retrieved November 5, 2011, from http://www.hc-sc.gc.ca/hl-vs/iyh-vsv/food-aliment/caffeine-eng.php.
24. Mesley, W., I. Colabrese, and S. Stevens. "Packing Drinks with a Punch." *CBC News Marketplace.* 2011. Retrieved November 5, 2011, from http://www.cbc.ca/marketplace/pre-2007/files/health/guarana/index.html.
25. CTV News. "New Research Links Soft Drinks to Type 2 Diabetes." 2010. Retrieved November 5, 2011, from http://www.ctv.ca/CTVNews/Health/20101027/soft-drinks-diabetes/.
26. Adan, A., and J.M. Serra-Grabulosa. "Effects of Caffeine and Glucose, Alone and Combined, on Cognitive Performance." *Human Psychopharmacology* 25, no. 4 (2010), pp. 310–17.
27. Scholey, A.B., and D.O. Kennedy. "Cognitive and Physiological Effects of an 'Energy Drink': An Evaluation of the Whole Drink and of Glucose, Caffeine and Herbal Flavouring Fractions." *Psychopharmacology (Berl)* 176, nos. 3–4 (2004), pp. 320–30.
28. Seidl, R., and others. "A Taurine and Caffeine-Containing Drink Stimulates Cognitive Performance

and Well-Being." *Amino Acids* 19, nos. 3–4 (2000), pp. 635–42.

29. Quertemont, E., and K.A. Grant. "Discriminative Stimulus Effects of Ethanol: Lack of Interaction with Taurine." *Behavioural Pharmacology* 15 (2004), pp. 495–501.
30. UK Food Standards Agency. *Statement on the Reproductive Effects of Caffeine.* 2001. Retrieved November 29, 2004, from www.food.gov.uk/science/ouradvisors/toxicity/statements/cotstatements2001/caffeine.
31. Centre for Addiction and Mental Health. *Do You Know . . . Caffeine.* 2009. Retrieved November 5, 2011, from http://www.camh.net/about_addiction_mental_health/drug_and_addiction_information/caffeine_dyk.html.
32. MADD Canada. *Youth, Alcohol and Energy Drinks.* 2007. Retrieved November 5, 2011, from http://www.madd.ca/english/news/pr/p20071120.htm.
33. Schmidt, S. "Canada Not Following U.S. Steps to Ban Alcoholic Energy Drinks." 2010. Retrieved November 5, 2011, from http://www.canada.com/health/Canada+following+steps+alcoholic+energy+drinks/3841736/story.html.
34. Yahoo Canada. "Family Sues Four Loko's Chicago Maker in Teen's Death. 'Blackout in a Can' Called Danger to Underage Drinkers at Prom Time." 2011. Retrieved November 5, 2011, from http://ca.finance.yahoo.com/news/Family-Sues-Four-Lokos-prnews-1918511263.html?x=0.
35. Statistics Canada. *Health Reports. Beverage Consumption of Canadian Adults.* 2008. Retrieved November 5, 2011, from http://www.statcan.gc.ca/pub/82-003-x/2008004/article/10716/6500244-eng.htm.
36. Griffiths, R.R., and others. "Human Coffee Drinking: Reinforcing and Physical Dependence Producing Effects of Caffeine." *Journal of Pharmacology and Experimental Therapeutics* 239 (1986), pp. 416–25.
37. Juliano, L.M., and R.R. Griffiths. "A Critical Review of Caffeine Withdrawal: Empirical Validation of Symptoms and Signs, Incidence, Severity, and Associated Features." *Psychopharmacology* 176 (2004), pp. 1–29.
38. Ozsungur, S., D. Brenner, and A. El-Sohemy. "Fourteen Well-Described Caffeine Withdrawal Symptoms Factor into Three Clusters." *Psychopharmacology (Berl)* 201, no. 4 (2009), pp. 541–48.
39. Hughes, J. R., and others. "Should Caffeine Abuse, Dependence, or Withdrawal Be Added to DSM-IV and ICD-10?" *American Journal of Psychiatry* 149 (1992), p. 33.
40. See http://www.dsm5.org/Pages/ RecentUpdates.aspx.
41. DSM-5 table, pp. 503–509.
42. Julien, R.M. *A Primer of Drug Action*, 10th ed. New York, NY: Worth, 2005.
43. Brain, M., and C.W. Bryant. *How Caffeine Works.* 2011. Retrieved November 5, 2011, from http://health.howstuffworks.com/wellness/drugs-alcohol/caffeine4.htm.
44. de Balzac, H. (paraphrasing Brillat-Savarin). *Traité des Excitants Modernes* (1838), translated from the French by R. Onopa. Quoted in Winston, A.P., E. Hardwick, and N. Jaberi. "Neuropsychiatric Effects of Caffeine." *Advances in Psychiatric Treatment* 11 (2005), pp. 432–39.
45. Drapeau, C., and others. "Challenging Sleep in Aging: The Effects of 200 mg of Caffeine during the Evening in Young and Middle-Aged Moderate Caffeine Consumers." *Journal of Sleep Research* 15, no. 2 (2006), pp. 133–41.
46. van de Sandt, J.J., and others. "In Vitro Predictions of Skin Absorption of Caffeine, Testosterone, and Benzoic Acid: A Multi-Centre Comparison Study." *Regulatory Toxicology and Pharmacology* 39, no. 3 (2004), pp. 271–81.
47. Sääksjärvi, K., and others. "Prospective Study of Coffee Consumption and Risk of Parkinson's Disease." *European Journal of Clinical Nutrition* 62, no. 7 (2008), pp. 908–15.
48. Ross, G.W. "Association of Coffee and Caffeine Intake with the Risk of Parkinson's Disease." *Journal of the American Medical Association* 283, no. 20 (2000), pp. 2674–79.
49. Canadian Diabetes Association. *Prevention of Type 2 Diabetes.* 2011. Retrieved November 5, 2011, from http://www.diabetescareguide.com/en/article_vol28.html.
50. Tunnicliffe, J.M., and J. Shearer. "Coffee, Glucose Homeostasis, and Insulin Resistance: Physiological Mechanisms and Mediators." *Applied Physiology, Nutrition, and Metabolism* 33, no. 6 (2008), pp. 1290–300.
51. Van Dam, R.M., and F.B. Hu. "Coffee Consumption and Risk of Type 2 Diabetes: A Systematic Review." *Journal of the American Medical Association* 294 (2005), pp. 97–104.
52. Wheeler, M. "Why Coffee Protects Against Diabetes." University of California–Los Angeles. *Science Daily.* 2011. Retrieved November 5, 2011, from http://www.sciencedaily.com/releases/2011/01/110113102200.htm.
53. Bowman, L. *Caffeine Can Improve Short-Term Memory.* 2005. Retrieved November 5, 2011, from http://www.seattlepi.com/lifestyle/health/article/Caffeine-can-improve-short-term-memory-1188727.php.
54. Mitchell, P.J., and J.R. Redman. "Effects of Caffeine, Time of Day, and User History on Study-Related Performance." *Psychopharmacology (Berl)* 109 (1992), p. 121.
55. Gilliland, K., and D. Andress. "Ad Lib Caffeine Consumption, Symptoms of Caffeinism, and Academic Performance." *American Journal of Psychiatry* 138, no. 4 (1981), pp. 512–14.
56. Ward, N., and others. "The Analgesic Effects of Caffeine in Headache." *Pain* 44 (1991), pp. 151–55.
57. Leon, M.R. "Effects of Caffeine on Cognitive, Psychomotor, and Affective Performance of Children with Attention Deficit/Hyperactivity Disorder." *Journal of Attention Disorders* 4 (2000), pp. 27–47.
58. Warzak, W., and others. "Caffeine Consumption in Young Children." *The Journal of Pediatrics* 158, no. 3 (2011), pp. 508–509.
59. Lieberman, H.R., and others. "Effects of Caffeine, Sleep Loss, and Stress on Cognitive Performance and Mood During U.S. Navy SEAL Training." *Psychopharmacology (Berl)* 164 (2002), pp. 250–61.
60. Fine, B.J., and others. "Effects of Caffeine or Diphenhydramine on Visual Vigilance." *Psychopharmacology (Berl)* 114 (1994), pp. 233–38.
61. Johnson, R.F., and D.J. Merullo. "Caffeine, Gender, and Sentry Duty: Effects of a Mild Stimulant on Vigilance

and Marksmanship." In *Pennington Center Nutrition Series Volume 10: Countermeasures for Battlefield Stressors,* K. Friedel, H.R. Lieberman, D.H. Ryan, and G.A. Bray, eds. Baton Rouge, LA: Louisiana State University Press, 2000, pp. 272–89.

62. McLellan, T.M., and others. "The Impact of Caffeine on Cognitive and Physical Performance and Marksmanship during Sustained Operations." *Canadian Military Journal.* 2004. Retrieved November 5, 2011, from http://www.journal.dnd.ca/vo4/no4/doc/military-meds-eng.pdf.
63. American Psychiatric Association. *Diagnostic and Statistical Manual of Mental Disorders,* 4th ed., text revision (DSM-IV-TR). Washington, DC: American Psychiatric Association, 2000, pp. 212–15, 708–09.
64. Stewart, S.A. "Caffeine Can Push the Panic Button." *USA Today,* October 23, 1985.
65. Hughes, R.N. "Drugs which Induce Anxiety: Caffeine." *New Zealand Journal of Psychology* 25, no. 1 (1996), pp. 36–42.
66. Coffee Association of Canada. *Cancer: Preventative Evidence Mounts.* (n.d.). Retrieved October 21, 2011, from http://www.coffeeandhealth.ca/cancer.htm.
67. Woolcott, C.G., W.D. King, and L.D. Marrett. "Coffee and Tea Consumption and Cancers of the Bladder, Colon and Rectum." *European Journal of Cancer Prevention* 11, no. 2 (2002), pp. 137–45.
68. LaCroix, A.Z., and others. "Coffee Consumption and the Incidence of Coronary Heart Disease." *New England Journal of Medicine* 315 (1986), pp. 977–82.
69. Cornelis, M.C., and A. El-Sohemy. "Coffee, Caffeine, and Coronary Heart Disease." *Current Opinion in Clinical Nutrition and Metabolic Care* 10 (2007), pp. 745–51.

Chapter 12

1. Department of Justice Canada. *Controlled Drugs and Substances Act: Regulations Respecting the Control of Narcotics (C.R.C., c. 1041) Enabling Statute.* 2011. Retrieved November 6, 2011, from http://laws.justice.gc.ca/en/C.R.C.-C.1041/FullText.html.
2. Health Canada. *Ipsos Reid Survey: Baseline Natural Health Products Survey among Consumers.* 2005. Retrieved November 6, 2011, from http://www.soscanada.net/doc/eng_cons_survey-eng.pdf.
3. CBC News. "Herbal Product Contamination 'Considerable,' DNA Tests Find." 2013. Retrieved June 14, 2014, from http://www.cbc.ca/news/health/herbal-product-contamination-considerable-dna-tests-find-1.1959278.
4. Linde, K., M.M. Berner, and L. Kriston. "St. John's Wort for Major Depression." *Cochrane Database Systematic Review* Oct 8, 2008, no. 4, CD000448.
5. Health Canada. *Risk of Important Drug Interactions between St. John's Wort and Prescription Drugs.* 2000. Retrieved November 6, 2011, from http://www.hc-sc.gc.ca/dhp-mps/medeff/advisories-avis/prof/_2000/hypericum_perforatum_hpc-cps-eng.php.
6. See http://www.enzyte.com.
7. MacKay, D. "Nutrients and Botanicals for Erectile Dysfunction: Examining the Evidence." *Alternative Medicine Review* 9 (2004), pp. 4–16.
8. See http://webprod.hc-sc.gc.ca/lnhpd-bdpsnh/index-eng.jsp.
9. Birks, J., and J. Grimley Evans. "Ginkgo Biloba for Cognitive Impairment and Dementia." *Cochrane Database Systematic Review* Jan 21, 2009, no. 1, CD003120.
10. Saleem, S., and others. "Ginkgo Biloba Extract Neuroprotective Action Is Dependent on Heme Oxygenase 1 in Ischemic Reperfusion Brain Injury." *Stroke* 39 (2008), pp. 3389–96.
11. Gruson, L. "A Controversy over Widely Sold Diet Pills." *New York Times,* February 13, 1982. Retrieved November 6, 2011, from http://query.nytimes.com/gst/fullpage.html?res=9D03E6D9123BF930A25751C0A964948260&sec=health&spon=&pagewanted=2.
12. Kernan, W.N., and others. "Phenylpropanolamine and the Risk of Hemorrhagic Stroke." *New England Journal of Medicine* 343 (2000), pp. 1826–32.
13. Boozer, C., and others. "Herbal Ephedra/Caffeine for Weight Loss: A 6-Month Randomized Safety and Efficacy Trial." *International Journal of Obesity and Related Metabolic Disorders* 26 (2002), pp. 593–604.
14. Health Canada. "Health Canada Requests Recall of Certain Products Containing Ephedra/Ephedrine." 2002. Retrieved February 21, 2011, from http://web.archive.org/web/20070206073244/http://www.hc-sc.gc.ca/ahc-asc/media/advisories-avis/2002/2002_01_e.html.
15. Haller, C., and N. Benowitz. "Adverse Cardiovascular and Central Nervous System Events Associated with Dietary Supplements Containing Ephedra Alkaloids." *New England Journal of Medicine* 343 (2000), pp. 1833–38.
16. Shochat, P., I. Haimov, and P. Lavie. "Melatonin: The Key to the Gate of Sleep." *Annals of Medicine* 30 (1998), pp. 109–114.
17. Ferracioli-Oda, E., A. Qawasmi, and M.H. Bloch. "Meta-Analysis: Melatonin for the Treatment of Primary Sleep Disorders." *PLOS ONE* 8 (2013), p. e63773.
18. Sarris, J., and G.J. Byrne. "A Systematic Review of Insomnia and Complementary Medicine." *Sleep Medicine Reviews* 15 (2011), pp. 99–106.
19. Lillehei, A.S., and L.L. Halcon. "A Systematic Review of the Effect of Inhaled Essential Oils on Sleep." *Journal of Alternative and Complementary Medicine* 20 (2014), pp. 441–51.
20. Zick, S.M., B.D. Wright, A. Sen, and J.T. Arnedt. "Preliminary Examination of the Efficacy and Safety of a Standardized Chamomile Extract for Chronic Primary Insomnia: A Randomized Placebo-Controlled Pilot Study." *BMC Complementary and Alternative Medicine* 11 (2011), p. 78.
21. CHP Canada. "Public Attitudes to Self-Care" *Ipsos-Reid Survey.* 2005. Retrieved November 6, 2011, from http://www.chpcanada.ca/index.cfm?fuseaction=main.dspFile&FileID=88.

22. Canadian Institute for Health Information. *Drug Expenditures in Canada, 1985 to 2004*. Ottawa: The Institute, 2005.
23. Health Canada. "Regulations Amending the Food and Drug Regulations (743–Non Medicinal Ingredients)." *Canada Gazette* 143, no. 23 (2009). Retrieved November 6, 2011, from www.gazette.gc.ca/rp-pr/pl/2009/2009-06-06/html/reg3-eng.html.
24. See http://webprod5.hc-sc.gc.ca/dpd-bdpp/index-eng.jsp.
25. Lynd, L., and others. "Prescription to Over-the-Counter Deregulation in Canada: Are We Ready for It, or Do We Need to Be?" *Canadian Medical Association Journal* 173 (2005), pp. 775–77.
26. CBC News. *Aspirin: The Versatile Drug*. 2010. Retrieved November 6, 2011, from http://www.cbc.ca/news/health/story/2009/05/28/f-aspirin-studies.html.
27. Boltri, M., and others. "Aspirin Prophylaxis in Patients at Low Risk for Cardiovascular Disease: A Systematic Review of All-Cause Mortality." *Journal of Family Practice* 51 (2002), pp. 700–705.
28. Moolten, S.E., and I.B. Smith. "Fatal Nephritis in Chronic Phenacetin Poisoning." *American Journal of Medicine* 28 (1960), p. 127.
29. Rapoport, A., L.W. White, and G.N. Ranking. "Renal Damage Associated with Chronic Phenacetin Overdosage." *Annals of Internal Medicine* 57 (1962), p. 970.
30. Prior, M.J., and others. "Acetaminophen Availability Increases in Canada with No Increase in the Incidence of Reports of Inpatient Hospitalizations with Acetamin ophen Overdose and Acute Liver Toxicity." *American Journal of Therapeutics* 11 (2004), pp. 443-52.
31. Bombardier, C., and others. "Comparison of Upper Gastrointestinal Toxicity of Rofecoxib and Naproxen in Patients with Rheumatoid Arthritis." *New England Journal of Medicine* 343 (2000), pp. 1520-28.
32. U.S. FDA Advisory Committee. *Cardiovascular Safety Review of Rofecoxib*. Rockville, MD: Food and Drug Administration, 2001. Retrieved March 7, 2011, from http://www.fda.gov/ohrms/dockets/ac/01/briefing/3677b2_06_cardio.pdf.
33. Editorial. "Vioxx: Lessons for Health Canada and the FDA." *Canadian Medical Association Journal* 172 (2005), p. 5.
34. MacDonald, N., and S.M. Macleod. "Has the Time Come to Phase Out Codeine?" *Canadian Medical Association Journal* 183 (2010), p. 1835.
35. Dickens, C. *The Collected Letters of Charles Dickens*. Chapman & Hall, 1880.
36. Klumpp, T.G. "The Common Cold–New Concepts of Transmission and Prevention." *Medical Times* 108, no. 11 (1980), pp. 98, 1s–3s.
37. Price, L.H., and J. Lebel. "Dextromethorphan-Induced Psychosis." *American Journal of Psychiatry* 157 (2000), p. 304.
38. Boak, A., and others. *Drug Use among Ontario Students, 1977–2013: Detailed OSDUHS Findings* (CAMH Research Document Series No. 36). Toronto: Centre for Addiction and Mental Health, 2013. Retrieved December 12, 2013, from http://www.camh.ca/en/research/news_and_publications/ontario-student-drug-use-and-health-survey/Documents/2013%20OSDUHS%20Docs/2013OSDUHS_Detailed_DrugUseReport.pdf.

Chapter 13

1. Baum, L.F. *The New Wizard of Oz*. New York: Grosset & Dunlap, 1944.
2. Scott, J.M. *The White Poppy: A History of Opium*. New York: Funk & Wagnalls, 1969.
3. Hamarneh, S. "Sources and Development of Arabic Medical Therapy and Pharmacology." *Sudhoffs Archiv fur Geschichte der Medizin und der Naturwissenschaften* 54 (1970), p. 34.
4. De Quincey, T. *Confessions of an English Opium-Eater*. London; New York: W. Scott Pub. Co., 1886.
5. Kramer, J.C. "Opium Rampant: Medical Use, Misuse and Abuse in Britain and the West in the 17th and 18th Centuries." *British Journal of Addiction*, 1979, p. 377.
6. Kramer, J.C. "Heroin in the Treatment of Morphine Addiction." *Journal of Psychedelic Drugs* 9, no. 3 (1977), pp. 193–97.
7. Dott, D.B., and R. Stockman. *Proceedings of the Royal Society of Edinburgh*, 1890, p. 321.
8. Manges, M. "A Second Report on the Therapeutics of Heroine." *New York Medical Journal* 71 (1900), pp. 51, 82–83.
9. Wilcox, R.W. *Pharmacology and Therapeutics*, 6th ed. Philadelphia: P. Blakiston's Son, 1905.
10. United Nations Office on Drugs and Crime (UNODC). *World Drug Report 2010. United Nations Publication, Sales No. E.10.XI.13)*. 2010. Retrieved October 13, 2011, from http://www.unodc.org/documents/wdr/WDR2010/World_Drug_Report_2010_lo-res.pdf.
11. Royal Canadian Mounted Police. Criminal Intelligence. *Report on the Illicit Drug Situation in Canada–2008*. 2009. Retrieved March 1, 2011, from http://www.rcmp-grc.gc.ca/drugs-drogues/2008/drug-drogue-2008-eng.pdf.
12. Royal Canadian Mounted Police. Criminal Intelligence. *Report on the Illicit Drug Situation in Canada–2009*. 2010. Retrieved March 1, 2011, from http://www.rcmp-grc.gc.ca/drugs-drogues/2009/drug-drogue-2009-eng.pdf.
13. Giffen, J., S. Endicott, and S. Lambert. *Panic and Indifference–The Politics of Canada's Drug Laws*. Ottawa: Canadian Centre on Substance Abuse, 1991.
14. Brands, B., and others. "Prescription Opioid Abuse in Patients Presenting for Methadone Maintenance Treatment." *Drug and Alcohol Dependence* 73 (2004), pp. 199–207.
15. Fischer, B., M.F. Cruz, and J. Rehm. "Illicit Opioid Use and Its Key Characteristics: A Select Overview and Evidence from a Canadian Multisite Cohort of Illicit

Opioid Users (OPICAN)." *Canadian Journal of Psychiatry* 51, no. 10 (2006), pp. 624–34. Review. PubMed PMID: 17052030.

16. Fischer, B., and others. "Changes in Illicit Opioid Use Profiles across Canada." *Canadian Medical Association Journal* 175 (2006), pp. 1–3.
17. Fischer, B., and others. "Comparing Heroin Users and Prescription Opioid Users in a Canadian Multi-Site Population of Illicit Opioid Users." *Drug and Alcohol Review* 27 (2008), pp. 625–32.
18. Haydon, E., and others. "Prescription Drug Abuse in Canada and the Diversion of Prescription Drugs into the Illicit Drug Market." *Canadian Journal of Public Health* 96, no. 6 (2005), pp. 459–61.
19. International Narcotics Control Board (INCB). *Narcotic Drugs: Estimated World Requirements for 2007: Statistics for 2005.* New York, NY: INCB, 2006.
20. International Narcotics Control Board (INCB). *Report of the International Narcotics Control Board for 2005.* Vienna, Austria: United Nations, 2006.
21. Martin, T.L., K.L. Woodall, and B.A. McLellan. "Fentanyl-Related Deaths in Ontario, Canada: Toxicological Findings and Circumstances of Death in 112 Cases (2002–2004)." *Journal of Analytical Toxicology* 30 (2006), pp. 603–10.
22. Popova, S., and others. "How Many People in Canada Use Prescription Opioids Nonmedically in General and Street Drug Using Populations?" *Canadian Journal of Public Health* 100, no. 2 (2009), pp. 104–108.
23. Brands, B., and others. "Prescription Opioid Abuse in Patients Presenting for Methadone Maintenance Treatment." *Drug and Alcohol Dependence* 73 (2004), pp. 199–207.
24. See http://www.ctvnews.ca/canada/illegal-fentanyl-linked-to-more-than-100-deaths-in-alberta-last-year-rcmp-1.2286229.
25. Picard, A. "Clement's Insite Attack Leaves WHO Red-Faced." *The Globe and Mail.* 2008. Retrieved from http://www.theglobeandmail.com/life/article701599.ece.
26. Centre for Addiction and Mental Health (CAMH). *Methadone Maintenance Treatment: Client Handbook.* 2009. Retrieved from http://www.camh.net/Care_Treatment/Resources_clients_ families_ friends/ Methadone_Maintenance_Treatment/mmt_clienthndbk_ch5.html.
27. McCaffery, M., and A. Beebe. *Pain: Clinical Manual for Nursing Practice.* St. Louis, MO: C.V. Mosby, 1989.
28. DuPen, A., D. Shen, and M. Ersek. "Mechanisms of Opioid-Induced Tolerance and Hyperalgesia: Opioid-Induced Hyperalgesia." *Pain Management Nursing* 8, no. 3 (2007), pp. 113–121. Retrieved from http://www.medscape.com/viewarticle/562216_4.
29. Canadian Centre on Substance Abuse. *Substance Abuse in Canada: Current Challenges and Choices.* 2005. Retrieved from http://www.ccsa.ca/2005%20CCSA%20Documents/ccsa-004032-2005.pdf.
30. Fischer, B., J. Rehm, J. Patra, and M.F. Cruz. "Changes in Illicit Opioid Use across Canada." *Journal of the Canadian Medical Association (CMAJ)* 175, no. 11 (2006), pp. 1385–1386.
31. Health Canada. *It's Your Health: Opioid Pain Medications.* 2009. Retrieved from http://www.hc-sc.gc.ca/hl-vs/iyh-vsv/med/opioid-faq-opioides-eng.php.
32. Health Canada. *Major Findings from the Canadian Alcohol and Drug Use Monitoring Survey (CADUMS) 2009.* 2010. Retrieved from http://www.hc-sc.gc.ca/hc-ps/drugs-drogues/stat/index-eng.php.
33. Zdeb, C. *Addiction often Starts in Hospital: Some Doctors Aggravate Prescription Drug Abuse.* Boyle McCauley Health Centre and Alberta Health Services. 2011. Retrieved from http://www.canada.com/health/Addiction+often+starts+hospital/1832972/story.html.
34. Pesut, B., and H. McDonald. "Connecting Philosophy and Practice: Implications of Two Philosophic Approaches to Pain for Nurses' Expert Clinical Decision Making." *Nursing Philosophy* 8 (2007), pp. 256–263.
35. Julien, R.M. *A Primer of Drug Action,* 10th ed. New York: Worth, 2005.
36. See http://vancouver.24hrs.ca/2014/11/06/life-saving-meds-not-reaching-users.
37. Siegel, S. "Morphine Analgesic Tolerance: Its Situation Specificity Supports a Pavlovian Conditioning Model." *Science* 193 (1976), pp. 323–25.
38. Siegel, S., and others. "Heroin 'Overdose' Death: Contribution of Drug-Associated Environmental Cues." *Science* 216 (1982), pp. 436–37.
39. Fifth Estate. *Report on Insite: Staying Alive.* 2009. Retrieved from http://www.cbc.ca/fifth/2008-2009/staying_alive/video.html.
40. Beirness, D.J., R. Jesseman, R. Notarandrea, and M. Perron. *Harm Reduction: What's in a Name?* 2008. Ottawa: Canadian Centre on Substance Abuse. Retrieved from http://www.ccsa.ca/2008%20CCSA%20Documents2/ccsa0115302008e.pdf.
41. Canadian Centre on Substance Abuse (CCSA). *Substance Abuse in Canada: Current Challenges and Choices.* 2005. Retrieved from www.ccsa.ca.
42. Lightfoot, B., C. Panessa, S. Hayden, M. Thumath, I. Goldstone, and B. Pauly. "Gaining Insight: Harm Reduction in Nursing Practice." *Canadian Nurse* 105, no. 4 (2009), pp. 16–22.
43. Pauly, B. "Harm Reduction through a Social Justice Lens." *International Journal of Drug Policy* 19 (2008), pp. 4–10.
44. Canadian Nurses Association. *Social Determinants of Health and Nursing. A Summary of the Issues.* 2005. Retrieved from http://www.cna-nurses.ca/CNA/documents/pdf/publications/BG8_Social_Determinants_e.pdf.
45. Kerr, T., J. Stoltz, M. Tyndall, K. Li, R. Zhang, J. Montaner, and E. Wood. "Impact of Medically Supervised Safer Injection Facility on Community Drug Use Patterns: A Before and After Study." *British Medical Journal* 332 (2006), pp. 220–222.

46. Pinkerton, S.D. "Is Vancouver Canada's Supervised Injection Facility Cost-Saving?" *Addiction* 105 (2010), pp. 1429–1436.
47. Kerr, T., J. Montaner, and E. Wood. "Supervised Injecting Facilities: Time for Scale-Up?" *The Lancet* 372 (2008), pp. 354–355.
48. Andresen, M., and N. Boyd. "A Cost-Benefit and Cost-Effectiveness Analysis of Vancouver's Supervised Injection Facility." *International Journal of Drug Policy* 21 (2010), pp. 70–76.
49. Kerr, T., M. Tyndall, C. Lai, J. Montaner, and E. Wood. "Drug-Related Overdoses within a Medically Supervised Safer Injection Facility." *International Journal of Drug Policy* 17 (2006), pp. 436–441.
50. Pauly, B. "Supervised Injection Site a Basic Health Service." *The Victoria Times Colonist*. July 18, 2010.
51. Wood, R., E. Wood, C. Lai, M. Tyndall, J. Montaner, and T. Kerr. "Nurse-Delivered Safer Injection Education among a Cohort of Injection Drug Users: Evidence from the Evaluation of Vancouver's Supervised Injection Facility." *International Journal of Drug Policy* 19 (2008), pp. 183–188.
52. Vancouver Coastal Health. *Supervised Injection Site*. 2010. Retrieved from http://supervisedinjection.vch.ca/.
53. Angus Reid Public Opinion. "Canadians Are Supportive of Insite and Oppose Moves to Shut It Down." July 31, 2010, pp. 1–6.
54. Keller, J. "'War on Drugs' Fuels HIV Epidemic as Governments Ignore Science, Experts Say." *The Globe and Mail*, July 19, 2010.
55. Oviedo-Joekes, E., and others. "The North American Opiate Medication Initiative (NAOMI): Profile of Participants in North America's First Trial of Heroin-Assisted Treatment." *Journal of Urban Health* 85, no. 6 (2008), pp. 812–25.
56. Rehm, J., and others. "Feasibility, Safety, and Efficacy of Injectable Heroin Prescription for Retractory Opioid Addicts: A Follow-Up Study." *Lancet* 358, no. 9291 (2001), pp. 1417–23.
57. Study to Assess Long-term Opioid Maintenance Effectiveness (SALOME). *SALOME Clinical Trial Questions and Answers*. Retrieved February 12, 2011, from http://www.naomistudy.ca/pdfs/SALOME_FAQs_v4.pdf; Inner Change Foundation. *Groundbreaking Addiction Research Trial Ramps Up in January. More Vancouver Participants Than Originally Anticipated*. 2011. Retrieved from http://www.innerchangefoundation.org/groundbreaking-addiction-research-trial-ramps-up-in-january.html.

Chapter 14

1. Schultes, R.E., and A. Hofmann. *Plants of the Gods*. New York, NY: McGraw-Hill, 1979.
2. Caporael, L.R. "Ergotism: The Satan Loosed in Salem." *Science* 192 (1976), pp. 21–26.
3. Gottlieb, J., and N.P. Spanos. "Ergotism and the Salem Village Witch Trials." *Science* 194 (1976), pp. 1390–94.
4. Hofmann, A. "Psychotomimetic Agents." In *Drugs Affecting the Central Nervous System* (Vol. 2), A. Burger, ed. New York, NY: Marcel Dekker, 1968.
5. Segal, J., ed. *Research in the Service of Mental Health, Research on Drug Abuse*. National Institute on Mental Health, Pub. No. (ADM) 75-236, U.S. Department of Health, Education, and Welfare. Washington, DC: U.S. Government Printing Office, 1975.
6. Griffiths, R.R., and C.S. Grob. "Hallucinogens as Medicine." *Scientific American* 303, no. 6 (2010), pp. 77–79.
7. Vollenweider, F.X., and M. Kometer. "The Neurobiology of Psychedelic Drugs: Implications for the Treatment of Mood Disorders." *Nature Reviews Neuroscience* 11 (2010), pp. 642–51.
8. Grob, C.S., and others. "Pilot Study of Psilocybin Treatment for Anxiety in Patients with Advanced-Stage Cancer." *Archives of General Psychiatry* 68 (2011), pp. 71–78.
9. Carstairs, C. "Psychedelic Psychiatry: LSD from Clinic to Campus." *Medical History* 54 (2010), pp. 561–62.
10. Dyck, E. "Land of the Living Sky with Diamonds: A Place for Radical Psychiatry?" *Journal of Canadian Studies* 41(2007), pp. 42–66.
11. Dyck, E. *Psychedelic Psychiatry: LSD from Clinic to Campus*. Baltimore, MD: Johns Hopkins University Press, 2008.
12. Dyck, E. "Hitting Highs at Rocks Bottom: LSD Treatment for Alcoholism, 1950–1970." *Social History of Medicine* 19 (2006), pp. 313–29.
13. Sealey, R. *Remembering Albert Hoffer*. Toronto: Sear Publications, 2009. Retrieved November 7, 2011, from http://www.searpubl.ca/Remembering_Abram_Hoffer.pdf.
14. Denson, R., and D. Sydiaha. "A Controlled Study of LSD Treatment in Alcoholism and Neurosis." *British Journal of Psychiatry* 116 (1970), pp. 443–45.
15. Dolan, E.W. "Study Finds LSD Treatment Is Not Effective." *PsyPost*, April 26, 2010. Retrieved November 7, 2011, from http://www.psypost.org/2010/04/lsd-treatment-not-effective-623.
16. Johnston, L. "Ford Signs Grant of $750,000 in LSD Death in CIA Test." *The New York Times*, October 14, 1976, p. C43.
17. Treaster, J.B. "Mind-Drug Test a Federal Project for Almost 25 Years." *The New York Times*, August 11, 1975, p. M42.
18. "CIA Considered Big LSD Purchase." *Washington Star*. August 4, 1975; Knight, M. "LSD Creator Says Army Sought Drug." *New York Times*. August 1, 1975.
19. United States Senate. *Project MK-ULTRA, The CIA's Program of Research into Behavioral Modification*. Joint Hearing before the Select Committee on Intelligence and the Subcommittee on Health and Scientific Research of the Committee on Human Resources, Ninety-Fifth Congress, First Session. Washington, DC: U.S. Government Printing Office, 1977. Retrieved February 18, 2011, from http://www.nytimes.com/packages/pdf/national/13inmate_ProjectMKULTRA.pdf.

20. Klein, N. *The Shock Doctrine: The Rise of Disaster Capitalism.* New York, NY: Picador, 2007.
21. Taylor, J.R., and W.N. Johnson. *Use of Volunteers in Chemical Agent Research.* Inspector General Report No. DAI-GIN 21-75. Washington, DC: U.S. Department of Army, 1976.
22. Weil, A.T. "The Strange Case of the Harvard Drug Scandal." *Look,* November 5, 1963, pp. 38–48.
23. Blumenthal, R. "Leary Drug Cult Stirs Millbrook." *New York Times.* June 14, 1967, p. 49.
24. New Yorker. "Celebration #1." *New Yorker* 42 (1966), p. 43.
25. Council on Mental Health and Committee on Alcoholism and Drug Dependence. "Dependence on LSD and Other Hallucinogenic Drugs." *Journal of the American Medical Association* 202 (1967), pp. 141–44.
26. Leary, T., and Liddy, G.G. "Debating Specialists." *New York Times,* September 3, 1981, p. B26.
27. Paglia-Boak, A., E.M. Adlaf, and R.E. Mann. *Drug Use among Ontario Students, 1977–2011: Detailed OSDUHS Findings* (CAMH Research Document Series No. 32). Toronto: Centre for Addiction and Mental Health, 2011. Retrieved October 29, 2013, from http://www.camh.ca/en/research/news_and_publications/ontario-student-drug-use-and-health-survey/Pages/default.aspx.
28. Adlaf, E.M., P. Begin, and E. Sawka, eds. *Canadian Addiction Survey (CAS): A National Survey of Canadians' Use of Alcohol and Other Drugs: Prevalence of Use and Related Harms: Detailed Report.* Ottawa: Canadian Centre on Substance Abuse, 2005.
29. American College Health Association. *National College Health Assessment II: Canadian Reference Group Data Report.* Spring 2013. Hanover, MD: American College Health Association, 2013.
30. Appel, J.B., and J.A. Rosecrans. "Behavioural Pharmacology of Hallucinogens in Animals: Conditioning Studies." In *Hallucinogens: Neurochemical, Behavioural and Clinical Perspectives,* B.L. Jacobs, ed. New York, NY: Raven Press, 1984.
31. Julien, R.M. *A Primer of Drug Action,* 10th ed. New York, NY: Worth, 2005.
32. Siegel, R.K. "The Natural History of Hallucinogens." In *Hallucinogens: Neurochemical, Behavioural and Clinical Perspectives,* B.L. Jacobs, ed. New York, NY: Raven Press, 1984.
33. Krippner, S. "Psychedelic Experience and the Language Process." *Journal of Psychedelic Drugs* 3, no. 1 (1970), pp. 41–51.
34. Levine, J., and A.M. Ludwig. "The LSD Controversy." *Comprehensive Psychiatry* 5, no. 5 (1964), pp. 318–19.
35. Forsch, W.A., E.S. Robbins, and M. Stern. "Untoward Reactions to Lysergic Acid Diethylamide (LSD) Resulting in Hospitalization." *New England Journal of Medicine* 273 (1965), pp. 1235–39.
36. Halpern, J.H., and others. "Hallucinogen Persisting Perceptual Disorder: What Do We Know after 50 Years?" *Drug & Alcohol Dependence* 69 (2003), pp. 109–19.
37. Zegans, L.S., J.C. Pollard, and D. Brown. "The Effects of LSD-25 on Creativity and Tolerance to Regression." *Archives of General Psychiatry* 16 (1967), pp. 740–49.
38. Spitzer, M., and others. "Increased Activation of Indirect Semantic Associations under Psilocybin." *Biological Psychiatry* 39 (1996), pp. 1055–57.
39. Hollister, L.E., J. Shelton, and G. Krieger. "A Controlled Comparison of Lysergic Acid Diethylamide (LSD) and Dextroamphetamine in Alcoholics." *American Journal of Psychiatry* 125 (1969), pp. 1352–57.
40. NIMH Research on LSD. *Extramural Programs Fiscal Year 1948 to Present.* September 1, 1975.
41. Manevski, N., and others. "Glucuronidation of Psilocin and 4-Hydroxyindole by the Human UDP-Glucuronosyltransferases." *Drug Metabolism and Disposition* 38 (2010), pp. 386–95.
42. The Canadian Biodiversity Web Site. *Distribution Map of Liberty Cap in Canada.* Retrieved March 10, 2011, from http://canadianbiodiversity.mcgill.ca/english/species/fungi/shroompages/psi_sem.htm.
43. Pahnke, W. "Drugs and Mysticism: An Analysis of the Relationship between Psychedelic Drugs and the Mystical Consciousness." Ph. D. thesis dissertation, Harvard University, 1963.
44. Griffiths R.R., W.A. Richards, U. McCann, and R. Jesse. "Psilocybin Can Occasion Mystical-Type Experiences Having Substantial and Sustained Personal Meaning and Spiritual Significance." *Psychopharmacology* 187 (2006), pp. 268–83.
45. Schultes, R.E., and A. Hofmann. *The Botany and Chemistry of Hallucinogens.* Springfield, IL: Charles C. Thomas, 1980.
46. Al-Assmar, S.E. "The Seeds of the Hawaiian Baby Woodrose Are a Powerful Hallucinogen [letter]." *Archives of Internal Medicine* 159 (1999), p. 2090.
47. Strassman, R.J., and others. "Differential Tolerance to Biological and Subjective Effects of Four Closely Spaced Doses of N,N-dimethyltryptamine in Humans." *Biological Psychiatry* 39 (1996), pp. 784–95.
48. Grob, C.S., and others. "Human Psychopharmacology of Hoasca, a Plant Hallucinogen Used in Ritual Context in Brazil." *Journal of Nervous and Mental Disease* 184 (1996), pp. 86–94.
49. Osmond, H. "Peyote Night." *Tomorrow* 9, no. 1 (1961). Retrieved November 7, 2011, from http://www.psychedelic-library.org/peyote.htm.
50. Dobkin de Rios, M., and M. Cardenas. "Plant Hallucinogens, Shamanism, and Nazca Ceramics." *Journal of Ethnopharmacology* 2 (1980), pp. 233–46.
51. De Ropp, R.S. *Drugs and the Mind.* New York, NY: Grove Press, 1957.
52. Ellis, H. "Mescal: A Study of a Divine Plant." *Popular Science Monthly* 61 (1902), pp. 59, 65.
53. Huxley, A. *The Doors of Perception.* New York, NY: Harper & Row, 1954.
54. "MDMA: Compound Raises Medical, Legal Issues." *Brain/Mind Bulletin* 10, no. 8 (1985).

55. Peroutka, S.J., and others. "Subjective Effects of 3,4-methylenedioxymethamphetamine in Recreational Users." *Neuropsychopharmacology* 1 (1988), pp. 273–77.
56. Moro, E.T., A.A.F. Ferraz, and N.S.P. Módolo. "Anesthesia and the Ecstasy User." *Revista Brasileira de Anestesiologia* 56 (2006), pp. 183–88. Retrieved October 4, 2011, from http://www.scielo.br/scielo.php?pid=S0034-7094 2006000200010&script=sci_arttext&tlng=en.
57. CBC News. "Whistler Ecstasy Death Highlights Risk: RCMP." 2009. Retrieved November 7, 2011, from http://www.cbc.ca/news/canada/british-columbia/story/2009/11/17/bc-whistler-ecstacy-overdoses.html.
58. Royal Canadian Mounted Police. *Synthetic Drugs: Report on the Illicit Drug Situation in Canada–2009.* Retrieved February 27, 2011, from www.rcmp-grc.gc.ca/drugs-drogues/2009/p8-eng.htm.
59. Luby, E., and others. "Study of a New Schizophrenomimetic Drug–Sernyl." *American Medical Association Archive of Neurological Psychiatry* 81 (1959), pp. 113–19.
60. Ricaurte, G.A., and others. "Severe Dopaminergic Neurotoxicity in Primates after a Common Recreational Dose Regimen of MDMA (Ecstasy)." *Science* 297 (2002), pp. 2260–63.
61. Ricaurte, G.A., J. Yuan, and U.D. McCann. "3,4-Methylenedioxymethamphetamine ('Ecstasy')-induced Serotonin Neurotoxicity: Studies in Animals." *Neuropsychobiology* 42 (2000), pp. 5–10.
62. Dworkin, S.I., S. Mirkis, and J.E. Smith. "Response-Dependent versus Response-Independent Presentation of Cocaine: Differences in the Lethal Effects of the Drug." *Psychopharmacology* 117 (1995), pp. 262–66.
63. Ricaurte, G.A., and others. "Retraction." *Science* 301 (2003), p. 1479.
64. Jevtovic-Todorovic, V., and others. "Ketamine Potentiates Cerebrocortical Damage Induced by the Common Anaesthetic Agent Nitrous Oxide in Adult Rats." *British Journal of Pharmacology* 130 (2000), pp. 1692–98.
65. Cosgrove, K.P., and M.E. Carroll. "Differential Effects of Bremazocine on Oral Phencyclidine (PCP) Self-Administration in Male and Female Rhesus Monkeys." *Experimental and Clinical Psychopharmacology* 12 (2004), pp. 111–17.
66. Overend, W. "Death in the 'Dust.'" *Los Angeles Times*, September 26, 1977.
67. Morris, B.J., S.M. Cochran, and J.A. Pratt. "From Pharmacology to Modeling Schizophrenia." *Current Opinion in Pharmacology* 5 (2005), pp. 101–6.
68. Genesis 30:14–16. *The New English Bible.* Oxford University Press and Cambridge University Press, 1970.
69. Schultes, R.E. "The Plant Kingdom and Hallucinogens (Part III)." *Bulletin on Narcotics* 22, no. 1 (1970), pp. 43–46.
70. Beverly, R. *The History and Present State of Virginia, 1705.* Chapel Hill, NC: University of North Carolina Press, 1947.
71. Allegro, J.M. *The Sacred Mushroom and the Cross.* New York, NY: Doubleday, 1970.
72. Wasson, R.G. "Fly Agaric and Man." In *Ethnopharmacologic Search for Psychoactive Drugs,* D.H. Efron, ed. Washington, DC: National Institute of Mental Health, 1967. See also Wasson, R.G. *Soma, Divine Mushroom of Immortality.* New York, NY: Harcourt Brace Jovanovich, 1971.
73. Columbia Law Review Association. "Hallucinogens." *Columbia Law Review* 68, no. 3 (1968), pp. 521–60.
74. Babu, K.M., C.R. McCurdy, and E.W. Boyer. "Opioid Receptors and Legal Highs: Salvia Divinorum and Kratom." *Clinical Toxicology* 46 (2008), pp. 146–52.
75. Sheffler, D.J., B.L. Roth, and A. Salvinorin. "The 'Magic Mint' Hallucinogen Finds a Molecular Target in the Kappa Opioid Receptor." *Trends in Pharmacological Sciences* 24 (2003), pp. 107–109.
76. Health Canada. *Canadian Alcohol and Drug Use Monitoring Survey, 2010.* Ottawa: Controlled Substances and Tobacco Directorate, 2010. Retrieved November 7, 2011, from http://www.hc-sc.gc.ca/hc-ps/drugs-drogues/stat/_2010/summary-sommaire-eng.php.

Chapter 15

1. Schultes, R.E., and A. Hofmann. *The Botany and Chemistry of Hallucinogens.* Springfield, IL: Charles C. Thomas, 1980.
2. Royal Canadian Mounted Police. Criminal Intelligence. *Report on the Illicit Drug Situation in Canada–2009.* 2010. Retrieved March 1, 2011, from http://www.rcmp-grc.gc.ca/drugs-drogues/2009/drug-drogue-2009-eng.pdf.
3. Mickel, E.J. *The Artificial Paradises in French Literature.* Chapel Hill, NC: University of North Carolina Press, 1969.
4. Baudelaire, C.P. *Artificial Paradises: On Hashish and Wine as Means of Expanding Individuality.* Translated by Ellen Fox. New York, NY: Herder & Herder, 1971.
5. Giffen, P.J., S. Endicott, and S. Lambert. *Panic and Indifference: The Politics of Canadian Drug Laws.* Toronto: The Canadian Centre on Substance Abuse, 1991.
6. Fischer, B. "Prohibition, Public Health and a Window of Opportunity: An Analysis of Canadian Drug Policy, 1985-1997." *Policy Studies* 20, no. 3 (1999), pp. 197–210.
7. Health Canada. *Canadian Alcohol and Drug Use Monitoring Survey: Detailed Tables for 2012.* 2013. Retrieved October 21, 2013 from http://www.hc-sc.gc.ca/hc-ps/drugs-drogues/cadums-esccad-eng.php.
8. Young, M.M., E. Saewyc, A. Boak, J. Jahrig, B. Anderson, Y. Doiron, S. Taylor, L. Pica, P. Laprise, and H. Clark. *Cross-Canada Report on Student Alcohol and Drug Use: Technical Report.* Ottawa: Canadian Centre on Substance Abuse, 2011. Retrieved March 13, 2014, from http://www.ccsa.ca/2011%20CCSA%20Documents/2011_CCSA_Student_Alcohol_and_Drug_Use_en.pdf.
9. Porath-Waller, A.J., J.E. Brown, A.P. Frigon, and H. Clark. *What Canadian Youth Think about Cannabis.* Ottawa: Canadian Centre on Substance Abuse, 2013.
10. Compassion Clubs. *Health Canada Recently Made an Important Announcement Regarding Compassion Clubs.* 2010. Retrieved February 13, 2011, from http://www.medicinalmarijuana.ca/learning-center/compassion-clubs.

11. Health Canada. *Health Canada Statement on Medicinal Marijuana Compassion Clubs.* 2010. Retrieved February 13, 2011, from http://www.hc-sc.gc.ca/ahc-asc/media/ftr-ati/_2010/2010_94-eng.php.
12. Government of Canada. "Marihuana for Medical Purposes Regulations." *Canada Gazette* 147 (2013). Retrieved October 26, 2013, from http://gazette.gc.ca/rp-pr/p2/2013/2013-06-19/html/sor-dors119-eng.php#archived.
13. DiMarzo, V., and others. "Formation and Inactivation of Endogenous Cannabinoid Anandamide in Central Neurons." *Nature* 372 (1994), p. 686.
14. Sim, L.I., and others. "Differences in G-protein Activation by Mu- and Delta-opioid, and Cannabinoid, Receptors in Rat Striatum." *European Journal of Pharmacology* 307 (1996), pp. 97–105.
15. Hart, C.L., and others. "Effects of Acute Smoked Marijuana on Complex Cognitive Performance." *Neuropsychopharmacology* 25 (2001), pp. 757–65.
16. Hart, C.L., and others. "Reinforcing Effects of Oral Δ9-THC in Male Marijuana Smokers in a Laboratory Choice Procedure." *Psychopharmacology* 181 (2005), pp. 237–43.
17. Jones, R.T. "Cardiovascular System Effects of Marijuana." *Journal of Clinical Pharmacology* 42, no. 11 (2002), pp. 585–635.
18. United Nations Office of Drugs and Crime. *World Drug Report 2009.* United Nations Publications: Sales No. E.09.XI.12, 2009.
19. Substance Abuse and Mental Health Services Administration. *Treatment Episode Data Set (TEDS): 1998–2008. National Admissions to Substance Abuse Treatment Services.* DASIS Series: S-55, DHHS Publication No. (SMA) 10-4613, Rockville, MD: Office of Applied Studies, 2010.
20. Justinova, Z., and others. "Self-Administration of Delta9-tetrahydrocannabinol (THC) by Drug Naive Squirrel Monkeys." *Psychopharmacology* 169 (2003), pp. 135–40.
21. Kelly, T.H., and others. "Effects of D9-THC on Marijuana Smoking, Dose Choice, and Verbal Report of Drug Liking." *Journal of the Experimental Analysis of Behaviour* 61 (1994), pp. 203–11.
22. Becker, H.S. "Becoming a Marijuana User." *American Journal of Sociology* 59 (1953), pp. 235–43.
23. Ward, A.S., and others. "The Effects of a Monetary Alternative on Marijuana Self-Administration." *Behavioural Pharmacology* 8 (1997), pp. 275–86.
24. Pope, H.G., and others. "Neuropsychological Performance in Long-Term Cannabis Users." *Archives of General Psychiatry* 58 (2001), pp. 909–15.
25. Eldreth, D.A., J.A. Matochik, J.L. Cadet, and K.I. Bolla. "Abnormal Brain Activity in Prefrontal Brain Regions in Abstinent Marijuana Users." *NeuroImage* 23 (2004), pp. 914–20.
26. Kanayama, G., J. Rogowska, H.G. Pope, S.A. Gruber, and D.A. Yugelun-Todd. "Spatial Working Memory in Heavy Cannabis Users: A Functional Magnetic Resonance Imaging Study." *Psychopharmacology* 176 (2004), pp. 239–47.
27. Jager, G., R.S. Kahn, W. Van Den Brink, J.M. Van Ree, and N.F. Ramsey. "Long-term Effects of Frequent Cannabis Use on Working Memory and Attention: An fMRI Study." *Psychopharmacology* 185 (2006), pp. 358–68.
28. Foltin, R.W., and M.W. Fischman. "Effects of Smoked Marijuana on Human Social Behaviour in Small Groups." *Pharmacology, Biochemistry, and Behavior* 30 (1988), pp. 539–41.
29. Health Canada. *Information for Health Care Professionals–Cannabis (Marihuana, Marijuana and the Cannabinoids).* 2013. Retrieved November 30, 2014, from http://www.hc-sc.gc.ca/dhp-mps/alt_formats/pdf/marihuana/med/infoprof-eng.pdf.
30. Hart, C.L. "Increasing Treatment Options for Cannabis Dependence: A Review of Potential Pharmacotherapies." *Drug and Alcohol Dependence* 80 (2005), pp. 147–159.
31. Substance Abuse and Mental Health Services Administration. *Results from the 2006 National Survey on Drug Use and Health: National Findings.* NSDUH Series H-32, DHHS Publication No. SMA 07-4293. Rockville, MD: Office of Applied Studies, 2007.
32. Aryana, A., and M.A. Williams. "Marijuana as a Trigger of Cardiovascular Events: Speculation or Scientific Certainty?" *International Journal of Cardiology* 118 (2007), pp. 141–44.
33. Beirness, D.J., and C.G. Davis. *Driving Under the Influence of Cannabis: Analysis Drawn from the 2004 Canadian Addiction Survey.* Ottawa: Canadian Centre on Substance Abuse, 2006.
34. Adlaf, E., R.E. Mann, and A. Paglia. "Drinking, Cannabis Use and Driving among Ontario Students." *Canadian Medical Association Journal* 168 (2003), 565–566.
35. Asbridge, M., C. Poulin, and A. Donato. "Motor Vehicle Collision Risk and Driving under the Influence of Cannabis: Evidence from Adolescents in Atlantic Canada." *Accident Analysis and Prevention* 37 (2005), pp. 1025–1034.
36. Beirness, D., and E.E. Beasley. *Alcohol and Drug Use among Drivers: British Columbia Roadside Survey 2008.* Ottawa: Canadian Centre on Substance Abuse, 2009.
37. Stoduto, G., E. Vingilis, B.M. Kapur, W.J. Sheu, B.A. McLellan, and C.B. Libanx. "Alcohol and Drug Use among Motor Vehicle Collision Victims Admitted to a Regional Trauma Unit: Demographic, Injury, and Crash Characteristic." *Accident Analysis and Prevention* 25 (1993), pp. 411–420.
38. Brault, M., C. Dussault, J. Bouchard, and A.M. Lemire. "The Contribution of Alcohol and Other Drugs among Fatally Injured Drivers in Quebec: Final Results." In *Proceedings of the 17th International Conference on Alcohol, Drugs and Traffic Safety* (CD ROM), 2004.
39. Beirness, D.J., E. Beasley, J. LeCavalier, P. Boase, and D. Mayhew. "Drug Use by Fatally Injured Drivers in Canada." In *Proceedings of the 19th Canadian Multidisciplinary Road Safety Conference,* Saskatoon, June 8–10, 2009.

40. Ramaekers, J.G., and others. "Dose-Related Risk of Motor Vehicle Crashes after Cannabis Use." *Drug & Alcohol Dependence* 73 (2004), pp. 109–19.
41. Smiley, A.M. "Marijuana: On Road and Driving Simulator Studies." *Alcohol, Drugs and Driving* 2 (1986), pp. 121–124.
42. Beirness, D., and A.J. Porath-Waller. *Cannabis Use and Driving. Clearing the Smoke on Cannabis.* Ottawa: Canadian Centre on Substance Abuse, 2009.
43. Tashkin, D.P. "Airway Effects of Marijuana, Cocaine and Other Inhaled Illicit Agents." *Current Opinion in Pulmonary Medicine* 7 (2001), pp. 43–61.
44. Tan, W.C., and others. Vancouver Burden of Obstructive Lung Disease (BOLD) Research Group. "Marijuana and Chronic Obstructive Lung Disease: A Population-based Study." *Canadian Medical Association Journal* 180 (2009), pp. 814–20.
45. Moir, D., and others. "A Comparison of Mainstream and Sidestream Marijuana and Tobacco Cigarette Smoke Produced under Two Machine Smoking Conditions." *Chemical Research and Toxicology* 21 (2008), pp. 494–502.
46. Schuel, H., and others. "Evidence that Anandamide-Signalling Regulates Human Sperm Functions Required for Fertilization." *Molecular Reproduction and Development* 63 (2002), pp. 376–87.
47. Shay, A.H., and others. "Impairment of Antimicrobial Activity and Nitric Oxide Production in Alveolar Macrophages from Smokers of Marijuana and Cocaine." *Journal of Infectious Diseases* 187 (2003), pp. 700–704.
48. Sidney, S., J.E. Beck, and G.D. Friedman. "Marijuana Use and Mortality." *American Journal of Public Health* 87 (1997), pp. 585–90.
49. Smith, D.E., and R.B. Seymour. "Clinical Perspectives on the Toxicology of Marijuana: 1967–1981." In *Marijuana and Youth: Clinical Observations on Motivation and Learning.* Washington, DC: U.S. Department of Health and Human Services, U.S. Government Printing Office, 1982.
50. Hampson, A.J., and others. "Neuroprotective Antioxidants from Marijuana." *Annals of the New York Academy of Sciences* 899 (2000), pp. 274–82.
51. Chan, G.C., and others. "Hippocampal Neurotoxicity of Delta9-tetrahydrocannabinol." *The Journal of Neuroscience* 18, no. 14 (1998), pp. 5322–32.
52. McLaren, J.A., and others. "Assessing Evidence for a Causal Link between Cannabis and Psychosis: A Review of Cohort Studies." *International Journal of Drug Policy* 21 (2010), pp. 10–19.
53. Van Winkel, R. "Family-Based Analysis of Genetic Variation Underlying Psychosis-Inducing Effects of Cannabis: Sibling Analysis and Proband Follow-Up." *Archives of General Psychiatry* 68 (2011), pp. 148–57.
54. Zammit, S., and others. "Genotype Effects of CHRNA7, CNR1 and COMT in Schizophrenia: Interactions with Tobacco and Cannabis Use." *British Journal of Psychiatry* 191 (2007), pp. 402–407.
55. Zammit, S., and others. "Cannabis, *COMT* and Psychotic Experiences." *British Journal of Psychiatry* 199 (2011), pp. 380–85.

Chapter 16

1. Donohue, T., and N. Johnson. *Foul Play: Drug Abuse in Sports.* Oxford, UK: Basil Blackwell, 1986.
2. Asken, M.J. *Dying to Win: The Athlete's Guide to Safe and Unsafe Drugs in Sports.* Washington, DC: Acropolis, 1988.
3. "AMA to Study Drugs in Sports; Use in Four-Minute Mile Hinted." *New York Times.* June 6, 1957.
4. Eichner, E.R. "Ergogenic Aids: What Athletes Are Using—and Why." *Physician and Sports Medicine* 25 (1997), pp. 70–83.
5. Goldman, B. *Death in the Locker Room.* South Bend, IN: Icarus Press, 1984.
6. Schmidt, M.S., and A. Schwarz. "Baseball Is Challenged on Rise in Stimulant Use." *The New York Times,* January 16, 2008.
7. Fainaru-Wada, M., and L. Williams. "Sports and Drugs: How the Doping Scandal Unfolded. Fallout from BALCO Probe Could Taint Olympics, Pro Sports." *San Francisco Chronicle.* December 21, 2003.
8. Canadian Centre for Ethics in Sports. "2011 Substance Classification Booklet." 2011. Retrieved March 7, 2011, from http://www.cces.ca/scb.
9. The World Anti-Doping Agency. "The World Anti-Doping Code; the 2010 Prohibited List International Standard." Retrieved March 2, 2011, from http://www.wada-ama.org/en/World-Anti-Doping-Program/Sports-and-Anti-Doping-Organizations/International-Standards/Prohibited-List/.
10. Smith, G.M., and H.K. Beecher. "Amphetamine Sulfate and Athletic Performance." *Journal of the American Medical Association* 170 (1959), pp. 542–57.
11. Laties, V.G., and B. Weiss. "The Amphetamine Margin in Sports." *Federation Proceedings* 40 (1981), pp. 2689–92.
12. Noble, B.J. *Physiology of Exercise and Sport.* St Louis, MO: Mosby, 1986.
13. Cohen, B.S., and others. "Effects of Caffeine Ingestion on Endurance Racing in Heat and Humidity." *European Journal of Applied Physiology* 73 (1996), pp. 358–63.
14. Bodley, H. "Medical Examiner: Ephedra a Factor in Bechler Death." *USA Today,* March 13, 2003.
15. Williams, M.H. *Ergogenic Aids in Sports.* Champaign, IL: Human Kinetics, 1983.
16. Marshall, E. "The Drug of Champions." *Science* 242 (1983), pp. 183–84.
17. Taylor, W.N. *Hormonal Manipulation: A New Era of Monstrous Athletes.* Jefferson, NC: McFarland & Co., 1985.
18. The Pharmacology Education Partnership. "Steroids and Athletes: Genes Work Overtime." 2003. Retrieved November 8, 2011, from http://www.thepepproject.net/Load/teacher/index.html?selUser=teacher&selHelp=true&y=49.
19. American College Health Association. *National College Health Assessment II: Canadian Reference Group Data Report.*

Spring 2013. Hanover, MD: American College Health Association, 2013. Retrieved December 12, 2013, from http://www.cacuss.ca/_Library/documents/NCHA-II_WEB_SPRING_2013_CANADIAN_REFERENCE_GROUP_DATA_REPORT.pdf.

20. Adlaf, E., P. Begin, and E. Sawka, eds. *Canadian Addiction Survey (CAS): A National Survey of Canadians' Use of Alcohol and Other Drugs. Prevalence of Use and Related Harms.* Detailed Report. Ottawa: Canadian Centre on Substance Abuse, 2005.
21. Pope, H.G., and D.L. Katz. "Affective and Psychotic Symptoms Associated with Anabolic Steroid Use." *American Journal of Psychiatry* 145 (1988), pp. 487–90.
22. Pope, H.G., E.M. Kouri, and J.L. Hudson. "Effects of Supraphysiologic Doses of Testosterone on Mood and Aggression in Normal Men: A Randomized Control Trial." *Archives of General Psychiatry* 57 (2000), pp. 133–40.
23. Lubell, A. "Does Steroid Abuse Cause–or Excuse–Violence?" *Physician and Sportsmedicine* 17 (1989), pp. 176–85.
24. Fultz, O. "'Roid Rage." *American Health* 10 (1991), p. 60.
25. National Institute on Drug Abuse. "NIDA InfoFacts: Steroids (Anabolic-Androgenic)." 2009. Retrieved November 8, 2011, from http://www.drugabuse.gov/infofacts/steroids.html.
26. Arnedo, M.T., and others. "Rewarding Properties of Testosterone in Intact Male Mice: A Pilot Study." *Pharmacology, Biochemistry, and Behavior* 65 (2000), pp. 327–32.
27. DiMeo, A.N., and R.I. Wood. "Self-Administration of Estrogen and Dihydrotestosterone in Male Hamsters." *Hormones and Behavior* 49 (2006), pp. 519–26.
28. Brower, K.J. "Anabolic Steroid Abuse and Dependence." *Current Psychiatry Reports* 4 (2002), pp. 377–87.
29. Burke, L., and others. "Supplements and Sports Foods." *Clinical Sports Nutrition*, 3rd ed., L. Burke and V. Deakin, eds. Sydney, Australia: McGraw-Hill, 2006, pp. 485–579. Retrieved November 8, 2011, from http://www.ais.org.au/nutrition/documents/16Complete.pdf.
30. Department of Justice. *Controlled Drugs and Substances Act.* Retrieved March 7, 2011, from http://laws.justice.gc.ca/en/ShowFullDoc/cs/C-38.8//20070425/en?command=home&caller=SI&fragment=anabolic&search_type=all&day=25&month=4&year=2007&search_domain=cs&showall=L&statuteyear=all&lengthannual=50&length=50.
31. Liu, H., and others. "Systematic Review: The Effects of Growth Hormone on Athletic Performance." *Annals of Internal Medicine* 148, no. 10 (2008), pp. 747–58.
32. Spann, S. "Effect of Clenbuterol on Athletic Performance." *Annals of Pharmacotherapy* 29 (1995), p. 75.
33. Lombardi, G., G. Banfi, G. Lippi, F. Sanchis-Gomar. "*Ex vivo* Erythrocyte Generation and Blood Doping." *Blood Transfusion* 11 (2013), pp. 161–163.
34. Marrocco, C., V. Pallotta, A. D'alessandro, G. Alves, and L. Zolla. "Red Blood Cell Populations and Membrane Levels of Peroxiredoxin 2 as Candidate Biomarkers to Reveal Blood Doping." *Blood Transfusion* 10 (2012), Suppl 2, pp. 71–7.
35. Morkeberg, J. "Detection of Autologous Blood Transfusions in Athletes: A Historical Perspective." *Transfusion Medicine Reviews* 26 (2012), pp. 199–208.
36. World Anti-Doping Agency–WADA. The World Anti-Doping Code. *The 2013 Prohibited List: International Standard.* Retrieved June 14, 2014, from http://www.wada-ama.org/en/Science-Medicine/Prohibited-List/.
37. De Oliveira, C.D., A.V. de Bairros, and M. Yonamine. "Blood Doping: Risks to Athletes' Health and Strategies for Detection." *Substance Use and Misuse.* (2014) [Epub ahead of print]

Chapter 17

1. Sehwan, K., and others. "Benefit-Cost Analysis of Drug Abuse Prevention Programs: A Macroscopic Approach." *Journal of Drug Education* 25 (1995), pp. 111–127.
2. Miller, T., and D. Hendrie. *Substance Abuse Prevention Dollars and Cents: A Cost-Benefit Analysis.* Center for Substance Abuse Prevention, Substance Abuse and Mental Health Services Administration, DHHS Pub. No. (SMA) 07-4298. Rockville, MD, 2008.
3. Lee, S., and others. *Return on Investment: Evidence-Based Options to Improve Statewide Outcomes.* Olympia: Washington State Institute for Public Policy, April 2012 (Document No. 12-04-1201).
4. DeBeck, K., and others. "Canada's New Federal 'National Anti-Drug Strategy': An Informal Audit of Reported Funding Allocation." *International Journal of Drug Policy* 20 (2009), pp. 188–191.
5. National Institute on Drug Abuse. *Drug Abuse Prevention for the General Population.* Washington, DC: U.S. Department of Health and Human Services, 1997.
6. Dr. Nora Volkow, "What Do We Know about Addictions?" Available at http://vimeo.com/30015129.
7. Think Big Interview with Nora Volkow. Available at http://www.youtube.com/watch?v=xoSARbXLjjo.
8. Blum, K., A.L.C. Chen, and others. "The Addictive Brain: All Roads Lead to Dopamine." *Journal of Psychoactive Drugs* 44 (2012), pp. 134–143.
9. Ross, S., and E. Peselow. "The Neurobiology of Addictive Disorders." *Clinical Neuropharmacology* 32 (2012), pp. 269–76.
10. Canadian Centre on Substance Abuse. *Substance Abuse in Canada: Youth in Focus.* Ottawa: Canadian Centre on Substance Abuse, 2007.
11. Health Canada. *Canadian Alcohol and Drug Use Monitoring Survey. Detailed Tables for 2012.* Ottawa: Controlled Substances and Tobacco Directorate, 2013. To obtain a copy, please send an e-mail request to CADUMS-ESC CAD@hc-sc.gc.ca.
12. Health Canada. *Canadian Alcohol and Drug Use Monitoring Survey: Summary of Results for 2011.* 2011. Retrieved January 29, 2014, from http://www.hc-sc.gc.ca/hc-ps/drugs-drogues/stat/_2011/summary-sommaire-eng.php.
13. Health Canada. *Supplementary Tables, Youth Smoking Survey 2010–11.* 2012. Retrieved January 29, 2014, from

http://www.hc-sc.gc.ca/hc-ps/tobac-tabac/research-recherche/stat/_survey-sondage_2010-2011/table-eng.php.

14. American College Health Association. *National College Health Assessment II: Canadian Reference Group Data Report.* Spring 2013. Hanover, MD: American College Health Association, 2013. Retrieved January 29, 2014, from http://www.cacuss.ca/_Library/documents/NCHA-II_WEB_SPRING_2013_CANADIAN_REFERENCE_GROUP_DATA_REPORT.pdf.
15. Health Officers Council of British Columbia. *A Public Health Approach to Drug Control in Canada: Discussion Paper.* October 2005. Retrieved January 28, 2014, from http://www.cfdp.ca/bchoc.pdf.
16. Goodstadt, M.S. "School-Based Drug Education in North America: What Is Wrong? What Can Be Done?" *Journal of School Health* 56 (1986), pp. 278–81.
17. Swisher, J.D., and others. "Drug Education: Pushing or Preventing?" *Peabody Journal of Education* 49 (1971), pp. 68–75.
18. Swisher, J.D., and others. "A Comparison of Four Approaches to Drug Abuse Prevention at the College Level." *Journal of College Student Personnel* 14 (1973), pp. 231–35.
19. Blum, R.H., E. Blum, and E. Garfield. *Drug Education: Results and Recommendations.* Lexington, MA: D.C. Heath, 1976.
20. Swisher, J.D. "Prevention Issues." In *Handbook on Drug Abuse,* R.I. DuPont, A. Goldstein, and J. O'Donnell, eds. Washington, DC: NIDA, U.S. Government Printing Office, 1979.
21. Canadian Home and School Federation. *Statement of Policy, Revised 2010.* 2010. Retrieved November 9, 2011, from http://www.canadianhomeandschool.com/CHSF/Policies_and_Forms_files/2010%20Policy%20Updated.pdf.
22. Schaps, E., and others. *The Napa Drug Abuse Prevention Project: Research Findings.* Washington, DC: DHHS Publication No. (ADM) 84-1339, U.S. Government Printing Office, 1984.
23. Department of Health and Human Services. "Prevention Research." In *Drug Abuse and Drug Abuse Research.* Washington, DC: DHHS Publication No. (ADM) 85-1372, U.S. Government Printing Office, 1984.
24. Government of Canada. *National Anti-Drug Strategy.* 2007. Retrieved November 9, 2011, from http://www.nationalantidrugstrategy.gc.ca/.
25. Bennett, W.J. *What Works: Schools without Drugs.* Washington, DC: U.S. Department of Education, 1987.
26. Evans, R.I. "Smoking in Children: Developing a Social Psychological Strategy of Deterrence." *Preventive Medicine* 5 (1976), pp. 122–27.
27. Flay, B.R. "What We Know about the Social Influences Approach to Smoking Prevention: Review and Recommendations." In *Prevention Research: Deterring Drug Abuse among Children and Adolescents,* C.S. Bell and R. Battjes, eds. Washington, DC: NIDA Research Monograph 63, DHHS Publication No. (ADM) 85-1334, U.S. Government Printing Office, 1985.
28. McCarthy, W.J. "The Cognitive Developmental Model and Other Alternatives to the Social Skills Deficit Model of Smoking Onset." In *Prevention Research: Deterring Drug Abuse among Children and Adolescents,* C.S. Bell and R. Battjes, eds. Washington, DC: NIDA Research Monograph 63, DHHS Publication No. (ADM) 85-1334, U.S. Government Printing Office, 1985.
29. Albaum, G., and others. "Smoking Behaviour, Information Sources, and Consumption Value of Teenagers: Implications for Public Policy and Other Intervention Failures." *Journal of Consumer Affairs* 36 (2002), pp. 50–76.
30. Canadian Centre on Substance Abuse. *Portfolio of Canadian Standards for Youth Substance Abuse Prevention.* 2010. Retrieved November 9, 2011, from http://www.ccsa.ca/Eng/Priorities/YouthPrevention/CanadianStandards/Pages/default.aspx.
31. Health Canada. *Major Findings from the Canadian Alcohol and Drug Use Monitoring Survey (CADUMS) 2009.* 2010. Retrieved November 9, 2011, from http://www.hc-sc.gc.ca/hc-ps/drugs-drogues/stat/index-eng.php.
32. Faggiano, F., and others. "School-Based Prevention for Illicit Drugs' Use." *Cochrane Database of Systematic Reviews* (2005) Issue 2, CD003020.
33. Tobler, N.S., and others. "School-Based Adolescent Drug Prevention Programs: 1998 Meta-Analysis." *Journal of Primary Prevention* 20 (2000), pp. 275–336.
34. Porath-Waller, A.J., E. Beasley, and D.J. Beirness. "A Meta-Analytic Review of School-Based Prevention for Cannabis Use." *Health Education and Behaviours* 37 (2010), pp. 709–23.
35. Thomas, R.F., and R. Perera. "School-Based Programs for Preventing Smoking." *Cochrane Database of Systematic Revirews* (2006) Issue 3, CD001293.
36. Pan, W., and H. Bai. "A Multivariate Approach to a Meta-Analytic Review of the Effectiveness of the D.A.R.E. Program." *International Journal of Environmental Research and Public Health* 6 (2010), pp. 267–277.
37. Ellickson, P.L., and R.M. Bell. "Drug Prevention in Junior High: A Multi-Site Longitudinal Test." *Science* 247 (1990), pp. 1299–1305.
38. Health Canada. *Preventing Substance Use Problems among Young People–A Compendium of Best Practices.* 2001. Retrieved November 9, 2011, from http://www.hc-sc.gc.ca/hc-ps/pubs/adp-apd/prevent/index-eng.php.
39. See http://nrepp.samhsa.gov.
40. CBC News. *Canada's Anti-Drug Strategy a Failure, Study Suggests.* 2007. Retrieved November 9, 2011, from http://www.cbc.ca/news/canada/story/2007/01/15/drug-strategy.html.
41. Ennett, S.T., and others. "Long-Term Evaluation of Drug Abuse Resistance Education." *Addictive Behaviours* 19 (1994), p. 113.
42. Ennett, S.T., and others. "How Effective Is Drug Abuse Resistance Education? A Meta-Analysis of Project DARE Outcome Evaluations." *American Journal of Public Health* 84 (1994), p. 1394.

43. Pan, W., and H. Bai. "A Multivariate Approach to a Meta-Analytic Review of the Effectiveness of the D.A.R.E. Program." *International Journal of Environmental Research and Public Health* 6 (2010), pp. 267–277.
44. Foxcroft, D.R., and A. Tsertsvadze. "Universal School-Based Prevention Programs for Alcohol Misuse in Young People." *Cochrane Database Systematic Reviews* (2011) Issue 5, CD009113.
45. Botvin, G.J., and S.P. Schinke. "Effectiveness of Culturally Focused and Generic Skills Training Approaches to Alcohol and Drug Abuse Prevention among Minority Adolescents: Two-Year Follow-up Results." *Psychology of Addictive Behaviours* 9 (1995), p. 183.
46. Sowden, A.J., and L.F. Stead. "Community Interventions for Preventing Smoking in Young People." *Cochrane Database for Systematic Reviews* (2003) Issue 1, CD001291.
47. Gates, S., and others. "Interventions for Prevention of Drug Use by Young People Delivered in Non-School Settings." *Cochrane Database of Systematic Reviews* (2006) Issue 1, CD005030.
48. Thomas, R.E., P.R.A. Baker, and D. Lorenzetti. "Family-Based Programs for Preventing Smoking by Children and Adolescents." *Cochrane Database of Systematic Reviews* (2007) Issue 1, CD004493.
49. Brinn, M.P., and others. "Mass Media Interventions for Preventing Smoking in Young People." *Cochrane Database of Systematic Reviews* (2010) Issue 11, CD001006.
50. Foxcroft, D., and others. "Primary Prevention for Alcohol Misuse in Young People." *Cochrane Database of Systematic Reviews* (2002) Issue 3, CD003024.
51. National Institute on Alcohol Abuse and Alcoholism. "Parent Education." In *Prevention Plus: Involving Schools, Parents, and the Community in Alcohol and Drug Education.* Washington, DC: DHHS Publication No. (ADM) 84-1256, U.S. Government Printing Office, 1984.
52. Center for Addiction and Mental Health. *Strengthening Families for the Future.* 2009. Retrieved November 9, 2011, from http://www.camh.net/Publications/Resources_for_Professionals/Strengthening_Families/sff_program_intro.htm.
53. National Institute on Drug Abuse. *Drug Abuse Prevention for At-Risk Groups.* Washington, DC: U.S. Department of Health and Human Services, 1997.
54. Anctil, M. *Nunavik Inuit Health Survey 2004, Qanuippitaa? How Are We? Survey Highlights.* Quebec, QC: Institut national de santé publique du Québec (INSPQ) and Nunavik Regional Board of Health and Social Services (NRBHSS), 2008. Retrieved November 9, 2011, from http://www.inspq.qc.ca/pdf/publications/774_ESISurveyHighlights.pdf.
55. Adlaf, E., P. Begin, and E. Sawka, eds. *Canadian Addiction Survey (CAS): A National Survey of Canadians' Use of Alcohol and Other Drugs. Prevalence of Use and Related Harms. Detailed Report.* Ottawa: Canadian Centre on Substance Abuse, 2005.
56. Elton-Marshall, T., S.T. Leatherdale, and R. Burkhalter. "Tobacco, Alcohol and Illicit Drug Use among Aboriginal Youth Living Off-Reserve: Results from the Youth Smoking Survey." *Canadian Medical Association Journal* 183 (2011), pp. E480–86.
57. Public Service Alliance of Canada. *Statement on National Aboriginal Peoples' Day, Making Aboriginal Poverty History; PSAC Fact Sheet.* 2008. Retrieved November 9, 2011, from http://psac.com/what/humanrights/june21factsheet1-e.shtml.
58. Statistics Canada. *Violent Victimization of Aboriginal People in the Provinces. 2011.* Retrieved November 9, 2011, from http://www.statcan.gc.ca/daily-quotidien/110311/dq110311c-eng.htm.
59. Health Canada. *National Native Alcohol and Drug Abuse Program.* 2006. Retrieved November 9, 2011, from http://www.hc-sc.gc.ca/fniah-spnia/substan/ads/nnadap-pnlaada-eng.php.
60. Government of Canada, Library of Parliament. *Drug Testing in the Workplace.* PRB 07-51E. 2008. Retrieved November 9, 2011, from http://www2.parl.gc.ca/Content/LOP/ResearchPublications/prb0751-e.pdf.

Chapter 18

1. Nova Scotia Addiction Services. *2009–2010 Annual Report.* 2011. Retrieved November 9, 2011, from http://www.gov.ns.ca/hpp/publications/Addiction-Services-Annual-Report-2009-2010.pdf.
2. Rhem, J., and others. *The Cost of Substance Abuse in Canada.* 2006. Canadian Centre on Substance Abuse. Retrieved November 9, 2011, from http://www.ccsa.ca.
3. Hall, W., and D.Z. Zador. "The Alcohol Withdrawal Syndrome." *Lancet* 349 (1997), pp. 1897–1900.
4. Victor, M. "The Alcohol Withdrawal Syndrome: Theory and Practice." *Postgraduate Medicine* 47 (1970), pp. 68–72.
5. Kosten, T.R., and P.G. O'Connor. "Management of Drug and Alcohol Withdrawal." *New England Journal of Medicine* 348 (2003), pp. 1786–95.
6. Chrousos, G.P., and P.W. Gold. "The Concepts of Stress and Stress System Disorders: Overview of Physical and Behavioural Homeostasis." *Journal of the American Medical Association* 267 (1992), pp. 1244–52.
7. Griffith, R.R., and B. Wolf. "Relative Abuse Liability of Different Benzodiazepines in Drug Abusers." *Journal of Clinical Psychopharmacology* 10 (1990), pp. 237–43.
8. Parr, J.M., and others. "Effectiveness of Current Treatment Approaches for Benzodiazepine Discontinuation: A Meta Analysis." *Addiction* 104 (2009), pp. 13–24.
9. Holden, J.D., I.M. Hughes, and A. Tree. "Benzodiazepine Prescribing and Withdrawal for 3234 Patients in 15 General Practices." *Family Practice* 11 (1994), pp. 358–62.
10. Lader, M. "Benzodiazepines. A Risk-Benefit Profile." *CNS Drugs* 1 (1994), pp. 377–87.
11. Kripke, D.F., and others. "Mortality Hazard Associated with Prescription of Hypnotics." *Biological Psychiatry* 43 (1998), pp. 687–93.
12. Hald, J., E. Jacobsen, and V. Larsen. "The Sensitizing Effect of Tetraethylthiuram Disulfide (Antabuse) to

Ethyl Alcohol." *Acta Pharmocologica et Toxicologica* 4 (1948), pp. 285–96.

13. O'Malley, S.S., and others. "Naltrexone and Coping Skills Therapy for Alcohol Dependence: A Controlled Study." *Archives of General Psychiatry* 49 (1992), pp. 894–98; Volpicelli, J., and others. "Naltrexone in the Treatment of Alcohol Dependence." *Archives of General Psychiatry* 49 (1992), pp. 867–80.
14. Sinclair, J.D. "Evidence about the Use of Naltrexone and for Different Ways of Using It in the Treatment of Alcoholism." *Alcohol* 36 (2001), pp. 2–10.
15. Dahchour, A., and P. De Witte. "Ethanol and Amino Acids in the Central Nervous System: Assessment of the Pharmacological Actions of Acamprosate." *Progress in Neurobiology* 60 (2000), pp. 343–62.
16. George, T.P., and S.S. O'Malley. "Current Pharmacological Treatments for Nicotine Dependence." *Trends in Pharmacological Sciences* 25 (2004), pp. 42–48.
17. Government of Canada. *Health Canada Advises Canadians Not to Use Electronic Cigarettes*. 2011. Retrieved June 16, 2014, from http://www.healthycanadians.gc.ca/recall-alert-rappel-avis/hc-sc/2009/13373a-eng.php.
18. Ascher, J.A., and others. "Bupropion: A Review of Its Mechanism of Antidepressant Activity." *Journal of Clinical Psychiatry* 56 (1995), pp. 395–401; Slemmer, J.E., B.R. Martin, and M.I. Damaj. "Bupropion Is a Nicotinic Antagonist." *Journal of Pharmacology Experimental Therapies* 295 (2000), pp. 321–27.
19. Piper, M.E., and others. "A Randomized Placebo Controlled Clinical Trial of 5 Smoking Cessation Pharmacotherapies." *Archives of General Psychiatry* 66, no. 11(2009), pp. 1253–62.
20. Stack, N.M. "Smoking Cessation: An Overview of Treatment Options with a Focus on Varenicline." *Pharmacotherapy* 27 (2007), pp. 1550–57.
21. Health Canada. *Health Canada Reviewing Stop Smoking Drug Champix (Varenicline Tartrate) and Potential Risk of Heart Problems in Patients with Heart Disease.* 2011. Retrieved November 7, 2001, from http://www.hc-sc.gc.ca/ahc-asc/media/advisories-avis/_2011/2011_84-eng.php.
22. Edens, E., A. Massa, and I. Petrakis. "Novel Pharmacological Approaches to Drug Abuse Treatment." *Current Topics in Behavioural Neurosciences* 3 (2010), pp. 343–86.
23. Cerny, E.H., and T. Cerny. "Anti-Nicotine Abuse Vaccines in the Pipeline: An Update." *Expert Opinion on Investigational Drugs* 17 (2008), pp. 691–96.
24. Cornuz, J., and others. "A Vaccine against Nicotine for Smoking Cessation: A Randomized Controlled Trial." *PLOS ONE* 3 (2008), p. e2547.
25. Latimer, D., and J. Goldberg. *Flowers in the Blood: The Story of Opium*. New York, NY: Arno Press, 1981.
26. Comer, S.D., and others. "Depot Naltrexone: Long-Lasting Antagonism of the Effects of Heroin in Humans." *Psychopharmacology* 159 (2002), pp. 351–60.
27. Health Canada. *Best Practices: Methadone Maintenance Treatment*. 2002. Retrieved March 1, 2011, from http://www.hc-sc.gc.ca/hc-ps/alt_formats/hecs-sesc/pdf/pubs/adp-apd/methadone-treatment-traitement/methadone-treatment-traitement-eng.pdf.
28. Suboxone News Release. First New Opioid Dependence Treatment in More Than 30 Years. Suboxone Approved by Health Canada and Available as New, Effective and Safe Treatment Option for Patients with Opioid Drug Dependence. 2007. Retrieved March 13, 2011, from http://metadame.org/suboxone/SUBOXONE-News-Release-Final-QC-ENt_10Dec07.pdf.
29. Foltin, R.W., and M.W. Fischman. "A Laboratory Model of Cocaine Withdrawal in Humans: Intravenous Cocaine." *Experimental and Clinical Psychopharmacology* 5 (1997), pp. 404–11.
30. Gawin, F.H., and H.D. Kleber. "Abstinence Symptomatology and Psychiatric Diagnosis in Cocaine Abusers. Clinical Observations." *Archives of General Psychiatry* 43 (1986), pp. 107–13.
31. Hart, C.L., and W.J. Lynch. "Developing Pharmacotherapies for Cannabis and Cocaine Use Disorders." *Current Neuropharmacology* 3 (2005), pp. 95–114.
32. Dackis, C.A., and others. "A Double-Blind, Placebo-Controlled Trial of Modafinil for Cocaine Dependence." *Neuropsychopharmacology* 30 (2005), pp. 205–11.
33. Hart, C.L., and others. "Smoked Cocaine Self-Administration Is Decreased by Modafinil." *Neuropsychopharmacology* 33 (2008), pp. 761–68.
34. Wisor, J.P., and K.S. Eriksson. "Dopaminergic-Adrenergic Interactions in the Wake Promoting Mechanism of Modafinil." *Neuroscience* 132 (2005), pp. 1027–34.
35. Madras, B.K., and others. "Modafinil Occupies Dopamine and Norepinephrine Transporters In Vivo and Modulates the Transporters and Trace Amine Activity In Vitro." *Journal of Pharmacology and Experimental Therapeutics* 319 (2006), pp. 561–9.
36. Ferraro, L., and others. "The Vigilance Promoting Drug Modafinil Increases Extracellular Glutamate Levels in the Medial Preoptic Area and the Posterior Hypothalamus of the Conscious Rat: Prevention by Local GABAA Receptor Blockade." *Neuropsychopharmacology* 20 (1999), pp. 346–56.
37. Anthony, J.C., L.A. Warner, and R.C. Kessler. "Comparative Epidemiology of Dependence on Tobacco, Alcohol, Controlled Substances, and Inhalants: Basic Findings from the National Comorbidity Survey." *Experimental and Clinical Psychopharmacology* 2 (1994), pp. 244–68.
38. Hart, C.L. "Increasing Treatment Options for Cannabis Dependence: A Review of Potential Pharmacotherapies." *Drug and Alcohol Dependence* 80 (2005), pp. 147–59.
39. Lichtman, A.H., J. Fisher, and B.R. Martin. "Precipitated Cannabinoid Withdrawal Is Reversed by Delta(9)-tetrahydrocannabinol or Clonidine." *Pharmacology, Biochemistry, and Behavior* 69 (2001), pp. 181–88.
40. Wong, S., Ordean, A., and Kahan, M., Maternal Fetal Medicine Committee; Family Physicians Advisory Committee; Medico-Legal Committee; Society of Obstetricians

and Gynaecologists of Canada. "Substance Use in Pregnancy." *Journal of Obstetricians and Gynaecologists of Canada* 33 (2011), pp. 367–84.

41. Simkin, D.R., and S. Grenoble. "Pharmacotherapies for Adolescent Substance Use Disorders." *Child and Adolescent Psychiatric Clinics of North America* 19 (2010), pp. 591–608.
42. Kaminer, Y. *Adolescent Substance Abuse: A Comprehensive Guide to Theory and Practice.* New York, NY: Plenum Press, 1994.
43. Wilens, T.E., and others. "Clinical Characteristics of Psychiatrically Referred Adolescent Outpatients with Substance Use Disorder." *Journal of the American Academy of Child and Adolescent Psychiatry* 36, no. 7 (1997), pp. 941–47.
44. Bukstein, O.G., and others. "Practice Parameter for the Assessment and Treatment of Children and Adolescents with Substance Use Disorders." *Journal of the American Academy of Child and Adolescent Psychiatry* 44, no. 6 (2005), pp. 609–21.
45. Wilens, T.E., J. Biederman, and T.J. Spencer. "Case Study: Adverse Effects of Smoking Marijuana while Receiving Tricyclic Antidepressants." *Journal of the American Academy of Child and Adolescent Psychiatry* 36, no. 1 (1997), pp. 45–48.
46. Rollnick, S., and W.R. Miller. "What Is Motivational Interviewing?" *Behavioural and Cognitive Psychotherapy* 23 (1995), pp. 325–34.
47. Polcin, D.L., and others. "The Case for High-Dose Motivational Enhancement Therapy." *Substance Use and Misuse* 39 (2004), pp. 331–43.
48. Higgins, S.T., S.H. Heil, and J.P. Lussier. "Clinical Implications of Reinforcement as a Determinant of Substance Use Disorders." *Annual Review of Psychology* 55 (2004), pp. 431–61.
49. Silverman, K., and others. "A Reinforcement-based Therapeutic Workplace for the Treatment of Drug Abuse: Three-year Abstinence Outcomes." *Experimental and Clinical Psychopharmacology* 10 (2002), pp. 228–40.
50. Carroll, K.M., and others. "One-Year Follow-Up of Psychotherapy and Pharmacotherapy for Cocaine Dependence. Delayed Emergence of Psychotherapy Effects." *Archives of General Psychiatry* 51 (1994), pp. 989–97.
51. Aharonovich, E., E. Nunes, and D. Hasin. "Cognitive Impairment, Retention and Abstinence among Cocaine Abusers in Cognitive-Behavioural Treatment." *Drug & Alcohol Dependence* 71 (2003), pp. 207–11.
52. Hart, C.L., and others. "Is Cognitive Functioning Impaired in Methamphetamine Users? A Critical Review." *Neuropsychopharmacology* 37 (2012), pp. 586–608.
53. Prochaska, J., and C. DiClemente. "Stages and Processes of Self-Change of Smoking: Toward an Integrative Model of Change." *Journal of Consulting and Clinical Psychology* 51, no. 3 (1983), pp. 390–95.
54. Vilela, F.A., and others. "The Transtheoretical Model and Substance Dependence: Theoretical and Practical Aspects." *Revista Brasileira de Psiquiatria* 31, no. 4 (2009), pp. 362–68.
55. The John Howard Society of Canada. *Perspectives on Canadian Drug Policy; Volume 1.* © Copyright 2003. All rights reserved. Reproduction of any article is permitted if source is cited. ISBN#: 0-9689335-2-1.
56. Des Jarlais, D.C. "Harm Reduction: A Framework for Incorporating Science into Drug Policy." *American Journal of Public Health* 85 (1995), pp. 10–12.
57. Lenton, S., and E. Single. "The Definition of Harm Reduction." *Drug and Alcohol Review* 17 (2004), pp. 213–20.
58. World Health Organization (WHO). *HIV/AIDS: Comprehensive Harm Reduction Package.* Geneva, Switzerland: WHO, 2009. Retrieved November 10, 2011, from http://www.who.int/hiv/topics/idu/harm_reduction/en/index.html.
59. Riley, D. *The Policy and Practice of Harm Reduction: The Application of Harm Reduction Measures in a Prohibitionist Society.* Ottawa: Canadian Centre on Substance Abuse, 1993.
60. Brissette, S. "Medical Prescription of Heroin: A Review." *Canadian HIV/AIDS Policy and Law Review* 6, nos. 1/2 (2001), pp. 1, 103–110. Retrieved February 27, 2011, from http://www.aidslaw.ca/publications/publicationsdocEN.php?ref=240.
61. Riley, D. *Drugs and Drug Policy in Canada: A Brief Review and Commentary.* Report Prepared for the Canadian Senate Special Committee on Illegal Drugs. 1998. Retrieved March 1, 2011, from http://www.parl.gc.ca/37/1/parlbus/commbus/senate/com-e/ille-e/library-e/riley-e.htm.
62. Riley, D. *Drugs and Drug Policy in Canada: A Brief Review and Commentary.* Report Prepared for the Senate Special Committee on Illegal Drugs. 1998.
63. Uchtenhagen, A., F. Gutzwiller, and A. Dobler-Mikola, eds. *Summary of the Synthesis Report, Programme for a Medical Prescription of Narcotics: Final Report of the Research Representatives.* Zurich, Switzerland: Institute for Social and Preventative Medicine at the University of Zurich, 1997. Retrieved February 28, 2011, from http://www.cfdp.ca/switz.html.
64. Uchtenhagen, A. *Heroin Assisted Treatment for Opiate Addicts: The Swiss Experience.* Ottawa: Parliament of Canada, 2001. Retrieved February 28, 2011, from http://www.parl.gc.ca/37/1/parlbus/commbus/senate/com-e/ille-e/presentatione/ucht1-e.htm.
65. Keizer, B. *The Netherlands' Drug Policy. Paper Presented to the Canadian Special Committee on Illegal Drugs.* Ottawa: Parliament of Canada, 2001. Retrieved February 28, 2011, from http://www.parl.gc.ca/37/1/parlbus/commbus/senate/com-e/ille -e/presentation-e/keizer-e.htm.
66. Pinkerton, S. "Is Vancouver Canada's Supervised Injection Facility Cost-Saving?" *Addiction* 105 (2010), pp. 1429–36.
67. Wood, R., and others. "Nurse-Delivered Safer Injection Education among a Cohort of Injection Drug Users:

Evidence from the Evaluation of Vancouver's Supervised Injection Facility." *International Journal of Drug Policy* 19 (2008), pp. 183–88.

68. Wood, E., and others. "Methodology for Evaluating Insite: Canada's First Medically Supervised Safer Injection Facility for Injection Drug Users." *Harm Reduction Journal* 1 (2004), p. 9.
69. Kerr, T., and others. "Drug-Related Overdoses within a Medically Supervised Safer Injection Facility." *International Journal of Drug Policy* 17 (2006), pp. 436–41.
70. Andresen, M., and N. Boyd. "A Cost-Benefit and Cost-Effectiveness Analysis of Vancouver's Supervised Injection Facility." *International Journal of Drug Policy* 21 (2010), pp. 70–76.
71. Canadian Centre on Substance Abuse. *Substance Abuse in Canada: Concurrent Disorders. Highlights: April 2010.* Ottawa: Canadian Centre on Substance Abuse, 2010. Retrieved July 28, 2011, from http://www.ccsa.ca/2010%20CCSA%20Documents/ccsa-011813-2010.pdf.
72. Rush, B., K. Urbanoski, D. Bassani, S. Castel, T.C. Wild, C. Strike, D. Kimberley, and J. Somers. "Prevalence of Co-Occurring Substance Use and Other Mental Disorders in the Canadian Population." *Canadian Journal of Psychiatry* 53, no. 12 (2008), pp. 800–9.
73. Health Canada. *Profile–Substance Abuse Treatment and Rehabilitation in Canada.* Ottawa: Minister of Public Works and Government Services Canada, 1999. Retrieved July 28, 2011, from http://www.hc-sc.gc.ca/hc-ps/alt_formats/hecs-sesc/pdf/pubs/adp-apd/profile-profil/profile.pdf.
74. Lewis, D.C. "More Evidence That Treatment Works." *The Brown University Digest of Addiction Theory and Application* 13 (1994), p. 12.
75. Williams, R.J., and S.Y. Chang. "A Comprehensive and Comparative Review of Adolescent Substance Abuse Treatment Outcome." *Clinical Psychology, Science and Practice* 7 (2000), pp. 138–66.
76. National Treatment Strategy Working Group. *A Systems Approach to Substance Use in Canada: Recommendations for a National Treatment Strategy.* Ottawa: National Framework for Action to Reduce the Harms Associated with Alcohol and Other Drugs and Substances in Canada, 2008. Retrieved July 28, 2011, from http://www.nationalframework-cadrenational.ca/uploads/files/TWS_Treatment/nts-report-eng.pdf.